W9-CDI-081

HESI Comprehensive Review for the

NCLEX-RN®
EXAMINATION

HESI

Comprehensive Review for the

NCLEX-RN® EXAMINATION

EDITION **3**

Editors

Mary M. Hinds, PhD, RN, NCS

Judy R. Hyland, MS, RN

Ann Lovric, MS, RN

Ainslie Nibert, PhD, RN

Sandra Upchurch, PhD, RN

ELSEVIER

ELSEVIER

3251 Riverport Lane
St. Louis, Missouri 63043

HESI Comprehensive Review for the NCLEX-RN® Examination,
Third Edition

ISBN: 978-0-323-06585-6

Copyright © 2011, 2008 by Elsevier Inc.

All rights reserved. No part of this publication may be reproduced or transmitted in any form or by any means, electronic or mechanical, including photocopying, recording, or any information storage and retrieval system, without permission in writing from the publisher. Details on how to seek permission, further information about the Publisher's permissions policies and our arrangements with organizations such as the Copyright Clearance Center and the Copyright Licensing Agency, can be found at our website: www.elsevier.com/permissions.

This book and the individual contributions contained in it are protected under copyright by the Publisher (other than as may be noted herein).

Notices

Knowledge and best practice in this field are constantly changing. As new research and experience broaden our understanding, changes in research methods, professional practices, or medical treatment may become necessary.

Practitioners and researchers must always rely on their own experience and knowledge in evaluating and using any information, methods, compounds, or experiments described herein. In using such information or methods they should be mindful of their own safety and the safety of others, including parties for whom they have a professional responsibility.

With respect to any drug or pharmaceutical products identified, readers are advised to check the most current information provided (i) on procedures featured or (ii) by the manufacturer of each product to be administered, to verify the recommended dose or formula, the method and duration of administration, and contraindications. It is the responsibility of practitioners, relying on their own experience and knowledge of their patients, to make diagnoses, to determine dosages and the best treatment for each individual patient, and to take all appropriate safety precautions.

To the fullest extent of the law, neither the Publisher nor the authors, contributors, or editors, assume any liability for any injury and/or damage to persons or property as a matter of products liability, negligence or otherwise, or from any use or operation of any methods, products, instructions, or ideas contained in the material herein.

NCLEX®, NCLEX-RN®, and NCLEX-PN® are registered trademarks of the National Council of State Boards of Nursing, Inc.

Nursing Diagnoses – Definitions and Classification 2009-2011. Copyright © 2009, 2007, 2005, 2003, 2001, 1998, 1996, 1994 by Nanda International. Used by arrangement with Wiley-Blackwell Publishing, a company of John Wiley and Sons, Inc. In order to make safe and effective judgments using NANDA-I nursing diagnoses it is essential that nurses refer to the definitions and defining characteristics of the diagnoses listed in this work.

Library of Congress Cataloging-in-Publication Data

HESI Comprehensive Review for the NCLEX-RN Examination / HESI; editors,
Donna Boyd ... [et al.]. – 3rd ed.
  p.; cm.
  Other title: Testing and remediation comprehensive review for the NCLEX-RN examination
  Rev. ed. of: Evolve Reach comprehensive review for the NCLEX-RN examination / HESI ; editors
Donna Boyd ... [et al.]. 2nd ed. c2008.
  Includes index.
  ISBN 978-0-323-06585-6 (pbk. : alk. paper)
  1. National Council Licensure Examination for Registered Nurses–Study guides.   2. Nursing–Examinations–Study guides.   3. Nursing–Examinations, questions, etc.   I. Boyd, Donna.   II. HESI (Firm)   III. Evolve Reach comprehensive review for the NCLEX-RN examination. IV. Title: Testing and remediation comprehensive review for the NCLEX-RN examination.
  [DNLM: 1. Nursing, Practical–Examination Questions.   2. Nursing, Practical–Outlines.   3. Nursing Care–Examination Questions.   4. Nursing Care–Outlines.   5. Nursing Process–Examination Questions.   6. Nursing Process–Outlines. WY 18.2 H584 2011]
  RT55.E96 2011
  610.73076–dc22

2010016826

Acquisitions Editor: Kristin Geen
Developmental Editor: Todd McKenzie
Marketing Manager: Fran Phillips

Publishing Services Manager: Jeff Patterson
Project Manager: Tracey Schriefer
Senior Designer: Amy Buxton

Working together to grow
libraries in developing countries

www.elsevier.com | www.bookaid.org | www.sabre.org

ELSEVIER | BOOK AID International | Sabre Foundation

Printed in the United States of America.

Last digit is the print number: 9 8 7 6 5 4 3

HESI Comprehensive Review for the

NCLEX-RN®
EXAMINATION

CONTENTS

INTRODUCTION TO TESTING AND THE NCLEX-RN® EXAM

Three cheers for you! You have made the wise decision to prepare, in a structured way, for the NCLEX-RN.

A. You have already successfully completed a basic nursing program and are well acquainted with your ability to take and pass tests and to perform successfully in the clinical area.

B. You have the basic knowledge required to pass the licensing exam. However, it is wise to:
   1. Organize your knowledge.
   2. Review content learned during the years of your basic nursing curriculum.
   3. Identify weaknesses in content knowledge so that you can focus your study time appropriately.
   4. Develop test-taking skills so you can demonstrate the knowledge you have.
   5. Reduce your level of anxiety by increasing your predictability.
   6. Know what to expect. Remember: Knowledge is power. You are powerful when you are well prepared and know what to expect.

Test-Taking Tips

There are no absolute ways to ensure that exam questions will always be answered correctly. These test-taking tips are guidelines to help the student study and understand the exam questions. On the NCLEX-RN exam, many different areas are tested with each question. For example, a question may on the surface be a medical/surgical or pediatric question but included in the question can be such topics as communication, nutrition, growth and development, medication, client and family education, and safety.

A. Understanding the question
   1. Determine if the question is written in a positive or negative style.
      a. A *positive* style may ask what the nurse should do or ask for the best or first action to implement.

HESI Hint • Most questions are written in a positive style.

      b. A *negative* style may ask what the nurse should avoid, which prescription the nurse should question, or which behavior indicates the need for re-teaching the client.

HESI Hint • Negative style questions will contain key words that denote the negative style.

EXAMPLES
1. "Which response indicates to the nurse a need to *re-teach* the client about...?" (Which information/ understanding by the client is incorrect?)
2. "Which prescription (order) should the nurse *question?*" (Which prescription is unsafe, not beneficial, inappropriate to this client situation, etc...?)

   2. Find the key words in the question.
      a. Ask yourself which words or phrases provide the critical information.
      b. This information may be the age of the client, the setting, the timing, a set of symptoms or behaviors, or any number of other factors.
      c. For example, the nursing actions for a 10-year-old 1 day postop are different than those for a 70-year-old 1 hour postop.
   3. Rephrase the question in your own words.
      a. This will help you eliminate nonessential information in the question and help you determine the correct answer.
      b. Ask yourself, "What is this question *really* asking?"
      c. While keeping the options covered, rephrase the question in your own words.

4. Rule out options.
   a. Based on your knowledge, you can probably identify one or two options that are clearly incorrect.
   b. Physically mark through those options on the test booklet if allowed. Mentally mark through those options in your head if using a computer.
   c. Now differentiate between the remaining options, considering your knowledge of the subject and related nursing principles, such as roles of the nurse, the nursing process, the ABCs (airway, breathing, and circulation), and Maslow's Hierarchy of Needs.

B. General guidelines about test taking
   1. Consider the content of the question and what the question is asking.
   2. Generally, an assessment of the client occurs before an action is taken.
   3. Identify the least invasion intervention before taking action.
   4. Have all the necessary information and take all possible relevant actions before calling the physician or health care provider.
   5. Determine which client to assess first (e.g., most at risk, most physiologically unstable).
   6. Identify opposites in the answers.
      a. Example: prone/supine; elevated/decreased
      b. Read *VERY* carefully; one is likely to be the answer, BUT not always
      c. If you do not know the answer, choose the most likely of the "opposites" and move on.
   7. Take into account a client's lifestyle, culture, and spiritual beliefs when answering a question.

C. Use CRITICAL THINKING, reasoning, and common sense to answer questions.
   1. DO respond based on...
      a. ABCs
      b. Scientific, behavioral, sociologic principles
      c. Principles of teaching/learning
      d. Maslow's Hierarchy of Needs
      e. Nursing process
      f. What's in the stem: no more, no less (Do not read more into the question than is already there.)
      g. NCLEX-RN ideal hospital
      h. Basic anatomy and physiology
   2. DON'T respond based on...
      a. *YOUR* past client care experiences or agency
      b. A familiar phrase or term
      c. "Of course, I would have already..."
      d. What YOU think is *REALISTIC*

   e. *YOUR* children, pregnancies, parents, elders, personal response to a drug, etc.
   f. The "what ifs"

D. Keep memorizing to a minimum.
   1. Growth and developmental milestones
   2. Death and dying stages
   3. Crisis intervention
   4. Immunizations schedule
   5. Principles of teaching/learning
   6. Stages of pregnancy and fetal growth
   7. Nurse Practice Act: Standards of Practice and Delegation

E. Know commonly used lab ranges (Appendix A), what variations mean, and the BEST nursing actions.
   1. H&H
   2. WBCs, RBCs, platelets
   3. Electrolytes: K^+, Na^+, Ca^{++}, Mg^{++}, Cl^-, PO_4^-
   4. BUN and creatinine
   5. Relationship of Ca^{++} and PO_4^-
   6. ABGs
   7. PT, INR, PTT (Don't get them confused.)

F. Nutrition
   1. Know commonly used nutrition information.
      a. High or low Na^+
      b. High or low K^+
      c. High PO_4
      d. Iron
      e. Vitamin K
      f. Proteins
      g. Carbohydrates
      h. Fats
   2. Foods and diets related to
      a. Gastrointestinal/genitourinary disturbances
      b. Chemotherapy diets and restrictions
      c. Pregnancy and fetal growth needs
   3. Remember concepts
      a. Introducing one food at a time (infants, allergies)
      b. Progression "AS TOLERATED" (What nursing assessment guides decisions regarding progression?)

G. Medications—SAFE medication administration is more than just knowing the name, classification, and action of the medication.
   1. "Six Rights" including techniques of skill execution
   2. Drug interactions
   3. Vulnerable organs
      a. What to assess
      b. Which lab values relate to specific organs
   4. Allergies
   5. Presence of suprainfections
   6. Concepts of *peak* and *trough*

7. How you would know
   a. The drug is working
   b. There's a problem
8. Nursing actions
9. Client education should include
   a. Safety
   b. Empowerment
   c. Compliance

The NCLEX-RN Licensing Exam

A. The main purpose of a licensing exam like the NCLEX-RN is to protect the public.
B. The NCLEX-RN:
   1. Was developed by the National Council of State Boards of Nursing (the Council; this abbreviation is used to refer to the NCSBN throughout this book)
   2. Is administered by the State Board of Nurse Examiners
   3. Is designed to test candidates'
      a. Capabilities for safe and effective nursing practice
      b. Essential nursing knowledge

Job Analysis Studies

A. Essential knowledge is determined by job analysis studies.

> **HESI Hint** • The Council wants to ensure that the licensing exam measures current entry-level nursing behaviors. For this reason, job analysis studies are conducted every 3 years. These studies determine how frequently various types of nursing activities are performed, how often they are delegated, and how critical they are to client safety, with criticality given more value than frequency.

B. Job analysis studies indicate that newly licensed registered nurses are using all five categories of the Nursing process and that such use is evenly distributed throughout the five Nursing process areas. Therefore, equal attention is given to each part of the Nursing process in selecting test items (Table 1-1).

NURSING DIAGNOSES

A. Nursing diagnoses are formulated during the analysis portion of the Nursing process. They give form and direction to the Nursing process, promote priority setting, and guide nursing actions (Table 1-2).

TABLE 1-1 The Nursing Process

Category	Activities Associated with Nursing Process
Assessment	• Gather objective and subjective data. • Verify data.
Analysis	• Interpret data. • Collect additional data when necessary. • Identify and communicate nursing diagnoses. • Determine health team's ability to meet client's needs.
Planning	• Determine and prioritize outcomes of care. Include client, significant others, and health team in setting outcomes. • Develop and modify plan for delivery of client's care.
Implementation	• Organize and manage the client's care, including assignment and delegation of tasks. • Perform or assist in performance of client's care. • Counsel and teach client, significant others, and health team. • Provide care specifically directed toward achieving outcomes.
Evaluation	• Compare actual outcomes with expected outcomes. • Evaluate compliance with the established regimen or plan. • Record and describe client's response to plan. • Modify plan as indicated and set priorities.

B. To qualify as a nursing diagnosis, the primary responsibility and accountability for recognition and treatment rest with the nurse.
C. The National Conference of the North American Nursing Diagnosis Association (NANDA) provided the following definition of a nursing diagnosis: "Nursing diagnosis is a clinical judgment about individual, family, or community responses to actual and potential health problems/life processes. Nursing diagnoses provide the basis for selection of nursing interventions to achieve outcomes for which the nurse is accountable" (Box 1-1).

TABLE I-2 Components of a Nursing Diagnosis

Component	Explanation
Response	• Includes potential or actual health response • Describes measurable outcomes that can be derived • Cites potential for changes based on nursing actions • *Example:* Alteration in comfort, pain
Etiology	• Includes potential or actual health response • Addresses independent, interdependent, and dependent nursing functions • *Example:* Related to fractured left ankle

D. NCLEX-RN questions regarding nursing diagnosis can take several forms:
  1. You may be given the nursing diagnosis in the stem and asked to select an appropriate nursing intervention based on the stated nursing diagnosis.
  2. You may be asked to select, from the four choices, an appropriate nursing diagnosis for the described case.
  3. You may be asked to choose, from four nursing diagnoses, the one that should have priority based on the data in the stem.

> **HESI Hint** • A nursing diagnosis is not a medical diagnosis. It must be subject to oversight by nursing management.
> The cause may or may not arise from a medical diagnosis.

CLIENT NEEDS

A. Job analysis studies have identified categories of care provided by nurses called Client Needs. The test plan is structured according to these categories (Table 1-3).

PRIORITIZING NURSING CARE

A. Many NCLEX-RN test items are designed to test your ability to set priorities—for example:
  1. Identify the *most important* client needs.
  2. Which nursing intervention is *most important?*
  3. Which nursing action should be done *first?*
  4. Which response is *best?*
B. Setting priorities
  1. What should be done first or next?

2. Those taking the NCLEX-RN should "Remember Maslow" (Table 1-4).
3. The Five Rights of Delegation (see Chapter 2, p. 17)

> **HESI Hint** • Answering NCLEX-RN questions correctly often depends on setting priorities properly, on making judgments about priorities, and on analyzing the case and formulating a decision about care (or the correct response) based on priorities. Using Maslow's Hierarchy of Needs can help you to set priorities.

The NCLEX-RN Computer Adaptive Testing

A. Computer adaptive testing (CAT) is used for implementation of the NCLEX-RN.
B. The CAT is administered at a testing center selected by the Council.
C. Pearson VUE is responsible for adapting the NCLEX-RN to the CAT format, processing candidate applications, and transmitting test results to its data center for scoring.
D. The testing centers are located throughout the United States.
E. The Council generates the NCLEX-RN test items.

THE WAY IT WORKS

A. The NCLEX-RN consists of 75 to 265 multiple-choice or alternative-format questions (15 of which are "pilot items") presented on a computer screen.
B. The candidate is presented with a test item and possible answers.
C. If the candidate answers the question correctly, a slightly more difficult item will follow, and the level of difficulty will increase with each item until the candidate misses an item.
D. If the candidate misses an item, a slightly less difficult item will follow, and the level of difficulty will decrease with each item until the candidate has answered an item correctly.
E. This process will continue until the candidate has achieved a definite pass or a definite fail score. There will be no borderline pass or fail scores because the adaptive testing method determines the candidate's level of performance before she or he has finished the exam.
F. The least number of items a candidate can answer to complete the exam is 75; 15 of them will be pilot items and will not count toward the pass or fail score; 60 of them will determine the candidate's score.

CONTRIBUTING AUTHORS

Mary Anderson, MSN, RN, CNS

Elizabeth Arnold, MSN, RN, CNS

Sara Bishop, PhD, RNC

Mary Ann Boyd, PhD, DNS, APRN, BC

Robin Britt, EdD, RNC

Mary Cassem, MS, RN

Rita D. Cinquemani, RN, MSN, FNP-BC

Darla M. Close, MSN, RN

Carol L. Collins, MS, RN

Pat Crotwell, MSN, RN

Debra Danforth, MS, RN, ARNP

Deborah Davenport, MSN, RN, CCRN

Judith Driscoll, MEd, RN, MSN

Karen F. Duncan, MS, RN

Laurie K. Erford, MSN, RN

Jean Flick, MS, RN

Judy Hammond, PhD, RNC

Mary M. Hinds, PhD, RN, CNS

Judy R. Hyland, MS, RN

Florence Jemes, RN, MSN, CS

Barbara Kearney, PhD, RN

Robin Lockhart, PhD(c), RN

Ann Lovric, RN, MSN

Mary Lou Martin, MSN, RN, CPNP

Jane Mathis, MSN, RNC, CCE

Susan Morrison, PhD, RN

Ainslie Nibert, PhD, RN

Cynthia K. Peterson, MSN, RN

Judy Siefert, MSN, RN

Betty Tracy, MN, RN

Mary Yoho, PhD, RN

REVIEWERS

Jacqueline B. Arnett, BSN, CPN
Registered Nurse, Staff Development Coordinator
Life Care Centers of America
Nursing Administration
Tucson, Arizona

Carolyn V. Daigneau, RN-CS, MSN, PNP-BC
Pediatric Nurse Practitioner
Formerly Department of Gastroenterology, Nutrition
  and Hepatology
Texas Liver Center – Pediatric Hepatology and Liver
  Transplant
The University of Texas Health Science Center at
  Houston
Houston, Texas

Cené L. Gibson, MSN, ARNP
Family Nurse Practitioner
Frontier School of Midwifery and Family Nursing
Regional Clinical Coordinator
Oklahoma City, Oklahoma

Marilyn L. Johnessee Greer, MS, RN
Associate Professor of Nursing
Rockford College
Rockford, Illinois

Sarah M. Howell, RN, MSN
Assistant Professor of Nursing
Mississippi University for Women
Columbus, Mississippi

Katherine Roberts, MSN, RN
Assistant Professor of Nursing
Lamar University
Department of Nursing
Beaumont, Texas

Denise Sevigny, RN, MSN
Adjunct Faculty
School of Nursing
Old Dominion University
Norfolk, Virginia

PREFACE

Welcome to *HESI Comprehensive Review for the NCLEX-RN® Examination* with online study exams, edited by HESI.

Congratulations! This outstanding review manual with online study exams is designed to prepare nursing students for what is very likely the most important examination they will ever take—the NCLEX-RN® Licensing Examination. As a graduate of an RN nursing program, the student has the basic knowledge required to pass tests and perform safely and successfully in the clinical area. *HESI Comprehensive Review for the NCLEX-RN Examination* allows the nursing student to prepare for the NCLEX-RN® licensure examination in a structured way.

- Organize nursing basic knowledge previously learned.

- Review content learned during basic nursing curriculum.

- Identify weaknesses in content knowledge so study effort can be focused appropriately.

- Develop test-taking skills so application of safe nursing practice from knowledge previously learned can be demonstrated.

- Reduce anxiety level by increasing predictability of ability to correctly answer NCLEX-type questions.

- Boost test-taking confidence by being well prepared and knowing what to expect.

Organization

Chapter 1, Introduction to Testing and the NCLEX-RN Exam, gives an overview of the NCLEX-RN licensing exam history and test plan for the examination. A review of the nursing process, updated with the latest NANDA-approved nursing diagnoses, client needs, and prioritizing nursing care, is also presented.

Chapter 2, Leadership and Management, reviews the legal aspects of nursing, leadership and management, and disaster nursing.

Chapter 3, Advanced Clinical Concepts, presents nursing assessment, analysis (nursing diagnoses), and

planning and intervention at the highest level of practice. Topics reviewed include respiratory failure, shock, disseminated intravascular coagulation (DIC), resuscitation, fluid and electrolyte balance, IV therapy, acid-base balance, ECG, perioperative care, HIV, pain, and death and grief.

Chapters 4 through 8, Medical-Surgical Nursing, Pediatric Nursing, Maternity Nursing, Psychiatric Nursing, and **Gerontologic Nursing**, are presented in traditional clinical groupings.

Each clinical area is divided into physiologic components, but essential knowledge about basic anatomy, growth and development, pharmacology and medication calculation, nutrition, communication, client and family education, acute and chronic care, leadership and management, and clinical decision making is threaded throughout the different components.

Open-ended style questions appear at the end of each chapter, which encourage the student to think in depth about the content that is presented throughout the particular chapter. When a variety of learning mechanisms are used, students have the opportunity to comprehensively prepare for the NCLEX exam; these strategies include:

- Reading the manual.

- Discussing content with others.

- Answering open-ended questions.

- Practicing with mock tests that simulate the licensure examination.

These learning experiences are all different ways that students should use to prepare for the NCLEX exam. The purpose of the open-ended questions appearing at the end of the chapter is not a focused practice session on managing NCLEX-style, multiple-choice questions, but rather this learning approach allows for more in-depth thinking about the particular topics in the chapter. Practice with multiple-choice questions alone cannot provide the depth of critical thinking and analysis possible with the short-answer questions at the end of the chapter. Additionally, open-ended questions presented at the end of the chapter provide a summary experience that helps students focus on the main topics that were covered in the chapter. Teachers use open-ended style questions to stimulate the critical thinking process, and **HESI Comprehensive Review for the NCLEX-RN Examination** facilitates the critical thinking process by posing the same type of questions the teacher might pose in this way.

When students need to practice multiple-choice questions, the online study exams on Evolve offer extensive opportunities for practice and skill-building to improve their test-taking abilities. The online study exams include six content-specific exams (Medical-Surgical Nursing, Pharmacology, Pediatrics, Fundamentals, Maternity, and Psychiatric-Mental Health Nursing) and one comprehensive exam patterned after categories on the NCLEX-RN® exam. The online study exams on Evolve can be accessed as many times as necessary, and the questions from one practice exam are not contained on another practice exam. For instance, the Medical-Surgical practice exam does not contain questions that are on the Pediatrics practice exam. The purpose of providing these mock exams is to provide practice and exposure to the critical thinking–style questions that students will encounter on the NCLEX-RN exam. However, the mock exams should not be used to predict performance on the actual NCLEX exam. Only the HESI Exit Exam, a secure, computerized exam that simulates the NCLEX test plan and has evidence-based results from numerous research studies indicating a high level of accuracy in predicting NCLEX success, is offered as a true predictor exam. Students are allowed unlimited practice on each mock exam so that they can be sure to have the opportunity to review all of the rationales for the questions.

Additional assistance for students studying for the NCLEX-RN Licensing Examination can be obtained from a variety of online products in the Elsevier family. Many nursing schools have also adopted the following:

• *HESI Practice Test*—This is the ideal way to practice for the NCLEX exam. With more than 1200 practice questions included in this online test bank, nursing students can access practice exams 24 hours a day, 7 days a week! *HESI Practice Test* questions are written at the critical thinking level, so that students are tested not for memorization but for their skills in clinical application. That is an advantage unique to *HESI Practice Test!* NCLEX exam-style questions include multiple-choice and alternate-item formats and are accompanied by correct answers and rationales. Available exams vary in size and scope. Students select a test option, and *HESI Practice Test* automatically supplies a series of critical-thinking practice questions. Included are standard exams on specialties and a comprehensive exam from a single specialty or from randomized specialties.

• *HESI Examinations*—A comprehensive set of examinations was designed to prepare nursing students for the NCLEX exam and enables customized remediation from Mosby and Saunders textbooks, which saves time for faculty and students. Each student is given an individualized report detailing exam results and is allowed to view questions and rationales for items that were answered incorrectly. The electronic remediation, a complementary feature of the specialty and exit exams, can be filed according to the subject matter in which the student did not answer a question correctly.

• *HESI Case Studies*—These prepare students to manage complex patient conditions and make sound clinical judgments. These online case studies cover a broad range of physiologic and psychosocial alterations, plus related management, pharmacology, and therapeutic concepts.

• *HESI Patient Reviews*—A live review course is presented by an expert faculty member who has been trained by the director of curriculum, Elsevier Assessment. Students are presented with a workbook and practice NCLEX-style questions that are used during the course.

• *Evolve eBooks*—Online versions of all of the Mosby and Saunders textbooks used in the student's nursing curriculum are presented. Search across titles, highlight, make notes, and more—all on your computer.

• *Elsevier Simulations*—Three virtual versions simulate the clinical environment. These multilayered, complex, supplemental experiences enable faculty to make clinical assignments without the need for actual clinical space.

• *Elsevier Courses*—Created by experts using instructional design principles, this interactive content engages students with reading, animation, video, audio, interactive exercises, and assessments.

BOX 1-1 *NANDA-Approved Nursing Diagnoses*

Sleep/Rest	Sexuality/Reproductive	Value/Belief
• Sleep deprivation • Disturbed sleep patterns • Readiness for enhanced sleep	• Sexual dysfunction • Ineffective sexuality patterns	• Readiness for enhanced religiosity • Risk for impaired religiosity • Spiritual distress • Risk for spiritual distress

Activity/Exercise	Nutrition/Metabolism
• Activity intolerance • Risk for activity intolerance • Ineffective airway clearance • Autonomic dysreflexia • Risk for autonomic dysreflexia • Ineffective breathing pattern • Decreased cardiac output • Risk for delayed development • Risk for disuse syndrome • Deficient diversional activity • Adult failure to thrive • Fatigue • Impaired gas exchange • Delayed growth and development • Risk for disproportionate growth • Impaired home maintenance • Disorganized infant behavior • Risk for disorganized infant behavior • Readiness for enhanced organize infant behavior • Impaired bed mobility • Impaired physical mobility • Impaired wheelchair mobility • Sedentary lifestyle • Risk for peripheral neurovascular dysfunction • Bathing/hygiene self-care deficit • Dressing/grooming self-care deficit • Feeding self-care deficit • Toileting self-care deficit • Delayed surgical recovery • Ineffective tissue perfusion (specify type) • Impaired transfer ability • Impaired spontaneous ventilation • Dysfunctional ventilatory weaning response • Impaired walking	• Risk for aspiration • Risk for imbalanced body temperature • Effective breastfeeding • Ineffective breastfeeding • Interrupted breastfeeding • Impaired dentition • Readiness for enhanced fluid balance • Deficient fluid volume • Excess fluid volume • Risk for deficient fluid volume • Risk for imbalanced fluid volume • Hyperthermia • Hypothermia • Nausea • Readiness for enhanced nutrition • Imbalanced nutrition: less than body requirements • Imbalanced nutrition: more than body requirements • Risk for imbalanced nutrition: more than body requirements • Ineffective infant feeding pattern • Impaired oral mucous membrane • Impaired skin integrity • Risk for impaired skin integrity • Impaired tissue integrity • Ineffective thermoregulation • Impaired swallowing

Health Perception/Health Management	Role/Relationship
• Latex allergy response • Risk for latex allergy response • Risk for sudden infant death syndrome • Disturbed energy field • Risk for falls • Health-seeking behaviors (specify)	• Risk for impaired parent/infant/child attachment • Caregiver role strain • Risk for caregiver role strain • Impaired verbal communication • Readiness for enhanced communication • Parental role conflict

(Continued)

BOX 1-1 NANDA-Approved Nursing Diagnoses—cont'd

Health Perception/Health Management—cont'd	Role/Relationship—cont'd
• Ineffective health maintenance • Risk for infection • Risk for injury • Risk for perioperative positioning injury • Deficient knowledge (specify) • Readiness for enhanced knowledge (specify) • Noncompliance (specify) • Risk for poisoning • Ineffective protection • Risk for suffocation • Ineffective family therapeutic regimen management • Risk for trauma • Wandering	• Dysfunctional family processes: alcoholism • Interrupted family processes • Readiness for enhanced family processes • Grieving • Complicated grieving • Risk for complicated grieving • Impaired parenting • Risk for impaired parenting • Readiness for enhanced parenting • Relocation stress syndrome • Risk for relocation stress syndrome • Social isolation • Chronic sorrow • Risk for other-directed violence • Risk for self-directed violence
Self-perception	**Elimination**
• Anxiety • Death anxiety • Disturbed body image • Fear • Hopelessness • Disturbed personal identity • Risk for loneliness • Powerlessness • Risk for powerlessness • Chronic low self-esteem • Situational low self-esteem • Risk for situational low self-esteem • Self-mutilation • Risk for self-mutilation	• Bowel incontinence • Perceived constipation • Constipation • Risk for constipation • Diarrhea • Functional urinary incontinence • Reflex urinary incontinence • Stress urinary incontinence • Urge urinary incontinence • Risk for urge urinary incontinence • Readiness for enhanced urinary elimination • Impaired urinary elimination • Urinary retention
Cognitive/Perceptual	**Coping/Stress Tolerance**
• Impaired comfort • Chronic pain • Decisional conflict (specify) • Acute confusion • Chronic confusion • Decreased intracranial adaptive capacity • Impaired memory • Unilateral neglect • Acute pain • Disturbed sensory perception (specify)	• Compromised family coping • Defensive coping • Disabled family coping • Ineffective coping • Ineffective community coping • Readiness for enhanced coping • Readiness for enhanced community coping • Readiness for enhanced family coping • Ineffective denial • Post-trauma syndrome • Risk for post-trauma syndrome • Risk for suicide

From North American Nursing Diagnosis Association International. (2009). *Nursing diagnoses: Definitions and classification 2009-2011*. Philadelphia: NANDA International.

TABLE 1-3   Client Needs

Category of Client Needs	NCLEX-RN (%)	Activities
Safe and Effective Care Environment • Management of care • Safety and infection control	16 to 22 8 to 14	• Coordination of care; quality assurance; goal-oriented care; environmental safety • Preparation for treatments and procedures • Safe and effective treatments and procedures
Health Promotion and Maintenance	6 to 12	• Continued growth and development • Self-care • Integrity of support systems • Prevention and early treatment of health problems
Psychosocial Integrity	6 to 12	• Promotion and support of emotional, mental, and social well-being
Physiological Integrity • Basic care and comfort • Pharmacologic and parenteral therapies • Reduction of risk potential • Physiologic adaptation	6 to 12 13 to 19 10 to 16 11 to 17	• Physiologic adaptation • Reduction for risk potential • Activities of daily living • Care room temperature, medication administration, and parental therapies • Provision of basic comfort and care

Note: The percentage of test questions assigned to each Client Needs category and subcategory of the 2010 NCLEX-RN Test Plan is based on the results of the Report of Findings from the 2008 RN Practice Analysis (2009). Linking the NCLEX-RN Examination to Practice: NCSBN.
Adapted from National Council of State Boards of Nursing. *Test plan for the NCLEX-RN examination.* Copyright ©2010, National Council of State Boards of Nursing, Inc., Chicago, IL.

G. The number of the item the candidate is currently answering will appear on the upper right area of the screen.

H. When the candidate has answered enough items to determine a definite pass or fail score, a message will appear on the screen notifying the candidate that he or she has completed the exam.

I. The most number of items a candidate can answer is 265, and the longest amount of time the candidate can take to complete the exam is 6 hours.

J. Candidates will have up to 6 hours to complete the NCLEX-RN examination; total examination time includes a short tutorial, two preprogrammed optional breaks, and any unscheduled breaks they may take. The first optional break is offered after 2 hours of testing. The second optional break is offered after 3½ hours of testing. The computer will automatically tell candidates when these scheduled breaks begin.
1. All breaks count against testing time.
2. When candidates take breaks, they must leave the testing room, and they will be required to provide a fingerprint before and after the breaks.

K. If a candidate has not obtained a pass/fail score at the end of the 6 hours and has not completed all 265 items in the 6-hour limit but has answered all of the last 60 questions presented correctly, he or she will pass the exam.

L. If a candidate has not obtained a pass/fail score at the end of the 6 hours, has not completed all 265 items in the 6-hour limit, and has not answered correctly all of the last 60 questions presented, he or she will fail the exam.

M. A specific passing score is recommended by the Council. All states require the same score to pass, so that if you pass in one state, you are eligible to practice nursing in any other state. However, states do differ in their requirements regarding the number of times a candidate can take the NCLEX-RN.

N. Although the Council has the ability to determine a candidate's score at the time of completion of the exam, it has been decided that it would be best for candidates to receive their scores from their individual Board of Nurse Examiners. The Council does not want the testing center to be in a position of having to deal with candidates' reactions to scores, nor does the Council want those waiting to take their exams to be influenced by such reactions.

O. You must answer each question in order to proceed. You cannot omit a question or return to an item presented earlier. There is no going back; this works in your favor!

P. The examination is written at a 10th grade reading level.

TABLE I-4 Maslow's Hierarchy of Needs

Need	Definition	Nursing Implications
Physiologic	Biologic needs for food, shelter, water, sleep, oxygen, sexual expression	The priority biologic need is breathing, i.e., an open airway. Review Table 1-3, Client Needs activities associated with physiologic integrity. If you were asked to identify the *most important* action, you would identify needs associated with physiologic integrity (e.g., providing an open airway) as the most important nursing action.
Safety	Avoiding harm; attaining security, order, and physical safety	Review Table 1-3, the activities associated with Safe and Effective Care Environment. Ensuring that the client's environment is safe is a priority (e.g., teaching an older client to remove throw rugs that pose a safety hazard when ambulating would have a greater priority than teaching him or her how to use a walker). The first priority is safety, then coping skills.
Love and Belonging Esteem and Recognition	Giving and receiving affection; companionship; and identification with a group Self-esteem and respect of others; success in work; prestige	Although these needs are important (described in Table 1-3, Client Needs, activities associated with psychosocial integrity), they are less important than physiologic or safety needs. For example, it is more important for a client to have an open airway and a safe environment for ambulating than it is to assist him or her to become part of a support group. However, assisting the client in becoming a part of a support group would have higher priority than assisting him or her in developing self-esteem. The sense of belonging would come first, and such a sense might help in developing self-esteem.
Self-actualization Aesthetic	Fulfillment of unique potential Search for beauty and spiritual goals	It is important to understand the last two needs in Maslow's Hierarchy. They could deal with Client Needs associated with Health Promotion and Maintenance, such as continued growth and development and self-care, as well as those associated with Psychosocial Integrity. However, you will probably not be asked to prioritize needs at this level. Remember, it is the goal of the Council to ensure *safe* nursing practice, and such practice does not usually deal with the client's self-actualization or aesthetic needs.

Q. There is no penalty for guessing; with four choices, you have a 25% chance of guessing the correct answer.

R. The NCSBN Candidate Bulletin is available at http://www.ncsbn.org. Select NCLEX Examinations/Candidates/Basic Information/Bulletin.

> **HESI Hint** • One or more of the choices are likely to be very wrong. You will usually be able to rule out two of the four choices rather quickly. Reread the question and choices again if necessary. Ask yourself which choice answers the question being asked. Even if you have absolutely no idea what the correct answer is, you will have a 50/50 chance of guessing the right answer if you follow this process. Your first response will provide an educated guess and will usually be the correct answer. Go with your gut response!
>
> Pace yourself from the beginning of the test. Allow approximately 1.5 minutes per question.

EXAM ITEM FORMATS

A. There are six types of exam items presented on the NCLEX-RN examination.
   1. The majority of the questions are multiple-choice items with four choices (answers) from which to choose one correct answer.
   2. Multiple-response items require the candidate to select one or more responses from five to seven choices. The item will instruct the candidate to choose all that apply.
   3. Fill-in-the-blank questions require the candidate to calculate the answer and type in the numbers. A drop down calculator is provided.
   4. Hot-spot items require the candidate to identify an area on a picture or graph and click on the area.
   5. Chart or exhibit formats present a chart or exhibit that the candidate must read to be able to solve the problem.
   6. Drop-and-drag items require a candidate to rank order or move options to provide the correct order of actions or events.

B. There is no set percentage of alternative items on the NCLEX-RN examination. All examination items are scored either right or wrong. There is no partial credit in scoring any examination questions.

Gentle Reminders of General Principles

Take care of yourself. Follow these golden rules for NCLEX-RN success.

A. Eat well: Consume a high-carbohydrate, high-protein, and low-fat diet.

B. Sleep well: Get a good night's sleep the night before the test. This is not the time to cram or to party. You have done your job. Now enjoy the process.

C. Eliminate alcohol and other mind-altering drugs: It goes without saying that such substances can inhibit your performance on the exam.

D. Schedule study time: Between now and the exam, review nursing content, focusing on areas that you have identified as your weak points when taking the practice tests (review your computer scoring sheets). Use a study schedule to block out the time needed for study. Then be good to yourself, and use that blocked time for yourself: study.

E. Be prepared: Assemble all necessary materials the night before the exam (admission ticket, directions to the testing center, identification, money for lunch, glasses or contacts).
   1. Approved items: Candidates are allowed to bring only identification forms into the testing room. Watches, candy, chewing gum, food, drinks, purses, wallets, pens, pencils, beepers, cellular phones, Post-It notes, study materials or aids, and calculators are not allowed. A test administrator will provide each candidate with an erasable note board that may be replaced as needed while testing. Candidates may not take their own note boards, scratch paper, or writing instruments into the exam. A calculator on the computer screen will be available for use.
   2. Allow plenty of time: Arrive early; it is better to be early than late. Allow for traffic jams and so forth. The candidate may want to consider spending the night in a hotel or motel near the testing center the night before the exam.
   3. Dress comfortably: Dress in layers so that you can take off a sweater or jacket if you become too warm or wear it if you become too cold.

F. Avoid negative people: From now until you have completed the exam, stay away from those who share their anxieties with you or project their insecurities onto you. Sometimes this is a fellow classmate or even your best friend. The person will still be there when the exam is over. Right now you need to take care of yourself. Avoid the negative; look for the positive.

G. Do not discuss the exam: Avoid talking about the exam during breaks and while waiting to take the exam.

H. Avoid distractions: Take earplugs with you and use them if you find that those around you are distracting you, such as those chewing gum, rattling paper, or getting up to leave the exam.

I. Think positively: Use the affirmation "I am successful." Obtain a relaxation and affirmation tape and use it hs (hour of sleep) and prn (as needed) from now until you take the exam. Use the relaxation tape at night (not on the way to the exam or during breaks while taking the exam; you might

fall asleep!). Use the affirmation on the way to the exam or any time you feel the need to boost your confidence. Think, "I have the knowledge to successfully complete the NCLEX-RN."

HESI Hint • The night before taking the NCLEX-RN, allow only 30 minutes of study time. This 30-minute period should be designated for review of test-taking strategies only. Practice these strategies with various practice test items if you wish (for 30 minutes only; do not take an entire test). Spend the night before the exam doing something you enjoy, something that promotes stress reduction, something that does not involve alcohol or other mind-altering drugs. Only you can identify the special something that will work for you. Remember, you can be successful!

2

LEADERSHIP AND MANAGEMENT

Legal Aspects of Nursing

LAWS GOVERNING NURSING

A. Nurse Practice Acts provide the laws that control the practice of nursing in each state. Mandatory Nurse Practice Acts authorize that, under the law, only licensed professionals can practice nursing. All states now have mandatory Nurse Practice Acts.

B. Nurse Practice Acts govern the nurse's responsibility in making assignments.
   1. Assignments should be commensurate with the nursing personnel's educational preparation, experience, and knowledge.
   2. The nurse should supervise the care provided by nursing personnel for which he or she is administratively responsible.
   3. Sterile or invasive procedures should be assigned to or supervised by a professional nurse (registered nurse [RN]).

TORTS

Description: An act involving injury or damage to another (except breech of contract) resulting in civil liability (i.e., the victim can sue) instead of criminal liability (see Crime).

Unintentional Torts

A. Negligence and malpractice
   1. Negligence: Performing an act that a reasonable and prudent person would not perform. The measure of negligence is "reasonableness" (i.e., would a reasonable and prudent nurse act in the same manner under the same circumstances?).
   2. Malpractice: Negligence by professional personnel (e.g., professional misconduct or unreasonable lack of skill in carrying out professional duties)

B. Four elements are necessary to prove negligence or malpractice; if any one element is missing, they cannot be proved.
   1. Duty: Obligation to use due care (what a reasonable, prudent nurse would do); failure to care for and/or to protect others against unreasonable risk. The nurse must *anticipate* foreseeable risks. Example: If a floor has water on it, the nurse is responsible for anticipating the risk for a client's falling.
   2. Breach of duty: Failure to perform according to the established standard of conduct in providing nursing care.
   3. Injury/damages: Failure to meet standard of care, which causes actual injury or damage to the client, either physical or mental.
   4. Causation: A connection exists between conduct and the resulting injury referred to as "proximate cause" or "remoteness of damage."

C. Hospital policies provide a guide for nursing actions. They are not laws, but courts generally rule against nurses who have violated the employer's policies. Hospitals can be liable for poorly formulated or poorly implemented policies.

D. Incident reports alert administration to possible liability claims and the need for investigation; they do not protect against legal action being taken for negligence or malpractice.

E. Examples of negligence or malpractice
   1. Burning a client with a hot water bottle or heating pad
   2. Leaving sponges or instruments in a client's body after surgery
   3. Performing incompetent assessments
   4. Failing to heed warning signs of shock or impending myocardial infarction
   5. Ignoring signs and symptoms of bleeding
   6. Forgetting to give a medication or giving the wrong medication

Intentional Torts

A. Assault and battery
   1. Assault: Mental or physical threat (e.g., forcing [without touching] a client to take a medication or treatment)
   2. Battery: Touching, with or without the intent to do harm (e.g., hitting or striking a client). If a mentally competent adult is forced to have a treatment he or she has refused, battery occurs.
B. Invasion of privacy: Encroachment or trespassing on another's body or personality
   1. False imprisonment: Confinement without authorization
   2. Exposure of a person: Exposure or discussion of a client's case. After death, a client has the right to be unobserved, excluded from unwarranted operations, and protected from unauthorized touching of the body.
   3. Defamation: Divulgence of privileged information or communication (e.g., through charts, conversations, or observations)
C. Fraud: Willful and purposeful misrepresentation that could cause, or has caused, loss or harm to a person or property. Examples of fraud include:
   1. Presenting false credentials for the purpose of entering nursing school, obtaining a license, or obtaining employment
   2. Describing a myth regarding a treatment (e.g., telling a client that a placebo has no side effects and will cure the disease, or telling a client that a treatment or diagnostic test will not hurt, when indeed pain is involved in the procedure)

CRIME

A. An act contrary to a criminal statute. Crimes are wrongs punishable by the state, committed against the state, with intent usually present. The nurse remains bound by all criminal laws.
B. Commission of a crime involves the following behaviors:
   1. A person commits a deed contrary to criminal law.
   2. A person omits an act when there is a legal obligation to perform such an act (e.g., refusing to assist with the birth of a child if such a refusal results in injury to the child).
   3. Criminal conspiracy occurs when two or more persons agree to commit a crime.
   4. Assisting or giving aid to a person in the commission of a crime makes that person equally guilty of the offense (awareness must be present that the crime is being committed).
   5. Ignoring a law is not usually an adequate defense against the commission of a crime (e.g., a nurse who sees another nurse taking narcotics from the unit supply and ignores this observation is not adequately defended against committing a crime).
   6. Assault is justified for self-defense. However, to be justified, only enough force can be used as to maintain self-protection.
   7. Search warrants are required prior to searching a person's property.
   8. It is a crime *not* to report suspected child abuse (i.e., the nurse's legal responsibility is to report suspected child abuse).

NURSING PRACTICE AND THE LAW

Psychiatric Nursing

A. Civil procedures: Methods used to protect the rights of psychiatric clients
B. Voluntary admission: Client admits himself or herself to an institution for treatment and retains civil rights
C. Involuntary admission: Someone other than the client applies for the client's admission to an institution.
   1. This requires certification by a health care provider that the person is a danger to self or others. (Depending on the state, one or two health care provider certifications are required.)
   2. Individuals have the right to a legal hearing within a certain number of hours or days.
   3. Most states limit commitment to 90 days.
   4. Extended commitment is usually no longer than 1 year.
D. Emergency admission: Any adult may apply for emergency detention of another. However, medical or judicial approval is required to detain anyone beyond 24 hours.
   1. A person held against his or her will can file a writ of habeas corpus to try to get the court to hear the case and release the person.
   2. The court determines the sanity and alleged unlawful restraint of a person.
E. Legal and civil rights of hospitalized clients
   1. The right to wear their own clothes and to keep personal items and a reasonable amount of cash for small purchases
   2. The right to have individual storage space for one's own use
   3. The right to see visitors daily
   4. The right to have reasonable access to a telephone and the opportunity to have private conversations by telephone
   5. The right to receive and send mail (unopened)
   6. The right to refuse shock treatments and lobotomy

F. Competency hearing: Legal hearing that is held to determine a person's ability to make responsible decisions about self, dependents, or property.
   1. Persons declared incompetent have the legal status of a minor—they cannot:
      a. Vote
      b. Make contracts or wills
      c. Drive a car
      d. Sue or be sued
      e. Hold a professional license
   2. A guardian is appointed by the court for an incompetent person. Declaring a person incompetent can be initiated by the state or the family.

G. Insanity: Legal term meaning the accused is not criminally responsible for the unlawful act committed because he or she is mentally ill

H. Inability to stand trial: Person accused of committing a crime is not mentally capable of standing trial. He or she:
   1. Cannot understand the charge against himself or herself
   2. Must be sent to psychiatric unit until legally determined to be competent for trial
   3. Once mentally fit, must stand trial and serve any sentence, if convicted

HESI Hint • Often an NCLEX-RN® question asks who should explain a surgical procedure to the client. The answer is the provider. This is probably the only question in which you refer to the health care provider. Remember, nurses are proud people; nurses wrote the test items, and they expect nurses to handle most client situations. Also remember that it is the nurse's responsibility to be sure that the operative permit is signed and is on the chart. It is not the nurse's responsibility to explain the procedure to the client.

Patient Identification

A. The Joint Commission has implemented new patient identification requirements to meet safety goals.

B. Use at least two patient identifiers whenever taking blood samples, administering medications, or administering blood products.

C. The patient room number may *not* be used as a form of identification.

Surgical Permit

A. Consent to operate (surgical permit) must be obtained prior to any surgical procedure, however minor it might be.

B. Legally, the surgical permit must be:
   1. Written.
   2. Obtained voluntarily.
   3. Explained to the client (i.e., informed consent must be obtained).

C. Informed consent means the operation has been fully explained to the client, including:
   1. Possible complications and disfigurements
   2. Removal of any organs or parts of the body

D. Surgery permits must be obtained as follows:
   1. They must be witnessed by an authorized person, such as the health care provider or a nurse.
   2. They protect the client against unsanctioned surgery, and they protect the health care provider and surgeon, hospital, and hospital staff against possible claims of unauthorized operations.
   3. Adults and emancipated minors may sign their own operative permits if they are mentally competent.
   4. Permission to operate on a minor child or an incompetent or unconscious adult must be obtained from a responsible family member or guardian.

Consent

A. The law does not *require* written consent to perform medical treatment.
   1. Treatment can be performed if the client has been fully informed about the procedure.
   2. Treatment can be performed if the client voluntarily consents to the procedure.
   3. If informed consent cannot be obtained (e.g., client is unconscious) and immediate treatment is required to save life or limb, the emergency laws can be applied. (See the subsequent section, Good Samaritan Act.)

B. Verbal or written consent
   1. When verbal consent is obtained, a notation should be made.
      a. It describes in detail how and why verbal consent was obtained.
      b. It is placed in the client's record or chart.
      c. It is witnessed and signed by two persons.
   2. Verbal or written consent can be given by:
      a. Alert, coherent, or otherwise competent adults
      b. A parent or legal guardian
      c. A person in loco parentis (a person standing in for a parent with a parent's rights, duties, and responsibilities) in cases of minors or incompetent adults

C. Consent of minors
   1. Minors 14 years of age and older must agree to treatment along with their parents or guardians.
   2. Emancipated minors can consent to treatment themselves. Be aware that the definition of an emancipated minor may change from state to state.

Emergency Care

A. Good Samaritan Act: Protects health practitioners against malpractice claims for care provided in emergency situations (e.g., the nurse gives aid at the scene to an automobile accident victim).

B. A nurse is required to perform in a "reasonable and prudent manner."

> **HESI Hint** • Often questions are asked regarding the Good Samaritan Act, which is the means of protecting a nurse when she or he is performing emergency care.

PRESCRIPTIONS AND HEALTH CARE PROVIDERS OR PHYSICIANS

A. A nurse is required to obtain a prescription (order) to carry out medical procedures from a health care provider or physician.

B. Although verbal telephone prescriptions should be avoided, the nurse should follow the agency's policy and procedures. Failure to follow such rules could be considered negligence. The Joint Commission requires that organizations implement a process for taking verbal or telephone orders that includes a read-back of critical values. The employee receiving the prescription should write the verbal order or critical value on the chart or record it in the computer and then read back the order or value to the health care provider.

C. If a nurse questions a health care provider's or physician's prescription because he or she believes that it is wrong (e.g., the wrong dosage was prescribed for a medication), the nurse should do the following:
  1. Inform the health care provider or physician.
  2. Record that the health care provider or physician was informed and record the health care provider's or physician's response to such information.
  3. Inform the nursing supervisor.
  4. Refuse to carry out the prescription.

D. If the nurse believes that a health care provider's or physician's prescription was made with poor judgment (e.g., the nurse believes the client does not need as many tranquilizers as the health care provider or physician prescribed), the nurse should:
  1. Record that the health care provider or physician was notified and that the prescription was questioned.

  2. Carry out the prescription because nursing judgment cannot be substituted for a health care provider's or physician's medical judgment.

E. If a nurse is asked to perform a task for which he or she has not been prepared educationally (e.g., obtain a urine specimen from a premature infant by needle aspiration of the bladder) or does not have the necessary experience (e.g., a nurse who has never worked in labor and delivery is asked to perform a vaginal exam and determine cervical dilation), the nurse should do the following:
  1. Inform the health care provider or physician that he or she does not have the education or experience necessary to carry out the prescription.
  2. Refuse to carry out the prescription.

> **HESI Hint** • If the nurse carries out a health care provider's or physician's prescription for which he or she is not prepared and does not inform the health care provider or physician of his or her lack of preparation, the nurse is solely liable for any damages.
>
> If the nurse informs the health care provider or physician of his or her lack of preparation in carrying out a prescription and carries out the prescription anyway, the nurse *and* the health care provider or physician are liable for any damages.

F. The nurse cannot, without a health care provider's or physician's prescription, alter the amount of drug given to a client. For example, if a health care provider or physician has prescribed pain medication in a certain amount and the client's pain is not, in the nurse's judgment, severe enough to warrant the dosage prescribed, the nurse cannot reduce the amount without first checking with the health care provider or physician. Remember, nursing judgment cannot be substituted for medical judgment.

> **HESI Hint** • Assignments are often tested on the NCLEX-RN. The Nurse Practice Acts of each state govern policies related to making assignments. Usually, when determining who should be assigned to do a sterile dressing change, for example, a licensed nurse should be chosen; that is, an RN or licensed practical nurse (LPN) who has been checked off on this procedure.

Restraints

A. Clients may be restrained only under the following circumstances:
1. In an emergency
2. For a limited time
3. For the purpose of protecting the client from injury
B. Nursing responsibilities with regard to restraints
1. The nurse must notify the health care provider or physician immediately that the client has been restrained.
2. The nurse should document the facts regarding the rationale for restraining the client.
C. When restraining a client, the nurse should do the following:
1. Use restraints (chemical or physical) after exhausting all reasonable alternatives.
2. Apply the restraints correctly and in accordance with facility procedures.
3. Check frequently to see that the restraints do not impair circulation or cause pressure sores or other injuries.
4. Remove restraints as soon as possible.
5. Document the need for and application, monitoring, and removal of restraints.

HESI Hint • Restraints of any kind may constitute false imprisonment.
Freedom from unlawful restraint is a basic human right and is protected by law.

Health Insurance Portability and Accountability Act of 1996

Congress passed the Health Insurance Portability and Accountability Act of 1996 (HIPAA) to create a national patient-record privacy standard.

A. HIPAA privacy rules pertain to health care providers, health plans, and health clearinghouses and their business partners who engage in computer-to-computer transmission of health care claims, payment and remittance, benefit information, and health plan eligibility information and who disclose personal health information that specifically identifies an individual and is transmitted electronically, in writing, or verbally.
B. Patient privacy rights are of key importance. Patients must provide written approval of the disclosure of any of their health information for almost any purpose. Health care providers and physicians must offer specific information to patients that explain how their personal health information will be used. Patients must have access to their medical records, and they can receive copies of them and request that changes be made if they identify inaccuracies.
C. Health care providers and physicians who do not comply with HIPAA regulations or make unauthorized disclosures risk civil and criminal liability. According to the U.S. Department of Health and Human Services (DHHS), civil penalties can be assessed as high as $25,000 per year, and criminal penalties can be assessed at $50,000 with 1 year in prison to as much as $250,000 and 10 years in prison.
D. For further information, use this link to the DHHS Website, Office of Civil Rights, which contains frequently asked questions about HIPAA Standards for Privacy of Individually Identifiable Health Information (July, 2001): http://aspe.hhs.gov/admnsimp/final/pvcguide1.htm

Review of Legal Aspects of Nursing

1. What types of procedures should be assigned to professional nurses?
2. Negligence is measured by reasonableness. What question might the nurse ask when determining such reasonableness?
3. List the four elements that are necessary to prove negligence.
4. Define an *intentional tort*, and give one example.
5. Differentiate between voluntary and involuntary admission.
6. List five activities a person who is declared incompetent cannot perform.
7. Name three legal requirements of a surgical permit.
8. Who may give consent for medical treatment?
9. What law protects the nurse who provides care or gives aid in an emergency situation?
10. What actions should the nurse take if he or she questions a health care provider's or physician's prescription—that is, believes the prescription is wrong?
11. Describe the nurse's legal responsibility when asked to perform a task for which he or she is unprepared.
12. Describe nursing care of the restrained client.
13. Describe six patient rights guaranteed under HIPAA regulations that nurses must be aware of in practice.

Answers to Review

1. Sterile or invasive procedures
2. Would a reasonable and prudent nurse act in the same manner under the same circumstances?
3. Duty: Failure to protect client against unreasonable risk. Breach of duty: Failure to perform according to established standards. Causation: A connection exists between conduct of the nurse and the resulting damage. Damages: Damage is done to the client, physical or mental.
4. Conduct causing damage to another person in a *willful* or *intentional* way *without* just cause. Example: Hitting a client out of anger, not in a manner of self-protection.
5. Voluntary: Client admits self to an institution for treatment and retains his or her civil rights; he or she may leave at any time. Involuntary: Someone other than client applies for the client's admission to an institution (a relative, a friend, or the state); requires certification by one or two health care providers or physicians that the person is a danger to self or others; the person has a right to a legal hearing (habeas corpus) to try to be released, and the court determines the justification for holding the person.
6. Vote, make contracts or wills, drive a car, sue or be sued, hold a professional license
7. Voluntary, informed, written
8. Alert, coherent, or otherwise competent adults; a parent or legal guardian; a person in loco parentis of minors or incompetent adults
9. The Good Samaritan Act
10. Inform the health care provider or physician; record that the health care provider or physician was informed and the health care provider's or physician's response to such information; inform the nursing supervisor; refuse to carry out the prescription
11. Inform the health care provider or physician or person asking the nurse to perform the task that he or she is unprepared to carry out the task; refuse to perform the task
12. Apply restraints properly; check restraints frequently to see that they are not causing injury and *record* such monitoring; remove restraints as soon as possible; use restraints *only* as a last resort
13. A patient must give written consent before health care providers can use or disclose personal health information; health care providers and physicians must give patients notice about providers' responsibilities regarding patient confidentiality; patients must have access to their medical records; providers who restrict access must explain why and must offer patients a description of the complaint process; patients have the right to request that changes be made in their medical records to correct inaccuracies; health care providers must follow specific tracking procedures for any disclosures made that ensure accountability for maintenance of patient confidentiality; patients have the right to request that health care providers and physicians restrict the use and disclosure of their personal health information, though the provider may decline to do so.

Leadership and Management

Description: Nurses act in both leadership and management roles.

A. A leader is an individual who influences people to accomplish goals.

B. A manager is an individual who works to accomplish the goals of the organization.

C. A nurse manager acts to achieve the goals of safe, effective client care within the overall goals of a health care facility.

SKILLS OF THE NURSE MANAGER

Refer to Box 2-1.

Communication Skills

Assertive communication:

A. Includes clearly defined goals and expectations

B. Includes verbal and nonverbal messages that are congruent

C. Is critical to the directing aspect of management

> **HESI Hint** • Assertive communication starts with "I need" rather than with "You must."

> **HESI Hint** • Motivation comes from within an individual. A nurse leader can provide an environment that will promote motivation through positive feedback, respect, and seeking input. Look for responses that demonstrate these behaviors.

Organizational Skills

Organizational skills encompass management of:

A. People

B. Time

C. Supplies

Delegation Skills

A. The authority, accountability, and responsibility of the RN are based on the state Nurse Practice

BOX 2-1 *Skills and Characteristics of the Nurse Manager*

Skills of the Nurse Manager	Characteristics of the Nurse Manager
Communication Act as a liaison between clients and others. Engage in conflict resolution as needed with staff.	Authority
Organization Plan overall strategies to address client problems. Review management outcomes.	Accountability
Delegation Identify roles/responsibilities of health care team members.	Responsibility
Supervision Supervise care provided by others (e.g., LPN/VN, assistive personnel, other RNs).	Leadership
Critical thinking Serve as resource person to other staff.	Commitment to quality

HESI Hint • NCLEX-RN questions often include examples of nursing interventions that do or do not demonstrate these skills and characteristics.

Classic Leadership Styles	Behavior Associated With Leadership Styles
Democratic (participative)	Assertive
Authoritarian (autocratic)	Aggressive
Laissez-faire (permissive)	Passive

HESI Hint • Effective leadership involves assertive management skills. Look for responses that demonstrate that the nurse is using assertive communication skills.

Act, standards of professional practice, the policies of the health care organization, and ethical-legal models of behavior.

B. Definitions
  1. *Delegation* is the process by which responsibility and authority are transferred to another individual.
  2. *Responsibility* is the obligation to complete a task.
  3. *Authority* is the right to act or command the actions of others.
  4. *Accountability* is the ability and willingness to assume responsibility for actions and related consequences.

C. The nurse transfers responsibility and authority for the completion of delegated tasks, but the nurse retains accountability for the delegation process. This accountability involves ensuring that the five rights of delegation have been achieved.

D. Five Rights of Delegation (as defined by the National Council of State Boards of Nursing)
  1. Right task: Is this a task that can be delegated by a nurse?
  2. Right circumstance: Considering the setting and available resources, should delegation take place?
  3. Right person: Is the task being delegated by the right person to the right person?
  4. Right direction/communication: Is the nurse providing a clear, concise description of the task, including limits and expectations?
  5. Right supervision: Once the task has been delegated, is appropriate supervision maintained?

Supervision Skills

A. Direction/guidance
  1. Clear, concise directions
  2. Expected outcome
  3. Time frame
  4. Limitations
  5. Verification of assignment

B. Evaluation/monitoring
  1. Frequent check-in
  2. Open communication lines
  3. Achievement of outcome

C. Follow-up
  1. Communication of evaluation findings to the LPN or unlicensed assistive personnel (UAP) and other appropriate personnel
  2. Need for teaching or guidance

Critical Thinking Skills

A. Nurses are accustomed to using the nursing process as the model for problem solving in client care situations.

B. Use this model to think critically in leadership and management situations.
  1. Assessment: What are the needs or problems?
  2. Analysis: What has the highest priority?
  3. Planning
    a. What outcomes and goals must be accomplished?
    b. What are the available resources?
      (1) Nursing staff
      (2) Interdisciplinary team members
      (3) Time
      (4) Equipment
      (5) Space (client rooms, home environment, etc.)

4. Implementation
   a. Communicating expectations
   b. Is documentation complete?
5. Evaluation
   a. Were the desired outcomes achieved?
   b. Was safe, effective care provided?

HESI Hint • Delegating to the right person requires that the nurse be aware of the qualifications of the delegatee: appropriate education, training, skills, experience, and demonstrated and documented competence.

HESI Hint • Remember nursing process: assessments, analysis, diagnosis, planning, and evaluation (any activity requiring nursing judgment) may not be delegated to UAP. Delegated activities fall within the implementation phase of the nursing process.

HESI Hint • UAPs generally do not perform invasive or sterile procedures.

HESI Hint • The RN is accountable for adhering to the three basic aspects of supervision when delegating to other health care personnel, such as LPNs, graduate nurses, inexperienced nurses, student nurses, and UAPs.

HESI Hint • Priorities often center on which client should be assessed first by the nurse. Ask yourself: Which client is the most critically ill? Which client is most likely to experience a significant change in condition? Which client requires assessment by an RN?

HESI Hint • The nurse manager must analyze all the desired outcomes involved when assigning rooms for clients or assigning client care responsibilities. A client with an infection should not be assigned to share a room with a surgical or immunocompromised client. A nurse's client care management should be based on the nurse's abilities, the individual client's needs, and the needs of the entire group of assigned clients. Safety and infection control are high priorities.

TABLE 2-1 Nurse Leaders and Managers as Change Agents

Lewin's Change Theory	Nurses Act as Change Agents, Which Involves:
Unfreezing	Initiation of a change
Moving	Motivation toward a change
Refreezing	Implementation of a change

SKILLS NEEDED BY CHANGE AGENTS

A. Problem solving
B. Decision making
C. Interpersonal relationships (Table 2-1)

Nurse Leaders and Managers as Collaborators

A. Collaborative health care teams require:
   1. Shared goals, commitment, and accountability
   2. Open and clear communication
   3. Respect for the expertise of all team members
B. Critical pathways:
   1. Are interdisciplinary plans of care
   2. Are used for diagnoses and care that can be standardized
   3. Are guides to track client progress
   4. Do *not* replace individualized care
C. Case management:
   1. Is the coordination of care provided by an interdisciplinary team
   2. Manages resources effectively
   3. Uses critical pathways to organize care
D. Quality assurance:
   1. Involves continuous quality improvement (CQI)/total quality management (TQM)
   2. Is an organized approach to the improvement of:
      a. Outcome achievement
      b. Quality of care provided

HESI Hint • Change causes anxiety. An effective nurse change agent uses problem-solving skills to recognize factors such as anxiety that contribute to resistance to change and uses decision making and interpersonal skills to overcome that resistance. Interventions that demonstrate these skills include seeking input, showing respect, valuing opinions, and building trust.

Review of Leadership and Management

1. By what authority may RNs delegate nursing care to others?
2. A UAP may perform care that falls within which component of the nursing process?
3. Which type of communication skills is necessary to implement a democratic leadership style?
4. What are the five rights of delegation?
5. Which tasks can be delegated to a UAP?
   A. Inserting a Foley catheter
   B. Measuring and recording the client's output through a Foley catheter
C. Teaching a client how to care for a catheter after discharge
D. Assessing for symptoms of a urinary tract infection
6. What are the essential steps of effective supervision?
7. Which of the following is an example of assertive communication?
   A. "You need to improve the way you spend your time so that all of your care gets performed."
   B. "I've noticed that many of your clients did not get their care today."

Answers to Review

1. State Nurse Practice Act
2. Implementation
3. Assertive communication skills
4. Right task, right circumstance, right person, right direction or communication, and right supervision
5. Delegation is as follows:
   A. Is a sterile invasive procedure and should not be delegated to a UAP
   B. Falls within the implementation phase of the nursing process and does not require nursing judgment. Evaluation of the I&O must be done by the nurse.
   C. Client teaching requires the abilities of a nurse and should not be delegated. The UAP may be instructed to report anything unusual that is observed and any symptoms reported by the client, but this does not replace assessment by the nurse.
   D. Assessment must be performed by the nurse, and should not be delegated. The UAP may be instructed to report anything unusual that is observed, or any symptoms reported by the client, but this does not replace assessment by the nurse.
6. Direction, evaluation, and follow-up
7. Examples:
   A. This is an aggressive communication, which causes anger, hostility, and a defensive attitude.
   B. Assertive communication begins with "I" rather than "you" and clearly states the problem.

Disaster Nursing

A. The role of the nurse takes place at all three levels of disaster management:
   1. Disaster preparedness
   2. Disaster response
   3. Disaster recovery
B. To achieve effective disaster management:
   1. Organization is the key.
   2. All personnel must be trained.
   3. All personnel must know their roles.

LEVELS OF PREVENTION IN DISASTER MANAGEMENT

A. Primary prevention
   1. Participate in the development of a disaster plan.
   2. Train rescue workers in triage and basic first aid.
   3. Educate personnel about shelter management.
   4. Educate the public about the disaster plan and personal preparation for disaster.
B. Secondary prevention
   1. Triage
   2. Treatment of injuries
   3. Treatment of other conditions, including mental health
   4. Shelter supervision
C. Tertiary prevention
   1. Follow-up care for injuries
   2. Follow-up care for psychological problems
   3. Recovery assistance
   4. Prevention of future disasters and their consequences

TRIAGE

A. A French word meaning "to sort or categorize"
B. Goal: Maximize the number of survivors by sorting the injured according to treatable and

TABLE 2-2 Triage Color Code System

	Red	Yellow	Green	Black
Urgency	Most urgent, first priority	Urgent, second priority	Third priority	Dying or dead
Injury type	Life-threatening injuries	Injuries with systemic effects and complications	Minimal injuries with no systemic complications	Catastrophic injuries
May delay treatment?	NO	For 30 to 60 minutes	Several hours	No hope for survival, no treatment

untreatable victims (Table 2-2, Triage Color Code System).

C. Primary criteria used
1. Potential for survival
2. Availability of resources

Nursing Interventions and Roles in Triage

A. Triage duties using a systematic approach such as the START method (Figure 2-1)

B. Treatment of injuries
1. Render first aid for injuries.
2. Provide additional treatment as needed in definitive care areas.

C. Treatment of other conditions, including mental health
1. Determine health needs other than injury.
2. Refer for medical treatment as required.
3. Provide treatment for other conditions based on medically approved protocols.

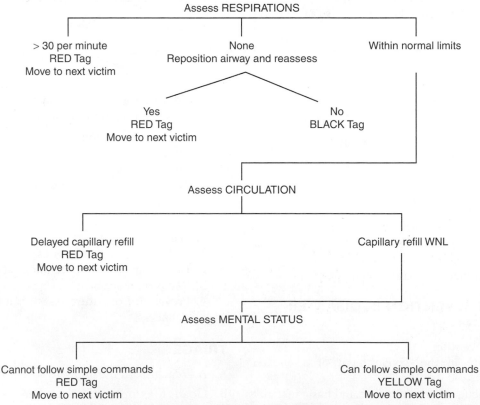

First: Separate the walking wounded – Move to a safe area – Evaluate later/GREEN Tag
Next: Three step evaluation of non-walking victims – ONE VICTIM AT A TIME

FIGURE 2-1 Simple triage and rapid treatment (START) method for triage.

Shelter Supervision

A. Coordinate activities of shelter workers.

B. Oversee records of victims admitted and discharged from shelter.

C. Promote effective interpersonal and group interactions among victims in shelter.

D. Promote independence and involvement of victims housed in the shelter.

BIOTERRORISM

A. Learn the symptoms of illnesses that are associated with exposure to likely biological and chemical agents.

B. Understand that they could appear days or weeks after exposure.

C. Nurses and other health care providers and physicians would be the first responders when victims seek medical evaluation after symptoms manifest. First responders are critical in identifying an outbreak, determining cause of outbreak, identifying risk factors, implementation of measures to control and minimize the outbreak.

D. Possible agents (Table 2-3, Signs, Symptoms, and Treatments of Biologic and Chemical Agents and Radiation)
   1. Biologic agents
      a. Anthrax
      b. Pneumonic plague
      c. Botulism
      d. Smallpox
      e. Inhalation tularemia
      f. Viral hemorrhagic fever
   2. Chemical agents
      a. Biotoxin agents: ricin
      b. Nerve agents: sarin
   3. Radiation

> **HESI Hint** • It is important to remember that in disaster and bioterrorism management, the nurse must consider both the individual and the community.

Nursing Assessment

A. Community-disaster risk assessment

B. Measures to mitigate disaster effect

C. Exposure symptom identification

Analysis (Nursing Diagnosis)

A. *Deficient knowledge (specify)* related to…

B. *Risk for poisoning* related to…

C. *Risk for trauma* related to…

D. *Risk for suffocation* related to…

E. *Anxiety* related to…

F. *Fear* related to…

G. *Ineffective community coping* related to…

H. *Risk for post-trauma syndrome* related to…

Nursing Plans and Interventions

A. Participate in development of disaster plan.

B. Educate the public on disaster plan and personal preparation for disaster.

C. Train rescue workers in triage and basic first aid.

D. Educate personnel for shelter management.

E. Practice triage.

F. Treat injuries and illness.

G. Treat other conditions, including mental health.

H. Supervise shelters.

I. Arrange for follow-up care for injuries.

J. Arrange for follow-up care for psychological problems.

K. Assist in recovery.

L. Work to prevent future disasters and their consequences.

TABLE 2-3   **Signs, Symptoms, and Treatments of Biologic and Chemical Agents and Radiation**

	BIOLOGIC AGENTS		
	Anthrax	**Pneumonic Plague**	**Botulism**

Agent	• *Bacillus anthracis*
	• Bacterium that forms spores
	• Three types:
	  Cutaneous
	  Inhalation
	  Digestive
		• *Yersinia pestis*
		• Bacterium found in rodents and their fleas
			• *Clostridium botulinum*
			• Toxin made by a bacterium

Transmission	• Inhalation of powder form • Inhalation of spores from infected animal products (e.g., wool) • Handling of infected animals • Eating of undercooked meat from infected animals • Not spreadable from person to person	• Aerosol release into the environment • Respiratory droplets from an infected person (6-foot range) • Untreated bubonic plague sequelae	• Food: a person ingests preformed toxin • Wound: infection by *C. botulinum* that secretes the toxin • Not spreadable from person to person
Incubation period	• Within 7 days (all types) • Inhalation incubation: period extends to 42 days	• 1 to 6 days	• A few hours to a few days • Food-borne: most commonly 12 to 36 hours, but range is 6 hours to 2 weeks
Signs and symptoms	• Cutaneous: sores that develop into painless blisters, then ulcers with black centers • Gastrointestinal: nausea, anorexia, bloody diarrhea, fever, severe stomach pain • Inhalation: cold and flu symptoms, including sore throat, mild fever, muscle aches, cough, chest discomfort, shortness of breath, tiredness, muscle aches	• Fever • Weakness • Rapidly developing pneumonia • Bloody or watery sputum • Nausea, vomiting • Abdominal pain • Without early treatment will see shock, respiratory failure, and rapid death	• Double and/or blurred vision • Drooping eyelids • Slurred speech • Difficulty swallowing • Descending muscle weakness
Treatment	• Prevention after exposure consists of the use of antibiotics, such as ciprofloxacin, doxycycline, or penicillin, and vaccination • Treatment after infection is usually a 60-day course of antibiotics • Success of treatment after infection depends on the type of anthrax and how soon the treatment begins	• If close contact with infected person and within 7 days of exposure, treatment is with antibiotics prophylactically • Recommended antibiotic treatment within 24 hours of first symptom and treat for at least 7 days • Oral: tetracyclines, fluoroquinolones • IV: Streptomycin or gentamycin	• Antitoxin to reduce severity of disease (most effective when administered early in course of disease) • Supportive care • May require mechanical ventilation

TABLE 2-3   Signs, Symptoms, and Treatments of Biologic and Chemical Agents and Radiation—cont'd

BIOLOGIC AGENTS		
	Anthrax	**Pneumonic Plague**	**Botulism**
Miscellaneous	• Vaccine available, but not to the general public • Given to those who may be exposed such as certain members of the U.S. Armed Forces, laboratory workers, and workers who enter or reenter contaminated areas	• Easily destroyed by sunlight and drying • In air can survive up to 1 hour • No vaccine available	• No vaccine available
	Smallpox	**Inhalation Tularemia**	**Viral Hemorrhagic Fever**
Agent	• Variola virus • Orthopoxvirus	• *Francisella tularensis* • Highly infectious bacterium	• Five families of viruses (examples: Ebola, Lassa, dengue, yellow, Marburg) • RNA viruses enveloped in a lipid coating
Transmission	• Aerosol release into the environment • Contact with infected person (direct and prolonged, face-to-face) • Bodily fluids • Contaminated objects • Air in enclosed settings (rare)	• Insect (usually tick or deerfly) bites • Handling of sick or dead infected animals • Consuming of contaminated food or water • Inhalation of airborne bacterium • Cannot be spread from person to person	• From viral reservoirs such as rodents and arthropods or an animal host; some hosts remain unknown • May be transmitted person to person via close contact or bodily fluids • Objects contaminated by bodily fluids
Incubation period	• 7 to 17 days	• Most commonly 3 to 5 days, but may range from 1 to 14 days	• 2 to 21 days (varies according to virus)
Signs and symptoms	• High fever • Head and body aches • Vomiting • Rash that progresses to raised bumps and pus-filled blisters that crust and scab, then fall off in about 3 weeks, leaving a pitted scar	• Skin ulcers • Swollen and painful lymph glands • Sore throat • Mouth sores • Diarrhea • Pneumonia • If inhaled: abrupt onset of fever and chills, headache, muscle aches, joint pain, dry cough, and progressive weakness • If pneumonia develops: may exhibit chest pain, difficulty breathing, bloody sputum, and respiratory failure	• Varies by individual virus but common symptoms exist • Marked fever • Exhaustion • Muscle aches • Loss of strength • As disease worsens more severe symptoms emerge • Bleeding under skin, in internal organs, or from body orifices (mouth, eyes, ears) • Shock • Central nervous system malfunction • Seizures • Coma • Renal failure

(Continued)

TABLE 2-3 **Signs, Symptoms, and Treatments of Biologic and Chemical Agents and Radiation—cont'd**

	BIOLOGIC AGENTS		
	Smallpox	**Inhalation Tularemia**	**Viral Hemorrhagic Fever**
Treatment	• No proven treatment • Supportive therapy • Antibiotic treatment for secondary infections • Research being done with antivirals	• Antibiotics for 10 to 14 days • Oral: tetracyclines, fluoroquinolones IM or IV: streptomycin, gentamicin	• Supportive therapy • Generally no established cure • May use ribavirin with Lassa fever
Miscellaneous	• A fragile virus; if aerosolized, die within 24 hours (quicker if in sunlight) • Vaccine available	• Can remain alive in water and soil for 2 weeks • No vaccine available	• Need a reservoir to survive; humans are not the natural reservoir but once infected by the host, can transmit to one another • Once geographically restricted to where the host lived; increasing international travel brings outbreaks to places where the viruses have never been seen before • No vaccines available except for Argentine and yellow fever

	CHEMICAL AGENTS AND RADIATION		
	Ricin	**Sarin**	**Radiation**
Agent	• Poison made from waste left over from processing castor beans • Forms include powder, mist, pellet • Dissolved in water or weak acid	• Human-made chemical • Similar to but far more potent than organophosphate pesticides • Clear, odorless, and tasteless liquid that can evaporate into a gas and spread into the environment	• Form of energy both manmade and natural
Transmission	• Deliberate act of poisoning by inhalation or injection (need minuscule amount [500 mcg] to kill) • Deliberate act of contamination of food and water supply (requires greater amount to kill) • Cannot be spread from person to person through casual contact	• Agent in air: exposed through skin, eyes, inhalation • Ingested in water or food • Clothing can release sarin for approximately 30 minutes after contact	• External exposure comes from the sun or from human-made sources such as x-rays, nuclear bombs, and nuclear disasters (e.g., Chernobyl) • Small quantities in air, water, food cause internal exposure

TABLE 2-3   Signs, Symptoms, and Treatments of Biologic and Chemical Agents and Radiation—cont'd

CHEMICAL AGENTS AND RADIATION			
	Ricin	**Sarin**	**Radiation**
Incubation period	• Inhalation: within 8 hours • Ingestion: <6 hours	• Vapor: a few seconds • Liquid: a few minutes to 18 hours	• Exposure is cumulative; low-dose exposure effects may not be seen for several years • High dose received in a matter of minutes results in acute radiation syndrome (ARS)
Signs and symptoms	• Inhalation: respiratory distress, fever, nausea, tightness in chest, heavy sweating, pulmonary edema, decreased blood pressure, respiratory failure, death • Ingestion: vomiting and diarrhea that becomes bloody, severe dehydration, decreased blood pressure, hallucinations, seizures, hematuria; within several days, liver, spleen, and kidney failure occur • Skin and eyes: redness and pain	• Runny nose • Watery eyes • Pinpoint pupils • Eye pain and blurred vision • Drooling • Excessive sweating • Respiratory symptoms • Diarrhea • Altered level of consciousness (LOC) • Nausea and vomiting • Headache • Decreased or increased blood pressure • In large doses: loss of consciousness, convulsions, paralysis, respiratory failure, death	• ARS: nausea, vomiting, diarrhea; then bone marrow depletion, weight loss, loss of appetite, flu symptoms, infection, and bleeding • Mild effects include skin reddening • May lead to cancers (with low dose and in those surviving ARS)
Treatment	• Supportive care	• Remove from body as soon as possible • Supportive care • Antidote available: most effective if given as soon as possible after exposure	• Dependent on dose and type of radiation • Supportive care
Miscellaneous	• Stable agent; not affected by very hot or very cold temperatures • Death usually occurs in about 36 to 72 hours • If survive for 3 to 5 days, victim usually recovers • No vaccine available	• A heavy vapor, this agent sinks to low-lying areas • Mildly or moderately exposed people usually recover completely • Severely exposed people usually do not survive • May experience neurologic problems lasting 1 to 2 weeks after exposure	• Survival dependent on dose • Full recovery may take a few weeks to a few years

Note: For further information, go to www.bt.cdc.gov/index.asp.

Review of Disaster Nursing

1. List the three levels of disaster management.
2. List examples of the three levels of prevention in disaster management.

3. Define *triage*.
4. Identify three bioterrorism agents.

Answers to Review

1. Disaster preparedness, disaster response, disaster recovery
2. Primary: develop plan, train and educate personnel and public; secondary: triage, treatment-shelter supervision; tertiary: follow-up, recovery assistance, prevention of future disasters

3. To sort or categorize
4. Anthrax, pneumonic plague, botulism, smallpox, inhalation tularemia, viral hemorrhagic fever, ricin, sarin, radiation

For more review, go to **http://evolve.elsevier.com/HESI/RN** for HESI's online study exams.

ADVANCED CLINICAL CONCEPTS

Respiratory Failure

ACUTE RESPIRATORY DISTRESS SYNDROME (ARDS)

Description: The exchange of oxygen for carbon dioxide in the lungs is inadequate for oxygen consumption and carbon dioxide production within the body's cells.

A. ARDS is characterized by:
1. Hypoxemia that persists even when 100% oxygen is given
2. Decreased pulmonary compliance
3. Dyspnea
4. Non-cardiac-associated bilateral pulmonary edema
5. Dense pulmonary infiltrates on radiography

> **HESI Hint** • ARDS is an unexpected, catastrophic pulmonary complication occurring in a person with no previous pulmonary problems. The mortality rate is high (50%).

B. No abnormal lung sounds are present on auscultation because the edema of ARDS occurs first in the interstitial spaces, not in the airways.

> **HESI Hint** • In ARDS, a common laboratory finding is a lowered Po_2. However, these clients are not very responsive to high concentrations of oxygen and often require intubation and mechanical ventilation with positive end-expiratory pressure (PEEP).

> **HESI Hint** • Think about the physiology of the lungs by remembering "PEEP": Positive end-expiratory pressure is the instillation and maintenance of small amounts of air into the alveolar sacs to prevent them from collapsing each time the client exhales. The amount of pressure can be set by the ventilator and is usually around 5 to 10 cm H_2O.

C. Common causes of respiratory failure include:
1. Chronic obstructive pulmonary disease (COPD)
2. Pneumonia
3. Tuberculosis
4. Contusion
5. Aspiration
6. Inhaled toxins
7. Emboli
8. Drug overdose
9. Fluid overload
10. Disseminated intravascular coagulation (DIC)
11. Shock

Nursing Assessment

A. Dyspnea, hyperpnea
B. Intercostal retractions
C. Cyanosis, pallor
D. Hypoxemia: Po_2 <50 mm Hg with Fio_2 >60%
E. Diffuse pulmonary infiltrates seen on chest radiograph as "white-out" appearance
F. Verbalized anxiety, restlessness

Analysis (Nursing Diagnoses)

A. *Impaired gas exchange* related to…
B. *Risk for deficient fluid volume* related to…
C. *Ineffective breathing pattern* related to…
D. *Risk for injury* related to…
E. *Risk for infection* related to…

Nursing Plans and Interventions

A. Position client for maximal lung expansion.
B. Monitor client for signs of hypoxemia and oxygen toxicity.

> **HESI Hint** • Suction only when secretions are present.

C. Monitor breath sounds for pneumothorax, especially when PEEP is used to keep small airways open.

TABLE 3-1 Arterial Blood Gases

Blood Gases	Normal Values
pH	7.35 to 7.45
PCO_2	35 to 45 mm Hg
HCO_3	21 to 28 mEq/L
Po_2	80 to 100 mm Hg
O_2 Saturation	95% to 100%
O_2 Content	15 to 20 vol %
Base Excess	0 ± 2 mEq/L

D. Provide emotional support to decrease anxiety and allow ventilator to "work" the lungs.

E. Monitor client hemodynamically with essential vital signs and cardiac monitor.

F. Monitor arterial blood gases (ABGs) routinely.

G. Monitor vital organ status: central nervous system (CNS), level of consciousness, renal system output, and myocardium (apical pulse, blood pressure [BP]).

H. Monitor fluid and electrolyte balance.

I. Monitor metabolic status through routine lab work (Table 3-1).

> **HESI Hint** • Before drawing a sample for ABGs from the radial artery, perform the Allen test to assess collateral circulation. Make the client's hand blanch by obliterating both the radial and the ulnar pulses. Then release the pressure over the ulnar artery only. If flow through the ulnar artery is good, flushing will be seen immediately. The Allen test is then positive, and the radial artery can be used for puncture. If the Allen test is negative, repeat on the other arm. If this test is also negative, seek another site for arterial puncture. The Allen test ensures collateral circulation to the hand if thrombosis of the radial artery should follow the puncture.

RESPIRATORY FAILURE IN CHILDREN

Description: Common causes of respiratory failure in children include:

A. Congenital heart disease
B. Respiratory distress syndrome
C. Infection, sepsis
D. Neuromuscular diseases
E. Trauma and burns
F. Aspiration
G. Fluid overload and dehydration
H. Anesthesia and narcotic overdose

Nursing Assessment

A. "Bad-looking" child
B. Very slow or very rapid respiratory rate (tachypnea), dyspnea, apnea, gasping
C. Tachycardia
D. Cyanosis, pallor, or mottled color (connotes deterioration of systemic perfusion)
E. Irritability and later, lethargy (connotes a deteriorating level of consciousness)
F. Retractions, nasal flaring, poor air movement
G. Hypoxemia, hypercapnia, respiratory acidosis
H. Laboratory data: Values should be evaluated, keeping in mind the percentage of oxygen the child is receiving.

> **HESI Hint**
> - Pco_2 >45 or Po_2 <60 on 50% O_2 signifies respiratory failure.
> - A child in severe distress should be on 100% O_2.

Review of Respiratory Failure

1. What Po_2 value indicates hypoxemia?
2. What blood value indicates hypercapnia?
3. Identify the condition that exists when the Po_2 is less than 50 mm Hg and FiO_2 is greater than 60%.
4. List three symptoms of respiratory failure in adults.
5. List four common causes of respiratory failure in children.
6. What percentage of O_2 should a child in severe respiratory distress receive?

Answers to Review

1. Below 50 mm Hg
2. P_{CO_2} above 45 mm Hg
3. Hypoxemia
4. Dyspnea/tachypnea; intercostal and sternal retractions; cyanosis
5. Congenital heart disease; infection or sepsis; respiratory distress syndrome; aspiration; fluid overload or dehydration
6. 100%

Shock

Description: Widespread, serious reduction of tissue perfusion (lack of O_2 and nutrients) that, if prolonged, leads to generalized impairment of cellular functioning

A. Arterial pressure is the driving force of blood flow through all the organs.
   1. It is dependent on cardiac output to perfuse the body.
   2. It is dependent on peripheral vasomotor tone to return blood and other fluids to the heart.
   3. It is dependent on the amount of circulating blood.
   4. Marked reduction in either cardiac output or peripheral vasomotor tone, without a compensatory elevation in the other, results in system hypotension.
   5. Those at risk for development of shock include:
      a. Very young and very old clients
      b. Post–myocardial infarction (MI) clients
      c. Clients with severe dysrhythmia
      d. Clients with adrenocortical dysfunction
      e. Persons with a history of recent hemorrhage or blood loss
      f. Clients with burns
      g. Clients with massive or overwhelming infection

HESI Hint • Early signs of shock are agitation and restlessness resulting from cerebral hypoxia.

B. Types of shock
   1. Hypovolemic—related to external or internal blood or fluid loss (the most common cause of shock; Table 3-2)
   2. Cardiogenic—related to ischemia or impairment in tissue perfusion resulting from MI, serious arrhythmia, or heart failure. All of these cause decreased cardiac output.
   3. Vasogenic—related to allergens (anaphylaxis), spinal cord injury, or peripheral neuropathies, all resulting in venous pooling and decreased blood return to the heart, which decreases cardiac output over time
   4. Septic—related to endotoxins released by bacteria, which cause vascular pooling, diminished venous return, and reduced cardiac output

HESI Hint • If cardiogenic shock exists in the presence of pulmonary edema (i.e., from pump failure), position client to reduce venous return (high Fowler position with legs down) to decrease further venous return to the left ventricle.

MEDICAL TREATMENT FOR SHOCK

A. Rapid infusion of volume-expanding fluids
   1. Whole blood, plasma, plasma substitutes (colloid fluids). Note that although whole blood is an acceptable volume expander, it is rarely used because of a high risk for transfusion reactions.
   2. Isotonic, electrolyte intravenous solutions such as Ringer's lactate solution and normal saline
B. If shock is cardiogenic in nature, the infusion of volume-expanding fluids may result in pulmonary edema.
   1. Restoration of cardiac function should take priority.
   2. Administration of cardiotonic drugs (such as digitalis) may increase cardiac contractility.
   3. Other drugs that enhance contractility include dopamine (Intropin).
   4. Vasoconstricting agents such as dopamine (Intropin) and norepinephrine (Levophed) may be used in cardiogenic shock.
C. Central venous pulmonary artery catheters are inserted in the operating room (OR) to monitor cardiogenic versus hypovolemic shock.
D. Serial measurements of central venous pressure (CVP), urine output, heart rate, and the clinical and mental state of the client are taken every 5 to 15 minutes.

TABLE 3-2 **Stages of Hypovolemic Shock**

Stage	Signs and Symptoms	Clinical Description
Stage I: • Initial Stage • Blood loss of less than 10% • Compensatory mechanisms triggered	• Apprehension and restlessness (first signs of shock) • Increased heart rate • Cool, pale skin • Fatigue	• Arteriolar constriction • Increased production of antidiuretic hormone (ADH) • Arterial pressure maintained • Cardiac output usually normal (for healthy individuals) • Selective reduction in blood flow to skin and muscle beds
Stage II: • Compensatory Stage • Blood volume reduced by 15% to 25% • Decompensation begins	• Flattened neck veins and delayed venous filling time • Increased pulse and respirations • Pallor, diaphoresis, and cool skin • Decreased urinary output • Sunken, soft eyeballs • Confusion	• Marked reduction in cardiac output • Arterial pressure decline (despite compensatory arteriolar vasoconstriction) • Massive adrenergic compensatory response, resulting in tachycardia, tachypnea, cutaneous vasoconstriction, and oliguria • Decreased cerebral perfusion
Stage III: • Progressive Stage	• Edema • Increased blood viscosity • Excessively low BP • Dysrhythmia, ischemia, and myocardial infarction • Weak, thready, or absent peripheral pulses	• Rapid circulatory deterioration • Decreased cardiac output • Decreased tissue perfusion • Reduced blood volume
Stage IV: • Irreversible Stage	• Profound hypotension, unresponsiveness to vasopressor drugs • Severe hypoxemia, unresponsiveness to O_2 administration • Anuria, renal shut down • Heart rate slows, BP falls, with consequent cardiac and respiratory arrest	• Cell destruction so severe that death is inevitable • Multiple organ system failure • It is the nurse's responsibility to recognize the signs and symptoms of shock. Every effort should be made to prevent the devastating clinical course that the progression of shock can take.

HESI Hint • Severe shock leads to widespread cellular injury and impairs the integrity of the capillary membranes. Fluid and osmotic proteins seep into the extravascular spaces, further reducing cardiac output.

A vicious circle of decreased perfusion to all cellular level activities ensues. All organs are damaged, and if perfusion problems persist, the damage can be permanent.

E. Following immediate attention to improvement of perfusion, attention is directed toward treating the underlying cause of the condition.

F. Administration of drugs is usually withheld until circulating volume has been restored.

G. Oxygen is administered.

Nursing Assessment

A. Vital signs
  1. Tachycardia (pulse >100 bpm)
  2. Tachypnea (respirations >24 min)
  3. BP decrease (systolic <80 mm Hg)

B. Mental status
  1. Early shock: restless, hyperalert
  2. Late shock: decreased alertness, lethargy, coma

C. Skin changes
  1. Cool, clammy skin (warm skin in vasogenic and early septic shock)
  2. Diaphoresis
  3. Paleness

D. Fluid status (acute renal tubular necrosis can happen quickly in shock)
  1. Urine output decreases, or an imbalance between intake and output occurs.

TABLE 3-3 Arterial Pressure

Concept	Definition
Mean arterial pressure (MAP)	• Level of pressure in the central arterial bed measured indirectly by BP measurement • MAP = cardiac output × total peripheral resistance = systolic blood pressure + 2 (diastolic blood pressure)/3 • In adults, usually approaches 100 mm Hg • Can be measured directly through arterial catheter insertion
Cardiac output (CO)	• Volume of blood ejected by the left ventricle per unit of time • Stroke volume (amount of blood ejected per beat) × heart rate (normal: 4 to 6 L/min)
Peripheral resistance (PR)	• Resistance to blood flow offered by the vessels in the peripheral vascular bed
Central venous pressure (CVP)	• Pressure within the right atrium (normal = 4 to 10 cm H_2O)

  2. CVP is abnormal (<4 cm H_2O).
  3. A urine specific gravity >1.020 indicates hypovolemia.

Analysis (Nursing Diagnoses)

A. *Deficient fluid volume* related to…

B. *Decreased cardiac output* related to…

C. *Anxiety (family and individual)* related to…

Nursing Plans and Interventions

A. Monitor arterial pressure by understanding the concepts related to arterial pressure (Table 3-3).

B. Monitor BP, pulse, respirations, and arrhythmias every 15 minutes or more often, depending on stability of client.

C. Assess urine output every hour to maintain at least 30 ml/hr.

D. Notify health care provider if urine output drops below 30 ml/hr (reflects decreased renal perfusion and may result in permanent renal damage).

E. Administer fluids as prescribed by provider: blood, colloids, or electrolyte solutions until designated CVP is reached. (In shock situations, the health care provider often orders fluids so as to elevate CVP to 16 to 19 cm H_2O as compensation for decreased cardiac output; Table 3-4.)

F. Place client in modified Trendelenburg position (feet up 45 degrees, head flat).

G. Administer medications IV (*not* IM or subcutaneous) until perfusion improves in muscles and subcutaneous tissue.

H. Keep client warm; increase heat in room or put warm blankets (not too hot) on client.

I. Keep side rails up during all procedures; clients in shock experience mental confusion and may easily be injured by falls.

J. Obtain blood for lab work as prescribed: complete blood count (CBC), electrolytes, blood urea nitrogen (BUN), creatinine (renal damage), and blood gases (oxygenation).

K. When administering vasopressors or adrenergic stimulants, such as epinephrine (Bronkaid), dopamine (Intropin), dobutamine (Dobutrex), norepinephrine (Levophed), or isoproterenol (Isuprel):
  1. Administer through volume-controlled pump.
  2. Monitor BP every 5 to 15 minutes.
  3. Watch intravenous site carefully for extravasation and tissue damage.
  4. Ask health care provider for target mean systolic BP (usually 80 to 90 mm Hg).

L. When administering vasodilators, such as hydralazine (Apresoline), nitroprusside (Nipride), or labetalol hydrochloride (Normodyne, Trandate) to counteract effects of vasopressors:
  1. Wait for precipitous decrease or increase in BP if prescribed together.
  2. If drop in BP occurs, decrease vasodilator infusion rate first; then increase vasopressor.
  3. If BP increases precipitously, decrease vasopressor rate first; then increase rate of vasodilator.
  4. Obtain blood work as prescribed: CBC, electrolytes, BUN, creatinine (renal damage), and blood gases (oxygenation).

HESI Hint • All vasopressor and vasodilator drugs are potent and dangerous and require that the client be weaned onto and off them. Do not change both infusion rates simultaneously.

M. Provide family support:
  1. Notify appropriate support persons for families waiting during crisis—call spiritual advisor,

TABLE 3-4 **Administration of Blood Products**

Component therapy has replaced the use of whole blood, which accounts for less than 10% of all transfusions.

BLOOD PRODUCTS

Description	Special Considerations	Indications for Use
Packed red blood cells (RBCs)	Less danger of fluid overload	Acute blood loss
Frozen RBCs: prepared from RBCs using glycerol for protection and then frozen	Must be used within 24 hr of thawing	Auto transfusion: infrequently used because filters remove most of white blood cells
Platelets: pooled—300 ml One unit contains single donor—200 ml	Bag should be agitated periodically.	Bleeding caused by thrombocytopenia
Fresh-frozen plasma (FFP): liquid portion of whole blood is separated from cells and frozen	The use of FFP is being replaced by albumin plasma expanders.	Bleeding caused by deficiency in clotting factors
Albumin: prepared from plasma and is available in 5% and 20% solutions	Albumin 25 g/L00 ml is osmotically equal to 500 ml of plasma.	Hypovolemic shock, hypoalbuminemia
Cryoprecipitates and commercial concentrates: prepared from fresh-frozen plasma with 10 to 20 ml/bag	Used in treating hemophilia	Replacement of clotting factors, especially factor VIII and fibrinogen

TRANSFUSION REACTIONS

Reactions/Complications	Assessment	Nursing Interventions
Acute hemolytic	Chills, fever, low back pain, flushing, tachycardia, hypotension progressing to acute renal failure, shock, and cardiac arrest	*Stop transfusion* Change tubing, then continue saline IV Treat for shock if present Draw blood samples for serologic testing Monitor hourly urine output Give diuretics as prescribed
Febrile nonhemolytic (most common)	Sudden chills and fever, headaches, flushing, anxiety, and muscle pain	Give antipyretics as prescribed
Mild allergic	Flushing, itching, urticaria (hives)	Give antihistamine as directed
Anaphylactic and severe allergic	Anxiety, urticaria, wheezing, progressive cyanosis leading to shock and possible cardiac arrest	Initiate CPR
Circulatory overload	Cough, dyspnea, pulmonary congestion, headache, hypertension	Place client in upright position with feet in dependent position and administer diuretics, oxygen, morphine
Sepsis	Rapid onset of chills, high fever, vomiting, marked hypotension, or shock	Ensure a patent airway, obtain blood for culture, administer prescribed antibiotics, take vital signs every 5 minutes until stable

TABLE 3-4 Administration of Blood Products—cont'd

NURSING SKILLS
• Obtain venous access; use central venous catheter or 19-gauge needle.
• Use only blood administration tubing to infuse blood products.
• Run blood products with saline solutions only. Dextrose solutions and Ringer's lactate solution will induce RBC hemolysis.
• Run infusion at prescribed rate, and remain with client for the first 15 to 30 minutes of infusion.
• The blood should be administered as soon as it is brought to the client.
• Check vital signs frequently before, during, and immediately following infusion; note any increase in temperature.
• Follow agency policy regarding specific timetable for blood infusion.
• Check and double-check the product before infusing to see that it is the:
• Correct product, as prescribed; double-check with a second licensed person.
• Correct blood type and Rh factor, matched with the client, and note expiration date.

other family members, or anyone the family thinks will be supportive.

2. At intervals, notify family of actions and progress or lack of progress in realistic terms.
3. Collaborate with health care provider before notifying family of medical interventions.

HESI Hint • A client is brought into the hospital suffering shock symptoms as a result of a bee sting. What is the first priority? Maintaining an open airway (the allergic reaction damages the lining of the airways, causing edema). Also, keep the client warm and free of constricting clothing; keep client's legs elevated (but not in the Trendelenburg position because the weight of the lower organs restricts breathing).

Epinephrine: 1:1000, 0.2 to 0.5 ml subcutaneous for mild cases

or

Epinephrine: 1:10,000, 5 ml IV for severe cases

Volume-expanding fluids are usually given to clients in shock. However, if the shock is cardiogenic, pulmonary edema may result.

Drugs of choice for shock:
• Digitalis preparations. They increase the contractility of the heart muscle.
• Vasoconstrictors (Levophed, Dopamine). Generalized vasoconstriction provides more blood to the heart to help maintain cardiac output.

Disseminated Intravascular Coagulation (DIC)

Description: Coagulation disorder with paradoxical thrombosis and hemorrhage

A. DIC is an acute complication of conditions such as hypotension and septicemia. It is suspected when there is blood oozing from two or more unexpected sites.

B. The first phase involves abnormal clotting in the microcirculation, which uses up clotting factors and results in the inability to form clots, so hemorrhage occurs.

C. The diagnosis is based on laboratory findings.
1. Prothrombin time (PT): prolonged
2. Partial thromboplastin time (PTT): prolonged
3. Fibrinogen: decreased
4. Platelet count: decreased
5. Fibrin degradation (split) products (FDP): increased

NURSING ASSESSMENT

A. Petechiae, purpura, hematomas
B. Oozing from IV sites, drains, gums, and wounds
C. Gastrointestinal and genitourinary bleeding
D. Hemoptysis
E. Mental status change
F. Hypotension, tachycardia
G. Pain

ANALYSIS (NURSING DIAGNOSES)

A. *Risk for injury* related to…
B. *Ineffective tissue perfusion (specific type)* related to…

NURSING PLANS AND INTERVENTIONS

A. Monitor client for bleeding.
B. Monitor vital signs.
C. Monitor PT/INR.
D. Protect client from injury and bleeding.
1. Provide gentle oral care with mouth swabs.
2. Minimize needle sticks; use smallest gauge needle possible.

3. Turn client frequently to eliminate pressure points.
4. Minimize number of BP measurements taken by cuff.
5. Use gentle suction to prevent trauma to mucosa.

6. Apply pressure to any oozing site.

E. Administer heparin IV during the first phase to inhibit coagulation.

F. Provide emotional support to decrease anxiety.

> **HESI Hint** • You are caring for a woman who was in a severe automobile accident several days earlier. She has several fractures and internal injuries. The exploratory laparotomy was successful in controlling the bleeding. However, today you find that this client is bleeding from her incision, is short of breath, and has a weak, thready pulse, cold and clammy skin, and hematuria.
>
> What do you think is wrong with the client, and what would you expect to do about it?
>
> These are typical signs and symptoms of DIC crisis. Expect to administer IV heparin to block the formation of thrombin (Coumadin does not do this). However, the client described is already past the coagulation phase and into the hemorrhagic phase. Her care would include administration of clotting factors, along with palliative treatment of the symptoms as they arise. (Her prognosis is poor.)

Review of Shock and DIC

1. Define *shock*.
2. What is the most common cause of shock?
3. What causes septic shock?
4. What is the goal of treatment for hypovolemic shock?
5. What intervention is used to restore cardiac output when hypovolemic shock exists?
6. It is important to differentiate between hypovolemic and cardiogenic shock. How might the nurse determine the existence of cardiogenic shock?
7. If a client is in cardiogenic shock, what might result from administration of volume-expanding fluids, and what intervention can the nurse expect to perform in the event of such an occurrence?
8. List five assessment findings that occur in most shock victims.

9. What is the normal CVP for an adult?
10. Once circulating volume is restored, vasopressors may be prescribed to increase venous return. List the main drugs that are used.
11. What is the established minimum renal output per hour?
12. List four measurable criteria that are the major expected outcomes of a shock crisis.
13. Define *DIC*.
14. What is the effect of DIC on PT, PTT, platelets, and FSPs (FDPs)?
15. What drug is used in the treatment of DIC?
16. Name four nursing interventions to prevent injury in clients with DIC.

Answers to Review

1. Widespread, serious reduction of tissue perfusion, which leads to generalized impairment of cellular function
2. Hypovolemia
3. Release of endotoxins by bacteria, which act on nerves in vascular spaces in the periphery, causing vascular pooling, reduced venous return, and decreased cardiac output and result in poor systemic perfusion
4. Quick restoration of cardiac output and tissue perfusion
5. Rapid infusion of volume-expanding fluids
6. History of MI with left ventricular failure or possible cardiomyopathy, with symptoms of pulmonary edema

7. Pulmonary edema; administer cardiotonic drugs such as digitalis preparations
8. Tachycardia; tachypnea; hypotension; cool, clammy skin; decrease in urinary output
9. 4 to 10 cm H_2O
10. Epinephrine (Bronkaid), dopamine (Intropin), dobutamine (Dobutrex), norepinephrine (Levophed), or isoproterenol (Isuprel)
11. 30 ml/hr
12. BP mean of 80 to 90 mm Hg; Po_2 >50 mm Hg; CVP >6 cm H_2O; urine output at least 30 ml/hr

13. A coagulation disorder in which there is paradoxical thrombosis and hemorrhage
14. PT, prolonged; PTT, prolonged; platelets, decreased; FSPs, increased
15. Heparin

16. Gently provide oral care with mouth swabs. Minimize needle sticks and use the smallest-gauge needle possible when injections are necessary. Eliminate pressure by turning the client frequently. Minimize the number of BP measurements taken by cuff. Use gentle suction to prevent trauma to mucosa. Apply pressure to any oozing site.

Resuscitation

CARDIOPULMONARY ARREST

A. Usually caused by MI; necrosis of the heart muscle caused by inadequate blood supply to heart
B. MIs usually occur at rest or with moderate activity, contrary to the belief that they occur with strenuous activity.
C. Symptoms immediately preceding MI:
   1. Chest pain or discomfort at rest or with ordinary activity
   2. Change in previous stable anginal pain—an increase in frequency or severity or rest angina occurring for the first time
   3. Chest pain in a client with known coronary heart disease that is unrelieved by rest or nitroglycerin

> **HESI Hint** • NCLEX-RN® questions on cardiopulmonary resuscitation (CPR) often deal with prioritization of actions.
> Question: What actions are required for each of the following situations?
> • A 24-year-old motorcycle accident victim with a ruptured artery of the leg who is pulseless and apneic
> • A 36-year-old first-time pregnant woman who arrests during labor
> • A 17-year-old with no pulse or respirations who is trapped in an overturned car that is starting to burn
> • A 40-year-old businessman who arrests 2 days after a cervical laminectomy

D. O_2 is necessary for survival; all other injuries are secondary except for removal of any source of imminent danger such as a fire.
E. Chest pain in MI:
   1. Is usually described as crushing, pressing, constricting, oppressive, or heavy
   2. Tends to increase in intensity over a few minutes

3. May be substernal or more diffused
4. May radiate to one or both shoulders and arms or to neck, jaw, or back

F. Occasions for cardiopulmonary resuscitation are often unwitnessed cardiac arrests.

> **HESI Hint** • When to seek emergency medical services (EMS):
> • The symptoms of anterior myocardial infarction (AMI) characteristically last more than 15 minutes and are more intense than angina.
> • The American Heart Association's guidelines recommend that those at risk for acute coronary syndrome (ACS) should activate the EMS system if chest discomfort worsens or is unimproved 5 minutes after taking one tablet or spray of nitroglycerin.

MANAGEMENT OF CARDIAC ARREST

Out-of-Hospital (Unwitnessed) Cardiac Arrest

> **HESI Hint** • It is important for the nurse to stay current with the American Heart Association's guidelines for basic life support (BLS) by being certified every 2 years, as required.

A. Position person supine, tap, and call out, "Are you okay?"
B. If no response occurs, call for help or ask someone to call the local emergency number, usually 911. Obtain an automated external defibrillator (AED) if one is available.
C. Establish an airway by extending neck with the head-tilt, chin-lift maneuver or the jaw-thrust maneuver. Clear airway of foreign body, if visible.
D. Assess breathing by the look-listen-feel method.
   1. Look for chest excursion.
   2. Listen for breathing sounds through the mouth and nose.
   3. Feel for breath on your own cheek.

4. Differentiate between agonal breathing (ineffective gasps) and regular, effective breathing.
E. If no breathing is noted:
   1. Ventilate with two mouth-to-mouth breaths over 1 second and make the chest rise.
   2. Assess circulation by palpating carotid pulse for no more than 10 seconds.
   3. If no pulse, initiate cardiac compressions by depressing sternum at a rate of 100/min ("push hard, push fast").
   4. Continue CPR until spontaneous respirations and pulse return.

HESI Hint • CPR is performed at a 30:2 ratio of compression to ventilations, at the compression rate of 100/min, continuously without pauses for ventilation. After five cycles, reassess for breathing and pulse. The compressor role should be rotated about every 2 minutes without interruption of the compression rate.

HESI Hint • At 20 weeks' gestation and beyond, the gravid uterus should be shifted to the left by placing the woman in a 15- to 30-degree angled left lateral position or by using a wedge under her right side to tilt her to her left.

In-Hospital Cardiac Arrest

HESI Hint • Initiate CPR with BLS guidelines immediately; then move on to advanced cardiac life support (ACLS) guidelines.

A. Determine responsiveness by tapping the client and shouting, "Are you all right?"
   1. If no response occurs, call a "code," or cardiac arrest, in order to initiate response of cardiac arrest team.
   2. Position client on cardiac board.
   3. Ventilate with 100% O_2 with oral airway and mouth-to-mask or use a bag-mask device.
   4. Initiate chest compressions.
B. Team leader arrives and assesses client, directs team members, and obtains history and precipitating events to arrest.
   1. Without interrupting CPR, apply cardiac portable monitor "quick-look" paddles to determine whether defibrillation is necessary or whether asystole has occurred.
   2. Rapid defibrillation is indicated in ventricular fibrillation or pulseless ventricular tachycardia.

3. Resume CPR, beginning with compressions, immediately after defibrillations.

HESI Hint • When significant arterial acidosis is noted, try to reduce Pco$_2$ by increasing ventilation, which will correct arterial, venous, and tissue acidosis.
Bicarbonate may exacerbate acidosis by producing CO_2. ACLS guidelines have recommended that bicarbonate *not* be used unless hyperkalemia, tricyclic antidepressant overdose, or preexisting metabolic acidosis is documented.

PEDIATRIC RESUSCITATION

Neonatal
See Maternity Nursing.
A. Ventilations are done over mouth and nose, using a size 1 mask for a term neonate, a size 0 for a preterm neonate.
B. With neonates, an initial ventilation with peak inflating pressures of 30 to 40 cm H_2O at a rate of 40 to 60/min is usually successful in unresponsive term infants.
C. Palpate brachial pulse in infant less than 1 year old to assess heart rate.
D. If the heart rate is under 60, compressions are done with thumbs side by side over the lower third of the sternum, to a depth of one-third the anteroposterior chest diameter, with a compression-to-ventilation ratio of 3:1 to achieve 120 events per minute (90 compressions plus 30 breaths).
E. Compressions can also be accomplished with one hand under the back and two fingers over the midsternum.

Child Aged 1 to 8 Years
A. Ventilations (mouth-to-mouth) should make the chest rise. Mouth and nose should be used for infants (under 1 year).
B. The chest is compressed 1 inch with one palm at a rate of 100/min; "Push hard, push fast."
C. A ratio of 2 ventilations to 30 compressions, if there is one rescuer (or 2:15 if there are two rescuers) without pauses for ventilations (8 to 10/min) should be maintained.
D. The most common rhythm in pediatrics is asystole and bradycardia.
E. Epinephrine is the drug of choice given IV at 0.01 mg/kg body weight using a 1:10,000 solution.

HESI Hint • In the pulseless arrest algorithm (PALS), the search for and treatment of possible contributing factors should include checking for hypovolemia, hypoxia, hydrogen ion acidosis, hypokalemia and hyperkalemia, hypoglycemia, hypothermia, toxins, tamponade (cardiac), tension pneumothorax, thrombosis (cardiac, pulmonary), and trauma.

MANAGEMENT OF FOREIGN BODY AIRWAY OBSTRUCTION (FBAO)

Adults and Children 1 Year and Older

A. If unable to ventilate the person during CPR, suspect a foreign body in airway.

B. If person is conscious, stand behind person, grasp around waist with clenched fist (halfway between navel and xiphoid), and exert palmar thrust inward at epigastrium (Heimlich maneuver) in rapid sequence.

C. Chest thrust should be used in obese or pregnant patients.

D. Continue until object is expelled or person falls to ground unconscious; then activate EMS and begin CPR.

E. Use a finger sweep only if the object is seen obstructing the airway.

Infants and Children

A. Open a conscious child's mouth and attempt to clear obstruction manually if the object can be seen (*no* blind sweeps; they may push the foreign object farther down the throat).

B. For a child, perform subdiaphragmatic abdominal thrusts (Heimlich maneuver) in rapid sequence until the obstruction is relieved.

C. If the infant is able to cry, cough, or breathe, do *not* interfere.

D. If the infant is conscious and *cannot* cry, cough, or breathe:
1. Place infant facedown, head lower than trunk, with legs straddling your arm and chest supported by your upturned hand.
2. Give five firm blows to back with heel of hand (compresses rib cage between two hands).
3. Position face upward and give five chest thrusts as you would for cardiac massage.
4. Repeat until the object is expelled or the infant becomes unresponsive.

E. If unresponsive, begin CPR:
1. Using tongue-jaw lift (use your thumbs to pull down the jaw, lowering the jaw in order to do a visual inspection), open the mouth. If the foreign object is seen, take it out.
2. Open airway (tilt the infant's head and lift the chin) and perform mouth-to-mouth/nose breathing: cover the infant's mouth and nose with your mouth and give the infant two breaths; follow with chest compressions.

Review of Resuscitation

1. What is the first priority when a client with an unwitnessed cardiac arrest is found?
2. Define *myocardial infarction*.
3. What criteria should alert a client with known angina who takes nitroglycerin tablets sublingually to call EMS?
4. After calling out for help and asking someone to dial for emergency services, what is the next action in CPR?
5. True or False? In feeling for presence of a carotid pulse, no more than 5 seconds should be used.
6. During one-rescuer CPR, what is the ratio of compressions to ventilations for an adult? During one-rescuer CPR, what is the ratio of compressions to ventilations for a child?
7. What is the first drug most likely to be used for an in-hospital cardiac arrest?
8. A client in cardiac arrest is noted on bedside monitor to be in pulseless ventricular tachycardia. What is the first action that should be taken?
9. True or False? A precordial thump is a routine activity for an in-hospital cardiac arrest.
10. How would the nurse assess the adequacy of compressions during CPR? How would the nurse assess the adequacy of ventilations during CPR?
11. If a person is choking, when should the rescuer intervene?
12. One should never make blind sweeps into the mouth of a choking child or infant. Why?
13. Why do the ACLS guidelines recommend a decreased reliance on the use of bicarbonate during adult CPR?

Answers to Review

1. Begin CPR.
2. Necrosis of the heart muscle due to poor perfusion of the heart
3. Unrelieved chest pain after nitroglycerin
4. Call for help and begin CPR. For unresponsive infants and children, CPR should be performed for 1 minute before placing a 911 call for help.
5. False. Palpate for no more than 10 seconds, recognizing that arrhythmias or bradycardia could be occurring.
6. 30:2 × 5 cycles; 15:2 for a child or neonate with two rescuers
7. Epinephrine
8. Defibrillation
9. False. A thump is indicated only in pulseless VT or VF or when ventricular asystole on monitor responds to a thump with a QRS complex.
10. Check for a pulse. Watch for chest excursion and auscultate bilaterally for breath sounds.
11. When the person points to his or her throat and can no longer cough, talk, or make sounds
12. Because the object might be pushed farther down into the throat
13. Because acidosis should be relieved with improved ventilation; bicarbonate can actually contribute to increased CO_2.

Fluid and Electrolyte Balance

HOMEOSTASIS

Description: Process of maintaining a relative state of equilibrium

A. Homeostasis occurs in relation to maintenance of the composition of fluids.

B. Fluid composition involves a number of variables (Table 3-5).

> **HESI Hint** • Changes in osmolarity cause shifts in fluid. The osmolarity of the extracellular fluid (ECF) is almost entirely due to sodium. The osmolarity of intracellular fluid (ICF) is related to many particles, with potassium being the primary electrolyte. The pressures in the ECF and the ICF are almost identical. If either ECF or ICF changes in concentration, fluid shifts from the area of lesser concentration to the area of greater concentration.

> **HESI Hint** •
> - Dextrose 10% is a hypertonic solution and should be administered IV.
> - Normal saline is an isotonic solution and is used for irrigations, such as bladder irrigations or IV flush lines with intermittent IV medication.
> - Use only isotonic (neutral) solutions in irrigations, infusions, etc., unless the specific aim is to shift fluid to intracellular or extracellular spaces.

ORGAN FUNCTION

A. Kidneys
   1. Selectively maintain and excrete body fluids.
   2. Selectively retain needed substances and excrete unneeded substances, such as electrolytes.
   3. Regulate pH by excreting or maintaining hydrogen ions and bicarbonate.
   4. Excrete metabolic wastes and toxic substances.
B. Lungs
   1. Rid the body of approximately 300 ml of fluid per day and play a role in acid-base balance.
   2. Regulate carbon dioxide concentration.
C. Heart
   1. Pumps blood with sufficient force to perfuse the kidneys, allowing the kidneys to work effectively.
D. Adrenal glands
   1. Secrete aldosterone, which causes sodium retention (resulting in water retention) and potassium excretion.
E. Parathyroid glands
   1. Regulate calcium and phosphorus balance.
F. Pituitary gland
   1. Secretes antidiuretic hormone (ADH), which causes the body to retain water.

ELECTROLYTE IMBALANCE

Nursing Assessment
Refer to Table 3-6.

Nursing Plans and Interventions
Refer to Table 3-6.

> **HESI Hint** • Potassium imbalances are potentially life-threatening; they must be corrected immediately. A low magnesium level often accompanies a low K+, especially with the use of diuretics.

TABLE 3-5 Fluid Volume

Variable	Deficit	Excess
Description	• Occurs when the body loses water and electrolytes isotonically, that is, in the same proportion as exists in the normal body fluid • Serum electrolyte levels remain normal • Dehydration: state in which the body loses water and serum sodium levels increase	• Occurs when the body retains water and electrolytes isotonically • Water intoxication: state in which the body retains water and serum sodium levels decrease
Causes	• Vomiting • Diarrhea • GI suctioning • Sweating • Inadequate fluid intake • Massive edema, as in initial stage of major burns • Ascites • Elderly forgetting to drink	• Heart failure (HF) • Renal failure • Cirrhosis, liver failure • Excessive ingestion of table salt • Overhydration with sodium-containing fluid • Poorly controlled IV therapy, especially in young and old clients
Symptoms	• Weight loss (1 pint of fluid loss is equal to 1 pound of weight loss) • Decreased skin turgor • Oliguria (concentrated urine) • Dry and sticky mucous membranes • Postural hypotension or weak, rapid pulse	• Peripheral edema • Increased bounding pulse • Elevated BP • Distended neck and hand veins • Dyspnea; moist crackles heard when lungs auscultated • Attention loss, confusion, aphasia • Altered level of consciousness
Lab findings	• Elevated BUN and creatinine • Increased serum osmolarity • Elevated hemoglobin and hematocrit	• Decreased BUN • Decreased hemoglobin and hematocrit • Decreased serum osmolality • Decreased urine osmolality and specific gravity
Treatment and nursing care	• Strict I&O • Replacement of fluids isotonically, preferably orally • *Water is a hypotonic fluid* • If intravenous hydration is needed, isotonic fluids are used	• Diuretics • Fluid restriction • Strict I&O • Sodium-restricted diet • Weighed daily • K^+ serum monitored

HESI Hint • FLUID VOLUME DEFICIT: DEHYDRATION

• Elevated blood urea nitrogen (BUN): The BUN measures the amount of urea nitrogen in the blood. Urea is formed in the liver as the end product of protein metabolism. The BUN is directly related to the metabolic function of the liver and the excretory function of the kidneys.
• Creatinine, as with BUN, is excreted entirely by the kidneys and is therefore directly proportional to renal excretory function. However, unlike BUN, the creatinine level is affected very little by dehydration, malnutrition, or hepatic function. The daily production of creatinine depends on muscle mass, which fluctuates very little. Therefore, it is a better test of renal function than is the BUN. Creatinine is generally used in conjunction with the BUN test, and they are normally in a 1:20 ratio.
• Serum osmolality measures the concentration of particles in a solution. It refers to the fact that the same amount of solute is present, but the amount of solvent (fluid) is decreased. Therefore, the blood can be considered "more concentrated."
• Urine osmolality and specific gravity increase.

TABLE 3-6 **Electrolyte Imbalances**

Abnormalities and Common Causes	Signs and Symptoms	Treatment
Hyponatremia (↓Na) • Diuretics • GI fluid loss • Hypotonic tube feeding • D$_5$W or hypotonic IV fluids • Diaphoresis	• Anorexia, nausea, vomiting • Weakness • Lethargy • Confusion • Muscle cramps, twitching • Seizures • Na <135 mEq/L	• Restrict fluids (safer) • If IV saline solutions prescribed, administer very slowly; use if fluid restriction not effective
Hypernatremia (↑Na) • Water deprivation • Hypertonic tube feeding • Diabetes insipidus • Heatstroke • Hyperventilation • Watery diarrhea • Renal failure • Cushing syndrome	• Thirst • Hyperpyrexia • Sticky mucous membranes • Dry mouth • Hallucinations • Lethargy • Irritability • Seizures • Na >145 mEq/L	• Restrict sodium in the diet • Beware of hidden sodium in foods and medications • Increase water intake
Hypokalemia (↓K) • Diuretics • Diarrhea • Vomiting • Gastric suction • Steroid administration • Hyperaldosteronism • Amphotericin B • Bulimia • Cushing syndrome	• Fatigue • Anorexia • Nausea, vomiting • Muscle weakness • Decreased GI motility • Dysrhythmias • Paresthesia • Flat T waves on ECG • K <3.5 mEq/L	• Administer potassium supplements orally or IV • Oral forms of potassium are unpleasant tasting and are irritating to the GI tract (do not give on empty stomach; dilute) • *Never* give IV bolus; *must* be well diluted • Assess renal status, i.e., urinary output, prior to administering • Encourage foods high in potassium (e.g., bananas, oranges, cantaloupes, avocados, spinach, potatoes)
Hyperkalemia (↑K) • Hemolyzed serum sample produces pseudohyperkalemia • Oliguria • Acidosis • Renal failure • Addison disease • Multiple blood transfusions	• Muscle weakness • Bradycardia • Dysrhythmias • Flaccid paralysis • Intestinal colic • Tall T waves on ECG • K >5.0 mEq/L	• Eliminate parenteral potassium from IV infusions and medications • Administer 50% glucose with regular insulin • Administer cation exchange resin (Kayexalate) • Monitor ECG • Administer calcium gluconate to protect the heart • IV loop diuretics may be prescribed • Renal dialysis may be required
Hypocalcemia (↓Ca) • Renal failure • Hypoparathyroidism • Malabsorption • Pancreatitis • Alkalosis	• Diarrhea • Numbness • Tingling of extremities • Convulsions • Positive Trousseau sign • Positive sign • Ca <8.5 mEq/L • At risk for tetany	• Administer calcium supplements orally 30 minutes before meals • Administer calcium IV slowly; infiltration can cause tissue necrosis • Increase calcium intake (e.g., dairy products, greens)

TABLE 3-6 Electrolyte Imbalances—cont'd

Abnormalities and Common Causes	Signs and Symptoms	Treatment
Hypercalcemia ($\uparrow$Ca) • Hyperparathyroidism • Malignant bone disease • Prolonged immobilization • Excess calcium supplementation	• Muscle weakness • Constipation • Anorexia • Nausea, vomiting • Polyuria • Polydipsia • Neurosis • Dysrhythmias • Ca >10.5 mEq/L	• Eliminate parenteral calcium • Administer agents to reduce calcium such as calcitonin • Avoid calcium-based antacids • Renal dialysis may be required
Hypomagnesemia ($\downarrow$Mg) • Alcoholism • Malabsorption • Diabetic ketoacidosis • Prolonged gastric suction • Diuretics	• Anorexia, distention • Neuromuscular irritability • Depression • Disorientation • Mg <1.5 mEq/L	• Administer $MgSO_4$ IV • Encourage foods high in magnesium (e.g., meats, nuts, legumes, fish, and vegetables)
Hypermagnesemia ($\uparrow$Mg) • Renal failure • Adrenal insufficiency • Excess replacement	• Flushing • Hypotension • Drowsiness, lethargy • Hypoactive reflexes • Depressed respirations • Bradycardia • Mg >2.5 mEq/L	• Avoid magnesium-based antacids and laxatives • Restrict dietary intake of foods high in magnesium
Hypophosphatemia ($\downarrow$Ph) • Refeeding after starvation • Alcohol withdrawal • Diabetic ketoacidosis • Respiratory alkalosis	• Paresthesias • Muscle weakness • Muscle pain • Mental changes • Cardiomyopathy • Respiratory failure • Ph <2.0 mEq/L	• Correct underlying cause • Administer oral replacement of phosphates with vitamin D
Hyperphosphatemia ($\uparrow$Ph) • Renal failure • Excess intake of phosphorus	• Short-term: tetany symptoms • Long-term: phosphorus precipitation in nonosseous sites • Ph >4.5 mEq/L	• Administer aluminum hydroxide with meals to bind phosphorus • Dialysis may be required if renal failure is underlying cause

INTRAVENOUS (IV) THERAPY

Description: IV solutions are used to supply electrolytes, nutrients, and water (Table 3-7).

Administration of IV Therapy

A. The purpose and duration of the IV therapy determine the type of equipment, such as IV tubing and size of needle, that should be used (e.g., administration of blood requires a 19-gauge needle or larger [e.g., 18 or 16 gauge]).

B. Gloves *must* be worn during venipuncture and when discontinuing an IV line.

C. Assess the IV site frequently (minimum of every 2 hours). It is the nurse's legal responsibility to observe the client, to report any reactions, and to take measures necessary to prevent complications.

D. Intermittent IV therapy may be given through a saline lock; regular flushing maintains patency.

E. IV tubing and dressing should be changed according to hospital policy (usually every 72 hours).

F. When the IV is discontinued, apply pressure to the site for 1 to 3 minutes after the needle is removed.

Complications Associated With IV Administration

A. Occlusion/catheter damage
  1. Assess for:
    a. Pinholes, leaks, and tears
    b. Drainage after flushing
    c. Blood return
    d. Inability to infuse fluid
    e. Needle placement, if a port
    f. Pain in shoulder, neck, or arm
    g. Neck or shoulder edema
    h. Suture damage

TABLE 3-7 **Types of IV Solutions**

Isotonic	Hypotonic	Hypertonic

• Have an osmolality close to the extracellular fluid (ECF)
• Do not cause red blood cells to swell or shrink
• Indicated for intravascular dehydration
• Isotonic solutions
  → Normal saline (0.9% NS)
  → Lactated Ringer's solution (LR)
  → 5% dextrose in water (D_5W is on the low end of isotonic; some sources classify it as hypotonic)
• Used to treat intravascular dehydration (not enough fluid in vascular system)
• Common type of dehydration
• Examples: dehydration caused by running, labor, fever, etc.
	• Have an osmolality lower than the ECF
	• Cause fluid to move from ECF to intracellular fluid (ICF)
	• Indicated for cellular dehydration
	• Hypotonic solutions
	  → 0.5% normal saline (HNS or 0.45% NS)
	  → 2.5% dextrose in 0.45% saline ($D_{2.5}$ 45% NS)
	• Used to treat intracellular dehydration (cells have too many osmoles, need to drive fluid into the cells)
	• Not a common occurrence
	• Examples: dehydration caused by prolonged dehydration (may also see in clients who are on TPN for prolonged periods)
		• Have an osmolality higher than the ECF
		• Indicated for intravascular dehydration with interstitial or cellular overhydration
		• To be used with extreme caution
		• High concentrations of dextrose are given for caloric replacement such as intravenous hyperalimentation into a central vein for rapid dilution
		• Hypertonic saline solutions are available but used only when serum osmolality is dangerously low
		• Hypertonic solutions
		  → 5% dextrose in lactated Ringer (D_5LR)
		  → 5% dextrose in 0.45% saline (D5 ½ NS)
		  → 5% dextrose in 0.9% saline (D_5NS)
		• Used to treat intravascular dehydration with cellular or interstitial overhydration
		• Examples: dehydration resulting from surgery: blood loss causes intravascular dehydration, but the tissue cuts inflame and pull fluid into the area, causing interstitial overhydration; may also see with ascites and third-spacing

FLOW RATE CALCULATION

• Several formulas exist for calculating intravenous flow rates.
• Infusion pumps are used when measurement of exact flow is necessary.
• Using the following steps for IV calculation will ensure proper calculation:
  1. ml/hr: Total ml fluid to be given/Total hrs. to be administered = ml/hr (rate for IV infusions on a pump)
  2. gtts/min: Total ml fluid to be given/Total min to be administered × gtts/ml = gtts/min (rate for IV infusions by gravity)

ECF, extracellular fluid; ICF, intracellular fluid.

HESI Hint • Check the IV tubing container to determine the drip factor because drip factors vary. The most common drip factors are 10, 12, 15, and 60 drops per milliliter. A microdrip is 60 drops per milliliter.

2. Interventions
   a. Do not use syringes that are less than 5 ml to irrigate.
   b. Do not irrigate forcefully.
B. Infection/phlebitis
   1. Assess:
      a. Site for redness, drainage, edema, or tenderness
      b. Vital signs
      c. Laboratory findings
   2. Interventions
      a. Use aseptic and antiseptic techniques when starting an IV line and when caring for IV site.
      b. Inspect all fluids and containers before use to be sure they have not been opened or otherwise contaminated.
      c. Change administration sets according to hospital policy (usually every 72 hours).
      d. Use a catheter that is smaller than the vein.
C. Dislodgment/migration/incorrect placement
   1. Assess:
      a. Length of catheter
      b. Edema, drainage, and coiling of catheter
      c. Neck distention or distended neck veins
      d. Client complaints of gurgling sounds
      e. Change in patency of catheter
      f. Chest radiograph
      g. Cardiac dysrhythmias
      h. Hypotension
   2. Interventions
      a. Provide enough tubing length for client movement.
      b. Anchor the catheter well.
      c. Measure and record length of catheter.
D. Skin erosion/hematomas/scar tissue formation over port/infiltration/extravasation
   1. Assess:
      a. Loss of tissue or separation at exit site
      b. Drainage at exit site
      c. Erythema and edema at exit site
      d. Spongy feeling at exit site
      e. Labored breathing
      f. Complaints of pain
   2. Interventions
      a. Dilute medications adequately.
      b. Follow institutional protocol for administration of vesicant drugs.
      c. Change IV line within the time frame outlined in institutional protocol.
      d. Provide gentle skin care at exit site.
      e. Avoid selecting site over joint.
      f. Anchor the catheter well.
E. Pneumothorax/hemothorax/air emboli/hydrothorax
   1. Assess for:
      a. Subcutaneous emphysema
      b. Chest pain
      c. Dyspnea and hypoxia
      d. Tachycardia
      e. Hypotension
      f. Nausea
      g. Confusion
   2. Interventions
      a. Use clot filters when infusing blood and blood products.
      b. Avoid using veins in the lower extremities.
      c. Prevent fluid containers from becoming empty.
      d. Check valves and micropore filters on vented Y-type infusions or piggyback infusions, which allow solutions to run simultaneously. Air may be introduced into the line if the containers become empty.

HESI Hint • Flushing a saline lock efficiently requires approximately 1½ times the amount of fluid the tubing will hold. Remember to use sterile technique to prevent complications, such as infiltration, emboli, and infection.

ACID-BASE BALANCE

Description: An acid-base balance must be maintained in the body because alterations can result in alkalosis or acidosis.

A. Maintaining the acid-base balance is imperative and involves three systems:
   1. Chemical buffer system
   2. Kidneys
   3. Lungs
B. Acid-base balance is determined by the hydrogen ion concentration in body fluids.
   1. Normal range is 7.35 to 7.45 expressed as the pH (Figure 3-1).
   2. A pH level below 7.35 indicates acidosis.
   3. A pH level above 7.45 indicates alkalosis.
   4. Measurement is made by examining ABGs (Table 3-8).

Chemical Buffer System

A. Chemical buffers act quickly to prevent major changes in body fluid pH by removing or releasing hydrogen ions.
B. The main chemical buffer is the bicarbonate-carbonic acid (HCO_3-H_2CO_3) system.
   1. Normally there are 20 parts of bicarbonate to 1 part carbonic acid. If the 20:1 ratio is altered, the pH is changed (ratio is important, not absolute values).
   2. Carbonic acid (H_2CO_3) is formed when carbon dioxide (CO_2) combines with water (H_2O).

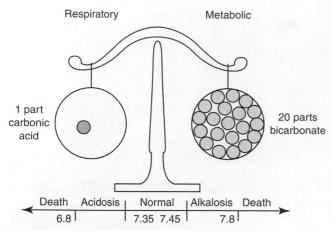

FIGURE 3-1   **Relationship of sodium bicarbonate to carbonic acid.** (From Potter PA, Perry AG: *Fundamentals of nursing,* ed 7. St. Louis, Mosby, 2009.)

TABLE 3-8   Arterial Blood Gas Comparisons

Acid-Base Conditions	pH	Pco$_2$ (mm Hg)	HCO$_3$ (mEq/L)
Normal	7.35 to 7.45	35 to 45	22 to 26
Respiratory acidosis	↓	↑	Normal
Respiratory alkalosis	↑	↓	Normal
Metabolic acidosis	↓	Normal	↓
Metabolic alkalosis	↑	Normal	↑

3. Excess CO_2 in the body alters the ratio and creates an imbalance. Other buffer systems involve:
   a. Phosphate
   b. Protein
   c. Hemoglobin

Lungs

A. Control CO_2 content through respirations (carbonic acid content).
B. Control, to a small extent, water balance (CO_2 + H_2O = H_2CO_3).
C. Release excess CO_2 by increasing respiratory rate.
D. Retain CO_2 by decreasing respiratory rate.

Kidneys

A. Regulate bicarbonate levels by retaining and reabsorbing bicarbonate as needed.

B. Provide a very slow compensatory mechanism (can require hours or days).
C. Cannot help with compensation when metabolic acidosis is created by renal failure.

Determining Acid-Base Disorders

A. In uncompensated acid-base disturbances, it is easy to determine when a disorder exists. Arrows are used to indicate whether the pH, P_{CO_2}, or HCO_3 is high (↑), low (↓), or within normal limits (WNL) (←——→).
B. When pH is high (↑), alkalosis is present.
C. In respiratory disorders, the HCO_3 is normal, and the arrows for pH and P_{CO_2} point in opposite directions.
D. In metabolic disorders, the P_{CO_2} is normal, and the arrows for pH and HCO_3 point in the same direction or are equal (Table 3-9).

TABLE 3-9   Analysis of Arterial Blood Gases

Component	Description	Values
pH	• Measures hydrogen ion (H$^+$) concentration • ↑ in ions (acidosis) reflects in pH • ↓ in ions (alkalosis) reflects in pH	• 7.35 to 7.45 • <7.35 • >7.45
Pco$_2$	• Partial pressure of CO_2 in arteries • Respiratory component of acid-base regulation • Hypercapnia (respiratory acidosis) • Hyperventilation (respiratory alkalosis)	• 35 to 45 mm Hg • >45 mm Hg • <35 mm Hg
HCO$_3$	• Measures serum bicarbonate • May reflect primary metabolic disorder or compensatory mechanism to respiratory acidosis • Metabolic acidosis • Metabolic alkalosis	• Normal 22 to 26 mEq/L • <22 mEq/L • >26 mEq/L

TABLE 3-10 Potential Causes of Acid-Base Conditions

Condition	Primary Cause	Contributing Causes
Respiratory acidosis	• Hypoventilation	• COPD (primary cause) • Pulmonary disease • Drugs • Obesity • Mechanical asphyxia • Sleep apnea
Metabolic acidosis	• Addition of large amounts of fixed acids to body fluids	• Lactic acidosis (circulatory failure) • Ketoacidosis (diabetes, starvation) • Phosphates and sulfates (renal disease) • Acid ingestion (salicylates) • Secondary to respiratory alkalosis • Adrenal insufficiency
Respiratory alkalosis	• Hyperventilation	• Overventilation on a ventilator • Response to acidosis • Bacteremia • Thyrotoxicosis • Fever • Hepatic failure • Response to hypoxia • Hysteria
Metabolic alkalosis	• Retention of base or removal of acid from body fluids	• Excessive gastric drainage • Vomiting • Potassium depletion (diuretic therapy) • Burns • Excessive $NaHCO_3$ administration

E. The body will begin to compensate in acid-base disorders to bring the pH back within the normal range of 7.35 to 7.45.

F. Example: For a client with a pH of 7.29 (↓), a P_{CO_2} of 50 (↑), and an HCO_3 of 26 (←———→):
1. Determine the pH: acidosis.
2. Determine the P_{CO_2}: respiratory.
3. Determine HCO_3: not metabolic.
4. Respiratory acidosis is the disorder (Table 3-10).

HESI Hint • The acronym ROME can help you remember: **r**espiratory, **o**pposite, **m**etabolic, **e**qual.

Review of Fluid and Electrolyte Balance

1. List four common causes of fluid volume deficit.
2. List four common causes of fluid volume overload.
3. Identify two examples of isotonic IV fluids.
4. List three systems that maintain acid-base balance.
5. Cite the normal ABGs for the following:
   A. pH
   B. P_{CO_2}
   C. HCO_3
6. Determine the following acid-base disorders:
   A. pH 7.50, P_{CO_2} 30, HCO_3 26
   B. pH 7.30, P_{CO_2} 42, HCO_3 20
   C. pH 7.48, P_{CO_2} 42, HCO_3 32
   D. pH 7.29, P_{CO_2} 55, HCO_3 26

Answers to Review

1. Gastrointestinal causes: vomiting, diarrhea, GI suctioning; decrease in fluid intake; increase in fluid output such as sweating; massive edema, ascites
2. Heart failure, renal failure; cirrhosis; excess ingestion of table salt or overhydration with sodium-containing fluids
3. Ringer's lactate; normal saline
4. Lungs; kidneys; chemical buffers
5. Normal values

A. 7.35 to 7.45 pH
B. 35 to 45 mm Hg Pco_2
C. 22 to 26 mEq/L HCO_3
6. Disorders
A. Respiratory alkalosis
B. Metabolic acidosis
C. Metabolic alkalosis
D. Respiratory acidosis

Electrocardiogram (ECG or EKG)

Description: Visual representation of the electrical activity of the heart reflected by changes in the electrical potential at the skin surface

---

HESI Hint • Review the order of blood flow through the heart:

Unoxygenated blood flows from the superior and inferior vena cava into the right atrium, then to the right ventricle. It flows out of the heart through the pulmonary artery, to the lungs for oxygenation. The pulmonary vein delivers oxygenated blood back to the left atrium, then to the left ventricle (largest, strongest chamber), and out the aorta.

Review the three structures that control the one-way flow of blood through the heart:
Valves
  Atrioventricular valves
    Tricuspid (right side)
    Mitral (left side)
  Semilunar valves
    Pulmonic (in pulmonary artery)
    Aortic (in aorta)
  Chordae tendinae
  Papillary muscles

A. The visual representation of an ECG can be recorded as a tracing on a strip of graph paper or seen on an oscilloscope.
B. The following conditions can interfere with normal heart functioning:
  1. Disturbances of rate or rhythm
  2. Disorders of conductivity
  3. Enlarged heart chambers
  4. Presence of myocardial infarction
  5. Fluid and electrolyte imbalances
C. Each ECG should include identifying information:
  1. Client's name and identification number
  2. Location, time, and date of recording
  3. Client's age, sex, and cardiac and noncardiac medications currently being taken
  4. Height, weight, and BP
  5. Clinical diagnosis and current clinical status
  6. Any unusual position of the client during the recording
  7. If present, thoracic deformities, respiratory distress, and muscle tremor
D. The standard ECG is the 12-lead ECG.
E. Bedside monitoring through telemetry is more commonly seen in the clinical setting.
  1. Telemetry uses three or five leads transmitted to an oscilloscope.
  2. Graphic information is printed either on request or at any time the set parameters are transcended.
F. A portable continuous monitor (Holter monitor) can be placed on the client to provide a magnetic tape recording. While wearing a Holter monitor, the client is instructed to keep a diary concerning:
  1. Activity
  2. Medications
  3. Chest pains
G. The ECG graph paper consists of small and large squares (Figure 3-2).
  1. The small squares represent 0.04 second each; five of these small squares combine to form one large square.
  2. Each large square represents 0.20 second (0.04 second × 5). Five large squares represent 1 second. Calculation of heart rate uses the 6-second rule (Box 3-1):
    a. It is the easiest means of calculating the heart rate.
    b. It cannot be used when the heart rate is irregular.
    c. Thirty large squares equal one 6-second time interval.
    d. Count the number of RR intervals in the 30 large squares and multiply by 10 to determine the heart rate for 1 minute (the R is the high peak on the strip; Figure 3-3).

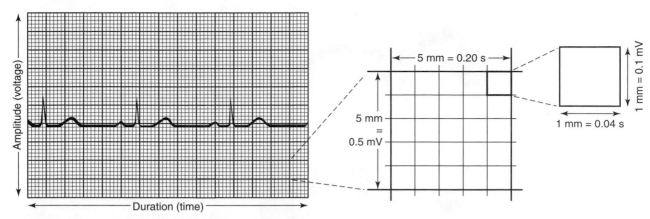

FIGURE 3-2   Composition of ECG paper. Electrocardiograph's waveforms are measured in amplitude (voltage) and duration (time).
(From Ignatavicius DD, Workman ML: *Medical-surgical nursing: Patient-centered collaborative care*, ed 6. St. Louis, Saunders, 2010.)

H. Composition of the ECG:
  1. P wave: atrial systole
     a. Represents depolarization of the atrial muscle
     b. Should be rounded and without peaking or notching

  2. QRS complex: ventricular systole
     a. Represents depolarization of the ventricular muscle
     b. Normally follows the P wave
     c. Is measured from the beginning of the

BOX 3-1   *Methods of Estimating Heart Rate Using an Electrocardiogram Tracing*

1. Measure the interval between consecutive QRS complexes, determine the number of small squares, and divide 1500 by that number. This method is used only when the heart rhythm is regular.

2. Measure the interval between consecutive QRS complexes, determine the number of large squares, and divide 300 by that number. This method is used only when the heart rhythm is regular.

3. Determine the number of RR intervals within 6 seconds and multiply by 10. The ECG paper is conveniently marked at the top with slashes that represent 3-second intervals. This method can be used when the rhythm is irregular. If the rhythm is extremely irregular, an interval of 30 to 60 seconds should be used.

4. Count the number of big blocks between the same point in any two successive QRS complexes (usually R wave to R wave) and divide into 300 because there are 300 big blocks in 1 minute. It is easiest to use a QRS that falls on a dark line. If little blocks are left over when counting big blocks, count each little block as 0.2, add this to the number of big blocks, and then divide by 300.

5. The memory method relies on memorization of the following sequence: 300, 150, 100, 75, 60, 50, 43, 37, 33, 30. Find a QRS complex that falls on the dark line representing 0.2 second or a big block, and count backward to the next QRS complex. Each dark line is a memorized number. This is the method most widely used in hospitals for calculating heart rates for regular rhythms.

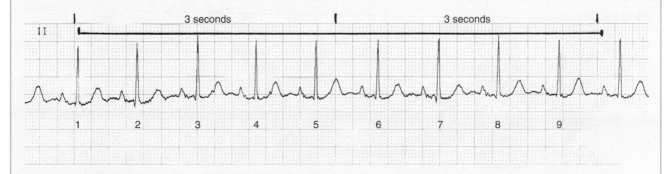

Calculation of heart rate. In this example, the heart rate using the big block method is 300÷4 big blocks (between QRS complexes), or 75 beats/min. The memory method is also demonstrated with a heart rate of 75 beats/min. (From Ignatavicius DD, Workman ML: *Medical-surgical nursing: patient-centered collaborative care*, ed 6. St. Louis, Saunders, 2010.)
Adapted from Monahan F, Sands J, Neighbors M, Marek J, Green C: *Phipps' medical-surgical nursing: Health and illness perspectives*, ed 8. St. Louis, Mosby, 2007; and Ignatavicius DD, Workman ML: *Medical-surgical nursing: Patient-centered collaborative care*, ed 6. St. Louis, Saunders, 2010.

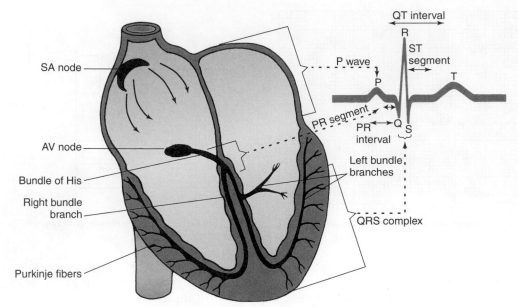

FIGURE 3-3   The cardiac conduction system. (From Ignatavicius DD, Workman ML: *Medical-surgical nursing: Patient-centered collaborative care,* ed 6. St. Louis, Saunders, 2010.)

QRS to the end of the QRS (normal <0.11 second)
d. T wave: ventricular diastole
  (1) Represents repolarization of the ventricular muscle
  (2) Follows the QRS complex
  (3) Usually is slightly rounded, without peaking or notching

> **HESI Hint** • The T wave represents repolarization of the ventricle, so this is a critical time in the heartbeat. This action represents a resting and regrouping stage so that the next heartbeat can occur. If defibrillation occurs during this phase, the heart can be thrust into a life-threatening dysrhythmia.

3. ST segment
  a. Represents early ventricular repolarization
  b. Is measured from the end of the S wave to the beginning of the T wave
4. PR interval
  a. Represents the time required for the impulse to travel from the atria (sinoatrial [SA] node), through the atrioventricular (AV) node, to the Purkinje fibers in the ventricles
  b. Is measured from the beginning of the P wave to the beginning of the QRS complex
  c. Represents AV nodal function (normal 0.12 to 0.20 second)

5. U wave
  a. Is not always present
  b. Is most prominent in the presence of hypokalemia
6. QT interval
  a. Represents the time required to completely depolarize and repolarize the ventricles
  b. Is measured from the beginning of the QRS complex to the end of the T wave
7. RR interval
  a. Reflects the regularity of the heart rhythm
  b. Is measured from one QRS to the next QRS

> **HESI Hint** • Observe the client for tolerance of the current rhythm. This information is the most important data the nurse can collect on a client with an arrhythmia.

> **HESI Hint** • NCLEX-RN questions are likely to relate to early recognition of abnormalities and associated nursing actions. Remember to monitor the client as well as the machine! If the ECG monitor shows a severe dysrhythmia but the client is sitting up quietly watching television without any sign of distress, assess to determine if the leads are attached properly.

Review of Electrocardiogram (ECG or EKG)

1. Identify the waveforms found in a normal ECG.
2. In an ECG reading, which wave represents depolarization of the atrium?
3. In an ECG reading, what complex represents depolarization of the ventricle?
4. What does the PR interval represent?
5. If the U wave is most prominent, what condition might the nurse suspect?

6. Describe the calculation of the heart rate using an ECG rhythm strip.
7. What is the most important assessment data for the nurse to obtain in a client with an arrhythmia?
8. Calculate the rate of this rhythm strip.

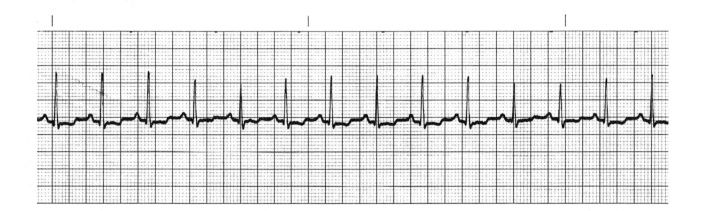

Answers to Review

1. P wave, QRS complex, T wave, ST segment, PR interval
2. Represented by the P wave
3. QRS complex
4. The time required for the impulse to travel from the atria through the AV node

5. Hypokalemia
6. Count the number of RR intervals in the 30 large squares and multiply by 10 to determine the heart rate for 1 minute.
7. Ability of the client to tolerate the arrhythmia
8. 120 beats per minute (bpm)

Perioperative Care

Description: The perioperative period includes client care before surgery (preoperative), during surgery (intraoperative), and after surgery (postoperative).

A. The nurse's role is to
1. Demystify the experience
2. Reduce anxiety
3. Promote an uncomplicated perioperative period for the client and family

B. Surgery is performed under aseptic conditions, in a hospital or an alternative hospital setting (ambulatory surgical center or health care provider's office).

C. Many changes in perioperative care have occurred since 1983 as a result of Medicare mandates for outpatient care. These mandates tend to result in changes to all health care insurance coverage.

SURGICAL RISK FACTORS

A. Age: the very young and very old are greater surgical risks than children and adults.

B. Nutrition: obesity and malnutrition increase surgical risk.

C. Fluid and electrolyte status: dehydration and hypovolemia increase surgical risk because of imbalances in calcium, magnesium, potassium, and phosphorus.

D. General health: any infection or pathology increases surgical risk.
1. Cardiac conditions: angina, MIs, hypertension, heart failure; well-controlled cardiac problems pose little risk.
2. Blood coagulation disorders can lead to severe bleeding, hemorrhage, and shock.
3. Upper respiratory tract infections (surgery is usually delayed when the client has an upper

respiratory infection) and chronic obstructive pulmonary disease are exacerbated by general anesthesia and adversely affect pulmonary function.
4. Renal disease, such as a renal insufficiency, impairs fluid and electrolyte regulation.
5. Diabetes mellitus predisposes clients to wound infection and delayed healing.
6. Liver disease impairs the liver's ability to detoxify medications used during surgery to produce prothrombin or to metabolize nutrients for wound healing.
7. Obesity exacerbates risk.
E. Current medications: prescription and over-the-counter drugs; medications that increase surgical risk include:
1. Anticoagulants (increase blood coagulation time)
2. Tranquilizers (may cause hypotension)
3. Heroin (decreases CNS response)
4. Antibiotics (may be incompatible with anesthetics)
5. Diuretics (may precipitate electrolyte imbalance)
6. Steroids
7. Over-the-counter herbal preparations
8. Vitamin E

PREOPERATIVE CARE

Description: Care provided from the time the client and family make the decision to have surgery until the client is taken to the operative suite

Data to Obtain When Taking a Preoperative Nursing History

A. Age
B. Allergies to medications, foods, and topical antiseptics (especially iodine)
C. Current medications; prescriptions, over-the-counter, and herbal preparations
D. History of medical and surgical problems
E. Previous surgical experiences
F. Previous experience with anesthesia
G. Tobacco, alcohol, and drug abuse
H. Understanding of surgical procedure
I. Coping resources
J. Cultural and ethnic factors that may affect surgery

Key Components of Preoperative Teaching Plans

A. Regulations concerning valuables, jewelry, dentures
B. Food and fluid restrictions such as NPO after midnight
C. Invasive procedures such as urinary catheters, IVs, nasogastric (NG) tubes, enemas, douches
D. Preoperative medications
E. Operating room, transportation, skin preparation, postanesthesia
F. Postoperative procedures:
1. Respiratory care, such as ventilator, incentive spirometer, deep breather, splinting
2. Activity, such as range of motion (ROM), leg exercises, early ambulation, turning
3. Pain control, such as IM medications, patient-controlled analgesia (PCA)
4. Dietary restrictions
5. Intensive care unit or postanesthesia care unit (PACU) orientation (recovery room)

Preoperative Checklist Information

A. Informed consent, surgical consent, signed and witnessed consent to treatment within 24 hours; signature must be obtained prior to administration of any narcotics or other medications affecting client cognition.
B. Accurate height and weight have been charted.
C. History and physical examination (by health care provider) are noted in chart.
D. Chest radiograph, ECG, and urinalysis have been performed, when prescribed.
E. Hemoglobin, hematocrit, electrolytes, glucose, and type/crossmatch for blood have been determined, if prescribed.
F. Old chart is on hand.
G. Identification band is on client and includes allergies.
H. Client identification information is clear (hard copy charting may use an addressograph card).
I. Contact lenses, glasses, dentures, partial plates, wigs, jewelry, artificial eyes, prostheses, makeup, and nail polish have been removed per institutional policy or as prescribed by health care provider.
J. Client has voided or been catheterized.
K. Client is in hospital gown.
L. Vital signs: BP, temperature, pulse, and respirations have been taken.
M. Premedication has been given; type and time have been noted.
N. Skin preparation has been performed (if prescribed by health care provider or physician):
1. Wash skin with soap and water.
2. Shave skin using a razor that is new and sharp because skin must not be broken.

3. Follow shave with scrub or shower with povidone-iodine or another antibacterial solution.

O. Signature of nurse certifies completion.

> **HESI Hint** • Marking the operative site is required for procedures involving right/left distinctions, multiple structures (fingers, toes), and levels (spinal procedures). Site marking should be done with the involvement of the client.

INTRAOPERATIVE CARE

Description: From the time the client is received in the operative suite until admission to the PACU, an operating room nurse is in charge of care.

A. Maintain quiet during induction.

B. Maintain safety:
1. Conduct client identification: right client, right procedure, right anatomic site.
2. Ensure that sponge, needle, and instrument counts are accurate.
3. Position client during procedure to prevent injury.
4. Apply grounding device to client if electrocautery is to be used.
5. Strictly adhere to asepsis during all intraoperative procedures.
6. Ensure adequate functioning suction setups are in place.
7. Take responsibility for correct labeling, handling, and deposition of any and all specimens.

C. Monitor physical status:
1. If excessive blood loss occurs, calculate effect on client.
2. Report changes in pulse, temperature, respirations, and blood pressure to surgeon, in conjunction with anesthesiologist/CRNA.

D. Provide psychological support:
1. Provide emotional support to client and family immediately prior to, during, and after surgery.
2. Arrange with physician to provide information to the family if surgery is prolonged or complications or unexpected findings occur.
3. Communicate emotional state of client to other health care team members.

POSTOPERATIVE CARE

Description: From admission to PACU, until client has recovered

A. Initially, the client goes to the PACU.

B. On arrival, the client is assessed for vital signs (BP, pulse, respirations, temperature), level of consciousness, skin color and condition, dressing location and condition, intravenous fluids, drainage tubes, position, and oxygen saturation levels.

C. When client has been stabilized, and it has been prescribed by the health care provider, the client is then transferred to the general nursing unit or the intensive care unit.

D. Immediate postoperative nursing care should include:
1. Monitoring for signs of shock and hemorrhage: hypotension, narrow pulse pressure, rapid weak pulse, cold moist skin, increased capillary filling time (Table 3-11)
2. Positioning client on side (if not contraindicated) to prevent aspiration and to allow client to cough out airway; side rails should be up at all times
3. Providing warmth with heated blanket
4. Managing nausea and vomiting with antiemetic drugs and NG suctioning
5. Managing pain with intravenous analgesics
6. Checking with anesthesiologist about intraoperative medications before administering pain medications
7. Determining intraoperative irrigations and instillations with drains to help evaluate amount of drainage on dressing and in drainage collection devices

> **HESI Hint** • NCLEX-RN items focus on the nurse's role in terms of the entire perioperative process.
> • Example: A 43-year-old mother of two teenage daughters enters the hospital to have her gallbladder removed in a same-day surgery using an endoscope instead of an incision. What nursing needs will dominate each phase of her short hospital stay?
> • Preparation phase: education about postoperative care, including NPO, assistance with meeting family needs
> • Operative phase: assessment, management of the operative suite
> • Postanesthesia phase: pain management, postanesthesia precautions
> • Postoperative phase: prevention of complications, assessment for pain management, and teaching about dietary restrictions and activity levels

TABLE 3-11 Common Postoperative Complications

Postoperative Complication	Occurrence	Interventions for Prevention
Urinary retention	8 to 12 hr postoperatively	• Monitor hydration status and encourage oral intake if allowed. • Offer bedpan or assist to commode.
Pulmonary problems • Atelectasis • Pneumonia • Embolus	1 to 2 days postoperatively	• Assist client to turn, cough, deep breathe every 2 hr. • Keep client hydrated. • Enable early ambulation. • Provide early incentive spirometer.
Wound-healing problems	5 to 6 days postoperatively	• Teach splinting of incision when client coughs. • Monitor for signs of infection, malnutrition, dehydration. • Provide high-protein diet.

HESI Hint • Wound dehiscence is separation of the wound edges; it is more likely to occur with vertical incisions. It usually occurs after the early postoperative period, when the client's own granulation tissue is "taking over" the wound, after absorption of the sutures has begun. Evisceration of the wound is protrusion of intestinal contents (in an abdominal wound) and is more likely in clients who are older, diabetic, obese, or malnourished and have prolonged paralytic ileus.

Urinary tract infections	5 to 8 days postoperatively	• Oral fluid intake • Emptying of bladder every 4 to 6 hr • Monitor intake and output. • Avoid catheterization if possible.
Thrombophlebitis	6 to 14 days postoperatively	• Leg exercises every 8 hr while in bed • Early ambulation • Apply antiembolus (TED) stockings or sequential compression devices as prescribed; remove TEDs every 8 hr and reapply. • Avoid pressure that may obstruct venous flow; do not raise knee gatch on bed; do not place pillows beneath knees; client should avoid crossing legs at knees. • Low-dose heparin may be used prophylactically.
Decreased gastrointestinal peristalsis • Constipation • Paralytic ileus	2 to 4 days postoperatively	• NG tubing to decompress GI tract • Client to limit use of narcotic analgesics, which decrease peristalsis • Encourage early ambulation.

Review of Perioperative Care

1. List five variables that increase surgical risk.
2. Why is a client with liver disease at increased risk for operative complications?
3. Preoperative teaching should include demonstration and explanation of expected postoperative client activities. What activities should be included?
4. What items should the nurse assist the client in removing before surgery?
5. How is the client positioned in the immediate postoperative period, and why?
6. List three nursing actions that prevent postoperative wound dehiscence and evisceration.
7. Identify three nursing interventions that prevent postoperative urinary tract infections.
8. Identify nursing/medical interventions that prevent postoperative paralytic ileus.
9. List four nursing interventions that prevent postoperative thrombophlebitis.
10. During the intraoperative period, what activities should the operating room nurse perform to ensure safety during surgery?

Answers to Review

1. Age: very young and very old, obesity and malnutrition, preoperative dehydration/hypovolemia, preoperative infection, use of anticoagulants (aspirin) preoperatively
2. Impairs ability to detoxify medications used during surgery; impairs ability to produce prothrombin to reduce hemorrhage
3. Respiratory activities: coughing, breathing, use of spirometer; exercises: range-of-motion, leg exercises, turning; pain management: medications, splinting; dietary restrictions: NPO evolving to progressive diet; dressings and drains; orientation to recovery room environment
4. Contact lenses, glasses, dentures, partial plates, wigs, jewelry, prostheses, makeup, and nail polish
5. Usually on the side or with head to side to prevent aspiration of any emesis
6. Teaching client to splint incision when coughing; encouraging coughing and deep breathing in early postoperative period when sutures are strong; monitoring for signs of infection, malnutrition, and dehydration; encouraging high-protein diet
7. Avoiding postoperative catheterization; increasing oral fluid intake; emptying bladder every 4 to 6 hr; early ambulation
8. Early ambulation; limiting use of narcotic analgesics; NG tube decompression
9. Teaching performance of in-bed leg exercises; encouraging early ambulation; applying antiembolus stockings; teaching avoidance of positions and pressures that obstruct venous flow
10. Ascertain correct sponge, needle, and instrument count; position client to avoid injury; apply ground during electrocautery use; apply strict use of surgical asepsis

HIV Infection

Description: Infection with human immunodeficiency virus (HIV).

A. HIV was first documented in 1981. At that time, the constellation of symptoms was not known to be caused by a virus, and the disease was named in a manner that describes what is now known to be the end stage of a very long, chronic infection by a virus. The name given to symptoms was acquired immunodeficiency syndrome (AIDS).

B. It is now understood that the disease is caused by a retrovirus, which is attracted to CD4 T cells, lymphocytes, macrophages, and cells of the CNS.

C. The virus enters the cell and begins to replicate. An event, such as cofactors (herpes simplex and cytomegalovirus [CMV]), can stimulate this replication.

D. The destruction of the CD4 T cell causes depletion in the number of CD4 T cells and a loss of the body's ability to fight infection. Individuals with fewer than 200 CD4 T cells are at risk for opportunistic infections. (Normal CD4 T-cell count is 600 to 1200.)

E. Initially, an individual commonly suffers an acute infection that is quite similar to mononucleosis (Table 3-12).

F. Initial symptoms usually occur within 3 weeks of first exposure to HIV, after which the person becomes asymptomatic. Persons infected with HIV can transmit the virus to others anytime after infection has occurred, whether they are symptomatic or asymptomatic.

G. Current Centers for Disease Control and Prevention (CDC) definition of AIDS (end-stage infection) includes persons with specific serious opportunistic infections such as *Pneumocystis jiroveci* pneumonia (PCP), disseminated CMV, or Kaposi sarcoma.

H. Risk groups include the following:
   1. Homosexual or bisexual males
   2. IV drug abusers and those who have had tattoos or acupuncture
   3. Heterosexual partners of a risk-group member
   4. Recipients of blood products prior to blood product screening (e.g., those with hemophilia who were diagnosed and treated prior to 1985)
   5. Those taking medications such as steroids or other agents that cause immunosuppression
   6. Infants born to infected mothers
   7. Breast-feeding infants of infected mothers

NURSING ASSESSMENT

A. Laboratory testing
   1. Positive ELISA (enzyme-linked immunosorbent assay); false-positive results can occur.
   2. Confirmation by the Western blot test, which uses electrophoresis and evaluates virus-specific bands
   3. Polymerase chain reaction (PCR) test may be used to differentiate between HIV infection in the neonate and antibodies the neonate receives from the mother.
   4. Seroconversion to positive on these tests occurs usually within 6 weeks to 3 months but may take as long as 12 months.
   5. Prior to seroconversion to antibody-positive status, a P24 antigen assay will be positive. (This test detects the core antigen of the virus.)

TABLE 3-12 Stages of HIV

Stage	Description and Symptoms
Primary infection (acute HIV infection or acute HIV syndrome) CD4 T-cell counts of at least 800 cells/mm^3	• Flu-like symptoms, fever, malaise • Mononucleosis-like illness, lymphadenopathy, fever, malaise, rash • Symptoms usually occur within 3 weeks of initial exposure to HIV, after which the person becomes asymptomatic
HIV asymptomatic (CDC Category A) CD4 T-cell counts more than 500 cells/mm^3	• No clinical problems • Characterized by continuous viral replication • Can last for many years (10 years or longer)
HIV symptomatic (CDC Category B) CD4 T-cell counts between 200 and 499 cells/mm^3	• Persistent generalized lymphadenopathy • Persistent fever • Weight loss, diarrhea • Peripheral neuropathy • Herpes zoster • Candidiasis • Cervical dysplasia • Hairy leukoplakia, oral
AIDS (CDC Category C) CD4 T-cell counts less than 200 cells/mm^3	• Occurs when a variety of bacteria, parasites, or viruses overwhelm the body's immune system • Once classified as category C, the patient remains classified as category C; this has implications for entitlements (e.g., health benefits, housing, food stamps).

B. Symptoms
   1. Extreme fatigue
   2. Loss of appetite and unexplained weight loss of more than 10 pounds in 2 months
   3. Swollen glands
   4. Leg weakness or pain
   5. Unexplained fever for more than 1 week
   6. Night sweats
   7. Unexplained diarrhea
   8. Dry cough; may represent PCP
   9. White spots in the mouth and throat; may represent candidiasis
   10. Painful blisters; may represent shingles
   11. Painless purple-blue lesions on the skin
   12. Confusion, disorientation
   13. In women, recurrent vaginal infections that are resistant to treatment
C. Opportunistic infections
   Refer to Table 3-13.

HESI Hint • HIV clients with tuberculosis require respiratory isolation. Tuberculosis is the only real risk to nonpregnant caregivers that is not related to a break in standard precautions (e.g., needle sticks).

ANALYSIS (NURSING DIAGNOSES)

A. *Risk for infection* related to…

B. *Imbalanced nutrition: less than body requirements* related to…

C. *Impaired urinary elimination* related to…

D. *Ineffective breathing pattern* related to…

E. *Ineffective sexuality patterns* related to…

F. *Fatigue* related to…

G. *Risks for complicated grieving* related to…

NURSING PLANS AND INTERVENTIONS

A. Assess respiratory functioning frequently.

B. Avoid known sources of infection.

C. Use strict asepsis for all invasive procedures.

D. Obtain vital signs frequently.

E. Plan activities to allow for rest periods.

F. Elevate head of bed.

G. Refer client to nutritionist.

H. Offer small, frequent feedings.

I. Weigh daily.

J. Encourage client to avoid fatty foods.

TABLE 3-13 Opportunistic Infections

Pneumocystis Carinii Pneumonia	Kaposi's Sarcoma	Cryptosporidiosis	Candidiasis of Oral Cavity and Esophagus
• Fever • Dry cough • Dyspnea at rest • Chills	• Purple-blue lesions on skin, often arms and legs • Invasion of gastrointestinal tract, lymphatic system, lungs, and brain	• Severe watery diarrhea (may be 30 to 40 stools per day) • Abdominal cramps • Nausea • Electrolyte imbalance • Malaise	• Thick white exudate in the mouth • Unusual taste to food • Retrosternal burning • Oral ulcers
Cryptococcal Meningitis	**Cytomegalovirus (CMV) Retinitis**	**CMV Colitis**	**Disseminated CMV**
• Headache • Changes in level of consciousness • Nausea, vomiting • Stiff neck • Blurred vision	• Most common CMV infection in persons with AIDS • Impaired vision in one or both eyes • Can lead to blindness	• Diarrhea • Malabsorption of nutrients • Weight loss	• Malaise • Fever • Pancytopenia • Weight loss • Positive cultures from blood, urine, or throat
Perirectal Mucocutaneous Herpes Simplex Virus	**Lymphomas of Central Nervous System (CNS)**	**Tuberculosis**	**HIV Encephalopathy**
• Severe pain • Bleeding, rectal discharge • Ulceration in the rectal area	• Change in mental status • Apathy • Psychomotor slowing • Seizures	• Pulmonary and extrapulmonary • Lymphatic and hematogenous TB are common • Negative skin testing does not rule out TB	• Memory loss and impaired concentration • Apathy • Depression • Psychomotor slowing (most prominent symptom) • Incontinence • CT scan findings: diffuse atrophy and ventricular enlargement

K. Monitor for skin breakdown, and offer good skin care.
L. Use safety precautions for clients with neurologic symptoms or loss of vision.
M. Orient client who is confused.
N. Provide emotional support for grieving client who is losing all relationships and skills.
O. Provide emotional support for significant others: family, family of choice, lovers, friends.
P. Administer IV fluids for hydration, as prescribed.
Q. Administer total parenteral nutrition (TPN), as prescribed.
R. Administer agents that treat specific opportunistic infections and medications for HIV (Table 3-14).
S. Assist with pain management; administer prescribed narcotics or analgesics.

HESI Hint • Standard Precautions
• Wash hands, even if gloves have been worn to give care.
• Wear exam gloves for touching blood or body fluids or any nonintact body surface.
• Wear gowns during any procedure that might generate splashes (e.g., changing clients with diarrhea).
• Use masks and eye protection during activity that might disperse droplets (e.g., suctioning).
• Do not recap needles; dispose of in puncture-resistant containers.
• Use mouthpiece for resuscitation efforts.
• *Refrain from giving care* if you have open skin lesions.

TABLE 3-14 HIV Drugs

Drugs	Indications	Adverse Reactions	Nursing Implications
NRT inhibitors • Didanosine (Videx) • Lamivudine (Epivir) • Abacavir (Ziagen) • Zalcitabine (Hivid) • Zidovudine (Retrovir)	HIV infection Classifications used in various combinations to reduce viral load and slow development of resistance	• Peripheral neuropathies • Pancreatitis • ↑Triglycerides • Fever, rash, N/V, abdominal cramps	• Monitor for neuropathies. • Monitor amylase, lipase, triglycerides. • Give on empty stomach.
Protease inhibitors • Indinavir (Crixivan) • Amprenavir (Agenerase) • Saquinavir (Invirase) • Ritonavir (Norvir, Kaletra) • Nelfinavir (Viracept)		• Depression • Ketoacidosis • Seizures • Angioedema • Stevens-Johnson syndrome	• Many drug-drug interactions • High-fat, high-protein foods reduce absorption. • Give most of these *with* food. • Reduces contraceptive effects • Do not confuse ritonavir (Norvir) with trade name zidovudine (Retrovir).
Non-NRT inhibitors • Efavirenz (Sustiva) • Delavirdine (Rescriptor) • Nevirapine (Viramune) • Amprenavir (Agenerse)		• CNS changes • Nausea • Rash • ↑ Triglycerides • Hepatotoxicity	• Many drug-drug interactions • Monitor liver function tests. • Reduces contraceptive effects • Do not confuse Viramune with Viracept.
Combination products • Lamivudine + zidovudine (Combivir) • Zidovudine + lamivudine + abacavir (Trizivir)		• Monitor for side effects associated with the individual drugs	• Note implications of the individual drugs in the combination product.
Antiinfectives • Atovaquone (Mepron) • Trimethoprim/ sulfamethoxazole (Bactrim)	Mepron used for PCP in those unable to tolerate trimethoprim/ sulfamethoxazole prophylaxis	• CNS disturbances • Agranulocytosis • Phlebitis if IV • Renal calculi with Bactrim	• Enhances effects of oral hypoglycemics • Increases thrombocytopenia risk if given with thiazide diuretics • Check for allergy to sulfonamide.
• Enfuvirtide (Fuzeon)		• Infection risk and lipodystrophy if injection site is not rotated	• Monitor skin reactions at injection site.
Antivirals • Acyclovir sodium (Zovirax) • Ganciclovir (Cytovene)	Herpes simplex CMV retinitis	• Granulocytopenia • Thrombocytopenia	• Give with or without food. • Many incompatibilities IV PO, IV, topical • Monitor liver function tests.
Antifungals • Ampherotericin B (Fungizone)	IV: Cryptococcal meningitis PO: Oral candidiasis	• Nephrotoxicity • Hypotension • Hypokalemia • Febrile reaction • Muscle cramps • Circulatory problems	• Many drug-drug interactions • Vesicant: monitor IV site closely; premedicate with antipyretic; give slowly. • Swish as long as possible before swallowing PO form.
Antiprotozoals • Pentamidine isethionate (Pentam 300)	Prophylaxis for PCP Treatment of PCP	• Leukopenia • ECG abnormalities	• IV or aerosol; not oral • Use careful precautions against potential spread of TB.

Note: Client should have regular blood counts to track CD4 levels and viral load.

> **HESI Hint** • Caregivers who are pregnant may choose not to care for a client with cytomegalovirus (CMV).

> **HESI Hint** • Pediatric HIV is often evidenced by lymphoid interstitial pneumonitis, pulmonary lymphoid hyperplasia, and opportunistic infections.

Pediatric HIV Infection

Description: Infection with HIV in infants and children

A. Sources of infection in pediatric clients
  1. Perinatal transmission. Between 30% and 50% of children born to HIV-positive mothers will be infected unless the mother is treated with zidovudine during pregnancy and the neonate is treated after birth; then rate decreases to 4% to 8%.
  2. HIV-infected blood products
  3. Breast milk
  4. Sexual abuse
B. Although maternal antibodies may be present at birth in some children, the antibody tests will convert to negative before 18 months of age.

NURSING ASSESSMENT

A. Risk groups
  1. Infants born to mothers who are HIV positive
  2. Hemophiliacs
  3. Infants and children who have received blood transfusions
B. Symptoms
  1. Failure to thrive
  2. Lymphadenopathy
  3. Organomegaly
  4. Neuropathy
  5. Cardiomyopathy
  6. Chronic recurrent infections such as thrush
  7. Unexplained fevers

> **HESI Hint** • The focus of NCLEX-RN questions is likely to be assessment of early signs of the disease and management of complications associated with HIV.

ANALYSIS (NURSING DIAGNOSES)

A. All diagnoses for adults may be experienced by children, depending on the age of the child.
B. *Interrupted family processes* related to…
C. *Delayed growth and development* related to…

NURSING PLANS AND INTERVENTIONS

A. Avoid exposure to persons with infections, especially chickenpox.
B. Administer *no* live virus vaccines.
C. Teach the family to:
  1. Use gloves when diapering the child.
  2. Clean any soiled surfaces (wearing gloves) with a 10% bleach solution.
  3. Identify signs of opportunistic infections.
D. Monitor growth parameters.
E. Administer gamma globulin as prescribed, usually each month.
F. Support use of social services.
G. Support child's attending school as much as child is able.
H. See care plan for adult HIV client (p. 54).
I. Assist in community and school education programs.

Review of HIV Infection

1. Identify the ways HIV is transmitted.
2. Vertical transmission (from mother to fetus) occurs how often if the mother is not treated during pregnancy?
3. Describe universal precautions.
4. What are the side effects of amphotericin B?
5. What does the CD4 T-cell count describe?
6. Why does the CD4 T-cell count drop in HIV infections?
7. Describe the ways a pediatric client might acquire HIV infection.

Answers to Review

1. HIV is transmitted through blood and body fluids—e.g., unprotected sexual contact with an infected person, sharing needles with drug-abusing persons, infected blood products (rare), breast milk (mother-to-fetus transmission), and breaks in universal precautions (needle sticks or similar occurrences).
2. Vertical transmission occurs 30% to 50% of the time.
3. Protection from blood and body fluids is the goal of standard precautions. Standard precautions initiate barrier protection between caregiver and client through hand washing; using gloves; using gowns and masks; using eye protection as indicated, depending on activity of care and the likelihood of exposure; preventing needle sticks by not recapping needles.
4. Side effects of amphotericin B can be quite severe; they include anorexia, chills, cramping, muscle and joint pain, and circulatory problems.
5. CD4 T-cell count describes the number of infection-fighting lymphocytes the person has.
6. CD4 T-cell count drops because the virus destroys CD4 T cells as it invades them and replicates.
7. Pediatric acquisition may occur through infected blood products, through sexual abuse, and through breast milk.

Pain

Description: An individual's subjective experience

A. Clients' pain often goes unrecognized and untreated.
   1. Health care professionals are poorly educated about identifying, assessing, and managing pain.
   2. Health care professionals often cling to outdated beliefs and biases, including fear of addiction.
B. An individual's response to pain is influenced by several factors:
   1. Anxiety: reduction of anxiety can help to control pain.
   2. Past experience with pain: the more pain experienced in childhood, the greater the perception of pain in adulthood.
   3. Culture and religion: cultural and religious practices learned from one's family play an important role in determining how a person experiences and expresses pain.
   4. Gender affects the expression of pain.
C. Pain is classified as either acute or chronic.
   1. Acute pain
      a. Is temporary
      b. Occurs after an injury to the body
      c. Includes postoperative pain, labor pain, renal calculus pain
   2. Chronic pain may be
      a. Nonmalignant (e.g., low back pain, rheumatoid arthritis)
      b. Intermittent (e.g., migraine headaches)
      c. Malignant, associated with neoplastic diseases

THEORY OF PAIN

A. Gate control theory: pain impulses travel from the periphery to the gray matter in the dorsal horn of the spinal cord along small nerve fibers.
   1. A "gating" mechanism, called the substantia gelatinosa, either opens to or closes off the transmission of pain impulses to the brain.
   2. It is thought that the stimulation of large, fast-conducting sensory fibers opposes the input from small pain fibers, thus blocking pain transmission.
   3. Modalities used: stimulation of large fibers by massage, heat, cold, acupuncture, transcutaneous electrical nerve stimulation (TENS)
B. Endorphin/enkephalin theory:
   1. Endorphins: naturally occurring compounds that have morphine-like qualities; they modulate pain by preventing the conduction of pain impulses in the CNS.
   2. Enkephalins: specific neurotransmitters that bind with opiate receptors in the dorsal horn of the spinal cord; they modulate pain by closing the gate and stopping the pain impulse.
   3. Modalities used: stimulation of endogenous opiate release through acupuncture, placebos, TENS

NURSING ASSESSMENT

A. Location: pain may be localized, radiating, or referred.
B. Intensity: ask client to rate pain before and after an intervention such as medication (use scale such as 0 to 10, with 0 being no pain).
C. Comfort: often clients can describe what relieves pain better than they can describe the pain itself.
D. Quality: pain may be sharp, dull, aching, sore, etc.
E. Chronology: ask client when pain started, what time of day it occurs, how often it appears, how long it lasts, whether it is constant or intermittent, whether the intensity changes.
F. Subjective experience: determine what decreases or aggravates pain, what other symptoms are associated with pain, what interventions provide relief, what limitations the pain inflicts.

ANALYSIS (NURSING DIAGNOSES)

A. *Acute or chronic pain* related to…

B. *Ineffective coping* related to…

C. *Disturbed sleep pattern* related to…

D. *Activity intolerance* related to…

E. *Self-care deficit (specify)* related to…

NURSING PLANS AND INTERVENTIONS FOR PAIN MANAGEMENT

A. Pharmacologic interventions (Table 3-15)
1. Nonnarcotics, nonsteroidal antiinflammatory drugs (NSAIDs; see Table 4-28)
   a. Act by means of a peripheral mechanism at level of damaged tissue by inhibiting prostaglandin and other chemical mediator syntheses involved in pain
   b. Show antipyretic activity through action on the hypothalamic heat-regulating center to reduce fever
   c. Examples: salicylate-aspirin (Bayer), nonsalicylates, acetaminophen (Tylenol), ibuprofen (Motrin)
2. Narcotic agonists and antagonists
   a. Act as narcotics (agonists) that antagonize the "pure" agonists (counteract the narcotic effects)
   b. May cause withdrawal symptoms if administered after client has been receiving narcotics
   c. Produce side effects, including drowsiness, occasionally, nausea, and psychomimetic effects, such as hallucinations and euphoria
   d. Examples: butorphanol (Stadol), nalbuphine (Nubain)
3. Narcotics
   a. Act as opioids, binding with specific opiate receptors throughout the CNS to reduce pain perception
   b. Cause such side effects as nausea and vomiting, constipation, respiratory depression, and CNS depression
   c. Examples: dilaudid, morphine sulfate (Table 3-16)

TABLE 3-15   Routes of Administration for Analgesics

Route	Administration
Oral	• Preferred method of administration • Drug level peak: 1 to 2 hr
Intramuscular	• Acceptable method of managing acute short-term pain • Onset 30 min; peak effect 1 to 3 hr; duration of action: 4 hr
Rectal	• Useful for clients with nausea and inability to take analgesics by mouth • Useful for home care and for elderly clients as an alternative to PO and IV administration • Reduced effectiveness with constipation
IV bolus (IV push)	• Provides the most rapid onset (5 min) but has the shortest duration (1 hr) • Useful for acute pain, such as a client in labor
Patient-controlled analgesia (PCA)	• Ideal method of pain control; client is able to prevent pain by administering to self smaller doses of the narcotic (usually morphine) as soon as the first sign of discomfort arises • Usually administered IV • A predetermined dose and a set lockout interval (5 to 20 min) are prescribed by physician; pump is calibrated to deliver the specified dose whenever client hits the button. • Lock-out mechanism prevents overdose. • Pump can record number of times the client uses the pump and the cumulative dose delivered
Continuous subcutaneous narcotic infusion (CSI)	• Useful for clients who are NPO but require prolonged administration of parenteral narcotics • Provides a constant level of analgesia by continuous infusion of a narcotic • Site should be inspected every 8 hr and changed at least every 7 days.
Continuous epidural analgesia	• Catheter threaded into epidural space with continuous infusion of fentanyl citrate, morphine, or other narcotic analgesics • Risk for respiratory depression
Transdermal patches	• Applied to skin (self-adhesive or with overlay to secure patch) • Also used to deliver hormonal therapy, nitroglycerin, and nicotine • Sites for application and frequency of application are specific to each medication • Document removal of old patch, site and application date and time of new patch

TABLE 3-16 Onset of Commonly Administered Narcotics

Medication	Mode	Onset	Comments
Codeine	PO IM or SC	30 to 45 min 10 to 30 min	• Do *not* administer discolored injection solutions. • May also be prescribed as an antitussive or antidiarrheal
Hydromorphone (Dilaudid)	PO IM IV	30 min 15 min 10 to 15 min	• Fast-acting, potent narcotic • More likely to cause appetite loss than other narcotics
Morphine sulfate	PO IM IV	60 to 90 min 10 to 30 min 10 min	• Drug of choice in relieving pain associated with myocardial infarction • May cause transient decrease in blood pressure • Drug of choice for use with chronic cancer pain
Propoxyphene HCl (Darvon, Eration)	PO	15 to 60 min	• May cause false decreases in urinary steroid secretion tests
Fentanyl citrate (Duragesic)	IM IV Intradermal Intrabuccal Intrathecal	7 to 15 min Within 5 min Within 12 hr 5 to 15 min Immediate	• Synthetic narcotic, MSO_4-like • Acts quicker; less duration

HESI Hint • For narcotic-induced respiratory depression, naloxone (Narcan) may be adminstered as prescribed by the health care provider.

B. Adjuvants to analgesics
1. Are given in combination with an analgesic to potentiate or enhance the analgesic's effectiveness
2. Are helpful in controlling discomforts associated with pain, such as nausea, anxiety, and depression (e.g., promethazine [Phenergan])

HESI Hint • Use noninvasive methods for pain management when possible:
- Relaxation exercises
- Distraction
- Imagery
- Biofeedback
- Interpersonal skills
- Physical care: altering positions, touch, hot and cold applications

Nursing Assessment of Pain Relief Techniques

A. Pain (Table 3-17)
B. Response to pharmacologic intervention: tolerance to pharmacologic interventions may occur—i.e., the client physiologically requires increasingly larger doses to provide the same effect.
1. The first sign of tolerance is a decreased duration of drug effectiveness.
2. The need for increased doses can be the result of increased pain rather than tolerance (e.g., clients with advanced cancer).

HESI Hint • Narcotic analgesics are preferred for pain relief because they bind to the various opiate receptor sites in the CNS. Morphine is often the preferred narcotic (*remember*, it causes respiratory depression).

Other agonists are meperidine and methadone. Narcotic antagonists block the attachment of narcotics such as naloxone (Narcan) to the receptors. Once Narcan has been given, additional narcotics cannot be given until the Narcan effects have passed.

TABLE 3-17   Pain Relief Techniques

NONINVASIVE
Cutaneous stimulation that is useful alone or in combination with other pain management techniques • Heat and cold applications decrease pain and muscle spasm. • Transcutaneous electrical nerve stimulation (TENS) provides continuous mild electrical current to the skin via electrodes. • Massage provides a simple, inexpensive, and effective method of pain relief. • Distraction diverts client's attention from the pain, useful during short periods of pain or during painful procedures such as IV venipunctures. • Relaxation can be used as a distraction and to facilitate sedation or sleep; it rarely decreases pain sensation. • Biofeedback techniques enable control of autonomic responses (tachycardia, muscle tension) to pain through electrical feedback.

INVASIVE
Any procedure that invades the body and is used to relieve pain • Nerve blocks involve injection of anesthetic into or near a nerve to decrease pain pathways (e.g., deadening area for dental work, regional anesthesia used in obstetrics). • Neurosurgical procedures include surgical or chemical (alcohol) interruption of nerve pathways; it is commonly used in clients with cancer who have severe pain. • Acupuncture is the insertion of needles at various points in the body to relieve pain.

Review of Pain

1. What modalities are associated with the gate control pain theory?
2. How does past experience with pain influence current pain experience?
3. What modalities are thought to increase the production of endogenous opiates?
4. What six factors should the nurse include when assessing the pain experience?
5. What mechanism is involved in the reduction of pain through the administration of nonsteroidal antiinflammatory medications?
6. If narcotic agonist/antagonist drugs are administered to a client already taking narcotic drugs, what may be the result?
7. List four side effects of narcotic medications.
8. What is the antidote for narcotic-induced respiratory depression?
9. What is the first sign of tolerance to pain analgesics?
10. Which route of administration for pain medications has the quickest onset and the shortest duration?
11. List the six modalities that are considered noninvasive, nonpharmacologic pain relief measures.

Answers to Review

1. Massage, heat and cold, acupuncture, TENS
2. The more pain experienced in childhood, the greater is the perception of pain in adulthood or with current pain experience.
3. Acupuncture, administration of placebos, TENS
4. Location, intensity, comfort measures, quality, chronology, and subjective view of pain
5. NSAIDs act via a peripheral mechanism at the level of damaged tissue by inhibiting prostaglandin synthesis and other chemical mediators involved in pain transmission.
6. Initiation of withdrawal symptoms
7. Nausea/vomiting; constipation; CNS depression; respiratory depression
8. Narcan (naloxone)
9. Decreased duration of drug effectiveness
10. Intravenous push, or bolus
11. Heat and cold applications; TENS; massage; distraction; relaxation techniques; biofeedback techniques

Death and Grief

Description: Death is the last developmental task for an individual. It completes the life cycle. Grief is the process an individual goes through to deal with loss.

NURSING ASSESSMENT

A. Types of death
   1. Natural/expected
   2. Sudden/unexpected
   3. Suicide
B. Stages of preparing for an expected death
   1. Denial
      a. Coping style used to protect self/ego
      b. Noncompliance, refusal to seek treatment, ignoring of symptoms
      c. Changing the subject when speaking about illness
      d. Stating, "Not me, it must be a mistake."
   2. Anger
      a. Often directing it at family or health care team members
      b. Stating, "Why me? It's not fair."
   3. Bargaining
      a. Making a deal with God to prolong life
      b. Usually not sharing this with anyone, keeping it a very private experience
   4. Depression
      a. Results from the losses experienced because of health status and hospitalization
      b. Anticipating the loss of life
   5. Acceptance
      a. Accepting of the inevitable
      b. Beginning to separate emotionally
C. Stages of dealing with loss (grief)
   1. Shock, disbelief, rejection, or denial
      a. Anger and crying
      b. Conflicting emotions
      c. Anger toward the deceased
      d. Guilt
      e. Preoccupation with loss
   2. Resolution
      a. Process taking up to 1 year or more
      b. Renewed interest in activities
D. Complicated grief
   1. Unresolved grief
      a. Determine level of dysfunction
   2. Physical symptoms similar to those of the deceased
   3. Clinical depression
   4. Social isolation
   5. Failure to acknowledge loss

ANALYSIS (NURSING DIAGNOSES)

A. *Complicated grief* related to…
B. *Powerlessness* related to…

NURSING PLANS AND INTERVENTIONS

A. Encourage client to express anger in a supportive, nonthreatening environment.
B. Discourage rumination.
C. Assist client in giving up idealized perception of deceased; point out misrepresentations.
D. Encourage interaction with others.
E. Assist client with identification of support systems.
F. Consult spiritual leader as indicated by client need and preference.
G. Assist client toward a comfortable, peaceful death.

> **HESI Hint** • Do not take away the coping style used in a crisis state.
>   Denial is a very useful and needed tool for some at the initial stage. Support, do not challenge, unless it hinders or blocks treatment, endangering the patient.

Review of Death and Grief

1. Identify the five stages of death and dying.
2. A client has been told of a positive breast biopsy report. She asks no questions and leaves the health care provider's office. She is overheard telling her husband, "The doctor didn't find a thing." What coping style is operating at this stage of grief?
3. Your client, an incest survivor, is speaking of her deceased father, the perpetrator. "He was a wonderful man, so good and kind. Everyone thought so." What would be the most useful intervention at this time?
4. Your client feels responsible for his sister's death because he took her to the hospital where she died. "If I hadn't taken her there, they couldn't have killed her." It has been 1 month since her death. Is this response indicative of a normal or a complicated grief reaction?
5. Mrs. Green lost her husband 3 years ago. She has not disturbed any of his belongings and continues to set a place at the table for him nightly. Is this response indicative of a normal or a complicated grief reaction?

Answers to Review

1. Denial, anger, bargaining, depression, acceptance
2. Denial
3. Gently point out both the positive and negative aspects of her relationship with her father. Try to minimize the idealization of the deceased.
4. This is a normal expression of the anger and guilt that occur. Try to minimize rumination on these thoughts.
5. This is a dysfunctional grief reaction. Mrs. Green has never moved out of the denial stage of her grief work.

For more review, go to **http://evolve.elsevier.com/HESI/RN** for HESI's online study exams.

MEDICAL-SURGICAL NURSING

Respiratory System

PNEUMONIA

Description: Inflammation of the lower respiratory tract

A. Pneumonia can be caused by infectious agents.

B. Organisms that cause pneumonia reach the lungs by three methods.
1. Aspiration
2. Inhalation
3. Hematogenous spread

C. Pneumonia is generally classified according to causative agent.
1. Bacterial (gram-positive and gram-negative)
2. Viral
3. Fungal (rare)
4. Chemical

D. Pneumonia may be community-acquired or nosocomial (hospital/agency-acquired).

E. High-risk groups include individuals who are:
1. Debilitated by accumulated lung secretions
2. Cigarette smokers
3. Immobile
4. Immunosuppressed
5. Experiencing a depressed gag reflex
6. Sedated
7. Experiencing neuromuscular disorders

Nursing Assessment

A. Tachypnea: shallow respirations, often with use of accessory muscles

B. Abrupt onset of fever with shaking and chills (not reliable in older adults)

C. Productive cough with pleuritic pain

D. Rapid, bounding pulse

E. In older adults, symptoms include:
1. Confusion
2. Lethargy
3. Anorexia
4. Rapid respiratory rate

F. Pain and dullness to percussion over the affected lung area

G. Bronchial breath sounds, crackles

H. Chest radiograph indication of infiltrates with consolidation or pleural effusion

I. Elevated white blood cell (WBC) count

J. Arterial blood gas (ABG) indication of hypoxemia

K. On pulse oximetry, a drop in O_2 saturation (should be >90%, ideally >95%)

> **HESI Hint** • Fever can cause dehydration because of excessive fluid loss due to diaphoresis. Increased temperature also increases metabolism and the demand for O_2.

> **HESI Hint** • **HIGH RISK FOR PNEUMONIA**
> • Any person who has an altered level of consciousness, has depressed or absent gag and cough reflexes, or is susceptible to aspirating oropharyngeal secretions, including alcoholics, anesthetized individuals, those with brain injury, those in a state of drug overdose, and stroke victims, is at high risk.
> • When feeding, raise the head of the bed and position the client on his or her side, not on the back.

Analysis (Nursing Diagnoses)

A. *Impaired gas exchange* related to…

B. *Ineffective airway clearance* related to…

C. *Activity intolerance* related to…

D. *Risk for deficient fluid volume* related to…

E. *Ineffective breathing pattern* related to….

Nursing Plans and Interventions

A. Assess sputum for volume, color, consistency, and clarity.

B. Assist client to cough productively by:
   1. Deep breathing every 2 hours (may use incentive spirometer)
   2. Using humidity to loosen secretions (may be oxygenated)
   3. Suctioning the airway, if necessary

C. Provide fluids up to 3 L/day unless contraindicated (helps liquefy lung secretions).

D. Assess lung sounds before and after coughing.

E. Assess rate, depth, and pattern of respirations regularly (normal adult rate is 16 to 20 breaths/min).

F. Monitor ABGs (Po_2 >80 mm Hg; Pco_2 <45 mm Hg).

G. Monitor O_2 saturation with pulse oximetry (ideally >95%).

H. Assess skin color.

I. Assess mental status, restlessness, and irritability.

J. Administer O_2 as prescribed.

K. Monitor temperature regularly.

L. Provide adequate rest periods, including uninterrupted sleep.

M. Administer antibiotics as prescribed (Table 4-1).

N. Teach high-risk clients and their families about risk factors and include preventive measures.

O. Encourage at-risk groups to get annual pneumonia and influenza ("flu") immunizations.

HESI Hint • Bronchial breath sounds are heard over areas of density or consolidation. Sound waves are easily transmitted over consolidated tissue.

HESI Hint • **HYDRATION**
- Enables liquefaction of mucus trapped in the bronchioles and alveoli, facilitating expectoration
- Is essential for client experiencing fever
- Is important because 300 to 400 ml of fluid is lost daily by the lungs through evaporation

---

HESI Hint • Irritability and restlessness are early signs of cerebral hypoxia; the client's brain is not receiving enough O_2.

HESI Hint • **PNEUMONIA PREVENTIVES**
- Older adults: flu shots; pneumonia immunizations; avoiding sources of infection and indoor pollutants (dust, smoke, and aerosols); no smoking
- Immunosuppressed and debilitated persons: infection avoidance, sensible nutrition, adequate intake, balance of rest and activity
- Comatose and immobile persons: elevation of head of bed to feed and for 2 hours after feeding; frequently turning

---

CHRONIC AIRFLOW LIMITATION (CAL)

Description: Chronic lung disease includes chronic bronchitis, pulmonary emphysema, and asthma (Table 4-2).

A. Emphysema and chronic bronchitis termed as chronic obstructive pulmonary disease (COPD) are characterized by bronchospasm and dyspnea. The damage to the lung is not reversible and increases in severity.

HESI Hint • Exposure to tobacco smoke is the primary cause of COPD in the United States.

B. Asthma, unlike COPD, is an intermittent disease with reversible airflow obstruction and wheezing.

HESI Hint •
- Compensation occurs over time in clients with chronic lung disease, and ABGs are altered.
- As COPD worsens, the amount of O_2 in the blood decreases (hypoxemia) and the amount of carbon dioxide (CO_2) in the blood increases (hypercarbia), causing chronic respiratory acidosis (increased arterial carbon dioxide [$Paco_2$]), which results in metabolic alkalosis (increased arterial bicarbonate) as compensation.
- Not all clients with COPD are CO_2 retainers, even when hypoxemia is present, because CO_2 diffuses more easily across lung membranes than O_2.
- In advanced emphysema, due to the alveoli being affected, hypercarbia is a problem, rather than in bronchitis, where the airways are affected.
- It is imperative that baseline data be obtained for the client.

TABLE 4-1 Antiinfectives

Drugs	Indications	Adverse Reactions	Nursing Implications
Penicillins			
• Procaine penicillin G (Wycillin) • Benzathine penicillin (Bicillin L-A) • Penicillin V (Pen-Vee K)	• Antiinfectives • Used primarily for gram-positive infections	• Allergic reactions • Anaphylaxis • Phlebitis at IV site • Diarrhea • GI distress • Superinfection	• Use with caution in clients allergic to cephalosporins • Monitor for allergic reactions • Observe all clients for at least 30 minutes following parenteral administration • Oral penicillin G should be taken on an empty stomach • Probenecid decreases renal excretion, thereby resulting in an increased blood level of the drug • Alters contraceptive effectiveness
Semisynthetic			
• Oxacillin sodium • Nafcillin sodium • Cloxacillin sodium • Dicloxacillin sodium	• Antiinfectives • Used primarily for gram-positive infections	• Allergic reactions • Anaphylaxis • Superinfection • See *Penicillins*	• Cannot be used in clients allergic to penicillin • Caution in clients allergic to cephalosporins • Monitor for superinfection (sore mouth, vaginal discharge, diarrhea, cough) • See *Penicillins*
Antipseudomonal Penicillins and Combinations			
• Ampicillin • Ticarcillin + clavulanate (Timentin) • Piperacillin + tazobactam (Zosyn) • Ampicillin + sulbactam (Unasyn)	• Antiinfectives • Broad spectrums	• Similar to penicillin • Ampicillin rash	• Contraindicated in clients allergic to penicillin • See *Penicillins*
Tetracyclines			
• Tetracycline HCl • Doxycycline hyclate (Vibramycin)	• Antiinfectives	• Hypersensitivity reactions • Photosensitivity	• Decrease the effectiveness of oral contraceptives • Avoid concurrent use of antacids, milk products • Inspect IV site frequently • Monitor for superinfections • Avoid exposure to sunlight during use • Avoid use in pregnant clients and children under 8 years; can cause yellow-brown discoloration of teeth and growth retardation
Aminoglycocides			
• Gentamicin sulfate • Tobramycin sulfate (Nebcin) • Amikacin sulfate	• Antiinfectives • Used with gram-negative bacteria	• Neuromuscular blockade • Nephrotoxicity • Ototoxicity	• Monitor renal function, BUN, creatinine, and I&O • Monitor for ototoxicity: headache, dizziness, hearing loss, tinnitus • Monitor for superinfection

TABLE 4-1   Antiinfectives—cont'd

Drugs	Indications	Adverse Reactions	Nursing Implications
Miscellaneous Agents • Vancomycin hydrochloride • Metronidazole (Flagyl)			• Monitor for serum drug concentrations
Cephalosporins			
First Generation • Cefazolin (Kefzol) • Cephalexin (Keflex) **Second Generation** • Cefaclor (Ceclor) • Cefamandole (Mandol) • Cefuroxime (Ceftin, PO; Zinacef, IV) • Cefoxitin (Mefoxin) **Third Generation** • Cefotaxime (Claforan) • Ceftriaxone (Rocephin) • Ceftazidime (Fortaz) • Cefepime (Maxipime)	• Antiinfectives	• Allergic reactions • Thrombophlebitis • GI distress • Superinfection	• Use with caution in clients allergic to penicillin and cephalosporins • See *Penicillins*
Carbapenems			
• Imipenem (Primaxin) • Meropenem (Merrem) • Ertapenem (Invanz)			
Monobactam			
• Azactam	• *Pseudomonas aeruginosa* + many otherwise resistant organisms • Most effective against gram-negatives	• Phlebitis • Pseudo-membranous colitis • CNS changes • EEG changes • Headache, diplopia • Hypotension	• Monitor renal and hepatic function, especially in older adults • Carefully monitor for diarrhea • Assess motor sensory function and cardiac rhythm
Macrolides			
• Clarithromycin (Biaxin) • Azithromycin (Zithromax) • Erythromycin	• Biaxin (PO): URI, including streptococci; as adjunct treatment for *H. pylori* • Zithromax (IV): gram-negative and gram-positive organisms	• Pseudomembranous colitis • Phlebitis: a vesicant • Superinfections • Dizziness • Dyspnea	• Give Biaxin XL with food • Space MAO inhibitors 14 days before start and after end of Biaxin. • Report diarrhea, abdominal cramping (all macrolides) • Monitor liver, renal labs • PO Zithromax: give on empty stomach
Fluoroquinolones			
• Ciprofloxacin (Cipro) • Levofloxacin (Levaquin) • Gatifloxacin (Tequin)	• Used to treat respiratory infections, UTIs, skin, bone and joint infections	• Superinfections • CNS disturbances • Arroyos and cataracts possible with Cipro • Cipro: a vesicant	• Prompt onset • Crosses placenta and in breast milk • Can lower seizure threshold • Monitor liver, renal, and blood counts • Safety for children not known • Many drug-drug interactions

(Continued)

TABLE 4-1 **Antiinfectives—cont'd**

Drugs	Indications	Adverse Reactions	Nursing Implications
Fluoroquinolones			
	• Has been used as conjunctive treatment for TB and AIDS		
Lincosamides			
• Clindamycin (Cleocin)	• *Pneumocystis carinii* pneumonia (PCP) in AIDS • Severe infections resistant to penicillins and cephalosporins • Used in penicillin- and erythromycin-sensitive clients	• Agranulocytosis • Pseudomembranous colitis • Superinfections	• Highly toxic drug; use only when absolutely necessary • Periodic liver, renal, and blood count monitoring • Report diarrhea immediately
Streptogramin			
• Quinupristin/ dalfopristin (Synercid)	• Life-threatening vancomycin-resistant *Enterococcus* (VRE)	• Arthralgia, myalgia • Severe vesicant • Pseudomembranous colitis • Nausea/vomiting, diarrhea • Rash, pruritus	• Incompatible with any saline solutions or heparin • Functionally related to both macrolides and lincosamides • Monitor total bilirubin • Many drug-drug interactions
Oxazolidinone			
• Zyvox	• Life-threatening VRE and methicillin-resistant *Staphylococcus aureus* (MRSA)	• GI disturbances • Headache • Pancytopenia • Pseudomembranous colitis • Superinfections	• Monitor renal and liver labs and blood count. • May exacerbate hypertension, especially if ingests foods with tyramine • Report diarrhea immediately

MRSA, Methicillin-resistant staphylococcus aureus; N/V, Nausea and vomiting; PCP, Pneumocystic pneumonia; VRE, Vanconuycin-resistant enteracoccus.

Nursing Assessment

A. Changes in breathing pattern (e.g., an increase in rate with a decrease in depth)

B. Use of accessory breathing muscles (barrel chest)

C. Generalized cyanosis of lips, mucous membranes, face, nail beds ("blue bloater")

D. Cough (dry or productive)

E. Higher CO_2 than average

F. Low O_2, as determined by pulse oximetry

G. Decreased breath sounds

H. Coarse crackles in lung fields that tend to disappear after coughing, wheezing

I. Dyspnea, orthopnea

J. Poor nutrition

K. Activity intolerance

L. Anxiety concerning breathing; manifested by:
  1. Anger
  2. Fear of being alone
  3. Fear of not being able to catch breath

HESI Hint • Productive cough and comfort can be facilitated by semi-Fowler or high-Fowler position, which lessens pressure on the diaphragm by abdominal organs. Gastric distention becomes a priority in these clients because it elevates the diaphragm and inhibits full lung expansion.

TABLE 4-2 Chronic Airflow Limitation

Chronic Bronchitis	Emphysema	Asthma
Pathophysiology		
• Chronic sputum with cough production on a daily basis for a minimum of 3 months per year • Chronic hypoxemia, cor pulmonale • Increase in mucus, cilia production • Increase in bronchial wall thickness (obstructs air flow) • Reduced responsiveness of respiratory center to hypoxemic stimuli	• Reduced gas exchange surface area • Increased air trapping (increased AP diameter) • Decreased capillary network • Increased work, increased O_2 consumption	• Narrowing or closure of the airway due to a variety of stimulants
Precipitating Factors		
• Higher incidence in smokers	• Cigarette smoking • Environmental and/or occupational exposure • Genetic	• Mucosal edema • V/Q abnormalities • Increased work of breathing • Beta-blockers • Respiratory infection • Allergic reaction • Emotional stress • Exercise • Environmental or occupational exposure • Reflux esophagitis
Assessment		
• Generalized cyanosis • "Blue bloaters" • Right-sided heart failure • Distended neck veins • Crackles • Expiratory wheezes	• "Pink puffers" • Barrel chest • Pursed-lip breathers • Distant, quiet breath sounds • Wheezes • Pulmonary blebs on radiograph	• Dyspnea, wheezing, chest tightness • Assess precipitating factors. • Medication history
Nursing Plans and Interventions		
• Lowest FIO_2 possible to prevent CO_2 retention • Monitor for signs and symptoms of fluid overload • Maintain PaO_2 between 55 and 60. • Baseline ABGs • Teach pursed-lip breathing and diaphragmatic breathing • Teach tripod position	• Lowest FIO_2 possible to prevent CO_2 retention • Monitor for signs and symptoms of fluid overload • Maintain PaO_2 between 55 and 60 • Baseline ABGs • Teach pursed-lip breathing and diaphragmatic breathing • Teach tripod position	• Administer bronchodilators. • Administer fluids and humidification • Education (causes, medication regimen) • ABGs • Ventilatory patterns

HESI Hint • NORMAL ABG VALUES

Blood Gas	Adult	Child
pH	7.35 to 7.45	7.36 to 7.44
Pco_2	35 to 45 mm Hg	Same as adult
Po_2	80 to 100 mm Hg	Same as adult
HCO_3^-	21 to 28 mEq/L	Same as adult

HESI Hint • Pink puffer: Barrel chest is indicative of emphysema and is caused by use of accessory muscles to breathe. The person works harder to breathe, but the amount of O_2 taken in is adequate to oxygenate the tissues.

Blue bloater: Insufficient oxygenation occurs with chronic bronchitis and leads to generalized cyanosis and often right-sided heart failure (cor pulmonale).

Analysis (Nursing Diagnoses)

A. *Ineffective airway clearance* related to…

B. *Ineffective breathing pattern* related to…

C. *Impaired gas exchange* related to…

D. *Activity intolerance* related to…

HESI Hint • Cells of the body depend on O_2 to carry out their functions. Inadequate arterial oxygenation is manifested by cyanosis and slow capillary refill (<3 seconds). A chronic sign is clubbing of the fingernails, and a late sign is clubbing of the fingers.

Nursing Plans and Interventions

A. Teach client to sit upright and bend slightly forward to promote breathing.
   1. In bed: teach client to sit with arms resting on overbed table (tripod position).
   2. In chair: teach client to lean forward with elbows resting on knees (tripod position; Fig. 4-1).

B. Teach diaphragmatic and pursed-lip breathing. Teach prolonged expiratory phase to clear trapped air.

C. Administer O_2 at 1 to 2 L per nasal cannula (Table 4-3).

HESI Hint • Caution must be used in administering O_2 (not greater than 2 L of O_2) to a COPD client. The stimulus to breathe is hypoxia (hypoxic drive), not the usual hypercapnia, which is the stimulus to breathe for healthy persons. Therefore, if too much O_2 is given, the client may stop breathing!

D. Pace activities to conserve energy.

E. Maintain adequate dietary intake.
   1. Small, frequent meals
   2. Increase calories and protein
      a. Select foods that derive their calories from high fat rather than high carbohydrate levels because CO_2 that is a natural end product of carbohydrate metabolism and can elevate $Paco_2$ levels.

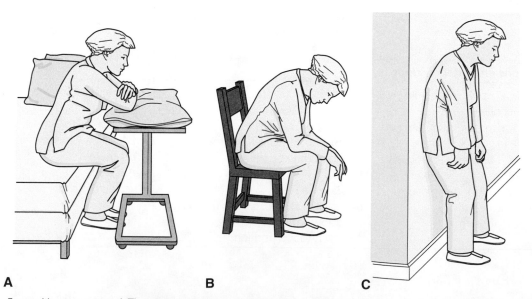

FIGURE 4-1 Forward-leaning position. *A,* The patient sits on the edge of the bed with arms folded on a pillow placed on the elevated bedside table. *B,* Patient in three-point position. The patient sits in a chair with the feet approximately 1 foot apart and leans forward with elbows on knees. *C,* The patient leans against a wall with feet spread apart, allowing shoulders to sag forward with arms relaxed. (From Monahan FD et al: *Phipps' medical-surgical nursing: Health and illness perspectives,* ed 8. St. Louis, 2007, Mosby.)

TABLE 4-3 Nursing Skills: Respiratory Client

SUCTIONING (TRACHEAL)

- Suction when adventitious breath sounds are heard, when secretions are present at endotracheal tube, and when gurgling sounds are noted.
- Use aseptic/sterile technique throughout procedure.
- Wear mask and goggles.
- Advance catheter until resistance is felt.
- Apply suction only when withdrawing catheter (gently rotate catheter when withdrawing).
- Never suction for more than 10 to 15 seconds, and pass the catheter only three or fewer times.
- Oxygenate with 100% O_2 for 1 to 2 minutes before and after suctioning to prevent hypoxia.

VENTILATOR SETTING MAINTENANCE

- Verify that alarms are on.
- Maintain settings and check often to ensure that they are specifically set as prescribed by health care provider.
- Verify functioning of ventilator at least every 4 hours.

OXYGEN ADMINISTRATION

- Nasal cannula: low O_2 flow for low O_2 concentrations (good for COPD)
- Simple face mask: low flow, but effectively delivers high O_2 concentrations; cannot deliver <40% O_2
- Nonrebreather mask: low flow, but delivers high O_2 concentrations (60% to 90%)
- Partial rebreather mask: low-flow O_2 reservoir bag attached; can deliver high O_2 concentrations
- Venturi mask: high-flow system; can deliver exact O_2 concentration

PULSE OXIMETRY

- Easy measurement of O_2 saturation
- Should be >90%, ideally above 95%
- Noninvasive, fastens to finger, toe, or earlobe
- No nail polish
- Must have good peripheral perfusion to be accurate

TRACHEOSTOMY CARE

- Aseptic technique (remove inner cannula only from stoma)
- Clean nondisposable inner cannula with H_2O_2; rinse with sterile saline
- 4 × 4 gauze dressing is butterfly-folded

RESPIRATORY ISOLATION TECHNIQUE

- Mask is required for anyone entering room.
- Private room is required with negative air pressure.
- Client must wear mask if leaving room.

PROPER USE OF AN INHALER

- Have client exhale completely.
- Grip mouthpiece (in mouth) only if client has a spacer; otherwise, keep the mouth open to bring in volume of air with misted medication. While inhaling slowly, push down firmly on the inhaler to release the medication.
- Use bronchodilator inhaler before steroid inhaler.
- Wait at least 1 minute minutes between puffs (inhaled doses).

3. Favorite foods
4. Dietary supplements
   a. For people continuing to smoke tobacco, additional vitamin C may be necessary.
   b. Magnesium and calcium, because of their role in muscle contraction and relaxation, may be important for people with COPD.

   c. Routine monitoring of magnesium and phosphorus levels is important because of their role related to bone mineral density (osteoporosis).
F. Provide an adequate fluid intake (minimum 3 L/day).
   a. Fluids should be taken between meals (rather than with them) to prevent excess stomach distention and to decrease pressure on the diaphragm.

TABLE 4-4 **Bronchodilators and Corticosteroids**

Drugs	Indications	Adverse Reactions	Nursing Implications
Adrenergics and Sympathomimetics			
• Epinephrine • Isoproterenol HCl (Isuprel) • Albuterol (Proventil) • Isoetharine (Bronuometer) • Terbutaline (Brethine) • Salmeterol (Serevent) • Metaproterenol (inhaled) (Alupent) • Levalbuterol (Xopenex)	• Bronchodilator	• Anxiety • Increased heart rate • Nausea, vomiting • Urinary retention	• Check heart rate • Monitor for urinary retention, especially in men over 40 • Instruct in proper use of inhaler • Use bronchodilator inhaler before steroid inhaler • May cause sleep disturbance
Methylxanthine			
• Aminophylline (IV) • Theophylline (PO)	• Bronchodilator	• GI distress • Sleeplessness • Cardiac dysrhythmias • Hyperactivity	• Administer oral forms with food • Avoid foods containing caffeine • Check heart rate. • Instruct in proper use of inhaler • Monitor therapeutic range of 10 to 20 mg/ml • Crosses placenta
Corticosteroids			
• Prednisone (PO) • Solu-Medrol (IV) • Beclomethasone dipropionate (inhaled) (Vanceril) • Budesonide (inhaled) (Pulmicort) • Fluticasone (inhaled) (Flovent) • Triamcinolone (inhaled) (Azmacort) • Flunisolide (inhaled) (AeroBid)	• Antiinflammatory	• Cardiac dysrhythmias occur with long-term steroid use	• See Endocrine Disorders in Medical-Surgical Nursing • Instruct in proper use of inhaler
Anticholinergics			
• Ipratropium (Atrovent)	• Bronchodilator • Control of rhinorrhea	• Dry mouth • Blurred vision • Cough	• Do not exceed 12 doses in 24 hours
Combination Products			
• Fluticasone + salmeterol (Advair) • Ipratropium + albuterol (Combivent)	• See individual drugs	• See individual drugs	• See individual drugs

G. Instruct client in relaxation techniques (teach when not in distress).

H. Teach prevention of secondary infections.

I. Teach about medication regimen (Table 4-4).

J. Smoking cessation is imperative.

K. Encourage health-promoting activities.

HESI Hint • HEALTH PROMOTION
- Eating consumes energy needed for breathing. Offer mechanically soft diets, which do not require as much chewing and digestion. Assist with feeding if needed.
- Prevent secondary infections; avoid crowds, contact with persons who have infectious diseases, and respiratory irritants (tobacco smoke).
- Teach client to report any change in characteristics of sputum.
- Encourage client to hydrate well (3 L/day) and decrease caffeine due to diuretic effect.
- Obtain immunizations when needed (flu and pneumonia).

HESI Hint • When asked to prioritize nursing actions, use the ABC rule:
- Airway first
- Then breathing
- Then circulation

HESI Hint • Look and listen! If breath sounds are clear but the client is cyanotic and lethargic, adequate oxygenation is not occurring.

HESI Hint • The key to respiratory status is assessment of breath sounds as well as visualization of the client. Breath sounds are better described, not named; e.g., sounds should be described as crackles, wheezes, or high-pitched whistling sounds rather than rales, rhonchi, etc., which may not mean the same thing to each clinical professional.

HESI Hint • Watch for NCLEX-RN® questions that deal with O_2 delivery. In adults, O_2 must bubble through some type of water solution so it can be humidified if given at >4 L/min or delivered directly to the trachea. If given at 1 to 4 L/min or by mask or nasal prongs, the oropharynx and nasal pharynx provide adequate humidification.

CANCER OF THE LARYNX

Description: Neoplasm occurring in the larynx, most commonly squamous cell in origin

A. Prolonged use of alcohol and tobacco is directly related to development.

B. Other contributing factors include:
1. Vocal straining
2. Chronic laryngitis
3. Family predisposition
4. Industrial exposure to carcinogens
5. Nutritional deficiencies
C. Men are affected eight times more often than are women.
D. Diagnosis usually occurs between the ages of 55 and 70.
E. The earliest sign is hoarseness or a change in vocal quality.
F. Medical management includes radiation therapy, often with adjuvant chemotherapy or surgical removal of the larynx (laryngectomy).

Nursing Assessment

A. Magnetic resonance imaging (MRI)
B. Direct laryngoscopy
C. Assessing for hoarseness of longer than 2 weeks (early changes)
D. Assessing for color changes in mouth or tongue

HESI Hint • With cancer of the larynx, the tongue and mouth often appear white, gray, dark brown, or black and may appear patchy.

E. Assessing for dysphagia, dyspnea, cough, hemoptysis, weight loss, neck pain radiating to the ear, enlarged cervical nodes, and halitosis (later changes)
F. Radiographs of head, neck, and chest
G. Computed tomography (CT) scan of neck and biopsy

Analysis (Nursing Diagnoses)

Client undergoing a laryngectomy:
A. *Anxiety* related to…
B. *Ineffective airway clearance* related to…
C. *Impaired verbal communication* related to…
D. *Ineffective breathing pattern* related to…

Nursing Plans and Interventions

A. Provide preoperative teaching.
1. Allow client and family to observe and handle tracheostomy tubes and suctioning equipment.
2. Explain how and why suctioning will take place after surgery.

3. Plan for acceptable communication methods after surgery.
4. Consider literacy level.
5. Refer client to speech pathologist.
6. Discuss the planned rehabilitation program.

B. Provide postoperative care.
1. Simplify communications.
2. Use planned alternative communication methods.
3. Keep call bell/light within reach at all times.
4. Ask client yes/no questions whenever possible.

C. Promote respiratory functioning.
1. Assess respiratory rate and characteristics every 1 to 2 hours.
2. Keep bed in semi-Fowler position at all times.
3. Keep laryngeal airway humidified at all times.
4. Auscultate lung sounds every 2 to 4 hours.
5. Provide tracheostomy care every 2 to 4 hours and PRN.

> **HESI Hint** • Tracheostomy care involves cleaning the inner cannula, suctioning, and applying clean dressings.

6. Administer tube feedings as prescribed.
7. Encourage ambulation as early as possible.
8. Refer for speech rehabilitation with artificial larynx or to learn esophageal speech.

> **HESI Hint** • Air entering the lungs is humidified along the nasobronchial tree. This natural humidifying pathway is gone for the client who has had a laryngectomy. If the air is not humidified before entering the lungs, secretions tend to thicken and become crusty.

> **HESI Hint** • A laryngectomy tube has a larger lumen and is shorter than the tracheostomy tube. Observe the client for any signs of bleeding or occlusion, which are the greatest immediate postoperative risks (first 24 hours).

> **HESI Hint** • Fear of choking is very real for laryngectomy clients. They cannot cough as they could earlier because the glottis is gone. Teach the glottal stop technique to remove secretions (take a deep breath, momentarily occlude the tracheostomy tube, cough, and simultaneously remove the finger from the tube).

TUBERCULOSIS

Description: Communicable lung disease caused by an infection by *Mycobacterium tuberculosis* bacteria

A. Transmission is airborne.
B. After initial exposure, the bacteria encapsulate (they form a Ghon lesion).
C. Bacteria remain dormant until a later time, when clinical symptoms appear.

Nursing Assessment

A. It is often asymptomatic.
B. Symptoms include:
1. Fever with night sweats
2. Anorexia, weight loss
3. Malaise, fatigue
4. Cough, hemoptysis
5. Dyspnea, pleuritic chest pain with inspiration
6. Cavitation or calcification as evidenced on chest radiograph
7. Positive sputum culture

> **HESI Hint** • **TUBERCULOSIS (TB) SKIN TEST**
> A positive TB skin test is exhibited by an induration 10 mm or greater in diameter 48 hours after the skin test. Anyone who has received a bacillus Calmette-Guérin (BCG) vaccine will have a positive skin test and must be evaluated with a chest radiograph.

Analysis (Nursing Diagnoses)

A. *Knowledge deficiency* (specify) related to…
B. *Risk for infection* related to…
C. *Imbalanced nutrition: less than body requirements* related to…

Nursing Plans and Interventions

A. Provide client teaching.
1. Cough into tissues and dispose of immediately into special bags.
2. Take all prescribed medications daily for 9 to 12 months.
3. Wash hands using proper handwashing technique.
4. Report symptoms of deteriorating condition, especially hemorrhage.

B. Collect sputum cultures as needed; client may return to work after three negative cultures.
C. Place client in respiratory isolation while hospitalized.
D. Administer anti-TB medications as prescribed (Table 4-5).

TABLE 4-5 Drug Therapy for Tuberculosis (TB)

Drug	Mechanisms of Action	Side Effects	Comments
FIRST-LINE DRUGS			
• Isoniazid (INH)	• Interferes with DNA metabolism of tubercle bacillus	• Nausea, vomiting, abdominal pain • Rare: neurotoxicity, optic neuritis, and hepatoxicity	• Metabolism primarily by liver and excretion by kidneys; pyridoxine (vitamin B$_6$) administration during high-dose therapy as prophylactic measure; use as single prophylactic agent for active TB in individuals whose PPD converts to positive; ability to cross blood-brain barrier
• Rifampin (Rifadin)	• Has broad-spectrum effects, inhibits RNA polymerase of tubercle bacillus	• Hepatitis, febrile reaction, GI disturbance, peripheral neuropathy, hypersensitivity	• Used in conjunction with at least one other antitubercular agent; low incidence of side effects; suppression of effect of birth control pills; possible orange urine
• Ethambutol (Myambutol)	• Inhibits RNA synthesis and is bacteriostatic for the tubercle bacillus	• Skin rash, GI disturbance, malaise, peripheral neuritis, optic neuritis	• Side effects uncommon and reversible with discontinuation of drug; most common use as substitute drug when toxicity occurs with isoniazid or rifampin
• Streptomycin	• Inhibits protein synthesis and is bactericidal	• Ototoxicity (eighth cranial nerve), nephrotoxicity, hypersensitivity	• Cautious use in older adults, those with renal disease, and pregnant women; must be given parenterally
• Pyrazinamide	• Bactericidal effect (exact mechanism is unknown)	• Fever, skin rash, hyperuricemia, jaundice (rare)	• High rate of effectiveness when used with streptomycin or capreomycin
SECOND-LINE DRUGS			
• Ethionamide (Trecator, SC)	• Inhibits protein synthesis	• GI disturbance, hepatotoxicity, hypersensitivity	• Valuable for treatment of resistant organisms; contraindicated in pregnancy
• Capreomycin (Capastat)	• Inhibits protein synthesis and is bactericidal	• Ototoxicity, nephrotoxicity	• Cautious use in older adults
• Kanamycin (Kantrex) and amikacin	• Interferes with protein synthesis	• Ototoxicity, nephrotoxicity	• Use in selected cases for treatment of resistant strains
• Para-aminosalicylic acid (PAS)	• Interferes with metabolism of tubercle bacillus	• GI disturbance (common), hypersensitivity, hepatotoxicity	• Interferes with absorption of rifampin; used uncommonly

(Continued)

TABLE 4-5 **Drug Therapy for Tuberculosis (TB)—cont'd**

Drug	Mechanisms of Action	Side Effects	Comments
SECOND-LINE DRUGS			
• Cycloserine (Seromycin)	• Inhibits cell-wall synthesis	• Personality changes, psychosis, rash	• Contraindicated in individuals with histories of psychosis; used in treatment of resistant strains

HESI Hint • Teaching is very important with the client with TB. Drug therapy is usually long term (9 months or longer). It is essential that the client take the medications as prescribed for the entire time. Skipping doses or prematurely terminating the drug therapy can result in a public health hazard.

HESI Hint • **TEACHING POINTS**
Rifampin: Reduces effectiveness of oral contraceptives; client should use other birth control methods during treatment; gives body fluids orange tinge; stains soft contact lenses.
Isoniazid (INH): Increased Dilantin levels
Ethambutol: Vision check before starting therapy and monthly thereafter; may have to take for 1 to 2 years
Teach rationale for combination-drug therapy to increase compliance. Resistance develops more slowly if several anti-TB drugs given, instead of just one drug at a time.

Data from Lewis S, Heitkemper M, Dirksen S, O'Brien P & Bucher L. *Medical-surgical nursing: Assessment and management of clinical problems,* ed 7. St. Louis, 2007, Mosby.

E. Refer client and high-risk persons to local or state health department for testing and prophylactic treatment.

LUNG CANCER

Description: Neoplasm occurring in the lung

A. Lung cancer is the leading cause of cancer-related death in the United States.

B. Cigarette smoking is responsible for 80% to 90% of all lung cancers.

C. Exposure to occupational hazards such as asbestos and radioactive dust poses significant risk.

D. Lung cancer tends to appear years after exposure; it is most commonly seen in persons in the fifth or sixth decade of life.

E. Lung cancer has a poor prognosis; 5-year survival rate is approximately 14%.

Nursing Assessment

A. Dry, hacking cough early, with cough turning productive as disease progresses

B. Hoarseness

C. Dyspnea

D. Hemoptysis; rust-colored or purulent sputum

E. Pain in the chest area

F. Diminished breath sounds, occasional wheezing

G. Abnormal chest radiograph

H. Positive sputum for cytology and for plural fluid

Analysis (Nursing Diagnoses)

A. *Chronic pain* related to…

B. *Ineffective breathing pattern* related to…

C. *Impaired gas exchange* related to…

D. *Imbalanced nutrition: less than body requirements* related to…

E. *Anxiety* related to…

Nursing Plans and Interventions

A. Nursing interventions are similar to those implemented for the client with COPD.

B. Place client in semi-Fowler position.

C. Teach pursed-lip breathing to improve gas exchange.

D. Teach relaxation techniques; client often becomes anxious about breathing difficulty.

E. Administer O_2 as indicated by pulse oximetry or ABGs.

F. Take measures to allay anxiety.
1. Keep client and family informed of impending tests and procedures.
2. Give client as much control as possible over personal care.
3. Encourage client and family to verbalize concerns.

G. Decrease pain to manageable level by administering analgesics as needed (within safety range for respiratory difficulty).

H. Surgery
1. Thoracotomy for clients who have a resectable tumor. (Unfortunately, detection commonly occurs so late that the tumor is no longer localized and is not amenable to resection.)
2. Pneumonectomy (removal of entire lung)
   a. Position client on operative side or back.
   b. Chest tubes are not usually used.
3. Lobectomy and segmental resection
   a. Position client on back.
   b. Check to ensure tubing is not kinked or obstructed.
   c. Chest tubes are usually inserted (Fig. 4-2).

> **HESI Hint** • Some tumors are so large that they fill entire lobes of the lung. When removed, large spaces are left. Chest tubes are not usually used with these clients because it is helpful if the mediastinal cavity, where the lung used to be, fills up with fluid. This fluid helps to prevent the shift of the remaining chest organs to fill the empty space.

4. Chest tubes
   a. Keep all tubing coiled loosely below chest level, with connections tight and taped.
   b. Keep water seal and suction control chamber at the appropriate water levels.
   c. Monitor the fluid drainage, and mark the time of measurement and the fluid level.
   d. Observe for air bubbling in the water seal chamber and fluctuations (tidaling).
   e. Monitor the client's clinical status.
   f. Check the position of the chest drainage system.
   g. Encourage the client to breathe deeply periodically.
   h. Do not empty collection container.
   i. Do not strip or milk chest tubes.
   j. Chest tubes are not clamped routinely. If the drainage system breaks, place the distal end of the chest tubing connection in a sterile water container at a 2 cm level as an emergency water seal.
   k. Maintain dry occlusive dressing.

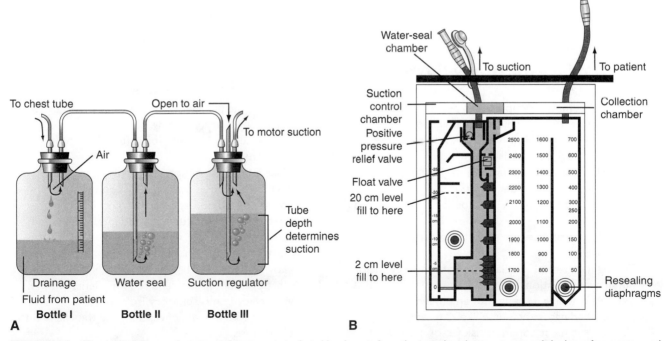

FIGURE 4-2 Chest tubes. Chest tubes are used to remove or drain blood or air from the intrapleural space, to expand the lung after surgery, and to restore subatmospheric pressure to the thoracic cavity. Many brands of commercial chest drainage systems are available; all are based upon the traditional three-bottle water-seal system. *A,* Three-bottle water-seal suction. Bottle I is the drainage bottle. A vertical piece of tape should be applied to the outer surface of the drainage bottle. The time and fluid level should be marked hourly on the tape. Bottle II is the water-seal bottle. Bottle III is the suction-control bottle. The length of tube below the water surface determines the amount of suction. *B,* Pleurevac disposable chest suction system **(displaying the wet suction control system).** (A, From Lewis SL, et al: *Medical-surgical nursing: Assessment and management of clinical problems,* ed 7, St Louis, 2007, Mosby. B, Courtesy of Deknatal, Inc., Fall River, MA.)

HESI Hint • CHEST TUBES
- If the chest tube becomes disconnected, do not clamp! Immediately place the end of the tube in a container of sterile saline or water until a new drainage system can be connected.
- If the chest tube is accidentally removed from the client, the nurse should apply pressure immediately with an occlusive dressing and notify the health care provider.

HESI Hint • NCLEX-RN CONTENT ON CHEST TUBES

Fluctuations (tidaling) in the fluid will occur if there is no external suction. These fluctuating movements are a good indicator that the system is intact; they should move upward with each inspiration and downward with each expiration. If fluctuations cease, check for kinked tubing, accumulation of fluid in the tubing, occlusions, or change in the client's position, because expanding lung tissue may be occluding the tube opening. Remember, when external suction is applied, the fluctuations cease. Most hospitals do not milk chest tubes as a means of clearing or preventing clots. It is too easy to remove chest tubes. Mediastinal tubes may involve orders to be stripped because of their location, compared to the larger thoracic cavity tubes.

I. Chemotherapy
1. Attend to immunosuppression factor. (See Oncology, p. 156.)
2. Administer antiemetics prior to administration of chemotherapy.
3. Take precautions in administrating antineoplastics. (See Oncology, p. 156.)

J. Radiation therapy
1. Provide skin care according to health care provider's request.
2. Instruct the client not to wash off the lines drawn by the radiologist.
3. Instruct client to wear soft cotton garments only.
4. Avoid use of powders and creams on radiation site unless specified by the radiologist.

HESI Hint • Various pathophysiologic conditions can be related to the nursing diagnosis *Ineffective breathing patterns*.
1. Inability of air sacs to fill and empty properly (emphysema, cystic fibrosis)
2. Obstruction of the air passages (carcinoma, asthma, chronic bronchitis)
3. Accumulation of fluid in the air sacs (pneumonia)
4. Respiratory muscle fatigue (COPD, pneumonia)

Review of Respiratory System

1. List four common symptoms of pneumonia the nurse might note on physical examination.
2. State four nursing interventions for assisting the client to cough productively.
3. What symptoms of pneumonia might the nurse expect to see in an older client?
4. What should the O_2 flow rate be for the client with COPD?
5. How does the nurse prevent hypoxia during suctioning?
6. During mechanical ventilation, what are three major nursing interventions?
7. When examining a client with emphysema, what physical findings is the nurse likely to see?
8. What is the most common risk factor associated with lung cancer?
9. Describe the preoperative nursing care for a client undergoing a laryngectomy.
10. List five nursing interventions after chest tube insertion.
11. What immediate action should the nurse take when a chest tube becomes disconnected from a bottle or suction apparatus? What should the nurse do if a chest tube is accidentally removed from the client?
12. What instructions should be given to a client following radiation therapy?
13. What precautions are required for clients with TB when placed on respiratory isolation?
14. List four components of teaching for the client with tuberculosis.

Answers to Review

1. Tachypnea, fever with chills, productive cough, bronchial breath sounds
2. Encourage deep breathing; increase fluid intake to 3 L/day; use humidity to loosen secretions; suction airway to stimulate coughing.
3. Confusion, lethargy, anorexia, rapid respiratory rate
4. Between 1 and 2 L per nasal cannula; too much O_2 may eliminate the COPD client's stimulus to breathe. A COPD client has a hypoxic drive to breathe.
5. Deliver 100% O_2 (hyperinflating) before and after each endotracheal suctioning.
6. Monitor client's respiratory status and secure connections; establish a communication mechanism with the client; keep airway clear by coughing and suctioning.
7. Barrel chest, dry or productive cough, decreased breath sounds, dyspnea, crackles in lung fields
8. Smoking
9. Involve family and client in manipulation of tracheostomy equipment before surgery; plan acceptable communication methods; refer to speech pathologist; discuss rehabilitation program.
10. Maintain a dry occlusive dressing on chest tube. Keep all tubing connections tight and taped. Monitor client's clinical status. Encourage the client to breathe deeply periodically. Monitor the fluid drainage, and mark the time of measurement and the fluid level.
11. Place the end of the tube in a sterile water container at a 2 cm level. Apply an occlusive dressing, and notify health care provider stat.
12. Do not wash off lines; wear soft cotton garments; avoid use of powders and creams on radiation site.
13. A mask for anyone entering room; private room; client must wear mask if leaving room.
14. Cough into tissues, and dispose of immediately in special bags. Long-term need for daily medication. Good handwashing technique. Report symptoms of deterioration, e.g., blood in secretions.

Renal System

ACUTE RENAL FAILURE (ARF)

Description: Abrupt deterioration of the renal system, a reversible syndrome

> **HESI Hint** • Normally, kidneys excrete approximately 1 ml of urine per kg of body weight per hour.
> For adults, total daily urine output ranges between 1500 and 2000 ml depending on the amount and type of fluid intake, amount of perspiration, environmental or ambient temperature, and the presence of vomiting or diarrhea.

A. ARF occurs when metabolites accumulate in the body and urinary output changes.
B. There are three major types of ARF (Table 4-6).
C. There are three phases of ARF.
   1. Oliguric phase
   2. Diuretic phase
   3. Recovery phase

Nursing Assessment

A. History of taking nephrotoxic drugs (salicylates, antibiotics, nonsteroidal antiinflammatory drugs [NSAIDs])
B. Alterations in urinary output
C. Edema, weight gain (ask if waistbands have suddenly become too tight)
D. Change in mental status

> **HESI Hint** • Electrolytes are profoundly affected by kidney problems (a favorite NCLEX-RN topic). There must be a balance between extracellular fluid and intracellular fluid to maintain homeostasis. A change in the number of ions or in the amount of fluid will cause a shift in one direction or the other. Sodium and chloride are the primary extracellular ions. Potassium and phosphate are the primary intracellular ions.

E. Diagnostic findings in the oliguric phase
   1. Increased blood urea nitrogen (BUN) and creatinine
   2. Increased potassium (hyperkalemia)
   3. Decreased sodium (hyponatremia)
   4. Decreased pH (acidosis)
   5. Fluid overload (hypervolemic)
   6. High urine specific gravity (>1.020 g/ml)
F. Diagnostic findings in the diuretic phase
   1. Decreased fluid volume (hypovolemia)
   2. Decreased potassium (hypokalemia)
   3. Further decrease in sodium (hyponatremia)
   4. Low urine specific gravity (<1.020 g/ml)
G. Diagnostic lab work returns to normal range in recovery phase.

TABLE 4-6 Acute Renal Failure

Types	Description	Causative Factors
• Prerenal	• Interference with renal perfusion	• Hemorrhage • Hypovolemia • Decreased cardiac output • Decreased renal perfusion
• Intrarenal	• Damage to renal parenchyma	• Prolonged prerenal state • Nephrotoxins • Intratubular obstruction • Infections (glomerulonephritis) • Renal injury • Vascular lesions • Acute pyelonephritis
• Postrenal	• Obstruction in the urinary tract anywhere from the tubules to the urethral meatus	• Calculi • Prostatic hypertrophy • Tumors

HESI Hint • In some cases, persons in ARF may not experience the oliguric phase but may progress directly to the diuretic phase, during which the urine output may be as much as 10 L per day.

Analysis (Nursing Diagnoses)

A. *Excess fluid volume* related to...

B. *Deficient fluid volume* related to...

C. *Anxiety* related to...

D. *Imbalanced nutrition: less than body requirements* related to...

Nursing Plans and Interventions

A. Monitor intake and output (I&O) accurately: give only enough fluids in oliguric phase to replace losses; usually 400 to 500 ml/24 hr.

B. Document and report any change in fluid volume status.

C. Monitor lab values of both serum and urine to assess electrolyte status, especially hyperkalemia indicated by serum potassium levels over 5 mEq/L and ECG changes.

D. Assess level of consciousness for subtle changes.

E. Weigh daily: in oliguric phase; client may gain up to 1 lb/day.

F. Prevent cross-infection.

G. Kayexalate may be prescribed if K+ is too high.

HESI Hint • Body weight is a good indicator of fluid retention and renal status. Obtain accurate weights of all clients with renal failure; obtain weight on the same scale at the same time every day.

HESI Hint • FLUID VOLUME ALTERATIONS

Excess fluid symptoms	Fluid-deficient symptoms
• Dyspnea	• Decreased urine output
• Tachycardia	• Reduction in body weight
• Jugular vein distention	• Decreased skin turgor
• Peripheral edema	• Dry mucous membranes
• Pulmonary edema	• Hypotension
• Weight gain	• Tachycardia
	• Weight loss

HESI Hint • Watch for signs of hyperkalemia: dizziness, weakness, cardiac irregularities, muscle cramps, diarrhea, and nausea.

HESI Hint • Potassium has a critical safe range (3.5 to 5.0 mEq/L) because it affects the heart, and any imbalance must be corrected by medications or dietary modification. Limit high-potassium foods (bananas, orange juice, cantaloupe, strawberries, avocados, spinach, fish) and salt substitutes, which are high in potassium.

HESI Hint • Clients with renal failure retain sodium. With water retention, the sodium becomes diluted and serum levels may appear near normal. With excessive water retention, the sodium levels appear decreased (dilution). Limit fluid and sodium intake in ARF clients.

H. Provide low-protein, moderate-fat, high-carbohydrate diet.

I. Monitor cardiac rate and rhythm (acute cardiac dysrhythmias are usually related to hyperkalemia).

J. Monitor drug levels and interactions.

> **HESI Hint** • During oliguric phase, minimize protein breakdown and prevent rise in BUN by limiting protein intake. When the BUN and creatinine return to normal, ARF is determined to be resolved.

CHRONIC RENAL FAILURE (CRF): END STAGE RENAL DISEASE (ESRD)

Description: Progressive, irreversible damage to the nephrons and glomeruli, resulting in uremia

A. Causes of chronic renal failure are multitudinous.

B. As renal function diminishes, dialysis becomes necessary.

C. Transplantation is an alternative to dialysis for some clients.

Nursing Assessment

A. History of high medication usage

B. Family history of renal disease

C. Increased blood pressure (BP) and/or chronic hypertension

D. Edema, pulmonary edema

E. Neurologic impairment (weakness, drowsiness)

F. Decreasing urinary function
  1. Hematuria
  2. Proteinuria
  3. Cloudy urine
  4. Oliguric (100 to 400 ml/day)
  5. Anuric (<100 ml/day)

> **HESI Hint** • Accumulation of waste products from protein metabolism is the primary cause of uremia. Protein must be restricted in CRF clients. However, if protein intake is inadequate, a negative nitrogen balance occurs, causing muscle wasting. The glomerular filtration rate (GFR) is most often used as an indicator of the level of protein consumption.

G. Jaundice

H. Gastrointestinal (GI) upsets

I. Metallic taste in mouth

J. Ammonia breath

K. Dialysis (Table 4-7)

> **HESI Hint** • **DIALYSIS COVERED BY MEDICARE**
> • All persons in the United States are eligible for Medicare as of their first day of dialysis under special ESRD funding.
> • Medicare card will indicate ESRD.
> • Transplantation is covered by Medicare procedure; coverage terminates 6 months postoperative if dialysis is no longer required.

L. Previous kidney transplant

M. Lab information
  1. Azotemia
  2. Increased creatinine and BUN
  3. Decreased calcium
  4. Elevated phosphorus and magnesium

Analysis (Nursing Diagnoses)

A. *Excess fluid volume* related to…

B. *Imbalanced nutrition: less than body requirements* related to…

C. *Decreased cardiac output* related to…

Nursing Plans and Interventions

A. Monitor serum electrolyte levels.

B. Weigh daily.

C. Monitor strict I&O.

D. Check for jugular vein distention (JVD) and other signs of fluid overload.

E. Monitor for edema and pulmonary edema.

F. Provide low-protein, low-sodium, low-potassium, low-phosphate diet.

> **HESI Hint** • Protein intake is restricted until blood chemistry shows ability to handle the protein catabolites, urea and creatinine. Ensure high calorie intake so protein is spared for its own work; give hard candy, jelly beans, or flavored carbohydrate powders.

G. Administer aluminum hydroxide antacids to bind phosphates because client is unable to excrete phosphates (no magnesium-based antacids). Timing is important!

H. Encourage client's protein intake to be of high biologic value (eggs, milk, meat) because the client is on a low-protein diet.

I. Alternate periods of rest with periods of activity.

J. Encourage strict adherence to medication regimen; teach client to obtain health care provider's permission before taking any over-the-counter medications.

TABLE 4-7   Renal Dialysis

Types of Dialysis	Description	Nursing Implications
• Hemodialysis	• Requires venous access (AV shunt, fistula, or graft) • Treatment is 3 to 8 hours in length, 3 times per week • Correction of fluid and electrolyte imbalance is rapid • Potential blood loss • Does not result in protein loss	• Heparinization is required • Requires expensive equipment • Rapid shifts of fluid and electrolytes can lead to disequilibrium syndrome (an unpleasant sensation and a potentially dangerous situation) • Potential hepatitis B and C • Do *not* take blood pressure or perform venipunctures on the arm with the AV shunt, fistula, or graft • Assess access site for thrill and bruit
• Continuous arteriovenous hemofiltration (CAVH)	• Requires vascular access: usually femoral or subclavian catheters • Slow process • Correction of fluid and electrolyte imbalance is slow • Does not cause blood loss • Does not result in protein loss	• Requires heparinization of filter tubing • Filters are costly • Equipment is simple to use but requires specialized training to monitor • Limited to special care units; not for home use • Filter may rupture, causing blood loss

• Peritoneal	• Surgical placement of abdominal catheter is required (Tenckhoff, Gore-Tex, column-disk)
	• Slow process up to 8 to 10 hours for repeated cycles
	• Correction of fluid and electrolyte imbalance is slow
	• Does not cause blood loss
	• Protein is lost in dialysate
		• Heparinization is not required
		• Fairly expensive
		• Simple to perform
		• Easy to use at home
		• Dialysate is similar to IV fluid and is prescribed for the individual client's electrolyte needs
		• Potential complications:
		  • Bowel or bladder perforation
		  • Exit-site and tunnel infection
		  • Peritonitis

HESI Hint • The major difference between dialysate for hemodialysis and peritoneal dialysis is the amount of glucose. Peritoneal dialysis dialysate is much higher in glucose. For this reason, if the dialysate is left in the peritoneal cavity too long, hyperglycemia may occur.

K. Observe for complications.
 1. Anemia (administer antianemic drug; Table 4-8)
 2. Renal osteodystrophy (abnormal calcium metabolism causes bone pathology)
 3. Severe, resistant hypertension
 4. Infection
 5. Metabolic acidosis

L. Living related or cadaver renal transplant (Table 4-9)
 1. Monitor for rejection.
 2. Monitor for infection.
 3. Teach client to maintain immunosuppressive drug therapy meticulously.

URINARY TRACT INFECTIONS (UTIs)

Description: Infection or inflammation at any site in the urinary tract (kidney, pyelonephritis; urethra, urethritis; bladder, cystitis; prostate, prostatitis)

A. Normally, the entire urinary tract is sterile.

B. The most common infectious agent is *Escherichia coli*.

C. Persons at highest risk for acquiring UTIs
 1. Diabetics
 2. Pregnant women
 3. Men with prostatic hypertrophy
 4. Immunosuppressed persons
 5. Catheterized clients
 6. Anyone with urinary retention, either short term or long term
 7. Older women (bladder prolapse)

D. Diagnosis
 1. Clean-catch midstream urine collection for culture to identify specific causative organism
 2. Intravenous pyelogram (IVP) to determine kidney functioning
 3. Cystogram to determine bladder functioning
 4. Cystoscopy to determine bladder or urethral abnormalities

TABLE 4-8 Antianemic: Biologic Response Modifier (BRM)

Drugs	Indications	Adverse Reactions	Nursing Interventions
• Erythropoietin (Epogen)	• Anemia due to decreased production of erythropoietin in end stage renal disease • Stimulates RBC production, increases Hgb, reticulocyte count, and Hct	• Use with caution in older adults because of increased risk for thrombosis	• Monitor Hct weekly; report levels over 30% to 33% and increases of more than 4 points in less than 2 weeks • Explain that pelvic and limb pain should dissipate after 12 hours • Do not shake vial; shaking may inactivate the glycoprotein • Discard unused contents; does not contain preservatives

HESI Hint • As kidneys fail, medications must often be adjusted. Of particular importance is digoxin toxicity because digitalis preparations are excreted by the kidneys. Signs of toxicity in adults include nausea, vomiting, anorexia, visual disturbances, restlessness, headache, cardiac dysrhythmias, and pulse <60 bpm.

TABLE 4-9 Postoperative Care: Kidney Surgery

Assessment	Nursing Interventions	Rationale
• Respiratory status	• Auscultate lung sounds to detect "wet" sounds indicating infection • Demonstrate method of splinting incision for comfort when coughing and deep breathing	• Flank incision causes pain with both inspiration and expiration. Therefore, client avoids deep breathing and coughing; this can lead to respiratory difficulties, including pneumonia
• Circulatory status	• Check vital signs to detect early signs of bleeding, shock • Monitor skin color and temperature (pallor and cold skin are signs of shock) • Monitor urinary output (decreases with circulatory collapse) • Monitor surgical site for frank bleeding	• The kidney is very vascular • Bleeding is a constant threat • Circulatory collapse will occur with hemorrhage and can occur very quickly
• Pain relief status	• Administer narcotic analgesics as needed to relieve pain	• Relief of pain will improve the client's cooperation with deep-breathing exercises • Relief of pain will improve client's cooperation with early ambulation
• Urinary status	• Check urinary output and drainage from all tubes inserted during the surgery • Maintain accurate intake and output	• Mechanical drainage of bladder will be implemented after surgery

Nursing Assessment

A. Signs of infection including fever and chills

B. Urinary frequency, urgency, or dysuria

C. Hematuria

D. Pain at the costovertebral angle

E. Elevated serum WBCs (>10,000)

Analysis (Nursing Diagnoses)

A. *Acute pain* related to...

B. *Impaired urinary elimination* related to...

C. *Deficient knowledge* (specify) related to...

Nursing Plans and Interventions

A. Administer antibiotics specific to infectious agent.

B. Instruct client in the appropriate medication regimen.

C. Encourage fluid intake of 3000 ml of fluid/day.

D. Maintain I&O.

E. Administer mild analgesics (phenazopyridine [Pyridium], acetaminophen, or aspirin).

F. Encourage client to void every 2 to 3 hours to prevent residual urine from stagnating in bladder.

HESI Hint • The key to resolving UTIs with most antibiotics is to keep the blood level of the antibiotic constant. It is important to tell the client to take the antibiotics around the clock and not to skip doses so that a consistent blood level can be maintained for optimal effectiveness.

G. Develop and implement a teaching plan:
  1. Take entire prescription as directed.
  2. Consume oral fluids up to 3 L/day (water, juices).
  3. Shower rather than bathe as a preventive measure. If bathing is necessary, never take a bubble or oil bath and avoid feminine hygiene sprays.
  4. Cleanse from front to back after toileting (women and girls).
  5. Avoid caffeine.
  6. Void immediately after intercourse (women).
  7. Void every 2 to 3 hours during the day.
  8. Wear cotton undergarments and loose clothing to help decrease perineal moisture.
  9. Practice good handwashing technique.
  10. Obtain follow-up care.

URINARY TRACT OBSTRUCTION

Description: Partial or complete blockage of the flow of urine at any point in the urinary system

A. Urinary tract obstruction may be caused by:
  1. Foreign body (calculi)
  2. Tumors
  3. Strictures
  4. Functional (e.g., neurogenic bladder)
B. When urinary tract obstruction occurs, urine is retained above the point of obstruction.
  1. Hydrostatic pressure builds, causing dilatation of the organs above the obstruction.
  2. If hydrostatic pressure continues to build, hydronephrosis develops, and it can lead to renal failure.

Nursing Assessment

A. Pain, usually quite severe, acute
B. Symptoms of obstruction
  1. Fever, chills
  2. Nausea, vomiting, diarrhea
  3. Abdominal distention
C. Change in voiding pattern
  1. Dysuria, hematuria
  2. Urgency, frequency, hesitancy, nocturia, dribbling
  3. Difficulty in starting a stream
  4. Incontinence

HESI Hint • Location of the pain can help to determine the location of the stone.
• Flank pain usually means the stone is in the kidney or upper ureter. If the pain radiates to the abdomen or scrotum, the stone is likely to be in the ureter or bladder.
• Excruciating spastic-type pain is called colic.
• During kidney stone attacks, it is preferable to administer pain medications at regularly scheduled intervals rather than PRN to prevent spasm and optimize comfort.

D. Those with the following conditions are at risk for developing calculi:
  1. Strictures
  2. Prostatic hypertrophy
  3. Neoplasms
  4. Congenital malformations
  5. History of calculi
  6. Family history of calculi

Analysis (Nursing Diagnoses)

A. *Acute pain* related to…
B. *Risk for infection* related to…
C. *Risk for injury* related to…

Nursing Plans and Interventions

A. Administer narcotic analgesics.
B. Apply moist heat to the painful area unless prescribed otherwise.
C. Encourage high oral fluid intake to help dislodge the stone.
D. Administer intravenous (IV) antibiotics if infection is present.
E. Strain all urine!
F. Send any stones found when straining to the laboratory for analysis.
G. Accurately document I&O.
H. Endourologic procedures
  1. Cystoscopy
  2. Cystolitholapaxy
  3. Ureteroscopy
  4. Percutaneous nephrolithotomy
I. Lithotripsy
  1. Ultrasonic
  2. Electrohydraulic
  3. Laser
  4. Extracorporeal shock-wave
J. Surgical therapy
  1. Nephrolithotomy
  2. Pyelothitomy
  3. Ureterolithotomy
  4. Cystotomy

HESI Hint • Percutaneous nephrostomy: A needle or catheter is inserted through the skin into the calyx of the kidney. The stone may be dissolved by percutaneous irrigation with a liquid that dissolves the stone or by ultrasonic sound waves (lithotripsy) that can be directed through the needle or catheter to break up the stone, which then can be eliminated through the urinary tract.

K. Develop and implement a teaching plan to include:
1. Pursue follow-up care, because stones tend to recur.
2. Maintain a high fluid intake of 3 to 4 L/day.
3. Follow prescribed diet (based on composition of stone).
4. Avoid long periods of remaining in supine position.

BENIGN PROSTATIC HYPERPLASIA (BPH)

Description: Enlargement or hypertrophy of the prostate (sometimes called hypertrophy of the prostate)

A. BPH tends to occur in men over 40 years of age.
B. Intervention is required when symptoms of obstruction occur.
C. The most common treatment is transurethral resection of the prostate gland (TURP). The prostate is removed by endoscopy (no surgical incision is made), allowing for a shorter hospital stay.

Nursing Assessment

A. Increased frequency of voiding, with a decrease in amount of each voiding
B. Nocturia
C. Hesitancy
D. Terminal dribbling
E. Decrease in size and force of stream
F. Acute urinary retention
G. Bladder distention

Analysis (Nursing Diagnoses)

A. *Chronic pain* related to…
B. *Risk for injury: hemorrhage* related to…
C. *Risk for injury: infection* related to…

Nursing Plans and Interventions

A. Preoperative teaching: include information concerning pain from bladder spasms that occurs postoperatively.

B. Maintain patent urinary drainage system (large three-way indwelling catheter with a 30-ml balloon) to decrease the spasms.
C. Provide pain relief as prescribed: analgesics, narcotics, and antispasmodics.

HESI Hint • Bladder spasms frequently occur after TURP. Inform the client that the presence of the oversized balloon on the catheter (30 to 45 ml inflated) will cause a continuous feeling of needing to void. The client should not try to void around the catheter because this can precipitate bladder spasms. Medications to reduce or prevent spasms should be given.

D. Minimize catheter manipulation by taping catheter to abdomen or leg.
E. Maintain gentle traction on urinary catheter.
F. Check the urinary drainage system for clots.
G. Irrigate bladder as prescribed (may be continuous or rarely intermittent). If continuous, keep Foley bag emptied to avoid retrograde pressure.

HESI Hint • Instillation of hypertonic or hypotonic solution into a body cavity will cause a shift in cellular fluid. Use only sterile saline for bladder irrigation after TURP because the irrigation must be isotonic to prevent fluid and electrolyte imbalance.

H. Observe the color and content of urinary output.
1. Normal drainage after prostate surgery is reddish pink, clearing to light pink within 24 hours after surgery. Some small to medium-sized blood clots may be present.
2. Monitor for bright-red bleeding with large clots and increased viscosity.
I. Monitor vital signs frequently for indication of circulatory collapse.
J. Monitor hemoglobin (Hgb) and hematocrit (Hct) for pattern of decreasing values that indicates bleeding.
K. After catheter is removed:
1. Monitor amount and number of times client voids.
2. Encourage fluids.
3. Have the client use urine cups to provide a specimen with each voiding.
4. Observe for hematuria after each voiding (urine should progress to clear yellow color by the fourth day).

5. Inform client that burning on urination and urinary frequency are usually experienced during the first postoperative week.
6. Generally the client is not impotent after surgery, but sterility may occur.
7. Instruct client to report any frank bleeding to physician immediately.

L. Instruct client to increase fluid intake to 3000 ml/day.

M. Prepare client for discharge with instructions to:
   1. Continue to drink 12 to 14 glasses of water a day.
   2. Avoid constipation, straining.

3. Avoid strenuous activity, lifting, intercourse, and engaging in sports during the first 3 to 4 weeks after surgery.
4. Schedule a follow-up appointment.

HESI Hint • Inform the client prior to discharge that some bleeding is expected after TURP. Large amounts of blood or frank bright bleeding should be reported. However, it is normal for the client to pass small amounts of blood as well as small clots during the healing process. He should rest quietly and continue drinking large amounts of fluid.

Review of Renal System

1. Differentiate between acute renal failure and chronic renal failure.
2. During the oliguric phase of renal failure, protein should be severely restricted. What is the rationale for this restriction?
3. Identify two nursing interventions for the client on hemodialysis.
4. What is the highest priority nursing diagnosis for clients in any type of renal failure?
5. A client in renal failure asks why he is being given antacids. How should the nurse reply?
6. List four essential elements of a teaching plan for clients with frequent urinary tract infections.
7. What are the most important nursing interventions for clients with possible renal calculi?
8. What discharge instructions should be given to a client who has had urinary calculi?
9. Following transurethral resection of the prostate gland (TURP), hematuria should subside by what postoperative day?
10. After the urinary catheter is removed in the TURP client, what are three priority nursing actions?
11. After kidney surgery, what are the primary assessments the nurse should make?

Answers to Review

1. Acute renal failure: often reversible, abrupt deterioration of kidney function. Chronic renal failure: irreversible, slow deterioration of kidney function characterized by increasing BUN and creatinine. Eventually dialysis is required.
2. Toxic metabolites that accumulate in the blood (urea, creatinine) are derived mainly from protein catabolism.
3. Do not take BP or perform venipuncture on the arm with the AV shunt, fistula, or graft. Assess access site for thrill and bruit.
4. Risk for imbalanced fluid volume
5. Calcium and aluminum antacids bind phosphates and help to keep phosphates from being absorbed into bloodstream, thereby preventing rising phosphate levels; must be taken with meals.
6. Fluid intake 3 L/day; good handwashing; void every 2 to 3 hours during waking hours; take all prescribed medications; wear cotton undergarments.
7. Straining all urine is the most important intervention. Other interventions include accurate intake and output documentation and administering analgesics as needed.
8. Maintain high fluid intake of 3 to 4 L/day. Pursue follow-up care (stones tend to recur). Follow prescribed diet based on calculi content. Avoid supine position.
9. The fourth day
10. Continued strict I&O. Continued observations for hematuria. Inform client burning and frequency may last for a week.
11. Respiratory status (breathing is guarded because of pain); circulatory status (the kidney is very vascular and excessive bleeding can occur); pain assessment; urinary assessment (most important, assessment of urinary output).

Cardiovascular System

HESI Hint • What is the relationship of the kidneys to the cardiovascular system?
- The kidneys filter about 1 L of blood per minute.
- If cardiac output is decreased, the amount of blood going through the kidneys is decreased; urinary output is decreased. Therefore, a decreased urinary output may be a sign of cardiac problems.
- When the kidneys produce and excrete 0.5 ml of urine/kg of body weight or average 30 ml/hr output, the blood supply is considered to be minimally adequate to perfuse the vital organs.

ANGINA

Description: Chest discomfort or pain that occurs when myocardial O_2 demands exceed supply

Common Causes

A. Atherosclerotic heart disease

B. Hypertension

C. Coronary artery spasm

D. Hypertrophic cardiomyopathy

Nursing Assessment

A. Pain
   1. Mild to severe intensity, described as heavy, squeezing, pressing, burning, choking, aching, and feeling of apprehension
   2. Substernal, radiating to left arm and/or shoulder, jaw, right shoulder
   3. Transient or prolonged, with gradual or sudden onset; typically of short duration
   4. Often precipitated by exercise, exposure to cold, a heavy meal, mental tension, sexual intercourse
   5. Relieved by rest and/or nitroglycerin

B. Dyspnea, tachycardia, palpitations

C. Nausea, vomiting

D. Fatigue

E. Diaphoresis, pallor, weakness

F. Syncope

G. Dysrhythmias

H. Diagnostic information
   1. ECG: is generally at client baseline unless taken during anginal attack, when ST-segment depression and T-wave inversion may occur
   2. Exercise stress test: shows ST-segment depression and hypotension
   3. Stress echocardiogram: looks for changes in wall motion (indicated in women)
   4. Coronary angiogram: detects coronary artery spasms
   5. Cardiac catheterization: detects arterial blockage

I. Risk factors
   1. Nonmodifiable
      a. Heredity
      b. Gender: male > female until menopause, then equal risk
      c. Ethnic background: African Americans
      d. Age
   2. Modifiable
      a. Hyperlipidemia
      b. Total serum cholesterol above 300 mg/dl: four times greater risk for developing coronary artery disease (CAD) than those with levels less than 200 mg/dl (desirable level)
      c. Low-density lipoprotein (LDL), "bad cholesterol": A molecule of LDL is approximately 50% cholesterol by weight (<100 mg/dl desirable).
      d. High-density lipoprotein (HDL), "good cholesterol": HDL is inversely related to the risk for developing CAD (>60 mg/dl is desirable). In fact, HDL may serve to remove cholesterol from tissues.
      e. Hypertension
      f. Cigarette smoking
      g. Obesity
      h. Physical inactivity
      i. Diabetes mellitus
      j. Stress

Analysis (Nursing Diagnoses)

A. *Acute pain* related to…

B. *Anxiety* related to…

Nursing Plans and Interventions

A. Monitor medications, and instruct client in proper administration.

B. Determine factors precipitating pain, and assist client and family in adjusting lifestyle to decrease these factors.

C. Teach risk factors, and identify client's own risk factors.

D. During an attack
   1. Provide immediate rest.
   2. Take vital signs.
   3. Record an ECG.
   4. Administer no more than three nitroglycerin tablets, 5 minutes apart (Table 4-10).
   5. Seek emergency treatment if no relief has occurred after taking nitroglycerin.

TABLE 4-10 **Antianginals**

Drugs	Indications/Actions	Adverse Reactions	Nursing Implications
Nitrates			
• Nitroglycerin (NTG) • Isosorbide dinitrate (Isordil) • Isosorbide mononitrate (Imdur)	• Anginal prophylaxis • Acute attack • Reduces vascular resistance	• Headache • Flushing • Dizziness • Weakness • Hypotension • Nausea	• Monitor relief • Have client rest • Monitor vital signs • Store medication in original container • Protect from light
Beta Blockers			
• Propranolol HCl (Inderal) • Atenolol (Tenormin) • Nadolol (Corgard)	• Anginal prophylaxis • Reduces O_2 demand	• Fatigue • Lethargy • Hallucinations • Impotence • Bradycardia • Hypotension • HF • Wheezing	• Monitor apical heart rate • Assess for decreased BP • Do not stop medication abruptly • Clients with HF, bronchitis, asthma, COPD, or renal or hepatic insufficiency have increased likelihood of incurring adverse reactions
Calcium Channel Blockers			
• Verapamil (Calan) • Nifedipine HCl (Procardia) • Diltiazem HCl (Cardizem, Norvasc)	• Anginal prophylaxis • Inhibits influx of calcium ions	• Dizziness • Hypotension • Fatigue • Headache • Syncope • Peripheral edema • Hypokalemia • Dysrhythmia • HF	• Clients with HF and older adults have an increased likelihood of incurring adverse reactions • Assess for decreased BP • Monitor serum potassium • Swallow pills whole • Store at room temperature • Do not stop abruptly • Take 1 hour before meals or 2 hours after meals

E. Physical activity
   1. Teach avoidance of isometric activity.
   2. Implement an exercise program.
   3. Teach that sexual activity may be resumed after exercise is tolerated, usually when able to climb two flights of stairs without exertion. Nitroglycerin can be taken prophylactically before intercourse.
F. Provide nutritional information about modifying fats (saturated) and sodium. Antilipemic medications may be prescribed to lower cholesterol levels (Table 4-11).
G. Medical interventions include:
   1. Percutaneous transluminal coronary angioplasty (PTCA). A balloon catheter is repeatedly inflated to split or fracture plaque, and the arterial wall is stretched, enlarging the diameter of the vessel. A rotoblade is used to pulverize plaque.
   2. Arthrectomy. A catheter with a collection chamber is used to remove plaque that is trapped in the chamber.
   3. Coronary artery bypass graft (CABG)
   4. Coronary laser therapy
   5. Coronary artery stent

MYOCARDIAL INFARCTION (MI)

Description: Disruption in or deficiency of coronary artery blood supply, resulting in necrosis of myocardial tissue.

Causes of MI

A. Thrombus or clotting
B. Shock or hemorrhage

Nursing Assessment

A. Sudden onset of pain in the lower sternal region (substernal)
   1. Severity increases until it becomes nearly unbearable.
   2. Heavy and viselike pain often radiates to the shoulders and down the arms and/or to the neck and jaw. Common locations for pain are substernal, retrosternal, or epigastric areas. Women

TABLE 4-11 Antilipemic

Drugs	Indications	Adverse Reactions	Nursing Implications
Bile Sequestrants			
• Colestipol HCL (Colestid) • Colesevelam (Welchol) • Cholestyramine (Questran)	• Treat type IIA hyperlipidemia (hyper-cholesterolemia) when dietary changes fail	• Abdominal pain, nausea and vomiting, distention, flatulence, belching, constipation • Reduced absorption of lipid-soluble vitamins: A, D, E, and K • Alteration in absorption of other oral medications	• Teach client to mix powder forms with adequate amounts of liquid or fruits high in moisture content such as applesauce to prevent accidental inhalation or esophageal distress • Monitor prothrombin times • Assess for visual changes and rickets • Administer other oral medications 1 hour before or 6 hours after giving bile sequestrants
HMG-CoA Reductase Inhibitors (statins)			
• Atorvastatin (Lipitor) • Fluvastatin (Lescol) • Pravastatin (Pravachol) • Simvastatin (Zocor) • Lovastatin (Mevacor)		• Side effects similar to bile sequestrants • May elevate liver enzymes • Hepatitis or pancreatitis • Rhabdomyolysis	• Obtain liver enzymes baseline and monitor every 6 months • Monitor CPK levels • Review specific drug-food interactions; avoid grapefruit juice • Timing with or without food varies with drug • Instruct client to report any muscle tenderness
Fibric Acid Derivatives			
• Gemfibrate (Lopid) • Fenofibrate (Tricor) • Clofibrate (Claripex)	• Used with diet changes to lower elevated cholesterol and triglycerides	• Abdominal and epigastric pain; diarrhea—most common • Flatulence, nausea and vomiting • Heartburn • Dyspepsia • Gallstones • Tricor: weakness, fatigue, headache • Myopathy	• Obtain baseline labs: liver function, CBC, and electrolytes; monitor every 3 to 6 months Administer: • Lopid: 30 minutes before breakfast and dinner • Tricor: with meals
Water-Soluble Vitamins			
• Niacin (Niaspan) • Nicotinic acid (Nicobid)	• Large doses decrease lipoprotein and triglyceride synthesis and increase HDL.	• Flushing of face and neck • Pruritus • Headache • Orthostatic hypotension • (ER form): Hepatotoxicity • Hyperglycemia • Hyperuricemia • Upper GI distress	• Give with milk or food to avoid GI irritation • Client to change positions slowly • Instruct client taking extended release (ER) form to report darkened urine, light-colored stools, anorexia, yellowing of eyes or skin, severe stomach pain

HESI Hint • Angina is caused by myocardial ischemia. Which cardiac medications would be appropriate for acute angina?

Digoxin: *not appropriate*; increases the strength and contractility of the heart muscle; the problem in angina is that the muscle is not receiving enough O_2. Digoxin will not help.

Nitroglycerin: *appropriate*; causes dilatation of the coronary arteries, allowing more O_2 to get to the heart muscle.

Atropine: *not appropriate*; increases heart rate by blocking vagal stimulation, which suppresses the heart rate; does not address the lack of O_2 to the heart muscle.

Propranolol (Inderal): *not appropriate* for acute angina attack; however, is appropriate for long-term management of stable angina because it acts as a beta-blocker to control vasoconstriction.

may also present with shortness of breath or fatigue.
3. It differs from angina pain in its sudden onset.
4. Pain is not relieved by rest.
5. Pain is not relieved by nitroglycerin.
6. Pain may persist for hours or days.
7. Client may not have pain (silent MI), especially those with diabetic neuropathy.

B. Rapid, irregular, and feeble pulse
C. Decreased level of consciousness indicating decreased cerebral perfusion
D. Left heart shift sometimes occurring post-MI
E. Cardiac dysrhythmias, occurring in about 90% of MI clients
F. Cardiogenic shock or fluid retention
G. Serum cardiac markers
1. Creatine kinase (CK) intracellular enzymes that are released into circulation after an MI
   a. Rise 3 to 12 hours after an MI
   b. Peak in 24 hours
   c. Return to normal within 2 to 3 days
2. CK-MB band is specific to myocardial cells and can help quantify myocardial damage.
3. Cardiac-specific troponin is a myocardial muscle protein released into circulation after MI injury with greater sensitivity and specificity for myocardial injury than CK-MB.
   a. Cardiac-specific troponin T (cTnT) and cardiac-specific troponin I (cTnI)
   b. Increase 3 to 12 hours after the onset of MI
   c. Peak at 10 to 24 hours
   d. Return to baseline over 5 to 14 days
H. Narrowed pulse pressure, e.g., 90/80 mm Hg
I. Bowel sounds are absent or high-pitched, indicating possibility of mesenteric artery thrombosis, which acts as an intestinal obstruction. (See Gastrointestinal System, p. 107.)
J. Heart failure indicated by wet lung sounds
K. ECG changes occur as early as 2 hours post-MI or as late as 72 hours post-MI (Table 4-12)

Analysis (Nursing Diagnoses)

A. *Ineffective tissue perfusion* (specify type) related to…
B. *Decreased cardiac output* related to…
C. *Activity intolerance* related to…
D. *Acute pain* related to…

Nursing Plans and Interventions

A. Administer medications as prescribed.
1. For pain and to increase O_2 perfusion, IV morphine sulfate (acts as a peripheral vasodilator and decreases venous return)
2. Other medications often prescribed include (see Table 4-10):
   a. Nitrates (e.g., nitroglycerin)
   b. Beta-blockers
   c. Calcium channel blockers
   d. Aspirin
   e. Antiplatelet aggregates
B. Obtain vital signs, including ECG rhythm strip regularly, per agency policy.
C. Administer O_2 at 2 to 6 L per nasal cannula.
D. Obtain cardiac enzymes as prescribed.
E. Provide a quiet, restful environment.
F. Assess breath sounds for rales (indicating pulmonary edema).
G. Maintain patent IV line for administration of emergency medications.
H. Monitor fluid balance.
I. Keep in semi-Fowler position to assist with breathing.
J. Maintain bed rest for 24 hours.
K. Encourage client to resume activity gradually.

TABLE 4-12 Post–Myocardial Infarction Cardiac Enzyme Elevations

Enzyme/Marker	Onset	Peak	Return to Normal
CK-MB (recognized indicator of MI by most clinicians)	2 to 4 hr	12 to 20 hr	48 to 72 hr
Myoglobin	1 to 4 hr (elevate prior to CK-MB)	4 to 8 hr	24 hr
Cardiac troponins	As early as 1 hr post injury	10 to 24 hr	5 to 14 days
LDH total	24 hr	3 to 6 days	10 to 14 days
LDH$_1$ (a higher LDH$_1$ than LDH$_2$ indicates MI)	12 to 24 hr	48 hr	10 days

L. Encourage verbalization of fears.

M. Provide information about the disease process and cardiac rehabilitation.

N. Consider medical interventions (see Angina, p. 87):
1. Thrombolytic agents, within 1 to 4 hours of MI (Table 4-13)
2. Intraaortic balloon pump (IABP) to improve myocardial perfusion

HYPERTENSION

Description: Persistent seated BP levels equal to or greater than 140/90 mm Hg

A. Essential (primary) hypertension has no known cause.

B. Secondary hypertension develops in response to an identifiable mechanism.

HESI Hint • Blood pressure is created by the difference in the pressure of the blood as it leaves the heart and the resistance it meets flowing out to the tissues. Therefore, any factor that alters cardiac output or peripheral vascular resistance will alter blood pressure. Diet and exercise, smoking cessation, weight control, and stress management can control many factors that influence the resistance blood meets as it flows from the heart.

Nursing Assessment

A. BP equal to or greater than 140/90 mm Hg on two separate occasions
1. Obtain BP while client is lying down, sitting, and standing.
2. Compare readings taken lying down, sitting, and standing. A difference of more than 10 mm Hg of either systolic or diastolic indicates postural hypotension. Take pressure in both arms.

B. Genetic risk factors (nonmodifiable)
1. Positive family history for hypertension
2. Gender (Men have a greater risk for being hypertensive at an earlier age than women.)
3. Age (Risk increases with increasing age.)
4. Ethnicity (African Americans are at greater risk than whites.)

C. Lifestyle and habits that increase risk for becoming hypertensive (modifiable)
1. Use of alcohol, tobacco, and caffeine
2. Sedentary lifestyle, obesity
3. Nutrition history of high salt and fat intake
4. Use of oral contraceptives or estrogens
5. Stress

HESI Hint • Remember the risk factors for hypertension: heredity, race, age, alcohol abuse, increased salt intake, obesity, and use of oral contraceptives.

D. Associated physical problems
1. Renal failure
2. Respiratory problems, especially COPD
3. Cardiac problems, especially valvular disorders

E. Pharmacologic history
1. Steroids (increase BP)
2. Estrogens (increase BP)

F. Assess for headache, edema, nocturia, nosebleeds, and vision changes (may be asymptomatic).

G. Assess level of stress and source of stress (related to job, economics, family).

H. Assess personality type (i.e., determine whether client exhibits type A behavior).

Analysis (Nursing Diagnoses)

A. *Deficient knowledge* related to...

B. *Noncompliance* related to...

C. *Ineffective tissue perfusion* (specify type) related to...

Nursing Plans and Interventions

A. Develop a teaching plan to include:
1. Information about disease process
   a. Risk factors
   b. Causes
   c. Long-term complications
   d. Lifestyle modifications
   e. Relationship of treatment to prevention of complications
2. Information about treatment plan
   a. How to take own BP
   b. Reasons for each medication (Tables 4-14 and 4-15)
   c. How and when to take each medication
   d. Necessity of consistency in medication regimen
   e. Need for ongoing assessment while taking antihypertensives

HESI Hint • The number one cause of a stroke in hypertensive clients is noncompliance with medication regimen. Hypertension is often symptomless, and antihypertensive medications are expensive and have side effects. Studies have shown that the more clients know about their antihypertensive medications, the more likely they are to take them; teaching is important!

TABLE 4-13 Fibrinolytic Agents

Drugs	Indications	Adverse Reactions	Nursing Implications
• Streptokinase (Streptase) (Kabikinase)	• Deep vein thrombosis • Pulmonary embolism • Arterial thrombosis and embolism • Coronary thrombosis • Dissolving clots in arteriovenous cannula	• Anaphylactic response ranging from breathing difficulties to bronchospasm, periorbital swelling, or angioneurotic edema • Increased risk for bleeding • Hemorrhagic infarction at site of myocardial damage • Reperfusion dysrhythmias	• Assess for bleeding at puncture site; apply pressure to control bleeding • Assess for allergic reactions and dysrhythmias during intracoronary perfusion • Immobilize client's leg for 24 hours after femoral coronary cannulation and perfusion; assess pedal pulses for adequate circulation • Monitor client's thrombin time after therapy. Do *not* administer heparin or oral anticoagulants until thrombin time is less than twice that of control • Do *not* shake vial when reconstituting; roll and tilt vial gently to mix
• Tenecteplase (TNKase) • Reteplase (Retavase)	• Acute management of coronary thrombosis	• Do not give if history of uncontrolled hypertension • Can cause hypotension	• Obtain baseline studies prior to administration: PT, PTT, CBC, fibrinogen level, renal studies, cardiac enzymes • Check for abnormal pulse, neurologic vital signs, and presence of skin lesions, which may indicate coagulation defects • Avoid needle punctures because of the possibility of bleeding; apply pressure for 10 minutes to venous puncture sites and for 30 minutes to arterial puncture sites; follow with pressure dressing • Be prepared to treat reperfusion dysrhythmias
• Urokinase (Abbokinase)	• Pulmonary embolism • Coronary thrombosis • IV catheter clearance	• Is nonantigenic and does not cause allergic reactions; otherwise has the same adverse reactions as those cited for streptokinase	• Infuse heparin and an oral anticoagulant following urokinase therapy to prevent rethrombosis • Is much more expensive than streptokinase but does not cause allergic reactions found with streptokinase therapy • Reconstitute immediately before use
• Alteplase (Activase) • Anistreplace (Eminase)	• Deep vein thrombosis • Pulmonary embolism • Coronary thrombosis	• Interacts with heparin, oral anticoagulants, and antiplatelet drugs to increase the risk for bleeding	• Alters coagulation only at the thrombus, *not* systemically (bleeding complications associated with streptokinase and urokinase are reduced with t-PA therapy) • Because t-PA is a human protein, allergic response is unlikely to occur • Half-life is 3 to 7 minutes; use immediately

TABLE 4-14 Diuretics

Drugs	Indications	Adverse Reactions	Nursing Implications
Thiazides			
• Chlorthalidone (Hygroton) • Hydrochlorothiazide (Esidrix, Microzide) • Indapamide (Lozol) • Metolazone (Zaroxolyn)	• To decrease fluid volume • Inexpensive • Effective • Useful in severe hypertension • Effective orally • Enhances other antihypertensives	• Hypokalemia symptoms include: → Dry mouth → Thirst → Weakness → Drowsiness → Lethargy → Muscle aches → Tachycardia • Hyperuricemia • Glucose intolerance • Hypercholesterolemia • Sexual dysfunction	• Observe for postural hypotension; can be potentiated by: → Alcohol → Barbiturates → Narcotics • Caution with: → Renal failure → Gout → Client taking lithium • Hypokalemia increases risk for digitalis toxicity • Administer potassium supplements
Loop			
• Furosemide (Lasix) • Torsemide (Demadex) • Bumetanide (Bumex)	• Rapid action • Potent for use when thiazides fail • Cause volume depletion	• Hypokalemia • Hyperuricemia • Glucose intolerance • Hypercholesterolemia • Hypertriglyceridemia • Sexual dysfunction • Weakness	• Volume depletion and electrolyte depletion are rapid • All nursing implications cited for thiazides
Potassium Sparing			
• Spironolactone (Aldactone) • Amiloride (Midamor)	• Volume depletion without significant potassium loss	• Hyperkalemia • Gynecomastia • Sexual dysfunction	• Watch for hyperkalemia and renal failure in those treated with ACE inhibitors or NSAIDs • Watch for increase in serum lithium levels • Give after meals to decrease GI distress
Combination Loops and Potassium Sparing			
• HCTZ and Triamterene (Maxidex) • HCTZ + Amiloride (Moduretic) • HCTZ + Spironolactone (Aldactazide)	• Decreases fluid volume while minimizing K⁺ loss	• Side effects of individual drug offset or minimized by its partner	• Caution client previously on a loop or thiazide alone not to overdo K⁺ foods now because of K⁺-sparing component in new drug • Follow scheduling doses to avoid sleep disruption

    f. Need to monitor serum electrolytes every 90 to 120 days for duration of treatment

    g. Need to monitor renal functioning (BUN and creatinine) every 90 to 120 days for duration of treatment

    h. Need to monitor BP and pulse rate, usually weekly

B. Encourage client to implement nonpharmacologic measures to assist with BP control, such as:

    1. Stress reduction

    2. Weight loss

    3. Tobacco cessation

    4. Exercise

C. Determine medication side effects experienced by client (see Table 14-15).

    1. Impotence

    2. Insomnia

D. Provide nutrition guidance, including a sample meal plan and how to dine out (low-salt, low-fat, low-cholesterol diet).

TABLE 4-15 **Antihypertensives**

Drugs	Indications	Adverse Reactions	Nursing Implications
Alpha-Adrenergic Blockers			
• Prazosin HCl (Minipress) • Terazosin (Hytrin) • Phentolamine mesylate (Regitine) • Doxazosin (Cardura)	• Used as peripheral vasodilator which acts directly on the blood vessels • Used in extreme hypertension of pheochromocytoma	• Orthostatic hypotension • Weakness • Palpitations	• Use cautiously in older clients. • Occasional vomiting and diarrhea • Warn clients of possible: → Drowsiness → Lack of energy → Weakness
Combined Alpha/Beta-Blockers			
• Labetalol (Normodyne) • Carvedilol (Coreg)	• Produces decrease in BP without reflex tachycardia or bradycardia	• HF • Ventricular dysrhythmias • Blood dyscrasias • Bronchospasm • Orthostatic hypotension	• Contraindicated with: → HF → Heart block → COPD
Beta-Blockers			
• Metoprolol tartrate (Lopressor) • Nadolol (Corgard) • Propranolol HCL (Inderal) • Timolol maleate (Blocadren) • Atenolol (Tenormin) • Bisoprolol (Zebeta) • Metoprolol (Lopressor, Toprol)	• Blocks the sympathetic nervous system, especially to the heart • Produces a slower heart rate • Lowers blood pressure • Reduces O_2 consumption during myocardial contraction	• Bradycardia • Fatigue • Insomnia • Bizarre dreams • Sexual dysfunction • Hypertriglyceridemia • Decreased HDL • Depression	• Check apical or radial pulse daily • Monitor for GI distress • Do not discontinue abruptly • Watch for shortness of breath; give cautiously with bronchospasm • Do not vary how taken (with or without food) • Do not vary time taken • May mask symptoms of hypoglycemia or may prolong a hypoglycemic reaction
Central-Acting Inhibitors			
• Clonidine (Catapres) • Guanabenz acetate (Wytensin) • Methyldopa (Aldomet)	• Decreases BP by stimulating central alpha receptors, resulting in decreased sympathetic outflow from the brain	• Drowsiness • Dry mouth • Fatigue • Sexual dysfunction	• Watch for rebound hypertension if abruptly discontinued • Use caution to make position changes slowly, avoid standing still and taking hot baths and showers
Vasodilators			
• Hydralazine HCl (Apresoline) • Minoxidil (Loniten)	• Decreases BP by decreasing peripheral resistance	• Headache • Tachycardia • Fluid retention (HF, pulmonary edema) • Postural hypotension	• Monitor BP, pulse routinely • Observe for peripheral edema • Monitor I&O • Weigh daily
Angiotensin II Receptor Antagonists			
• Losartan (Cozaar) • Valsartan (Diovan) • Irbesartan (Avapro)	• Blocks the vasoconstrictor and aldosterone-producing effects of angiotensin II at various sites (vascular smooth muscle and adrenal glands)	• Hypotension • Fatigue • Hepatitis • Renal failure • Hyperkalemia (rare)	• Monitor liver enzymes, electrolytes • Monitor for angioedema in those with history of it when on ACE inhibitors previously

TABLE 4-15 Antihypertensives—cont'd

Drugs	Indications	Adverse Reactions	Nursing Implications
Angiotensin-Converting Enzyme (ACE) Inhibitors			
• Captopril (Capoten) • Enalapril maleate (Vasotec) • Lisinopril (Zestril) • Ramipril (Altace) • Benazepril (Lotensin) • Quinapril (Accupril)	• Decreases BP by suppressing renin-angiotensin aldosterone system and inhibiting conversion of angiotensin I into angiotensin II • Useful with diabetics	• Proteinuria • Neutropenia • Skin rash • Cough	• Observe for acute renal failure (reversible) • Routine renal function tests • Remain in bed 3 hours after first dose
Calcium Channel Blockers			
• Diltiazem (Cardizem) • Nifedipine (Procardia, Adalat) • Verapamil HCl (Calan, Isoptin) • Nisoldipine (Sular)	• Inhibits calcium ion influx during cardiac depolarization • Decreases SA/AV node conduction	• Headache • Hypotension • Dizziness • Edema • Nausea • Constipation • Tachycardia • HF • Dry cough	• Check BP and pulse routinely • Limit caffeine consumption • Take medications before meals • Avoid grapefruit juice with these drugs; it increases serum levels, causing hypotension • High-fat meals elevate serum levels

PERIPHERAL VASCULAR DISEASE (PVD)

Description: Circulatory problems that can be due to arterial or venous pathology

Nursing Assessment

A. The signs, symptoms, and treatment of PVD can vary widely, depending on the source of pathology. Therefore, careful assessment is very important.
B. Predisposing factors
  1. Arterial
    a. Arteriosclerosis (95% of all cases are caused by atherosclerosis)
    b. Advanced age
  2. Venous
    a. History of deep vein thrombosis (DVT)
    b. Valvular incompetence
C. Associated diseases
  1. Arterial
    a. Raynaud disease (nonatherosclerotic, triggered by extreme heat or cold)
    b. Buerger disease (occlusive inflammatory disease, strongly associated with smoking)
    c. Diabetes
    d. Acute occlusion (emboli/thrombi)
  2. Venous
    a. Varicose veins
    b. Thrombophlebitis
    c. Venous stasis ulcers
D. Skin
  1. Arterial
    a. Smooth skin
    b. Shiny skin
    c. Loss of hair
    d. Thickened nails
  2. Venous
    a. Brown pigment around ankles
E. Color
  1. Arterial
    a. Pallor on elevation
    b. Rubor when dependent
  2. Venous—cyanotic when dependent
F. Temperature
  1. Arterial
    a. Cool
  2. Venous
    a. Warm
G. Pulses
  1. Arterial
    a. Decreased or absent
  2. Venous
    a. Normal
H. Pain
  1. Arterial
    a. Sharp
    b. Increases with walking and elevation
    c. Intermittent claudication: classic presenting symptom; occurs in skeletal muscles during exercise; is relieved by rest

d. Rest pain: occurs when the extremities are horizontal; may be relieved by dependent position; often appears when collateral circulation fails to develop
2. Venous
   a. Persistent, aching, full feeling, dull sensation
   b. Relieved when horizontal (Elevate and use compression stockings.)

I. Ulcers
1. Arterial
   a. Very painful
   b. Occur on lateral lower legs, toes, heels
   c. Demarcated edges
   d. Necrotic
   e. Not edematous
2. Venous
   a. Slightly painful
   b. Occur on medial legs, ankles
   c. Uneven edges
   d. Superficial
   e. Marked edema

Analysis (Nursing Diagnoses)

A. *Ineffective tissue perfusion* (specify type) related to…
B. *Activity intolerance* related to…
C. *Impaired skin integrity* related to…
D. *Risk for infection* related to…
E. *Acute pain* related to…

Treatment

A. Noninvasive treatment
1. Arterial
   a. Elimination of smoking
   b. Topical antibiotic
   c. Saline dressing
   d. Bed rest, immobilization
   e. Fibrinolytic agents if clots are the problem (not used for Raynaud or Buerger disease; see Table 4-13)
2. Venous
   a. Systemic antibiotics
   b. Compression dressing (snug) or alginate dressing if ulcerated
   c. Limb elevation
   d. For thrombosis: fibrinolytic agents (see Table 4-13) and anticoagulants (Table 4-16)
B. Surgery
1. Arterial
   a. Embolectomy: removal of clot
   b. Endarterectomy: removal of clot and stripping of plaque
   c. Arterial bypass: Teflon or Dacron graft or autograft
   d. Percutaneous transluminal angioplasty (PTA): compression of plaque

e. Amputation: removal of extremity
2. Venous
   a. Vein ligation
   b. Thrombectomy
   c. Débridement

Nursing Plans and Interventions

A. Monitor extremities at designated intervals.
   1. Color
   2. Temperature
   3. Sensation and pulse quality in extremities
B. Schedule activities within client's tolerance level.
C. Encourage rest at the first sign of pain.
D. Encourage client to keep extremities elevated (if venous) when sitting and to change position often.
E. Encourage client to avoid crossing legs and to wear nonrestrictive clothing.
F. Encourage client to keep the extremities warm by wearing extra clothing, such as socks and slippers, and not to use external heat sources such as electric heating pads.
G. Teach methods of preventing further injury.
   1. Change position frequently.
   2. Wear nonrestrictive clothing (no knee-high hose).
   3. Avoid crossing legs or keeping legs in a dependent position.
   4. Wear support hose or antiembolism stockings
   5. Wear shoes when ambulating.
   6. Obtain proper foot and nail care.

HESI Hint • Decreased blood flow results in diminished sensation in the lower extremities. Any heat source can cause severe burns before the client realizes the damage is being done.

H. Discourage cigarette smoking (causes vasoconstriction and spasm of arteries).
I. Provide preoperative and postoperative care if surgery is required.
   1. Preoperative: Maintain affected extremity in a level position (if venous) or in a slightly dependent position (if arterial; 15 degrees), at room temperature, and protect from trauma.
   2. Postoperative: Assess surgical site frequently for hemorrhage, and check peripheral pulses.
   3. Anticoagulants may be continued after surgery to prevent thrombosis of affected artery and to diminish development of thrombi at the initiating site.

TABLE 4-16 Anticoagulants

Drugs	Indications	Adverse Reactions	Nursing Implications
• Heparin sodium (Hepalean, Hep-Lock)	• Administered parenterally (SQ or IV) as an antagonist to thrombin and to prevent the conversion of fibrinogen to fibrin	• Hemorrhage • Agranulocytosis • Leukopenia • Hepatitis • Heparin-induced thrombocytopenia	• Assess PTT, Hgb, Hct, platelets • Assess stools for occult blood • Avoid IM injection • Notify anyone performing diagnostic testing of medication *Antagonist*: protamine sulfate
• Warfarin sodium (Coumadin, Coumarin, Panwarfin)	• Blocks the formation of prothrombin from vitamin K	• Hemorrhage • Agranulocytosis • Leukopenia • Hepatitis	• See *Heparin* • Given orally • Assess PT • Avoid sudden change in intake of foods high in vitamin K *Antagonist*: vitamin K
Antiplatelet agents • Ticlopidine (Ticlid) • Dipyridamole (Persantine) • Clopidogrel (Plavix)	• Short-term use after cardiac interventions • Reduce risk for thrombolytic stroke for those intolerant to aspirin • Prevention of thrombolytic disorders	• Neutropenia • Thrombocytopenia • Agranulocytosis • Leukopenia • Hemorrhage • GI irritation, bleeding • Pancytopenia	• Give PC or with food to decrease gastric irritation (Ticlid) • Advise not to take antacids within 2 hours of taking ticlopidine • Monitor CBC every 2 weeks for 3 months, and thereafter if signs of infection develop • Monitor for signs of bleeding • Give 1 hour AC (Persantine); (Plavix) no regard for meals
• Low-molecular-weight heparin, enoxaparin (Lovenox)	• Prevention of thrombolytic formation (deep vein)	• Hemorrhage • GI irritation, bleeding • Thrombocytopenia	• Monitor for signs of bleeding • Give subcutaneously • Monitor CBC • Use soft toothbrush; avoid cuts

ABDOMINAL AORTIC ANEURYSM (AAA)

Description: Dilatation of the abdominal aorta caused by an alteration in the integrity of its wall

A. The most common cause of AAA is atherosclerosis. It is a late manifestation of syphilis.

B. Without treatment, rupture and death will occur.

C. AAA is often asymptomatic.

D. The most common symptom is abdominal pain or low back pain, with the complaint that the client can feel his or her heart beating.

E. Those taking antihypertensive drugs are at risk for developing AAA.

HESI Hint • A client is admitted with severe chest pain and states that he feels a terrible tearing sensation in his chest. He is diagnosed with a dissecting aortic aneurysm. What assessments should the nurse obtain in the first few hours?

• Vital signs every hour
• Neurologic vital signs
• Respiratory status
• Urinary output
• Peripheral pulses

Nursing Assessment

A. Bruit (swooshing sound heard over a constricted artery when auscultated) heard over abdominal aorta, pulsation in upper abdomen

B. Abdominal or lower back pain

C. Abdominal radiograph (aortogram, angiogram, abdominal ultrasound) to confirm diagnosis if aneurysm is calcified

D. Symptoms of rupture: hypovolemic or cardiogenic shock with sudden, severe abdominal pain

Analysis (Nursing Diagnoses)

A. *Activity intolerance* related to…

B. *Impaired skin integrity* related to…

C. *Anxiety* related to…

Nursing Plans and Interventions

A. Assess all peripheral pulses and vital signs regularly.
   1. Radial
   2. Femoral
   3. Popliteal
   4. Posterior tibial
   5. Dorsalis pedis

B. Observe for signs of occlusion after graft.
   1. Change in pulses
   2. Severe pain
   3. Cool to cold extremities below graft
   4. White or blue extremities

C. Observe renal functioning for signs of kidney damage (artery clamped during surgery may result in kidney damage).
   1. Output of less than 30 ml/hr
   2. Amber urine
   3. Elevated BUN and creatinine (early signs of renal failure)

> **HESI Hint** • During aortic aneurysm repair, the large arteries are clamped for a period of time, and kidney damage can result. Monitor daily BUN and creatinine levels. Normal BUN is 10 to 20 mg/dl, and normal creatinine is 0.6 to 1.2 mg/dl. The ratio of BUN to creatinine is 20:1. When this ratio increases or decreases, suspect renal problems.

D. Observe for postoperative ileus.
   1. Nasogastric (NG) tube to low continuous suction for 1 to 2 days postoperative (may help to prevent ileus)
   2. Bowel sounds checked every shift

THROMBOPHLEBITIS

Description: Inflammation of the venous walls with the formation of a clot; also known as venous thrombosis, phlebothrombosis, DVT

Nursing Assessment

A. Calf pain if calf is involved, positive Homan sign (*Note:* Only about 10% of clients with phlebitis manifest this sign, and there are a lot of false positives.)

> **HESI Hint** • A positive Homan sign is considered an early indication of thrombophlebitis. However, it may also indicate muscle inflammation. If a DVT has been confirmed, a Homan sign should not be elicited because of the increased risk for embolization.

B. Functional impairment of extremity

C. Edema and warmth in extremity

D. Asymmetry
   1. Inspect legs from groin to feet.
   2. Measure diameters of calves.

E. Tender areas on affected extremity with very gentle palpation

F. Occlusion with diagnostic testing
   1. Venogram
   2. Doppler ultrasound
   3. Fibrinogen scanning

G. Risk factors
   1. Prolonged, strict bed rest
   2. General surgery
   3. Leg trauma
   4. Previous venous insufficiency
   5. Obesity
   6. Oral contraceptives
   7. Pregnancy
   8. Malignancy

Analysis (Nursing Diagnoses)

A. *Acute pain* related to…

B. *Ineffective tissue perfusion* related to…

> **HESI Hint** • Heparin prevents conversion of fibrinogen to fibrin and prothrombin to thrombin, thereby inhibiting clot formation. Because the clotting mechanism is prolonged, do not cause tissue trauma, which may lead to bleeding when giving heparin subcutaneously. Do not massage area or aspirate; give in the abdomen between the pelvic bones, 2 inches from umbilicus; rotate sites.

Nursing Plans and Interventions

A. Administer anticoagulant therapy as prescribed (see Table 4-16).

> **HESI Hint** • **ANTICOAGULANTS**
> *Heparin*
>   Antagonist: protamine sulfate
>   Lab: PTT or APTT determines efficacy
>   Keep 1.5 to 2.5 times normal control
> *Warfarin (Coumadin)*
>   Antagonist: vitamin K
>   Lab: PT determines efficacy
>   Keep 1.5 to 2.5 times normal control
>   INR (international normalized ratio): desirable therapeutic level usually 2 to 3 seconds (reflects how long it takes a blood sample to clot)

1. Observe for side effects, especially bleeding.
2. Teach client side effects of medications included in treatment regimen.
3. Monitor laboratory data to determine the efficacy of medications included in treatment regimen.
4. Note on all lab requests that client is receiving anticoagulants.
5. Partial thromboplastin time (PTT) determines efficacy of heparin.
6. Prothrombin time (PT)/international normalized ration determines efficacy of Coumadin.
7. Maintain pressure on venipuncture sites to minimize hematoma formation.
8. Notify physician of any unusual bleeding.
   a. Abnormal vaginal bleeding
   b. Nosebleeds
   c. Melena
   d. Hematuria
   e. Gums
   f. Hemoptysis
9. Advise client to use soft toothbrush, floss with waxed floss.
10. Advise client to wear medical alert symbol.
11. Advise client to avoid alcoholic beverages.
12. Advise client to avoid safety razors if taking Coumadin.
13. Advise client to avoid aspirin and aspirin products and NSAIDs.

B. Advise client to wear antiembolic stockings and to elevate extremity and use shock blocks at foot of bed.
C. Advise bed rest; strict, if prescribed, means no bathroom privileges! Advise client to avoid straining.
D. Monitor for decreasing symptomatology.
   1. Pain
   2. Edema
E. Monitor for pulmonary embolus (chest pain, shortness of breath).
F. Teach client that there is increased risk for DVT formation in the future.

DYSRHYTHMIAS

Description: Disturbance in heart rate or heart rhythm

A. Dysrhythmias are caused by a disturbance in the electrical conduction of the heart, not by abnormal heart structure.
B. Client is often asymptomatic until cardiac output is altered.
C. Common causes of dysrhythmias
   1. Drugs (e.g., digoxin, quinidine, caffeine, nicotine, alcohol)
   2. Acid-base and electrolyte imbalances (potassium, calcium, and magnesium)
   3. Marked thermal changes

4. Disease and trauma
5. Stress

Nursing Assessment

A. Change in pulse rate or rhythm
   1. Tachycardia: fast rates (>100 bpm)
   2. Bradycardia: slow rates (<60 bpm)
   3. Irregular rhythm
   4. Pulselessness
B. ECG changes
C. Complaints of:
   1. Palpitations
   2. Syncope
   3. Pain
   4. Dyspnea
D. Diaphoresis
E. Hypotension
F. Electrolyte imbalance

Analysis (Nursing Diagnoses)

A. *Ineffective tissue perfusion* related to...
B. *Activity intolerance* related to...

Selected Dysrhythmias

A. Atrial fibrillation (Fig. 4-3A)
   1. Description
      a. Chaotic activity in the AV node
      b. No true P waves visible
      c. Irregular ventricular rhythm
   2. Assessment and treatment
      a. Anticoagulant therapy due to risk for stroke
      b. Antidysrhythmic drugs
      c. Cardioversion to treat atrial dysrhythmias
B. Atrial flutter (see Fig. 4-3B)
   1. Description
      a. Saw-toothed waveform
      b. Fluttering in chest
      c. Ventricular rhythm states regular
   2. Assessment and treatment
      a. Cardioversion to treat atrial dysrhythmia
      b. Antidysrhythmic drugs
      c. Radiofrequency catheter ablation
C. Ventricular tachycardia (see Fig. 4-3C)
   1. Description
      a. Wide, bizarre QRS
   2. Assessment and treatment
      a. Pulse
      b. Impaired cardiac output
      c. Synchronized cardioversion if pulse present (if no pulse, treat as ventricular fibrillation)
      d. Antidysrhythmic drugs
D. Ventricular fibrillation (see Fig. 4-3D)
   1. Description
      a. Cardiac emergency

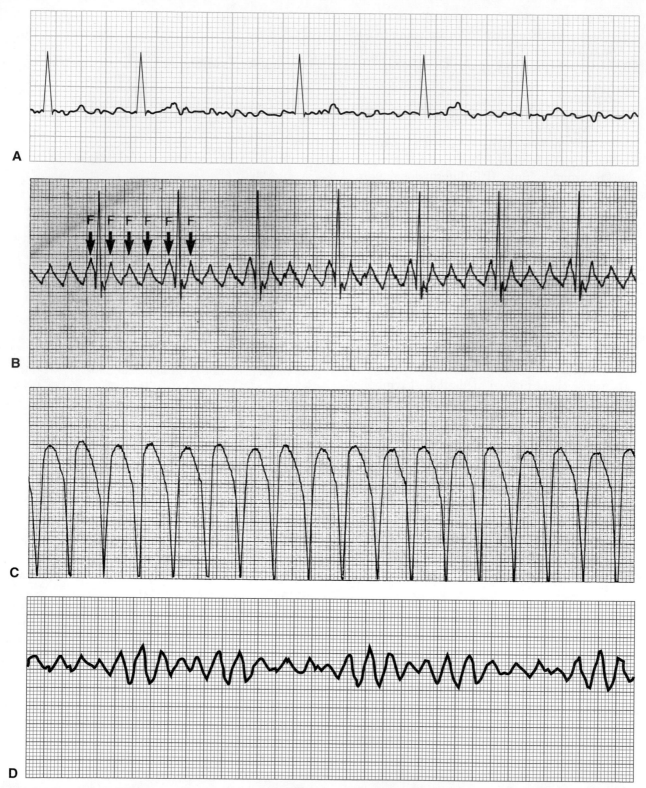

FIGURE 4-3 *A,* Atrial fibrillation. *B,* Atrial flutter (F) with 4:1 block. The atrial rate is 280 bpm; the ventricular rate is 70 bpm. *C,* Sustained ventricular tachycardia at a rate of 166 bpm. *D,* Coarse ventricular fibrillation. (A, From Huszar RJ: *Pocket guide to basic dysrhythmias,* ed 3. St. Louis, 2002, Mosby. B, C, D, From Ignatavicius DD, Workman ML: *Medical-surgical nursing: Patient-centered collaborative care,* ed 6. St. Louis, 2010, Saunders.)

b. Irregular undulations of varying amplitudes, from coarse to fine
c. No cardiac output
2. Assessment and treatment
   a. CPR
   b. Defibrillation as quickly as possible
   c. Antidysrhythmic drugs

Nursing Plans and Interventions

A. Determine medications client is currently taking.
B. Determine serum drug levels, especially digitalis.
C. Determine serum electrolyte levels, especially K^+ and Mg^{++}.
D. Obtain ECG reading on admission, and monitor continuously.

> **HESI Hint** • A Holter monitor offers continuous observation of the client's heart rate. To make assessment of the rhythm strips most meaningful, teach the client to keep a record of:
> • Medication times and doses
> • Chest pain episodes: type and duration
> • Valsalva maneuver (straining at stool, sneezing, coughing)
> • Sexual activity
> • Exercise and other activities

E. Approach client in a calm, reassuring manner.
F. Monitor client's activity, and observe for any symptoms occurring during activity.
G. Ensure proper administration of medications, and monitor for side effects (Table 4-17).
H. Be prepared for emergency measures, such as cardioversion or defibrillation.

> **HESI Hint** • Cardioversion is the delivery of synchronized electrical shocks to the myocardium.

I. Be prepared for pacemaker insertion.
   1. Temporary pacemaker: used temporarily in emergency situations. A pacing wire is threaded into the right ventricle via the superior vena cava, or an epicardial wire is put in place (through the client's chest incision) during cardiac surgery.
   2. Permanent internal pacemaker with pulse generator implanted in the abdomen or shoulder: may be single- or dual-chambered. Programmable pacemakers can be reprogrammed by placing a magnetic device over the generator.
   3. Instruct the client to:
      a. Report pulse rate lower than the set rate of the pacemaker.
      b. Avoid leaning over an automobile with the engine running.
      c. Stand 4 to 5 feet away from electromagnetic sources, such as operating microwave ovens and radar detectors that are operating.
      d. Avoid MRI diagnostic testing.

> **HESI Hint** • Difference in synchronous and asynchronous pacemakers:
> • Synchronous, or demand: Pacemaker fires only when the client's heart rate falls below a rate set on the generator.
> • Asynchronous, or fixed: Pacemaker fires at a constant rate.

J. Recognize and treat premature ventricular contractions (PVCs) as prescribed (they tend to be precursors of ventricular tachycardia and ventricular fibrillation; Fig. 4-4). A PVC is a contraction originating in an ectopic focus in the ventricles. It is the premature occurrence of a QRS complex that is wide and distorted in shape:
   1. If they occur more often than once in 10 beats.
   2. If they occur in groups of two or three.
   3. If they occur near the T wave.
   4. If they take on multiple configurations.

HEART FAILURE (HF)

Description: Inability of the heart to pump enough blood to meet the tissue's O_2 demands

A. Primary underlying conditions causing HF:
   1. Ischemic heart disease
   2. MI
   3. Cardiomyopathy
   4. Valvular heart disease
   5. Hypertension

Nursing Assessment

A. Observe for symptoms associated with left-sided or right-sided failure.
   1. Left-sided heart failure: pulmonary edema (left ventricular failure)
      a. Description: Results in pulmonary congestion due to the inability of the left ventricle to pump blood to the periphery

TABLE 4-17 Antidysrhythmics

Drugs	Indications	Adverse Reactions	Nursing Implications
Class I (A,B,C)			
• Quinidine • Disopyramide phosphate (Norpace) • Moricizine (Ethmozine) • Lidocaine HCl (Xylocaine) • Mexiletine (Mexitil) • Tocainide HCl (Tonocard) • Phenytoin sodium (Dilantin) • Propafenone (Rythmol) • Flecainide acetate (Tambocor)	• Premature beats • Atrial flutter, fibrillation • Contraindicated in heart block • Ventricular dysrhythmias • Unlabeled use: digitalis for induced dysrhythmias • Ventricular dysrhythmias	• Diarrhea • Hypotension • ECG changes • Cinchonism • Interacts with many common drugs • Hypotension • CNS effects • Seizures • GI distress • Bradycardia • Dizziness • Slurred speech • Ventricular dysrhythmias	• Instruct client to monitor pulse rate and rhythm • Monitor ECG • Monitor for tinnitus and visual disturbances • Lidocaine administered IV bolus and by infusion • Monitor for confusion, drowsiness, slurred speech, seizures with lidocaine • Administer oral drugs with food • May cause digoxin toxicity
Class II			
• Propranolol HCl (Inderal)	• Supraventricular and ventricular tachydysrhythmias	• Hypotension • Bradycardia • Bronchospasm	• Monitor vital signs • Contraindicated in asthma, COPD
Class III (Intropics)			
• Bretylium tosylate (Bretylol) • Amiodarone HCl (Cordarone) • Milrinone (Primacor) • Amrinone (Inocor) • Sotalol (Betapace)	• Ventricular dysrhythmias	• Dysrhythmias • Hypertension or hypotension • Muscle weakness, tremors • Photophobia	• Amiodarone is now one of the first-choice drugs • Monitor vital signs, ECG • Instruct client taking amiodarone to wear sunglasses and sunscreens when outside
Class IV			
• Verapamil HCL (Isoptin, Calan)	• Supraventricular dysrhythmias	• Hypotension • Bradycardia • Constipation	• Monitor BP and pulse • Instruct client to change positions slowly
Miscellaneous Agents			
• Atropine sulfate (Atropisol)	• Bradycardia	• Chest pain • Urinary retention • Dry mouth	• Monitor heart rate and rhythm • Assess for chest pain • Assess for urinary retention • Avoid use with glaucoma
• Digoxin (Lanoxin) • Digitoxin (Crystodigin)	• Supraventricular dysrhythmias • Atrial fibrillation	• Bradycardia • Dysrhythmias • Anorexia, nausea, vomiting, diarrhea, visual disturbances	• Monitor pulse rate and rhythm • Instruct client to report signs of toxicity • Hypokalemia increases the risk for toxicity • Causes hypercalcemia
• Epinephrine (adrenaline)	• Cardiac arrest	• Tachycardia • Hypertension	• Impaired renal function can cause toxicity; monitor BUN and creatinine • Monitor pulse return in asystole • Monitor vital signs

TABLE 4-17   Antidysrhythmics—cont'd

ADDITIONAL DRUGS THAT PROMOTE CARDIOVASCULAR PERFUSION IN THE FAILING HEART			
Drugs	**Indications**	**Adverse Reactions**	**Nursing Implications**
Vasopressors			
• Norepinephrine bitartrate (Levophed)	• Dilated coronary arteries and causes peripheral vasoconstriction for emergency hypotensive states not caused by blood loss, vascular thrombosis, or anesthesia using cyclopropane or halothane	• Can cause *severe* tissue necrosis, sloughing, and gangrene if infiltrates (blanching along vein pathway is preliminary sign of extravasation)	• Rapidly inactivated by various body enzymes; need to ensure IV patency • Use cautiously in previously hypertensive clients • Check BP every 2 to 5 minutes. • Use large veins to avoid complications of prolonged vasoconstriction • Pressor effects potentiated by many drugs; check drug-drug interactions • Have phentolamine (Regitine) diluted per protocol for local injection if infiltrates
Cardiotonic/Vasodilator (Human B-type natriuretic peptide: HBNP)			
• Nesiritide (Natrecor)	• Treatment of acutely decompensated HF in clients who have dyspnea at rest or with minimal activity • Reduces PCWP and reduces dyspnea	• Hypotension is primary side effect and can be dose limiting • Dysrhythmias • Headache, dizziness, insomnia, tremors, paresthesias • Abdominal pain, nausea and vomiting	• Many drug-drug interactions • Monitor BP and telemetry • As diuresis occurs, monitor electrolytes, especially K^+ • Watch for overresponse to treatment in older adults
Group IIa-IIIb Inhibitor (Platelet antiaggregate)			
• Eptifibatide (Integrilin)	• Acute coronary syndrome (unstable angina or non–Q wave MI) • Used in combination with heparin, aspirin, and, in selected situations, Ticlid and Plavix	• Bleeding, most frequent • Hypotension • Thrombocytopenia • Acute toxicity: decreased muscle tone, dyspnea, loss of righting reflex	• Check drug-drug interactions before giving other medications. • Obtain baseline PT/aPTT, Hgb, Hct, and platelet count, and monitor • Dose adjusted by weight for older adults • Same client teaching as with heparin; review activities to avoid • Watch for bleeding. • Quickly reversible, so emergency procedures may still be performed shortly after discontinuing infusion

PCWP, pulmonary capillary wedge pressure.

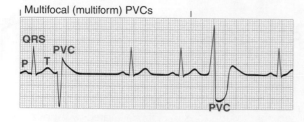

Multifocal (multiform) PVCs

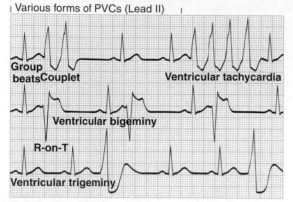

Various forms of PVCs (Lead II)

Group beats Couplet Ventricular tachycardia

Ventricular bigeminy

R-on-T

Ventricular trigeminy

FIGURE 4-4 Premature ventricular contractions (PVCs). (From Lewis SM, Heitkemper MM, Dirksen SR: *Medical-surgical nursing: Assessment and management of clinical problems,* ed 7. St. Louis, 2007, Mosby.)

b. Symptoms
  (1) Dyspnea
  (2) Orthopnea
  (3) "Wet" lung sounds
  (4) Cough
  (5) Fatigue
  (6) Tachycardia
  (7) Anxiety
  (8) Restlessness
  (9) Confusion
2. Right-sided heart failure: peripheral edema (right ventricular failure)
  a. Description: Results in peripheral congestion due to the inability of the right ventricle to pump blood out to the lungs; often results from left-sided failure or pulmonary disease
  b. Symptoms
    (1) Peripheral edema
    (2) Weight gain
    (3) Distended neck veins
    (4) Anorexia, nausea
    (5) Nocturia
    (6) Weakness
B. Enlargement of ventricles as indicated by chest radiograph

> **HESI Hint** • Restricting sodium reduces salt and water retention, thereby reducing vascular volume and preload.

Analysis (Nursing Diagnoses)

A. *Decreased cardiac output* related to…
B. *Impaired urinary elimination* related to…
C. *Activity intolerance* related to…
D. *Anxiety* related to…
E. *Ineffective tissue perfusion* related to…

Nursing Plans and Interventions

A. Monitor vital signs at least every 4 hours for changes.
B. Monitor apical heart rate with vital signs to detect dysrhythmias, S3 or S4.
C. Assess for hypoxia.
  1. Restlessness
  2. Tachycardia
  3. Angina
D. Auscultate lungs for indication of pulmonary edema (wet sounds or crackles).
E. Administer O_2 as needed.
F. Elevate head of bed to assist with breathing.
G. Observe for signs of edema.
  1. Weigh daily.
  2. Monitor I&O.
  3. Measure abdominal girth; observe ankles and fingers.
H. Limit sodium intake.
I. Elevate lower extremities while sitting.
J. Check apical heart rate prior to administration of digitalis; withhold medication and call physician if rate is <60 bpm (Table 4-18).
K. Administer diuretics in the morning if possible (see Table 4-14).
L. Provide periods of rest after periods of activity.

INFLAMMATORY AND INFECTIOUS HEART DISEASE

Description: Inflammatory and infectious process involving the endocardium and pericardium

A. Endocarditis is an inflammatory disease involving the inner surface of the heart, including the valves. Organisms travel through the blood to the heart, where vegetations adhere to the valve surface or endocardium and can break off and become emboli.
B. Causes of endocarditis
  1. Rheumatic heart disease
  2. Congenital heart disease
  3. IV drug abuse
  4. Cardiac surgery
  5. Immunosuppression

TABLE 4-18 Digitalis Preparations

Drugs	Indications	Adverse Reactions	Nursing Implications
• Digitoxin (Crystodigin, Purodigin) • Digoxin (Lanoxin, Lanoxicaps)	• HF • Increases the contractility of cardiac muscle • Slows heart rate and conduction	• Severe: AV block • Headache • Dysrhythmias • Nausea • Vomiting • Blurred vision • Yellow-green halos • Hypotension • Fatigue	• Monitor serum electrolytes; hypokalemia increases risk for digoxin toxicity • Monitor serum digitalis levels if any side effects are present • Check apical pulse prior to administration; call health care provider if rate is <60 bpm • Teach client to take radial pulse prior to administration and call health care provider if <60 bpm in adults • Therapeutic range: 0.5 to 2 mg
• Digoxin-immune Fab (Digibind)	• Antidote for digitalis toxicity • Binds with digitoxin or digoxin to prevent binding at their site of action	• Decreased cardiac output • Atrial tachydysrhythmias • Use with caution in children and older adults	• Use with 0.22-μm filter • Place client on continuous cardiac monitor • Have resuscitation equipment at bedside before giving first dose

HESI Hint • DIGITALIS
- Side effects of digitalis are increased when the client is hypokalemic.
- Digitalis has a negative chronotropic effect (i.e., it slows the heart rate). Hold the digitalis if the pulse rate is <60 or >120 bpm (<90 bpm in an infant) or has markedly changed rhythm.
- Bradycardia, tachycardia, and dysrhythmias may be signs of digitalis toxicity; these signs include nausea, vomiting, and headache in adults.
- If withheld, consult with physician.

6. Dental procedures
7. Invasive procedures

C. Pericarditis is an inflammation of the outer lining of the heart.

D. Causes of pericarditis
1. MI
2. Trauma
3. Neoplasm
4. Connective tissue disease
5. Heart surgery
6. Idiopathic
7. Infections

Nursing Assessment

A. Endocarditis
1. Fever
2. Chills, malaise, night sweats, fatigue
3. Murmurs
4. Symptoms of heart failure
5. Atrial embolization

B. Pericarditis
1. Pain: sudden, sharp, severe:
   a. Substernal, radiating to the back or arm
   b. Aggravated by coughing, inhalation, deep breathing
   c. Relieved by leaning forward
2. Pericardial friction rub
3. Fever

HESI Hint • Infective endocarditis damage to heart valves occurs with the growth of vegetative lesions on valve leaflets. These lesions pose a risk for embolization, erosion or perforation of the valve leaflets, or abscesses within adjacent myocardial tissue. Valvular stenosis or regurgitation (insufficiency), most commonly of the mitral valve, can occur, depending on the type of damage inflicted by the lesions, and can lead to symptoms of left- or right-sided heart failure (see Valvular Heart Disease, p. 106, and Heart Failure, p. 101).

HESI Hint • ACUTE AND SUBACUTE INFECTIVE ENDOCARDITIS
There are two types of infective endocarditis: acute, which often affects individuals with previously normal hearts and healthy valves and carries a high mortality rate; and subacute, which typically affects individuals with preexisting conditions, such as rheumatic heart disease, mitral valve prolapse, or immunosuppression. Intravenous drug abusers are at risk for both acute and subacute bacterial endocarditis. When this population develops subacute infective endocarditis, the valves on the right side of the heart (tricuspid and pulmonic) are typically affected because of the introduction of common pathogens that colonize the skin (*Staphylococcus epidermis* or *Candida* sp.) into the venous system.

HESI Hint • PERICARDITIS
The presence of a friction rub is an indication of pericarditis (inflammation of the lining of the heart). ST-segment elevation and T-wave inversion are also signs of pericarditis.

Analysis (Nursing Diagnoses)

A. *Decreased cardiac output* related to…
B. *Risk for injury: emboli* related to…

Nursing Plans and Interventions

A. Endocarditis
   1. Monitor hemodynamic status (vital signs, level of consciousness, urinary output).
   2. Administer antibiotics IV for 4 to 6 weeks. The American Heart Association recommends administration of erythromycin before dental or genitourinary procedures. Clients may be instructed in IV therapy for home health care.
   3. Teach clients about anticoagulant therapy if prescribed.
   4. Encourage client to maintain good hygiene.
   5. Instruct client to inform dentist and other health care providers of history.
B. Pericarditis
   1. Provide rest and maintain position of comfort.
   2. Administer analgesics and antiinflammatory drugs.

VALVULAR HEART DISEASE

Description: Heart valves that are unable to open fully (stenosis) or close fully (insufficiency or regurgitation)

A. Valve dysfunction most commonly occurs on the left side of the heart; the mitral valve is most commonly involved, followed by the aortic valve.

HESI Hint • In mitral valve stenosis, blood is regurgitated back into the left atrium from the left ventricle. In the early period, there may be no symptoms, but as the disease progresses, the client will exhibit excessive fatigue, dyspnea on exertion, orthopnea, dry cough, hemoptysis, or pulmonary edema. There will be a rumbling apical diastolic murmur, and atrial fibrillation is common.

B. Common causes of valvular disease
   1. Rheumatic fever
   2. Congenital heart diseases
   3. Syphilis
   4. Endocarditis
   5. Hypertension
C. Prevention of rheumatic heart disease would reduce the incidence of valvular heart disease.

Nursing Assessment

A. Fatigue
B. Dyspnea, orthopnea
C. Hemoptysis and pulmonary edema
D. Murmurs
E. Irregular cardiac rhythm
F. Angina

Analysis (Nursing Diagnoses)

A. *Decreased cardiac output* related to…
B. *Impaired gas exchange* related to…
C. *Activity intolerance* related to…

Nursing Plans and Interventions

A. See Heart Failure, p. 101.
B. Monitor client for atrial fibrillation with thrombus formation.
C. Teach the necessity for prophylactic antibiotic therapy before any invasive procedure, such as dental procedures, that is likely to produce gingival or mucosal bleeding: bronchoscopy, esophageal dilation, upper endoscopy, colonoscopy, sigmoidoscopy, or cystoscopy.
D. Prepare the client for surgical repair or replacement of heart valves.
E. Instruct clients receiving valve replacement of the need for lifelong anticoagulant therapy to prevent thrombus formation.

Review of Cardiovascular System

1. How do clients experiencing angina describe that pain?
2. Develop a teaching plan for a client taking nitroglycerin.
3. List the parameters of blood pressure for diagnosing hypertension.
4. Differentiate between essential and secondary hypertension.
5. Develop a teaching plan for a client taking antihypertensive medications.
6. Describe intermittent claudication.
7. Describe the nurse's discharge instructions to a client with venous peripheral vascular disease.
8. What is often the underlying cause of an abdominal aortic aneurysm?
9. What lab values should be monitored daily in a client with thrombophlebitis who is undergoing anticoagulant therapy?
10. When do PVCs (premature ventricular contractions) present a grave danger?
11. Differentiate between the symptoms of left-sided cardiac failure and right-sided cardiac failure.
12. List three symptoms of digitalis toxicity.
13. What condition increases the likelihood that digitalis toxicity will occur?
14. What lifestyle changes can the client who is at risk for hypertension initiate to reduce the likelihood of becoming hypertensive?
15. What immediate actions should the nurse implement when a client is having a myocardial infarction?
16. What symptoms should the nurse expect to find in a client with hypokalemia?
17. Bradycardia is defined as a heart rate below _____ bpm. Tachycardia is defined as a heart rate above _____ bpm.
18. What precautions should clients with valve disease take prior to invasive procedures or dental work?

Answers to Review

1. Described as squeezing, heavy, burning, radiates to left arm or shoulder, transient or prolonged
2. Take at first sign of anginal pain. Take no more than three, 5 minutes apart. Call for emergency attention if no relief in 10 minutes.
3. >140/90
4. Essential hypertension has no known cause; secondary hypertension develops in response to an identifiable mechanism.
5. Explain how and when to take medication, reason for medication, necessity of compliance, need for follow-up visits while on medication, need for certain lab tests, and vital sign parameters while initiating therapy.
6. Pain related to peripheral vascular disease; the pain occurs with exercise and disappears with rest.
7. Keep extremities elevated when sitting, rest at first sign of pain, keep extremities warm (but do not use heating pad), change position often, avoid crossing legs, wear unrestrictive clothing.
8. Atherosclerosis
9. PTT, PT, Hgb, Hct, platelets
10. When they begin to occur more often than once in 10 beats, occur in twos or threes, land near the T wave, or take on multiple configurations
11. Left-sided failure results in pulmonary congestion due to backup of circulation in the left ventricle. Right-sided failure results in peripheral congestion due to backup of circulation in the right ventricle.
12. Dysrhythmias, headache, nausea, and vomiting
13. Hypokalemia (which is more common when diuretics and digitalis preparations are given together)
14. Cease cigarette smoking, if applicable; control weight, exercise regularly, and maintain a low-fat, low-cholesterol diet.
15. Place the client on immediate strict bed rest to lower O_2 demands on heart; administer O_2 by nasal cannula at 2 to 5 L/min; take measures to alleviate pain and anxiety (administer PRN pain medications and antianxiety medications).
16. Dry mouth and thirst, drowsiness and lethargy, muscle weakness and aches, and tachycardia
17. 60 bpm; 100 bpm
18. Take prophylactic antibiotics.

Gastrointestinal System

HIATAL HERNIA AND GASTROESOPHA-GEAL REFLUX DISEASE (GERD)

A. Hiatal hernia is a herniation of the esophagogastric junction and a portion of the stomach into the chest through the esophageal hiatus of the diaphragm.
   1. Sliding hernia is the most common type, accounting for 75% to 90% of adult hiatal hernias.
B. GERD is the result of an incompetent lower esophageal sphincter that allows regurgitation of acidic gastric contents into the esophagus.

1. Multiple factors determine whether GERD is present.
   a. Efficiency of antireflux mechanism
   b. Volume of gastric contents
   c. Potency of refluxed material
   d. Efficiency of esophageal clearance
   e. Resistance of the esophageal tissue to injury and the ability to repair tissue
2. The client must have several episodes of reflux for GERD to be present.

Nursing Assessment

A. Heartburn after eating that radiates to arms and shoulders
B. Feeling of fullness and discomfort after eating
C. Positive diagnosis determined by fluoroscopy or barium swallow, gastroscopy

Analysis (Nursing Diagnoses)

A. *Acute pain* related to...
B. *Deficient knowledge* (specify) related to...
C. *Anxiety* related to...

Nursing Plans and Interventions

A. Determine an eating pattern that alleviates symptoms.
   1. Encourage small, frequent meals.
   2. Encourage elimination of foods that are determined to aggravate symptoms (these foods are client-specific but can include caffeine, catsup, strawberries, and chocolate).
   3. Encourage client to sit up while eating and remain in an upright position for at least 1 hour after eating.
   4. Encourage client to stop eating 3 hours before bedtime.
   5. Elevate the head of the bed on blocks.
   6. Teach about commonly prescribed medications (H$_2$ antagonists, antacids).

HESI Hint • A Fowler or semi-Fowler position is beneficial in reducing the amount of regurgitation as well as in preventing the encroachment of the stomach tissue upward through the opening in the diaphragm.

B. Teaching plan for client and family should include the following:
   1. Differentiate between the symptoms of hiatal hernia and those of MI.
   2. Be alert to the possibility of aspiration.
   3. Information about drugs used for treatment (Table 4-19).

PEPTIC ULCER DISEASE (PUD)

Description: Ulceration that penetrates the mucosal wall of the GI tract

A. Gastric ulcers tend to occur in the lesser curvature of the stomach.
B. Duodenal ulcers occur in the duodenum.
C. Esophageal ulcers occur in the esophagus.
D. The cause of some peptic ulcer disease is unknown. A significant number of gastric ulcers are caused by a bacterium, *Helicobacter pylori* (*H. pylori*), and can be successfully treated by drug therapy. Risk factors for the development of peptic ulcers include:
   1. Drugs (NSAIDs, corticosteroids)
   2. Alcohol
   3. Cigarette smoking
   4. Acute medical crisis or trauma
E. Symptoms common to all types of ulcers include the following:
   1. Belching
   2. Bloating
   3. Epigastric pain radiating to the back (not associated with the type of food eaten) and relieved by antacids

Nursing Assessment

A. Determine how food intake affects pain.
B. Take history of antacid or histamine antagonist use.
C. Determine presence of melena.
D. Determine presence and location of peptic ulcer as determined by:
   1. Barium swallow
   2. Upper endoscopy
   3. Gastric analysis indicating increased levels of stomach acid
E. Potential complications
   1. Hemorrhage
   2. Perforation (which always requires surgery)
   3. Obstruction

Analysis (Nursing Diagnoses)

A. *Acute pain* related to...
B. *Imbalanced nutrition: less than body requirements* related to...
C. *Deficient knowledge* related to...
D. *Risk for injury* related to...

Nursing Plans and Interventions

A. Determine symptom onset and how symptoms are relieved.
B. Monitor color, quantity, consistency of stools and emesis, and test for occult blood.

TABLE 4-19 Antiulcer Drugs

Drugs	Indications	Adverse Reactions	Nursing Implications
Antacids			
• Aluminum hydroxide/ Magnesium hydroxide (Maalox, Mylanta, Riopan, Gelusil II)	• Treatment of peptic ulcers • Work by neutralizing or reducing acidity of stomach contents • Differences in absorption rate	• Constipation • Diarrhea • Drug interactions	• Need to take several times a day • Administer after meals • Assess for history of renal diseases when client is taking magnesium products; electrolyte readjustment occurs and can result in renal insufficiency and calcinosis
Histamine₂ Antagonists			
• Ranitidine HCl (Zantac) • Cimetidine (Tagamet) • Famotidine (Pepcid) • Nizatidine (Axid)	• Treatment of peptic ulcers • Prophylactic treatment for clients at risk for developing ulcers (those on steroids or highly stressed)	• Multiple drug interactions	• Cigarette smoking interferes with drug action • Expensive
Mucosal Healing Agents			
• Sucralfate (Carafate)	• Treatment of peptic ulcers	• Constipation • Drug interaction with: • tetracycline • phenytoin sodium • digoxin • cimetidine	• Medication to be taken at least 1 hour before meals • Antacids interfere with absorption
Proton Pump Inhibitors			
• Lansoprazole (Prevacid) (PO only) • Pantoprazole (Protonix) (available PO and IV) • Esomeprazole (Nexium) (PO only) • Omeprazole (Prilosec) • Rabeprazole (Aciphex)	• Treatment of erosive esophagitis associated with GERD	• Constipation • Heartburn • Anxiety • Diarrhea • Abdominal pain, hepatocellular damage, pancreatitis, gastroenteritis • Tinnitus, vertigo, confusion, headache • Blurred vision, hypokinesia • Chest pain, dyspnea	• Taken before meals • Do not crush or chew Pantoprazole IV: • Resume oral therapy as soon as feasible • Long-lasting effects of drug may inhibit absorption of other drugs • Not removed by hemodialysis • Monitor for indications of adverse reactions
Additional Drugs			
• Prokinetic agents • Antimetics • Cough suppressants • Stool softeners	• Treatment of slow peristalsis and increased intraabdominal pressure in clients with GERD	• Diarrhea	• Monitor for indications of adverse reactions

C. Administer medications as prescribed, usually 1 to 2 hours after meals and at bedtime (see Table 4-19).

D. Administer mucosal healing agents at least 1 hour before meals, as prescribed (see Table 4-19).

E. Encourage small, frequent meals; no bedtime snacks; and avoidance of beverages containing caffeine.

F. Prepare client for surgery if uncontrolled bleeding, obstruction, or perforation occurs.
1. Gastric resection
2. Vagotomy
3. Pyloroplasty

G. Teach client that dumping syndrome may occur postoperatively.
1. Secondary to rapid entry of hypertonic food into jejunum (pulls water out of bloodstream)
2. Occurs 5 to 30 minutes after eating
3. Characterized by vertigo, syncope, sweating, pallor, tachycardia
4. Minimized by small, frequent meals: high-protein, high-fat, low-carbohydrate diet
5. Exacerbated by consuming liquids with meals; helped by lying down after eating
6. Can also be observed in clients on hypertonic tube feeding

H. Teach client to avoid medications that increase the risk for developing peptic ulcers.
1. Salicylates
2. NSAIDs such as ibuprofen
3. Corticosteroids in high doses
4. Reserpine (antihypertensive)
5. Anticoagulants

I. Teach client the importance of informing all health care personnel of ulcer history.

J. Teach client symptoms of GI bleeding.
1. Dark, tarry stools
2. Coffee-ground emesis
3. Bright-red rectal bleeding
4. Fatigue
5. Pallor
6. Severe abdominal pain, which should be reported immediately (could denote perforation)

K. Teach client importance of smoking cessation and stress management.

> **HESI Hint** • Stress can cause or exacerbate ulcers. Teach stress-reduction methods, and encourage those with a family history of ulcers to obtain medical surveillance for ulcer formation.

> **HESI Hint** • Clinical manifestations of GI bleeding:
> • Pallor: conjunctival, mucous membranes, nail beds
> • Dark, tarry stools
> • Bright-red or coffee-ground emesis
> • Abdominal mass or bruit
> • Decreased BP, rapid pulse, cool extremities (shock), increased respirations

INFLAMMATORY BOWEL DISEASES

Description: Consists of Crohn disease and ulcerative colitis

Crohn Disease (Regional Enteritis)

Description: Subacute, chronic inflammation extending throughout the entire intestinal mucosa (most commonly found in terminal ileum) with periods of remission interspersed with periods of exacerbation. Crohn disease occurs during the teenage years and early adulthood but has a second peak in the sixth decade. Capsule endoscopy has shown greater sensitivity than radiography when diagnosing Crohn disease. There is no known cause and no cure, so treatment relies on medications to treat the acute inflammation and maintain a remission. Surgery is reserved for patients who are unresponsive to medications or who develop life-threatening complications. In a total proctocolectomy (the colon and rectum are removed and the anus is closed), the terminal ileum is brought through the abdominal wall, and a permanent ileostomy is formed.

Nursing Assessment

A. Abdominal pain (unrelieved by defecation)

B. Diarrhea, steatorrhea (fatty diarrheal stools), and weight loss, with client becoming emaciated

C. Constant fluid loss

D. Low-grade fever

E. Perforation of the intestine occurring due to severe inflammation; constitutes a medical emergency

Analysis (Nursing Diagnoses)

A. *Risk for deficient fluid volume* related to…

B. *Chronic pain* related to…

C. *Imbalanced nutrition: less than body requirements* related to…

Nursing Plans and Interventions

A. Determine bowel elimination pattern, and control diarrhea with diet and medication as indicated.

B. Provide a nutritious, well-balanced, low-residue, low-fat, high-protein, high-calorie diet, with no dairy products.

C. Administer vitamin supplements and iron.

D. Advise client to avoid foods that are known to cause diarrhea, such as milk products and spicy foods.

E. Advise client to avoid smoking, caffeinated beverages, pepper, and alcohol.

F. Provide complete bowel rest with IV hyperalimentation if necessary.

G. Administer medications as prescribed: aminosalicylates, antimicrobials, corticosteroids, immunosuppressants, and biologic therapy

H. Monitor I&O and serum electrolytes.

I. Weigh at least twice a week.

J. Provide emotional support, and encourage use of support groups such as the Crohn's and Colitis Foundation of America.

K. Encourage client to talk with the enterostomal therapists before surgery.

L. If ileostomy is performed, teach stoma care (see Stoma Care, p. 114).

> **HESI Hint** • The GI tract usually accounts for only 100 to 200 ml of fluid loss per day, although it filters up to 8 L per day. Large fluid losses can occur if vomiting or diarrhea exists.

Ulcerative Colitis

Description: Disease that affects the superficial mucosa of the colon, causing the bowel to eventually narrow, shorten, and thicken due to muscular hypertrophy; occurs in the large bowel and rectum. Sigmoidoscopy and colonoscopy allow direct examination of the large intestine mucosa and are used for diagnosis of ulcerative colitis.

Nursing Assessment

A. Diarrhea

B. Abdominal pain and cramping

C. Intermittent tenesmus (anal contractions) and rectal bleeding

D. Liquid stools containing blood, mucus, and pus (may pass 10 to 20 liquid stools per day)

E. Weakness and fatigue

F. Anemia

Analysis (Nursing Diagnoses)

A. *Risk for deficient fluid volume* related to…

B. *Acute pain* related to…

C. *Imbalanced nutrition: less than body requirements* related to…

Nursing Plans and Interventions

A. Determine bowel elimination pattern, and control diarrhea with diet and medication as indicated.

B. Provide a nutritious, well-balanced, low-residue, low-fat, high-protein, high-calorie diet, with no dairy products.

C. Administer vitamin supplements and iron.

D. Advise client to avoid foods that are known to cause diarrhea, such as milk products and spicy foods.

E. Advise client to avoid smoking, caffeinated beverages, pepper, and alcohol.

F. Provide complete bowel rest with IV hyperalimentation if necessary.

G. Administer medications as prescribed, often steroids, antidiarrheals, sulfasalazine (Azulfidine).

H. Monitor I&O and serum electrolytes.

I. Weigh at least twice a week.

J. Provide emotional support, and encourage use of support groups such as the local Ileitis and Colitis Foundation.

K. Encourage client to talk with the enterostomal therapists before surgery.

L. If ileostomy is performed, teach stoma care (see Stoma Care, p. 114).

> **HESI Hint** • Opiate drugs tend to depress gastric motility. However, they should be given with care, and those receiving them should be closely monitored because a distended intestinal wall accompanied by decreased muscle tone may lead to intestinal perforation.

Diverticular Diseases

Description: Manifested in two clinical forms: diverticulosis and diverticulitis

A. Diverticulosis: bulging pouches in the GI wall (diverticula), which push the mucosa lining through the surrounding muscle

B. Diverticulitis: inflamed diverticula, which may cause obstruction, infection, and hemorrhage

> **HESI Hint** • Diverticulosis is the presence of pouches in the wall of the intestine. There is usually no discomfort, and the problem goes unnoticed unless seen on radiologic examination (usually prompted by some other condition). Diverticulitis is an inflammation of the diverticula (pouches), which can lead to perforation of the bowel.

Nursing Assessment

A. Left lower quadrant pain

B. Increased flatus

C. Rectal bleeding

D. Signs of intestinal obstruction:
1. Constipation alternating with diarrhea
2. Abdominal distention
3. Anorexia
4. Low-grade fever

E. Barium enema or colonoscopy positive for diverticular disease: obstruction, ileus, or perforation confirmed by abdominal radiograph (barium not used during acute phase of illness)

Analysis (Nursing Diagnoses)

A. *Ineffective tissue perfusion* related to…

B. *Acute pain* related to…

C. *Imbalanced nutrition: less than body requirements* related to…

Nursing Plans and Interventions

A. Provide a well-balanced, high-fiber diet unless inflammation is present, in which case client is NPO, followed by low-residue bland foods.

HESI Hint • A client admitted with complaints of severe lower abdominal pain, cramping, and diarrhea is diagnosed as having diverticulitis. What are the nutritional needs of this client throughout recovery?
• Acute phase: NPO, graduating to liquids
• Recovery phase: no fiber or foods that irritate the bowel
• Maintenance phase: high-fiber diet with bulk-forming laxatives to prevent pooling of foods in the pouches where they can become inflamed; avoidance of small, poorly digested foods such as popcorn, nuts, seeds, etc.

B. Include bulk-forming laxatives such as Metamucil in daily regimen.

C. Increase fluid intake to 3 L/day.

D. Monitor I&O and bowel elimination; avoid constipation.

E. Observe for complications.
1. Obstruction
2. Peritonitis
3. Hemorrhage (With ruptured diverticula, a temporary colostomy is performed and maintained for approximately 3 months to allow the bowel to rest.)
4. Infection

INTESTINAL OBSTRUCTION

Description: Partial or complete blockage of intestinal flow (fluids, feces, gas)

A. Mechanical causes of intestinal obstruction
1. Adhesions (most common cause).
2. Hernia (strangulates the gut).
3. Volvulus (twisting of the gut).
4. Intussusception (telescoping of the gut within itself).
5. Tumors; develop slowly; usually a mass of feces becomes lodged against the tumor

B. Neurogenic causes of intestinal obstruction
1. Paralytic ileus (usually occurs in postoperative clients)
2. Spinal cord lesion

C. Vascular cause of intestinal obstruction
1. Mesenteric artery occlusion (leads to gut infarct)

HESI Hint • BOWEL OBSTRUCTIONS
• Mechanical: Due to disorders outside the bowel (hernia, adhesions) caused by disorders within the bowel (tumors, diverticulitis) or by blockage of the lumen in the intestine (intussusception, gallstone)
• Nonmechanical: Due to paralytic ileus, which does not involve any actual physical obstruction but results from inability of the bowel itself to function

Nursing Assessment

A. Sudden onset of abdominal pain, tenderness, or guarding

B. History of abdominal surgeries

C. History of obstruction

D. Distention

E. Increased peristalsis when obstruction first occurs, then peristalsis becoming absent when paralytic ileus occurs

F. Bowel sounds that are high pitched with early mechanical obstruction and diminishes to absent with neurogenic or late mechanical obstruction

Analysis (Nursing Diagnoses)

A. *Impaired tissue perfusion* related to…

B. *Deficient volume* related to…

C. *Acute pain* related to…

HESI Hint • Blood gas analysis will show an alkalotic state if the bowel obstruction is high in the small intestine where gastric acid is secreted. If the obstruction is in the lower bowel where base solutions are secreted, the blood will be acidic.

Nursing Plans and Interventions

A. Maintain client NPO, with IV fluids and electrolyte therapy.

B. Monitor I&O; a Foley catheter maintains strict output.

C. Implement NG intubation.
1. Attach to low suction (intermittent 80 mm Hg).
2. Document output every 8 hours.
3. Irrigate with normal saline if policy dictates.

D. NG tube, Cantor, Miller-Abbott, or Harris tubes are passed through the nose and into the stomach, usually by the health care provider.
1. Advance tube every 1 to 2 hours.
2. Do not secure to nose until tube reaches specified position.
3. Reposition client every 2 hours to assist with placement of the tube.
4. Connect to suction.
5. Irrigate with air only.
6. Note amount, color, consistency, and any unusual odor of drainage.

E. Document pain; medicate as prescribed.

F. Assess abdomen regularly for distention, rigidity, change in status of bowel sounds.

G. If conservative medical interventions fail, surgery will be required to remove obstruction (see Perioperative Care, p. 49).

HESI Hint • A client admitted with complaints of constipation, thready stools, and rectal bleeding over the past few months is diagnosed with a rectal mass. What are the nursing priorities for this client?
- NPO
- NG tube (possibly an intestinal tube such as a Miller-Abbott)
- IV fluids
- Surgical preparations of bowel (if obstruction is complete)
- Foods and fluids are restricted for 8 to 10 hours before surgery if possible.
- If the patient has a bowel obstruction or perforation, bowel cleansing is contraindicated.
- Oral erythromycin and neomycin are given to further decrease the amount of colonic and rectal bacteria.
- If possible, all clients who require surgery for obstruction undergo NG intubation and suction before surgery. However, in cases of complete obstruction, surgery should proceed without delay
- Teaching (preoperative nutrition, etc.)

COLORECTAL CANCER

Description: Tumors occurring in the colon

A. Cancer of the colon is the fourth most common cancer in the United States.

B. This is second leading cause of cancer-related deaths in the United States.

C. Approximately 45% of cancerous tumors of the colon occur in the rectal or sigmoid area, 25% in the cecum and ascending colon, and 30% in the remainder of colon.

D. The highest incidence occurs in persons over 50 years of age.

E. A diet of high-fiber, low-fat foods, including cruciferous vegetables, may be a factor in prevention of colon cancer.

HESI Hint • Diet recommended by the American Cancer Society to prevent bowel cancer:
- Eat more cruciferous vegetables (those from the cabbage family, such as broccoli, cauliflower, Brussels sprouts, cabbage, and kale).
- Increase fiber intake.
- Maintain average body weight.
- Eat less animal fat.

F. Early detection is important.

HESI Hint • American Cancer Society recommendations for early detection of colon cancer:
- A digital rectal examination every year after 40.
- A stool blood test every year after 50.
- A colonoscopy or sigmoidoscopy examination every 3 to 5 years after the age of 50, based on the advice of a physician.

G. Usual treatment is surgical removal of the tumor, with adjuvant radiation or antineoplastic chemotherapy.

H. Diagnosis is made by digital examination, flexible fiberoptic sigmoidoscopy with biopsy, colonoscopy, and barium enema.

I. Carcinoembryonic antigen (CEA) serum level is used to evaluate effectiveness of chemotherapy.

Nursing Assessment

A. Rectal bleeding

B. Change in bowel habits

C. Sense of incomplete evacuation

D. Abdominal pain, nausea, vomiting

E. Weight loss, cachexia

F. Abdominal distention or ascites

G. Family history of cancer, particularly cancer of the colon

H. History of polyps

Analysis (Nursing Diagnoses)

A. *Deficient knowledge* related to…

B. *Ineffective coping* (specify) related to…

C. *Disturbed body image* related to…

Nursing Plans and Interventions

A. Prepare client for surgery (see Perioperative Care, p. 49).

B. Prepare client for bowel preparation, which may include laxatives and gut lavage with polyethylene glycol (Golytely).

C. If colostomy has been performed, teach stoma care (see Stoma Care).

D. Provide high-calorie, high-protein diet.

E. Promote prevention of constipation with high-fiber diet.

F. Encourage early detection by screening with Hemoccult (guaiac) tests.

> **HESI Hint** • An early sign of colon cancer is rectal bleeding. Encourage patients 50 years of age or older and those with increased risk factors to be screened yearly with fecal occult blood testing. Routine colonoscopy at 50 is also recommended.

Stoma Care

A. General information
1. The more distal the stoma is, the greater is the chance for continence.
2. An ileostomy drains liquid material; peristomal skin is prone to breakdown by enzymes.
3. The lower the stoma's location is in the GI tract, the more solid, or formed, is the effluence (stoma drainage).
4. The greatest chance for continence is with a stoma created from the sigmoid colon on the left side of the abdomen.
5. Consultation with an enterostomal therapist is essential.

B. Preoperative care
1. Client and family must be informed about what to expect postoperatively:
   a. Proposed location of the stoma
   b. Approximate size

c. What it will look like (Provide a picture, if indicated.)
2. The family should be included in teaching, but it should be emphasized that the client is ultimately responsible for his or her own care.

C. Pouch care
1. Ostomates often wear pouches.
2. The adhesive-backed opening, designed to cover the stoma, should provide about ⅛-inch clearance from the stoma.
3. A rubber band or clip is used to secure the bottom of the pouch and prevent leakage.
4. A simple squirt bottle is used to remove effluence from the sides of the bag. Pouch system is changed every 3 to 7 days.
5. Clients should maintain an extra supply of pouches so that they never run out and should change the pouch when bowel is inactive.
6. Pouch should be emptied when one third to one half full.

D. Irrigation
1. Those with descending-colon colostomies can irrigate to provide control over effluence.
   a. Clients should irrigate at approximately the same time daily.
   b. Clients should use warm water (cold or hot water causes cramping).
   c. Clients should wash around stoma with lukewarm water and a mild soap.
   d. Commercial skin barriers may be purchased for home use.
2. Odor control
   a. Commercial preparations are available.
   b. Foods in diet that cause offensive odors can be eliminated.

E. Diet
1. Ileostomy
   a. Clients should chew food thoroughly.
   b. High-fiber foods (popcorn, peanuts, unpeeled vegetables) can cause severe diarrhea and may have to be eliminated.
2. Colostomy
   a. Client should resume the regular diet gradually. Foods that were a problem preoperatively should be tried cautiously.

CIRRHOSIS

Description: Degeneration of liver tissue, causing enlargement, fibrosis, and scarring

A. Causes of cirrhosis include the following:
1. Chronic alcohol ingestion (Laennec cirrhosis)
2. Viral hepatitis
3. Exposure to hepatotoxins (including medications)
4. Infections

5. Congenital abnormalities
6. Chronic biliary tree obstruction
7. Chronic severe right-sided HF
8. Idiopathy
B. Initially, hepatomegaly occurs; later, the liver becomes hard and nodular.

Nursing Assessment

A. History of alcohol and street drug intake
B. Work history of exposure to toxic chemicals (pesticides, fumes, etc.)
C. Medication history of long-term use of hepatotoxic drugs
D. Family health history of liver abnormalities
E. Physical findings
1. Weakness, malaise
2. Anorexia, weight loss
3. Palpable liver (early); abdominal girth increases as liver enlarges
4. Jaundice
5. Fetor hepaticus (fruity or musty breath)

> **HESI Hint • CLINICAL MANIFESTATIONS OF JAUNDICE**
> • Yellow skin, sclera, or mucous membranes (bilirubin in skin)
> • Dark-colored urine (bilirubin in urine)
> • Chalky or clay-colored stools (absence of bilirubin in stools)

> **HESI Hint •** Fetor hepaticus is a distinctive breath odor of chronic liver disease. It is characterized by a fruity or musty odor that results from the damaged liver's inability to metabolize and detoxify mercaptan, which is produced by the bacterial degradation of methionine, a sulfurous amino acid.

6. Asterixis (hand-flapping tremor that often accompanies metabolic disorders)
7. Mental and behavioral changes
8. Bruising, erythema
9. Dry skin, spider angiomas
10. Gynecomastia (breast development), testicular atrophy
11. Ascites, peripheral neuropathy
12. Hematemesis
13. Palmar erythema (redness in palms of the hands)

> **HESI Hint •** For treatment of ascites, paracentesis and peritoneovenous shunts (La Veen and Denver shunts) may be indicated.

> **HESI Hint •** Esophageal varices may rupture and cause hemorrhage. Immediate management includes insertion of an esophagogastric balloon tamponade (a Blakemore-Sengstaken or Minnesota tube). Other therapies include vasopressors, vitamin K, coagulation factors, and blood transfusions.

F. Clotting defects noted in laboratory findings include:
1. Elevated bilirubin, AST, ALT, alkaline phosphatase, PT, and ammonia
2. Decreased Hgb, Hct, electrolytes, and albumin

> **HESI Hint •** Ammonia is not broken down as usual in the damaged liver; therefore, the serum ammonia level rises.
> The metabolism of drugs is slowed down so they remain in the system longer.

G. Complications include:
1. Ascites, edema
2. Portal hypertension
3. Esophageal varices
4. Encephalopathy
5. Respiratory distress
6. Coagulation defects

Analysis (Nursing Diagnoses)

A. *Excess fluid volume* related to…
B. *Risk for injury (bleeding)* related to…
C. *Pain* related to…
D. *Ineffective breathing pattern* related to…
E. *Imbalanced nutrition: less than body requirement* related to…
F. *Risk for infection* related to…

Nursing Plans and Interventions

A. Eliminate causative agent (alcohol, hepatotoxin).
B. Administer vitamin supplements (A, B complex, C, K), and teach client and family the need for continuing these supplements.
C. Observe mental status frequently (at least every 2 hours); note any subtle changes.
D. Avoid initiating bleeding, and observe for bleeding tendencies.
1. Avoid injections whenever possible.
2. Use small-bore needles for IV insertion.
3. Maintain pressure to venipuncture sites for at least 5 minutes.
4. Use electric razor.
5. Provide a soft-bristle toothbrush, and encourage careful mouth care.

6. Check stools and emesis for frank or occult blood.
7. Prevent straining at stool.
   a. Administer stood softeners as prescribed.
   b. Provide high-fiber diet.
E. Provide special skin care.
   1. Avoid soap, rubbing alcohol, and perfumed products (are drying to the skin).
   2. Apply moisturizing lotion or baby oil frequently.
   3. Observe skin for any lesions, including scratch marks.
   4. Turn frequently, and provide lotion to exposed skin.
F. Monitor fluid and electrolyte status daily.
   1. I&O (accurate output measurement may require Foley catheter).
   2. Observe for edema, pulmonary edema.
   3. Measure abdominal girth (determines increase or decrease of ascites).
   4. Weigh daily (determines increase or decrease of edema and ascites).
   5. Restrict fluids to 1500 ml/day (may help to reduce edema and ascites).
G. Monitor dietary intake carefully, especially protein intake. Restrict protein if client has hepatic coma; otherwise, encourage foods with high biologic protein.
H. Explain dietary restrictions: low sodium, low potassium, low fat, high carbohydrate.
I. If encephalopathy is present, lactulose is used (Table 4-20).
J. If esophageal varices are present, esophagogastric balloon tamponade (Blakemore tube), sclerotherapy, and/or portal systemic shunts may be used for treatment.

HEPATITIS

Description: Widespread inflammation of liver cells, usually caused by a virus (Table 4-21)

Nursing Assessment

A. Known exposure to hepatitis

B. Recent transfusions or hemodialysis
C. Individuals at risk for contracting hepatitis
   1. Homosexual males
   2. IV drug users (disease transmitted by dirty needles)
   3. Those who have recently had ears pierced or had tattoos drawn (disease transmitted by dirty needles)
   4. Those living in crowded conditions
   5. Health care workers employed in high-risk areas
      a. Labs
      b. Emergency departments
      c. Critical care units
      d. Hemodialysis units
      e. Oncology
      f. Centers for care of the mentally challenged
D. Fatigue, malaise, weakness
E. Anorexia, nausea, and vomiting
F. Jaundice, dark urine, clay-colored stools
G. Myalgia (muscle aches), joint pain
H. Dull headaches, irritability, depression
I. Abdominal tenderness in right upper quadrant
J. Fever (with hepatitis A)
K. Elevations of liver enzymes (ALT, AST, alkaline phosphatase), bilirubin

Analysis (Nursing Diagnoses)

A. *Activity intolerance* related to...
B. *Imbalanced nutrition: less than body requirements* related to...
C. *Risk for infection* related to...

Nursing Plans and Interventions

A. Assess client's response to activity, and plan periods of rest after periods of activity.
B. Assist client with care as needed; encourage client to get help with daily activities at home (caring for children, preparing meals, etc.).
C. Provide high-calorie, high-carbohydrate diet with moderate fats and proteins.
   1. Serve small, frequent meals.

TABLE 4-20 Ammonia Detoxicant/Stimulant Laxative

Drug	Implications	Adverse Reactions	Nursing Implications
• Lactulose (Cephulac)	• Encephalopathy • Used to decrease ammonia levels and bowel pH	• Diarrhea	• Instruct client regarding need for medication • Observe for diarrhea • Monitor ammonia levels

TABLE 4-21 Comparison of Three Types of Hepatitis

Characteristics	Hepatitis A (Infectious Hepatitis)	Hepatitis B (Serum Hepatitis)	Hepatitis C (Non-A, Non-B Hepatitis)
• Source of infection	• Contaminated food • Contaminated water or shellfish	• Contaminated blood products • Contaminated needles or surgical instruments • Mother to child at birth	• Contaminated blood products • Contaminated needles; IV drug use • Dialysis
• Route of infection	• Oral • Fecal • Parenteral	• Parenteral • Oral • Fecal • Direct contact • Breast milk • Sexual contact	• Parenteral • Sexual contact
• Incubation period	• 15 to 50 days	• 14 to 180 days	• Average: 14 to 180 days
• Onset	• Abrupt	• Insidious	• Insidious
• Seasonal variation	• Autumn • Winter	• All year	• All year
• Age group affected	• Children • Young adults	• Any age	• Any age
• Vaccine	• Yes	• Yes	• No
• Inoculation	• Yes	• Yes	• Yes
• Potential for chronic liver disease	• No	• Yes	• Yes
• Immunity	• Yes	• Yes	• No

2. Provide vitamin supplements.
3. Provide foods the client prefers.

D. Administer antiemetics as needed.

HESI Hint: • PROVIDE AN ENVIRONMENT CONDUCIVE TO EATING
For clients who are anorexic or nauseated:
• Remove strong odors immediately; they can be offensive and increase nausea.
• Encourage client to sit up for meals; this can decrease the propensity to vomit.
• Serve small, frequent meals.
• Give antiemetic prior to eating.

E. Teach client importance of adhering to personal hygiene, using individual drinking and eating utensils, toothbrushes, and razors. Prevention of spread to others must be emphasized.

F. Teach client to avoid hepatotoxic substances such as alcohol, aspirin, acetaminophen, and sedatives.

HESI Hint • Liver tissue is destroyed by hepatitis. Rest and adequate nutrition are necessary for regeneration of the liver tissue being destroyed by the disease. Many drugs are metabolized in the liver, so drug therapy must be scrutinized carefully. Caution the client that recovery takes many months, and previously taken medications and/or over-the-counter drugs should not be resumed without the health care provider's directions.

PANCREATITIS

Description: Nonbacterial inflammation of the pancreas

A. Acute pancreatitis occurs when there is digestion of the pancreas by its own enzymes, primarily trypsin.

B. Alcohol ingestion and biliary tract disease are major causes of acute pancreatitis.

C. Chronic pancreatitis is a progressive, destructive disease that causes permanent dysfunction.

D. Long-term alcohol use is the major factor in chronic pancreatitis.

E. Alcohol consumption should be stopped when acute pancreatitis is suspected and consumption completely avoided in chronic pancreatitis.

Nursing Assessment

A. Acute pancreatitis
   1. Severe mid-epigastric pain radiating to back; usually related to excess alcohol ingestion or a fatty meal
   2. Abdominal guarding; rigid, boardlike abdomen
   3. Nausea and vomiting
   4. Elevated temperature, tachycardia, decreased BP
   5. Bluish discoloration of flanks (Grey Turner sign) or periumbilical area (Cullen sign)
   6. Elevated amylase, lipase, and glucose levels

B. Chronic pancreatitis
   1. Continuous burning or gnawing abdominal pain
   2. Ascites
   3. Steatorrhea, diarrhea
   4. Weight loss
   5. Jaundice, dark urine
   6. Signs and symptoms of diabetes mellitus

Analysis (Nursing Diagnoses)

A. *Acute pain* related to…

B. *Chronic pain* related to…

C. *Imbalanced nutrition: less than body requirements* related to…

D. *Deficient fluid volume* related to…

Nursing Plans and Interventions

A. Acute pancreatitis
   1. Maintain NPO status.
   2. Maintain NG tube to suction; TPN is given.
   3. Administer meperidine (Demerol) or morphine as needed.
   4. Administer antacids, histamine-H$_2$, receptor–blocking drugs, anticholinergics, proton pump inhibitors.
   5. Assist client to assume position of comfort on side with legs drawn up to chest.
   6. Teach client to avoid alcohol, caffeine, and fatty and spicy foods.
   7. If severe, blood sugar monitoring and regular insulin coverage may be needed temporarily.
   8. Monitor for neuromuscular manifestations of hypocalcemia (e.g., tetany, muscle twitching, cramping, grimacing, seizure, altered deep tendon reflexes, and spasm).

HESI Hint • Acute pancreatic pain is located retroperitoneally. Any enlargement of the pancreas causes the peritoneum to stretch tightly. Therefore, sitting up or leaning forward reduces the pain.

B. Chronic pancreatitis
   1. Administer analgesics such as meperidine or morphine (narcotic tolerance and dependency may be a problem).
   2. Administer pancreatic enzymes such as pancreatin (Creon) or pancrelipase (Viokase) with meals or snacks. Powdered forms should be mixed with fruit juice or applesauce (mixing with proteins should be avoided).
   3. Monitor client's stools for number and consistency to determine effectiveness of enzyme replacement.
   4. Teach client about consuming a bland low-fat diet and to avoid rich foods, alcohol, and caffeine.
   5. Monitor for signs and symptoms of diabetes mellitus.

CHOLECYSTITIS AND CHOLELITHIASIS

Description: Cholecystitis: acute inflammation of the gallbladder; cholelithiasis: formation or presence of stones in the gallbladder

A. Incidence of these diseases is greater in females who are multiparous and overweight.

B. Treatment for cholecystitis consists of IV hydration, administration of antibiotics, and pain control with meperidine or morphine.

C. Treatment for cholelithiasis consists of nonsurgical removal of stones.
   1. Dissolution therapy (administration of bile salts; used rarely)
   2. Endoscopic retrograde cholangiopancreatography (ERCP)
   3. Lithotripsy (not covered by many insurance carriers, thereby limiting its use)

D. Cholecystectomy is performed if stones are not removed nonsurgically and inflammation is absent. It may be done through laparoscope.

HESI Hint • Following an ERCP, the client may feel sick. The scope is placed in the gallbladder, and the stones are crushed and left to pass on their own. These clients may be prone to pancreatitis.

Nursing Assessment

A. Pain, anorexia, vomiting, or flatulence precipitated by ingestion of fried, spicy, or fatty foods

B. Fever, elevated WBCs, and other signs of infection (cholecystitis)
C. Abdominal tenderness
D. Jaundice and clay-colored stools (blockage)
E. Elevated liver enzymes, bilirubin, and WBCs

Analysis (Nursing Diagnoses)

A. *Acute pain* related to…
B. *Deficient knowledge* (specify) related to…

Nursing Plans and Interventions

A. Administer analgesic for pain as needed.
B. Maintain NPO status.
C. Maintain NG tube to suction if indicated.
D. Administer IV antibiotics for cholecystitis, and administer antibiotics prophylactically for cholelithiasis.

E. Monitor I&O.
F. Monitor electrolyte status regularly.
G. Teach client to avoid fried, spicy, and fatty foods and to reduce intake of calories if indicated.

HESI Hint • Nonsurgical management of a client with cholecystitis includes:
• Low-fat diet
• Medications for pain and clotting if required
• Decompression of the stomach via NG tube

H. Provide preoperative and postoperative care if surgery is indicated. (See Perioperative Care, p. 49.)
I. Monitor T-tube drainage.

Review of Gastrointestinal System

1. List four nursing interventions for the client with a hiatal hernia.
2. List three categories of medications used in the treatment of peptic ulcer disease.
3. List the symptoms of upper and lower GI bleeding.
4. What bowel sound disruptions occur with an intestinal obstruction?
5. List four nursing interventions for postoperative care of a client with a colostomy.
6. List the common clinical manifestations of jaundice.
7. What are the common food intolerances for clients with cholelithiasis?

8. List five symptoms indicative of colon cancer.
9. In a client with cirrhosis, it Is Imperative to prevent further bleeding and observe for bleeding tendencies. List six relevant nursing interventions.
10. What is the main side effect of lactulose, which is used to reduce ammonia levels in clients with cirrhosis?
11. List four groups who have a high risk for contracting hepatitis.
12. How should the nurse administer pancreatic enzymes?

Answers to Review

1. Sit up while eating and for 1 hour after eating. Eat frequent, small meals. Eliminate foods that are problematic.
2. Antacids, H₂ receptor blockers, mucosal healing agents, proton pump inhibitors
3. Upper GI: melena, hematemesis, tarry stools; lower GI: bloody stools, tarry stools; common to both: tarry stools
4. Early mechanical obstruction: high-pitched sounds; late mechanical obstruction: diminished or absent bowel sounds
5. Irrigate daily at same time; use warm water for irrigations; wash around stoma with mild soap and water after each ostomy bag change; ensure that pouch opening extends at least ⅛ inch around the stoma.
6. Sclera-icteric (yellow sclera), dark urine, chalky or clay-colored stools

7. Fried, spicy, and fatty foods
8. Rectal bleeding, change in bowel habits, sense of incomplete evacuation, abdominal pain with nausea, weight loss
9. Avoid injections; use small-bore needles for IV insertion; maintain pressure for 5 minutes on all venipuncture sites; use electric razor; use soft-bristle toothbrush for mouth care; check stools and emesis for occult blood.
10. Diarrhea
11. Homosexual males, IV drug users, those who have had recent ear piercing or tattooing, and health care workers
12. Give with meals or snacks. Powder forms should be mixed with fruit juices.

Endocrine System

HYPERTHYROIDISM (GRAVES DISEASE, GOITER)

Description: Excessive activity of thyroid gland, resulting in an elevated level of circulating thyroid hormones

A. Hyperthyroidism can result from a primary disease state; from the use of replacement hormone therapy; or from excess thyroid-stimulating hormone (TSH) being produced by an anterior pituitary tumor.

B. Graves disease is thought to be an autoimmune process.

C. Diagnosis is made on the basis of serum hormone levels.

D. Common treatment for hyperthyroidism
1. Thyroid ablation by medication
2. Radiation
3. Thyroidectomy
4. Adenectomy of portion of anterior pituitary where TSH-producing tumor is located

E. All treatments make the client hypothyroid, requiring hormone replacement.

Nursing Assessment

A. Enlarged thyroid gland

B. Acceleration of body processes
1. Weight loss
2. Increased appetite
3. Diarrhea
4. Heat intolerance
5. Tachycardia, palpitations, increased BP
6. Diaphoresis, wet or moist skin
7. Nervousness, insomnia

C. Exophthalmos (Fig. 4-5)

D. T_3 elevated above 220

E. T_4 elevated above 12

F. Low level of TSH indicates primary disease; elevated T_4 level suppresses thyroid-releasing hormone (TRH), which suppresses TSH secretion. If source is anterior pituitary, both will be elevated.

G. Radioactive iodine uptake (^{131}I) (indicates presence of goiter)

H. Thyroid scan (indicating presence of goiter)

Analysis (Nursing Diagnoses)

A. *Decreased cardiac output* related to...

B. *Deficient knowledge* (specify) related to...

C. *Imbalanced nutrition: less than body requirements* related to...

D. *Risk for injury* related to...

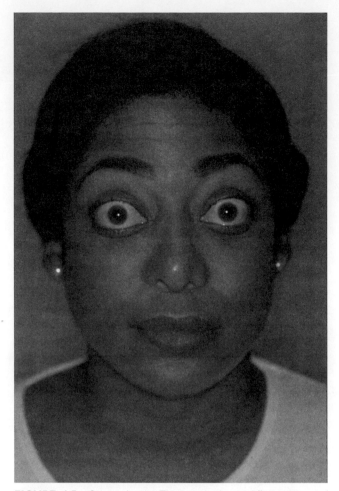

FIGURE 4-5 Graves disease. This woman has a diffuse goiter and exophthalmos. (From Lemmi FO, Lemmi CAE: *Physical assessment findings,* CD-ROM. Philadelphia, 2000, WB Saunders.)

Nursing Plans and Interventions

A. Provide a calm, restful atmosphere.

B. Observe for signs of thyroid storm (sudden oversecretion of thyroid hormone; is life-threatening).

HESI Hint • Thyroid storm is a life-threatening event that occurs with uncontrolled hyperthyroidism due to Graves disease. Symptoms include fever, tachycardia, agitation, anxiety, and hypertension. Primary nursing interventions include maintaining an airway and adequate aeration.

Propylthiouracil (PTU) and methimazole (Tapazole) are antithyroid drugs used to treat thyroid storm. Propranolol (Inderal) may be given to decrease excessive sympathetic stimulation.

C. Teach the following.
1. After treatment, resulting hypothyroidism will require daily hormone replacement.
2. Client should wear MedicAlert jewelry in case of emergency.

3. Signs of hormone-replacement overdosage are the signs for hyperthyroidism (see Nursing Assessment, Hyperthyroidism, p. 120).
4. Signs of hormone replacement underdosage are the signs for hypothyroidism (see Nursing Assessment, Hypothyroidism, p. 120).

D. Explain to client the recommended diet: high-calorie, high-protein, low-caffeine; low-fiber diet if diarrhea is present.
E. Perform eye care for exophthalmos.
   1. Artificial tears to maintain moisture
   2. Sunglasses when in bright light
   3. Annual eye examinations
F. Prepare client for treatment of hyperthyroidism.
   1. Thyroid ablation
      a. Propylthiouracil (PTU) and methimazole (Tapazole) act by blocking synthesis of T_3 and T_4.
      b. Dosage is calculated based on body weight and is given over several months.
      c. Client should take medication exactly as prescribed so that the desired effect can be achieved.
      d. The expected effect is to make the client euthyroid, often given to prepare the client for thyroidectomy.
   2. Radiation
      a. ^{131}I is given to destroy thyroid cells.
      b. ^{131} is very irritating to the GI tract.
      c. Clients commonly vomit (vomitus is radioactive).
      d. Place client on radiation precautions. Use time, distance, and shielding as means of protection against radiation (see Reproductive System, p. 166).
   3. Thyroidectomy

> **HESI Hint** • Postoperative thyroidectomy: Be prepared for the possibility of laryngeal edema. Put a tracheostomy set at the bedside along with O_2 and a suction machine; calcium gluconate should be easily accessible.

      a. Check frequently for bleeding.
      b. Support the neck when moving client (do not hyperextend).
      c. Check for laryngeal edema damage by watching for hoarseness or inability to speak clearly.
      d. Determine number of parathyroid glands that have been removed.
      e. Keep drainage devices compressed and empty.
   4. Adenectomy
      a. TSH-secreting pituitary tumors are resected using a transnasal approach (transsphenoidal hypophysectomy).

> **HESI Hint** • Normal serum calcium is 9.0 to 10.5 mEq/L. The best indicator of parathyroid problems is a decrease in the client's calcium compared to the preoperative value.

> **HESI Hint** • If two or more parathyroid glands have been removed, the chance of tetany increases dramatically:
> • Monitor serum calcium levels (9.0 to 10.5 mg/dl is normal range).
> • Check for tingling of toes and fingers and around the mouth.
> • Check Chvostek sign (twitching of lip after a tap over the parotid gland means it is positive; Fig. 4-6).
> • Check Trousseau sign (carpopedal spasm after BP cuff is inflated above systolic pressure means it is positive; see Fig. 4-6).

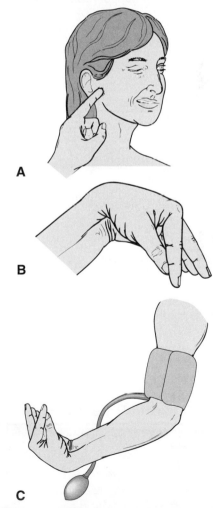

A

B

C

FIGURE 4-6   Tests for hypocalcemia. *A,* Chvostek sign is contraction of facial muscles in response to a light tap over the facial nerve in front of the ear. *B,* Trousseau sign is a carpal spasm induced by *C,* inflating a blood pressure cuff above the systolic pressure for a few minutes. (From Lewis SM, Heitkemper MM, Dirksen SR: *Medical-surgical nursing: Assessment and management of clinical problems,* ed 7. St Louis, 2007, Mosby.)

HYPOTHYROIDISM (HASHIMOTO DISEASE, MYXEDEMA)

Description: Hypofunction of the thyroid gland, with resulting insufficiency of thyroid hormone

A. Early symptoms of hypothyroidism are nonspecific but gradually intensify.

B. Hypothyroidism is treated by hormone replacement.

C. Endemic goiters occur in individuals living in areas where there is a deficit of iodine. Iodized salt has helped to prevent this problem.

> **HESI Hint** • Myxedema coma can be precipitated by acute illness, withdrawal of thyroid medication, anesthesia, use of sedatives, or hypoventilation (with the potential for respiratory acidosis and CO_2 narcosis). The airway must be kept patent and ventilator support used as indicated.

Nursing Assessment

A. Fatigue

B. Thin, dry hair; dry skin

C. Thick, brittle nails

D. Constipation

E. Bradycardia, hypotension

F. Goiter

G. Periorbital edema, facial puffiness

H. Cold intolerance

I. Weight gain

J. Dull emotions and mental processes

K. Diagnosis
1. Low T_3 (below 70)
2. Low T_4 (below 5)
3. Presence of T_4 antibody (indicating that T_4 is being destroyed by the body)

Analysis (Nursing Diagnoses)

A. *Deficient knowledge* related to…

B. *Noncompliance* related to…

C. *Activity intolerance* related to…

Nursing Plans and Interventions

A. Teach the following.
1. Medication regimen: daily dose of prescribed hormone
2. Medication effects and side effects (Table 4-22)
3. Ongoing follow-up to determine serum hormone levels
4. Signs and symptoms of myxedema coma (hypotension, hypothermia, hyponatremia, hypoglycemia, respiratory failure)

B. Develop a bowel-elimination plan to prevent constipation:
1. Fluid intake to be 3 L/day
2. High-fiber diet, including fresh fruits and vegetables
3. Increased activity
4. Little or no use of enemas and laxatives

C. Avoid sedating client; it can lead to respiratory difficulties.

ADDISON DISEASE (PRIMARY ADRENOCORTICAL DEFICIENCY)

Description: Autoimmune process commonly found in conjunction with other endocrine diseases of an autoimmune nature; a primary disorder

A. Sudden withdrawal from corticosteroids may precipitate symptoms of Addison disease (Table 4-23).

B. Addison disease is characterized by lack of cortisol, aldosterone, and androgens.

C. Definitive diagnosis is made using an ACTH stimulation test.

D. If ACTH production by the anterior pituitary has failed, it is considered secondary Addison disease.

TABLE 4-22 Thyroid Preparations

Drugs	Indications	Adverse Reactions	Nursing Implications
• Levothyroxine (Synthroid) • Liothyronine sodium (Cytomel) • Desiccated thyroid (Armour Thyroid)	• Action is to increase metabolic rates • Synthetic T_4	• Anxiety • Insomnia • Tremors • Tachycardia • Palpitations • Angina • Dysrhythmias	• Check serum hormone levels routinely • Check BP and pulse regularly • Weigh daily • Report side effects to health care provider • Avoid foods and products containing iodine • Initiate cautiously in clients with cardiovascular disease

TABLE 4-23 Corticosteroids

Drugs	Indications	Adverse Reactions	Nursing Implications
• Hydrocortisone • Prednisone • Dexamethasone	• Hormone replacement • Severe rheumatoid arthritis • Autoimmune disorders	• Emotional lability • Impaired wound healing • Skin fragility • Abnormal fat deposition • Hyperglycemia • Hirsutism • Moon face • Osteoporosis • All symptoms of Cushing syndrome if overdosage occurs	• Wean slowly (administer a high dose, then taper off); careful monitoring is required during withdrawal • Monitor serum potassium, glucose (can become diabetic), and sodium • Weigh daily; report weight gain of more than 5 lb per week • Administer with antiulcer drugs or food. • Use care to prevent injuries • Teach symptoms of Cushing syndrome • Monitor BP and pulse closely

---

HESI Hint • Many people take steroids for a variety of conditions. NCLEX-RN questions often focus on the need to teach clients the importance of following the prescribed regimen precisely. They should be cautioned against stopping the medications suddenly and should be informed that it is necessary to taper off the dosage when taking steroids.

Nursing Assessment

A. Fatigue, weakness

B. Weight loss, anorexia, nausea, vomiting

C. Postural hypotension

D. Hypoglycemia

E. Hyponatremia

F. Hyperkalemia

G. Hyperpigmentation (only if primary Addison disease; not seen in secondary Addison disease)

H. Signs of shock when in Addison crises (See Advanced Clinical Concepts, p. 29.)

I. Loss of body hair

J. Hypovolemia
  1. Hypotension
  2. Tachycardia
  3. Fever

Analysis (Nursing Diagnoses)

A. *Deficient fluid volume* related to...

B. *Deficient knowledge* related to...

Nursing Plans and Interventions

A. Take vital signs frequently (every 15 minutes if in crisis).

B. Monitor I&O and weigh daily.

C. Instruct client to rise slowly because of the possibility of postural hypotension.

D. During Addison crises, administer IV glucose with parenteral glucocorticoids; it requires large fluid volume replacement.

E. Monitor serum electrolyte levels.

F. Teach
  1. Need for lifelong hormone replacement
  2. Need for close medical supervision
  3. Need for MedicAlert jewelry
  4. Signs and symptoms of overdosage and underdosage of medication
  5. Diet requirements: high-sodium, low-potassium, and high-carbohydrate (complex carbohydrates)
  6. Fluid requirements: intake of at least 3 L of fluid per day

G. Provide ulcer prophylaxis.

HESI Hint • *Addison crisis is a medical emergency.* It is brought on by sudden withdrawal of steroids or a stressful event (trauma, severe infection).
• Vascular collapse: Hypotension and tachycardia occur; administer IV fluids at a rapid rate until stabilized.
• Hypoglycemia: Administer IV glucose.
• Essential to reversing the crisis: Administer parenteral hydrocortisone.
• Aldosterone replacement: Administer fludrocortisone acetate (Florinef) PO (available only as oral preparation) with simultaneous administration of salt (sodium chloride) if client has a sodium deficit.

CUSHING SYNDROME

Description: Excess adrenocorticoid activity

A. Cause is usually chronic administration of corticosteroids.

B. Cushing syndrome can also be caused by adrenal, pituitary, or hypothalamus tumors.

Nursing Assessment

A. Physical symptoms include
1. Moon face
2. Truncal obesity
3. Buffalo hump
4. Abdominal striae
5. Muscle atrophy
6. Thinning of the skin
7. Hirsutism in females
8. Hyperpigmentation
9. Amenorrhea
10. Edema, poor wound healing, easy bruising

B. Hypertension

C. Susceptibility to multiple infections

D. Osteoporosis

E. Peptic ulcer formation

F. Many false positives and false negatives in laboratory testing

G. Lab data often include the following findings:
1. Hyperglycemia
2. Hypernatremia
3. Hypokalemia
4. Decreased eosinophils and lymphocytes
5. Increased plasma cortisol
6. Increased urinary 17-hydroxycorticoids

Analysis (Nursing Diagnoses)

A. *Excess fluid volume* related to…

B. *Risk for infection* related to…

C. *Disturbed body image* related to…

Nursing Plans and Interventions

A. Encourage the client to protect himself or herself from exposure to infection.

B. Wash hands; use good handwashing technique.

C. Monitor client for signs of infection:
1. Fever
2. Oral infection by *Candida* sp.
3. Vaginal yeast infections
4. Adventitious lungs
5. Skin lesions
6. Elevated WBCs

D. Teach safety measures.
1. Position bed close to floor, with call light within easy reach.
2. Encourage use of side rails.
3. Be sure walkways are unobstructed.
4. Encourage wearing shoes when ambulating.

E. Provide low-sodium diet; encourage consumption of foods that contain vitamin D and calcium.

F. Provide good skin and perineal care.

G. Discuss possibility of weaning from steroids. (If weaning is done too quickly, symptoms of Addison disease will occur.)

H. Encourage selection of clothing that minimizes visible aberrations; encourage maintenance of normal physical appearance.

I. Monitor I&O and weigh daily.

J. Provide ulcer prophylaxis.

> **HESI Hint** • Teach clients to take steroids with meals to prevent gastric irritation. They should never skip doses. If they have nausea or vomiting for more than 12 to 24 hours, they should contact the physician.

DIABETES MELLITUS

Description: Metabolic disorder in which there is an absence of or an insufficient production of insulin

A. Diabetes mellitus is characterized by hyperglycemia.

B. Diabetes mellitus affects the metabolism of protein, carbohydrate, and fat.

C. The most recent diagnostic parameter is a fasting glucose level, either serum or capillary, of greater than 126 mg/dl.

D. The two major classifications of diabetes are:
1. Type 1: insulin-dependent diabetes mellitus (IDDM)
2. Type 2: non-insulin-dependent diabetes mellitus (NIDDM; Table 4-24)

E. Many type 2 diabetics use insulin but retain some degree of pancreatic function.

F. Obesity is a major factor in type 2 diabetes.

G. All diabetics develop diabetes-associated complications to some degree. The degree of pathologic change is related to the control of blood glucose levels.

Clinical Characteristics and Treatment of Diabetes Mellitus

A. Type 1 (IDDM)
1. Description
   a. Can become hyperglycemic relatively easily ("brittle diabetics")
   b. Can go into ketoacidosis

TABLE 4-24   **Variables Related to Diabetes Mellitus**

Variable	Type I (IDDM)	Type 2 (NIDDM)
• Age at onset	• Usually <30 years of age	• School age to older adult
• Insulin production	• Absent	• Present, but inadequate
• Onset	• Rapid	• Insidious
• Symptoms	• Polydipsia • Polyphagia • Polyuria • Weight loss • Weakness	• Often unnoticed • Same symptoms as type 1, plus blurred vision
• Weight	• Usually thin	• Usually obese, sometimes normal
• Ketosis	• Common	• Rare
• Genetics	• No overwhelming predisposition	• Strong predisposition
• Pathogenesis	• Viral, autoimmune	• Obesity, nutrition (major factor)
• Control	• Difficult, with wide glycemia swings	• Often only dietary restrictions and exercise required
• Meal planning	• Imperative	• Imperative
• Exercise	• Imperative	• Imperative
• Medication	• Insulin required by all	• Maybe none; oral hypoglycemics or insulin
• Long-term complications	• Common	• Common

2. Clinical characteristics
  a. Serum glucose of 350 and above
  b. Ketonuria in large amounts
  c. Venous pH of 6.8 to 7.2
  d. Serum bicarbonate below 15 mEq/dl
3. Treatment
  a. Usually with isotonic IV fluids
  b. Slow IV infusion by IV pump of regular insulin, with IM or SC bolus as needed with careful blood glucose monitoring
  c. Careful replacement of potassium, based on lab data
B. Type 2 (NIDDM)
  1. Description
    a. Rare development of ketoacidosis
    b. Development of nonketotic hyperosmolar hyperglycemia with extreme hyperglycemia
  2. Clinical characteristics
    a. Hyperglycemia
    b. Plasma hyperosmolality
    c. Dehydration
    d. Changed mental status
  3. Treatment
    a. Usually with isotonic IV fluid replacement and careful monitoring of potassium and glucose levels
    b. Intravenous insulin (not always necessary)

Nursing Assessment

A. Integument
  1. Breaks in skin, infections on skin
  2. Diabetic dermopathy (skin spots)
  3. Unhealed injection sites

HESI Hint • Why do diabetics have trouble with wound healing? High blood glucose contributes to damage of the smallest vessels, the capillaries. This damage causes permanent capillary scarring, which inhibits the normal activity of the capillary. This phenomenon causes disruption of capillary elasticity and promotes problems such as diabetic retinopathy, poor healing of breaks in the skin, cardiovascular abnormalities, etc.

B. Oral cavity
  1. Caries
  2. Periodontal disease
  3. Candidiasis (raised, white patchy areas on mucous membranes)
C. Eyes
  1. Cataracts
  2. Retinal problems

D. Cardiopulmonary system
   1. Angina
   2. Dyspnea
E. Periphery
   1. Hair loss on extremities, indicating poor perfusion
   2. Other signs of poor peripheral circulation:
      a. Coolness
      b. Skin shininess and thinness
      c. Weak or absent peripheral pulses
      d. Ulcerations on extremities
      e. Pallor
      f. Thick nails with ridges
F. Kidneys
   1. Edema of face, hands, and feet
   2. Symptoms of urinary tract infection (UTI): fatigue, pallor, and weakness
   3. Urinary retention
G. Neuromusculature
   1. Atrophy of hands and feet
   2. Neuropathies with symptoms of numbness, tingling, pain, burning
H. Gastrointestinal disturbances
   1. Nighttime diarrhea
   2. Emesis falling into a pattern (e.g., client vomits every night 1 hour after dinner)
   3. Gastroparesis (faulty absorption)
I. Reproductive
   1. Male impotence
   2. Vaginal dryness, frequent vaginal infections
   3. Menstrual irregularities
J. Glycosylated hemoglobin A1c (presence confirms existence of hyperglycemia in previous 4 months)

> **HESI Hint** • Glycosylated Hgb (Hgb A$_1$c):
> - Indicates glucose control over previous 120 days (life of red blood cells [RBCs])
> - Is a valuable measurement of diabetes control

Analysis (Nursing Diagnoses)

A. *Deficient knowledge* related to…
B. *Ineffective coping* related to…
C. *Risk for injury* related to…

Nursing Plans and Interventions

A. Determine baseline lab data.
   1. Serum glucose
   2. Electrolytes
   3. Creatinine
   4. BUN
   5. ABGs as indicated
B. Teach injection technique.
   1. Lift skin; use 90-degree angle.

   2. Identify the prescribed dose and type of insulin (Tables 4-25 and 4-26).
   3. Store unopened insulin vials in refrigerator; may be kept at room temperature for 28 days.
   4. May reuse syringes for same person: recap needle and store in refrigerator.
   5. Rotate injection sites (abdomen preferred for type 1).
   6. Draw regular insulin into syringe first when mixing insulins.
C. Teach about diet.
   1. Work with dietitian to reinforce specific meal plan.
   2. Encourage carbohydrate counting and the use of exchange list; can be used when dining out.
   3. Teach that meals should be timed according to medication peak times.
   4. Teach diet regimen.
      a. 55% to 60% carbohydrates
      b. 12% to 15% protein
      c. 30% or less fat
      d. Foods high in complex carbohydrates, high in fiber, and low in fat, whenever possible
      e. Alcoholic beverages: acceptable if proper exchanges are made
      f. Bedtime snack: can prevent insulin reactions due to long-acting insulin peak
   5. Teach about managing sick days (illness raises blood glucose).
      a. Teach client to keep taking insulin.
      b. Monitor glucose more frequently.
      c. Watch for signs of hyperglycemia.

> **HESI Hint** • The body's response to illness and stress is to produce glucose. Therefore, any illness results in hyperglycemia.

D. Teach exercise regimen because exercise decreases blood sugar levels.
   1. Get regular nonstrenuous exercise.
   2. Exercise after mealtime; either exercise with someone or let someone know where exercise will take place to ensure safety.
   3. A snack may be needed before or during exercise.
   4. Monitor blood glucose before, during, and after exercise when beginning a new regimen.
E. Teach signs and symptoms of hyperglycemia and hypoglycemia (Table 4-27).

> **HESI Hint** • If in doubt whether a client is hyperglycemic or hypoglycemic, treat for hypoglycemia.

TABLE 4-25 Oral Hypoglycemics

Drugs	Indications	Adverse Reactions	Nursing Implications
Sulfonylureas *First Generation* • Tolbutamide (Orinase) • Chlorpropamide (Diabinese) *Second Generation* • Glyburide (Micronase, DiaBeta) • Glipizide (Glucotrol) • Glimepiride (Amaryl)	• Lowers blood sugar by stimulating the release of insulin by the beta cells of the pancreas + causes tissues to take up and store glucose more easily • First generation is low potency and short acting • Second generation is high potency and longer acting	*First Generation* • Hypoglycemia • Nausea, heartburn, constipation, anorexia • Agranulocytosis • Allergic skin reactions *Second Generation* • Weight gain • Hypoglycemia, particularly in older adults	*First Generation* • Responsiveness may decline over time • Given once daily with first meal • Monitor blood sugar • Hard to detect hypoglycemia if older adult or also on beta-blockers *Second Generation* • Less likely to interact with other medications
Biguinides • Metformin (Glucophage)	• Lowers serum glucose levels by inhibiting hepatic glucose production and increasing sensitivity of peripheral tissue to insulin	• Abdominal discomfort • Diarrhea	• Many drug-drug interactions • Extended-release tablets should be taken with the evening meal • Use cautiously with preexisting renal or liver disease or HF • Wait 48 hours to restart dosage after diagnostic studies requiring IV iodine contrast media
Alpha-Glucosidase Inhibitors • Acarbose (Precose) • Miglitol (Glyset)	• Lowers blood glucose by blunting sugar levels after meals	• Hypoglycemia	• Optimally, must be taken with the FIRST bite of each meal • May be taken with other classes of oral hypoglycemics • Monitor blood sugar
Thiazolidinediones • Rosiglitazone (Avandia) • Pioglitazone (Actos)	• Lowers blood sugar by decreasing the insulin resistance of the tissues	• Hypoglycemia • Increased total cholesterol, weight gain • Edema, anemia	• Many drug-drug interactions • Skip dose if meal skipped • No known drug interactions • Monitor liver function • Caution with use in CAD; may precipitate HF
Meglitindes • Repaglinide (Prandin)	• Lowers blood sugar by stimulating beta cells in pancreas to release insulin; does this by closing K^+ channels and opening Ca^{++} channels	• Hypoglycemia • Angina, chest pain • Arthralgia, back pain • Nausea and vomiting, dyspepsia, constipation or diarrhea	• May be used with metformin • Give before meals; if a meal is skipped, skip the dose • Monitor blood sugar
Combinations • Glyburide and metformin (Glucovance)	• Lowers blood sugar by combining the advantages of two classes of hypoglycemics	• Note possible adverse reactions to both classes • Hypoglycemia (severe)	• Note implications of both classes of drugs

TABLE 4-26   Types and Action of Insulin

Type	Name	Onset	Peak Action	Nursing Implications
• Rapid acting	• Prompt zinc suspension insulin (Semilente) • Human insulin lispro (Humalog) • Insulin aspart (NovoLog)	• 0.5 to 1 hr • 0.5 to 1 hr • 5 to 15 min	• 2 to 3 hr • 2 to 4 hr • 0.75 to 1.5 hr	• Not to be given IV • Give within 15 min of a meal (Lispro and Aspart)
• Short acting	• Regular insulin (human)	• 30 to 60 min	• 2 to 3 hr	• Regular insulin may be given IV
• Intermediate acting	• Isophane insulin (NPH) (Iletin) • Insulin zinc suspension (Humulin L)	• 1 to 2 hr	• 6 to 12 hr	• Not to be given IV • Mixtures combine rapid-acting regular insulin with intermediate-acting NPH insulin in a 30% regular with 70% NPH proportion or at 50/50 combination
• Long acting	• Protamine zinc (PZI) (Iletin) • Extended zinc suspension (Ultralente) • Insulin glargine (Lantus)	• 4 to 8 hr • 1.1 hr	• 14 to 20 hr • 5 hr (some sources say there is no peak)	• Not to be given IV • Recommended: give once daily, SE, at bedtime. In some cases, given two times a day. Acts as basal insulin. Caution: Solution is clear, but bottle is distinctly different shape from regular insulin. *Do not confuse insulins.* Do not shake solution. Do not mix other insulins with Lantus. Use cautiously if patient is NPO.
• Premix	• Humalog 75/25 • Human 70/30 • NovoLog 70/30			• For all premixes: Offer when food readily available 25% Lispro/75% Humulin N (NPH) 30% Regular/70% NPH 30% Aspart/70% NPH

TABLE 4-27   Comparison of Hyperglycemia and Hypoglycemia

HYPERGLYCEMIA		HYPOGLYCEMIA	
Signs and Symptoms	Nursing Action	Signs and Symptoms	Nursing Action

• Polydipsia
• Polyuria
• Polyphagia
• Blurred vision
• Weakness
• Weight loss
• Syncope
	• Encourage water intake
	• Check blood glucose frequently
	• Assess for ketoacidosis:
	  → Urine ketones
	  → Urine glucose
	  → Administer insulin as directed
		• Headache
		• Nausea
		• Sweating
		• Tremors
		• Lethargy
		• Hunger
		• Confusion
		• Slurred speech
		• Tingling around mouth
		• Anxiety, nightmares
			• Usually occurs rapidly and is potentially life-threatening; treat immediately with complex CHO. Example: graham cracker and peanut butter twice, and if no response, seek medical attention
			• Check blood glucose (may seize if <40)

HESI Hint • Self-monitoring of blood glucose (SMBG):
- Provides tight glucose control, thereby decreasing the potential for long-term complications
- Uses techniques that are specific to each meter
- Requires monitoring before meals, at bedtime, and any time symptoms occur
- Requires recording results and reporting them to health care provider at time of visit

F. Teach about foot care.
   1. Feet should be checked daily for changes; signs of injury and breaks in skin should be reported to health care provider.
   2. Feet should be washed daily with mild soap and warm water; soaking is to be avoided; feet should be dried well, especially between toes.

3. Feet may be moisturized with a lanolin product, but not between the toes.
4. Well-fitting leather shoes should be worn; going barefoot and wearing sandals are to be avoided.
5. Clean socks should be worn daily.
6. Garters and tight elastic-topped socks should never be worn.
7. Corns and calluses should be removed by professional.
8. Nails should be cut or filed straight across.
9. Warm socks should be worn if feet are cold.

G. Encourage regular health care follow-ups.
   1. Refer to ophthalmologist.
   2. Refer to podiatrist.

H. Teach that immediate attention should be sought if any sign of infection occurs.

I. Refer client to the American Diabetes Association for information and emotional support.

Review of Endocrine System

1. What diagnostic test is used to determine thyroid activity?
2. What condition results from all treatments for hyperthyroidism?
3. State three symptoms of hyperthyroidism and three symptoms of hypothyroidism.
4. List five important teaching aspects for clients who are beginning corticosteroid therapy.
5. Describe the physical appearance of clients who have Cushing disease.
6. Which type of diabetic always requires insulin replacement?
7. Which type of diabetic sometimes requires no medication?
8. List five symptoms of hyperglycemia.
9. List five symptoms of hypoglycemia.
10. Name the necessary elements to include in teaching a new diabetic.
11. In fewer than 10 steps, describe the method of drawing up a mixed dose of insulin (regular with NPH).
12. Identify the peak action time of the following types of insulin: rapid-acting regular insulin; intermediate-acting insulin; long-acting insulin.
13. When preparing a diabetic for discharge, the nurse teaches the client the relationship between stress, exercise, bedtime snacking, and glucose balance. State the relationships among each of these.
14. When making rounds at night, the nurse notes that an insulin-dependent client is complaining of a headache, slight nausea, and minimal trembling. The client's hand is cool and moist. What is the client most likely experiencing?
15. Identify five foot-care interventions that should be taught to a diabetic client.

Answers to Review

1. T_3, T_4
2. Hypothyroidism, requiring thyroid replacement
3. Hyperthyroidism: weight loss, heat intolerance, diarrhea. Hypothyroidism: fatigue, cold intolerance, weight gain
4. Continue medication until weaning plan is begun by physician; monitor serum potassium, glucose, and sodium frequently; weigh daily, and report gain of >5 lb/wk; monitor BP and pulse closely; teach symptoms of Cushing syndrome.
5. Moon face, obesity in trunk, buffalo hump in back, muscle atrophy, and thin skin
6. Type 1, insulin-dependent diabetes mellitus (IDDM)
7. Type 2, non-insulin-dependent diabetes mellitus (NIDDM)
8. Polydipsia, polyuria, polyphagia, weakness, weight loss
9. Hunger, lethargy, confusion, tremors or shakes, sweating
10. The underlying pathophysiology of the disease; its management and treatment regimen; meal planning; exercise program; insulin administration; sick-day management; symptoms of hyperglycemia (not enough insulin); symptoms of hypoglycemia (too much insulin, too much exercise, not enough food)

11. Identify the prescribed dose and type of insulin per physician order; store unopened insulin in refrigerator. Opened insulin vials may be kept at room temperature for up to 28 days. Draw up regular insulin first; rotate injection sites; may reuse syringe by recapping and storing in refrigerator.
12. Rapid-acting regular insulin: 2 to 4 hours; immediate-acting insulin: 6 to 12 hours; long-acting insulin: 14 to 20 hours
13. Stress and stress hormones usually increase glucose production and increase insulin need; exercise can increase the chance of an insulin reaction; therefore, the client should always have a sugar snack available when exercising (to treat hypoglycemia); bedtime snacking can prevent insulin reactions while waiting for long-acting insulin to peak.
14. Hypoglycemia/insulin reaction
15. Check feet daily, and report any breaks, sores, or blisters to health care provider; wear well-fitting shoes; never go barefoot or wear sandals; never personally remove corns or calluses; cut or file nails straight across; wash feet daily with mild soap and warm water.

Musculoskeletal System

RHEUMATOID ARTHRITIS

Description: Chronic, systematic, progressive deterioration of the connective tissue (synovium) of the joints; characterized by inflammation

A. The exact cause is unknown, but it is classified as an immune complex disorder.
B. Joint involvement is bilateral and symmetrical.
C. Severe cases may require joint replacement (see Joint Replacement, p. 136).

HESI Hint • A client comes to the clinic complaining of morning stiffness, weight loss, and swelling of both hands and wrists. Rheumatoid arthritis is suspected. Which methods of assessment might the nurse use, and which methods would the nurse not use? Use inspection, palpation, and strength testing. Do not ROM (this activity promotes pain because ROM is limited).

Nursing Assessment

A. Fatigue
B. Generalized weakness
C. Weight loss
D. Anorexia
E. Morning stiffness
F. Bilateral inflammation of joints with the following symptoms:
1. Decreased ROM
2. Joint pain
3. Warmth
4. Edema
5. Erythema
G. Joint deformity

HESI Hint • In the joint, the normal cartilage becomes soft, fissures and pitting occur, and the cartilage thins. Spurs form and inflammation sets in. The result is deformity marked by immobility, pain, and muscle spasm. The prescribed treatment regimen is corticosteroids for the inflammation; splinting, immobilization, and rest for the joint deformity; and NSAIDs for the pain.

H. Diagnosis confirmed by the following:
1. Elevated erythrocyte sedimentation rate (ESR)
2. Positive rheumatoid factor (RF)
3. Presence of antinuclear antibody (ANA)
4. Joint-space narrowing indicated by arthroscopic examination (provides joint visualization)
5. Abnormal synovial fluid (fluid in joint) indicated by arthrocentesis
6. C-reactive protein (CRP) indicated by active inflammation

HESI Hint • Synovial tissues line the bones of the joints. Inflammation of this lining causes destruction of tissue and bone. Early detection of rheumatoid arthritis can decrease the amount of bone and joint destruction. Often the disease goes into remission. Decreasing the amount of bone and joint destruction reduces the amount of disability.

Analysis (Nursing Diagnoses)

A. *Chronic pain* related to…
B. *Impaired physical mobility* related to…
C. *Self-care deficit* (specify) related to…
D. *Ineffective coping* related to…

Nursing Plans and Interventions

A. Implement pain relief measures.
1. Use moist heat.
a. Warm, moist compresses

b. Whirlpool baths
c. Hot shower in the morning
2. Use diversionary activities.
   a. Imaging
   b. Distraction
   c. Self-hypnosis
   d. Biofeedback
3. Administer medications, and teach client about medications (Table 4-28; see Table 4-23).
B. Provide periods of rest after periods of activity.
   1. Encourage self-care to maximal level.
   2. Allow adequate time for the client to perform activities.
   3. Perform activities during time of day when client feels most energetic.
C. Encourage the client to avoid overexertion and to maintain proper posture and joint position.

> **HESI Hint** • What activity recommendations should the nurse provide a client with rheumatoid arthritis?
> • Do not exercise painful, swollen joints.
> • Do not exercise any joint to the point of pain.
> • Perform exercises slowly and smoothly; avoid jerky movements.

D. Encourage use of assistive devices.
   1. Elevated toilet seat
   2. Shower chair
   3. Cane, walker, and wheelchair
   4. Reachers

5. Adaptive clothing with Velcro closures
6. Straight-backed chair with elevated seat
E. Develop a teaching plan to include the following:
   1. Medication regimen
   2. Need for routine follow-up for evaluation of possible side effects
   3. ROM and stretching exercises tailored to specific client needs
   4. Safety tips and precautions about equipment use and environment

LUPUS ERYTHEMATOSUS

Description: Systemic inflammatory connective-tissue disorder

A. There are two classifications of lupus erythematosus:
   1. Discoid lupus erythematosus (DLE) affects skin only.
   2. Systemic lupus erythematosus (SLE) can cause major body organs and systems to fail.
B. SLE is more prevalent than DLE.
C. Lupus is an autoimmune disorder.
D. Kidney involvement is the leading cause of death in clients with lupus; it is followed by cardiac involvement as a leading cause of death.

> **HESI Hint** • NCLEX-RN questions often focus on the fact that avoiding sunlight is key in the management of lupus erythematosus; this is what differentiates it from other connective-tissue diseases.

TABLE 4-28 Nonsteroidal Antiinflammatory Drugs (NSAIDs)

Drugs	Indications	Adverse Reactions	Nursing Implications
• Aspirin (Anacin) • Ibuprofen (Motrin, Nuprin, Advil) • Indomethacin (Indocin) • Ketorolac tromethamine (Toradol) • Celecoxib (Celebrex) • Etodolac (Lodine) • Diclofenac (Voltaren) • Naproxen (Anaprox, Naprosyn)	• Used as antiinflammatory • Antipyretic • Analgesic • Can be used with other agents	• GI irritation, bleeding • Nausea, vomiting, constipation • Elevated liver enzymes • Prolonged coagulation time • Tinnitus • Thrombocytopenia • Fluid retention • Nephrotoxicity • Blood dyscrasias	• Teach to take with food or milk to reduce GI symptoms • Therapeutic serum salicylates level 20 to 25 mg% • Teach to watch for signs of bleeding • Teach to avoid alcohol • Teach to observe for tinnitus • Administer corticosteroids for severe rheumatoid arthritis (see Table 4-23) • NSAIDs reduce the effect of ACE inhibitors in hypertensive clients • Note name similarity of Celebrex with other drugs having one-letter difference in spelling • Encourage routine appointments to check liver/renal labs and CBC

E. Factors that trigger lupus:
   1. Sunlight
   2. Stress
   3. Pregnancy
   4. Drugs

Nursing Assessment

A. DLE: Dry, scaly rash on face or upper body (butterfly rash)
B. SLE
   1. Joint pain and decreased mobility
   2. Fever
   3. Nephritis
   4. Pleural effusion
   5. Pericarditis
   6. Abdominal pain
   7. Photosensitivity

Analysis (Nursing Diagnoses)

A. *Impaired skin integrity* related to…
B. *Chronic pain* related to…
C. *Disturbed body image* related to…

Nursing Plans and Interventions

A. Instruct client to avoid prolonged exposure to sunlight.
B. Instruct client to clean the skin with mild soap.
C. Monitor and instruct client in administration of steroids.

OSTEOARTHRITIS (OA) (FORMERLY KNOWN AS DEGENERATIVE JOINT DISEASE [DJD])

Description: Noninflammatory arthritis
A. OA is characterized by a degeneration of cartilage, a wear-and-tear process.
B. It usually affects one or two joints.
C. It occurs asymmetrically.
D. Obesity and overuse are predisposing factors.

Nursing Assessment

A. Joint pain that increases with activity and improves with rest
B. Morning stiffness
C. Asymmetry of affected joints
D. Crepitus (grating sound in the joint)
E. Limited movement
F. Visible joint abnormalities indicated on radiographs
G. Joint enlargement and bony nodules

Analysis (Nursing Diagnoses)

A. *Chronic pain* related to…
B. *Impaired physical mobility* related to…
C. *Deficient self-care* related to…
D. *Deficient knowledge* (specify) related to…

Nursing Plans and Interventions

(See Rheumatoid Arthritis, p. 130.)
A. Instruct in weight-reduction diet.
B. Remind client that excessive use of the involved joint aggravates pain and may accelerate degeneration.
C. Teach the client to:
   1. Use correct posture and body mechanics
   2. Sleep with rolled terry cloth towel under cervical spine if neck pain is a problem
   3. Relieve pain in fingers and hands by wearing stretch gloves at night
   4. Keep joints in functional position

OSTEOPOROSIS

Description: Metabolic disease in which bone demineralization results in decreased density and subsequent fractures

A. Many fractures in older adults occur as result of osteoporosis and often occur prior to the client's falling rather than as the result of a fall.
B. The cause of osteoporosis is unknown.
C. Postmenopausal women are at highest risk.

Nursing Assessment

A. Classic dowager's hump, or kyphosis of the dorsal spine (Fig. 4-7)
B. Loss of height, often 2 to 3 inches
C. Back pain, often radiating around the trunk
D. Pathologic fractures, often occurring in the distal end of the radius and the upper third of the femur
E. Compression fracture of spine: assess ability to void and defecate

HESI Hint • Postmenopausal, thin white women are at highest risk for development of osteoporosis. Encourage exercise, a diet high in calcium, and supplemental calcium. Tums are an excellent source of calcium, but they are also high in sodium, so hypertensive or edematous individuals should seek another source of supplemental calcium.

Analysis (Nursing Diagnoses)

A. *Risk for injury* related to…

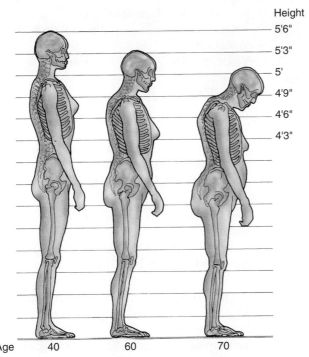

Height
- 5'6"
- 5'3"
- 5'
- 4'9"
- 4'6"
- 4'3"

Age   40   60   70

FIGURE 4-7 A normal spine at 40 years of age and osteoporotic changes at 60 and 70 years of age. These changes can cause a loss of as much as 6 inches in height and can result in the so-called dowager's hump (far right) in the upper thoracic vertebrae. (From Ignatavicius DD, Workman ML: *Medical-surgical nursing: Patient-centered collaborative care*, ed 6. St. Louis, 2010, Saunders.)

B. *Impaired physical mobility* related to…

C. *Deficient knowledge* related to…

Nursing Plans and Interventions

A. Create a hazard-free environment.

B. Keep bed in low position.

C. Encourage client to wear shoes or nonskid slippers when out of bed.

D. Encourage environmental safety.
1. Provide adequate lighting.
2. Keep floor clear.
3. Discourage use of throw rugs.
4. Clean spills promptly.
5. Keep side rails up at all times.

> **HESI Hint** • The main cause of fractures in older adults, especially in women, is osteoporosis. The main fracture sites seem to be hip, vertebral bodies, and Colles fracture of the forearm.

E. Provide assistance with ambulation.
1. Client may need walker or cane.
2. Client may need standby assistance when initially getting out of bed or chair.

F. Teach regular exercise program.
1. ROM exercise several times a day
2. Ambulation several times a day
3. Use of proper body mechanics

G. Provide diet that is high in protein, calcium, and vitamin D; discourage use of alcohol and caffeine.

H. Encourage preventive measures for females.
1. Hormone replacement therapy (HRT) has been used as a primary prevention strategy for reducing bone loss in the postmenopausal woman. However, recent studies demonstrated that HRT may increase a woman's risk of breast cancer, cardiovascular disease, and stroke. If using HRT, the benefits should outweigh the risks.
2. Take prescribed medications to prevent further loss of bone mineral density (BMD).
   a. Bisphosphonates: inhibits osteoclast-mediated bone resorption, thereby increasing BMD. Common side effects are anorexia, weight loss, and gastritis. Instruct the client to take with full glass of water, take 30 minutes before food or other medications, and remain upright for at least 30 minutes after taking.
      - alendronate (Fosamax)
      - clodronate (Bonefos)
      - etidronate (Didronel)
      - ibandronate (Boniva)
      - pamidronate (Aredia)
      - risedronate (Actonel)
      - tiludronate (Skelid)
   b. Selective estrogen receptor modulator: to mimic the effect of estrogen on bone by reducing bone resorption without stimulating the tissues of the breast or uterus. The most common side effects are leg cramps and hot flashes.
      - raloxifene (Evista)
      - teriparatide (Forteo)
3. High calcium and vitamin D intake beginning in early adulthood
4. Calcium supplementation after menopause (Tums are an excellent source of calcium.)
5. Weight-bearing exercise

I. Dual-energy x-ray absorptiometry (DEXA), which measures bone density in the spine, hips, and forearm, as a baseline after menopause, with frequency as recommended by health care provider

J. Osteopenia is defined as bone loss that is more than normal and has a T-score less than or equal to a range of −1 to −2.5 but is not yet at the level for a diagnosis of osteoporosis. BMD is commonly reported as a "T-score," which is the difference between the client's BMD and the BMD of "young normal adults" of the same gender. The difference between the client's score and the young adult norm is expressed as standard deviation (SD) below or above the average.

FRACTURE

Description: Any break in the continuity of the bone

> **HESI Hint** • NCLEX-RN questions focus on safety precautions. Improper use of assistive devices can be very risky. When using a nonwheeled walker, the client should lift and move the walker forward and then take a step into it. The client should avoid scooting the walker or shuffling forward into it; these movements take more energy and provide less stability than does a single movement.

A. Fractures are described by the type and extent of the break.
B. Fractures are caused by a direct blow, crushing force, a sudden twisting motion, or a disease such as cancer or osteoporosis.
1. Complete fracture: A break across the entire cross section of the bone
2. Incomplete fracture: A break across only part of the bone
3. Closed fracture: No break in the skin
4. Open fracture: Broken bone protrudes through skin or mucous membranes (much more prone to infection)
C. Five types of fractures
1. Greenstick: One side of a bone is broken; the other side is bent.
2. Transverse: Break occurs across the bone.
3. Oblique: Break occurs at an angle across the bone.
4. Spiral: Break twists around the bone.
5. Comminuted: Break has more than three fragments (Table 4-29).

> **HESI Hint** • What type of fracture is more difficult to heal: an extracapsular fracture (below the neck of the femur) or an intracapsular fracture (in the neck of the femur)?
>   The blood supply enters the femur below the neck of the femur. Therefore, an intracapsular fracture heals with greater difficulty, and there is a greater likelihood that necrosis will occur because the fracture is cut off from the blood supply.

Nursing Assessment

A. Signs and symptoms of fracture include:
1. Pain, swelling, tenderness
2. Deformity, loss of functional ability
3. Discoloration, bleeding at the site through an open wound
4. Crepitus: crackling sound between two broken bones
B. Fracture is evident on radiograph.
C. Therapeutic management is based on:
1. Reduction of the fracture
2. Maintenance of realignment by immobilization
3. Restoration of function
D. Observe client's use of assistive devices.
1. Crutches
a. There should be two to three finger widths between the axilla and the top of the crutch.
b. A three-point gait is most common. The client advances both crutches and the impaired leg at the same time. The client then swings the uninvolved leg ahead to the crutches.
2. Cane
a. It is placed on the unaffected side.
b. The top of the cane should be at the level of the greater trochanter.
3. Walker
a. Strength of upper extremity and unaffected leg is assessed and improved with exercises, if necessary, so that upper body is strong enough to use walker.
b. Client lifts and advances the walker and steps forward.
E. See Chapter 5, Pediatric Nursing, for cast care and care of a client in traction.

> **HESI Hint** • The risk for the development of a fat embolism, a syndrome in which fat globules migrate into the bloodstream and combine with platelets to form emboli, is greatest in the first 36 hours after a fracture. It is more common in clients with multiple fractures, fractures of long bones, and fractures of the pelvis. The initial symptom of a fat embolism is confusion due to hypoxemia (check blood gases for Po_2). Assess for respiratory distress, restlessness, irritability, fever, and petechiae. If an embolus is suspected, notify physician stat, draw blood gases, administer O_2, and assist with endotracheal intubation.

> **HESI Hint** • In clients with hip fractures, thromboembolism is the most common complication. Prevention includes passive ROM exercises, use of elastic stocking, elevation of the foot of the bed 25 degrees to increase venous return, and low-dose heparin therapy.

TABLE 4-29 Common Types of Fractures

Description	Illustration	Description	Illustration
• Burst: Characterized by multiple pieces of bone; often occurs at bone ends or in vertebrae		• Longitudinal: Fracture line extends in the direction of the bone's longitudinal axis	
• Comminuted: More than one fracture line; more than two bone fragments; fragments may be splintered or crushed		• Nondisplaced: Fragments aligned at fracture site	
• Complete: Break across the entire section of bone, dividing it into distinct fragments; often displaced		• Oblique: Fracture line occurs at approximately 45-degree angle across the longitudinal axis of the bone	
• Displaced: Fragments out of normal position at fracture site	Torsion	• Spiral: Fracture line results from twisting force; forms a spiral encircling the bone	
• Incomplete: Fracture occurs through only one cortex of the bone; usually nondisplaced		• Stellate: Fracture lines radiate from one central point	
• Linear: Fracture line is intact; fracture is caused by minor to moderate force applied directly to the bone		• Transverse: Fracture line occurs at a 90-degree angle to longitudinal axis of bone	

(Continued)

TABLE 4-29 Common Types of Fractures—cont'd

Description	Illustration	Description	Illustration
• Avulsion: Bone fragments are torn away from the body of the bone at the site of attachment of a ligament or tendon		• Colles': Fracture within the last inch of the distal radius; distal fragment is displaced in a position of dorsal and medial deviation	
• Compression: Bone buckles and eventually cracks as the result of unusual loading force applied to its longitudinal axis.		• Pott's: Fracture of the distal fibula, seriously disrupting the tibiofibular articulation; a piece of the medial malleolus may be chipped off as a result of rupture of the internal lateral ligament.	
• Greenstick: Incomplete fracture in which one side of the cortex is broken and the other side is flexed but intact.		• Impacted: Telescoped fracture, with one fragment driven into another.	

(From Black JM, Hawks JH: *Medical-surgical nursing: Clinical management for positive outcomes*, ed 8. St. Louis, 2009, WB Saunders.)

HESI Hint • Clients with fractures or edema in or casts on the extremities need frequent neurovascular assessment distal to the injury. Skin color, temperature, sensation, capillary refill, mobility, pain, and pulses should be assessed.

HESI Hint • Assess the 5 Ps of neurovascular functioning: pain, paresthesia, pulse, pallor, and paralysis.

JOINT REPLACEMENT

Description: Surgical procedure in which a mechanical device, designed to act as a joint, is used to replace a diseased joint

A. The most commonly replaced joints
   1. Hip
   2. Knee
   3. Shoulder
   4. Finger
B. Prostheses may be ingrown or cemented.
C. Accurate fitting is essential.
D. Client must have healthy bone stock for adequate healing.

E. Joint replacement provides excellent pain relief in 85% to 90% of the clients who have the surgery.
F. Infection is the concern postoperatively.

Nursing Assessment

A. Joint pathology
   1. Osteoarthritis
   2. Rheumatoid arthritis
   3. Fracture
B. Pain not relieved by medication
C. Poor ROM in the affected joint

Analysis (Nursing Diagnoses)

A. *Risk for infection* related to …
B. *Acute pain* related to …
C. *Chronic pain* related to …
D. *Risk for injury to affected limb* related to …

Nursing Plans and Interventions

A. Provide postoperative care for wound and joint.
   1. Monitor incision site.
      a. Assess for bleeding and drainage.

> **HESI Hint** • Orthopedic wounds have a tendency to ooze more than other wounds. A suction drainage device usually accompanies the client to the postoperative floor. Check drainage often.

    b. Assess suture line for erythema and edema.
    c. Assess suction drainage apparatus for proper functioning.
    d. Assess for signs of infection.

> **HESI Hint** • NCLEX-RN questions about joint replacement focus on complications. A big problem after joint replacement is infection.

    2. Monitor functioning of extremity.
      a. Check circulation, sensation, and movement of extremity distal to replacement.
      b. Provide proper alignment of affected extremity. (Client will return from the operating room with alignment for the initial postoperative period.)
      c. Provide abductor appliance (hip replacement) or continuous passive motion (CPM) device if indicated.
B. Monitor I&O every shift, including suction drainage.

> **HESI Hint** • Fractures of bone predispose the client to anemia, especially if long bones are involved. Check hematocrit every 3 to 4 days to monitor erythropoiesis.

C. Encourage fluid intake of 3 L per day.
D. Encourage client to perform self-care activities at maximal level.
E. Coordinate rehabilitation: work closely with health care team to increase client's mobility gradually.
    1. Get client out of bed as soon as possible.
    2. Keep client out of bed as much as possible.
    3. Keep abductor pillow in place while client is in bed (hip replacement).
    4. Use elevated toilet seat and chairs with high seats for those who have had hip or knee replacements (prevents dislocation).
    5. Do not flex hip more than 90 degrees (hip replacement).

> **HESI Hint** • After hip replacement, instruct the client not to lift the leg upward from a lying position or to elevate the knee when sitting. This upward motion can pop the prosthesis out of the socket.

F. Provide discharge planning that includes rehabilitation on an outpatient basis as prescribed.

> **HESI Hint** • Immobile clients are prone to complications: skin integrity problems; formation of urinary calculi (client's milk intake may be limited); and venous thrombosis (client may be on prophylactic anticoagulants).

AMPUTATION

Description: Surgical removal of a diseased part or organ
A. Causes for amputation include the following:
    1. Peripheral vascular disease, 80% (75% of these are diabetics)
    2. Trauma
    3. Congenital deformities
    4. Malignant tumors
    5. Infection
B. Amputation necessitates major lifestyle and body-image adjustments.

Nursing Assessment

A. Prior to amputation, symptoms of peripheral vascular disease include:
    1. Cool extremity
    2. Absent peripheral pulses
    3. Hair loss on affected extremity
    4. Necrotic tissue or wounds
      a. Blue or blue-gray, turning black
      b. Drainage possible, with or without odor
    5. Leathery skin on affected extremity
    6. Decrease of pain sensation in affected extremity
B. Inadequate circulation as determined by:
    1. Arteriogram
    2. Doppler flow studies

Analysis (Nursing Diagnoses)

A. *Acute pain* related to…
B. *Impaired physical mobility* related to…
C. *Self-care deficit* (specify) related to…
D. *Disturbed body image* related to…

Nursing Plans and Interventions

A. Provide wound care.
    1. Monitor surgical dressing for drainage.
      a. Mark dressing for bleeding, and check marking at least every 8 hours.
      b. Measure suction drainage every shift.
    2. Change dressing as needed (physician usually performs initial dressing change).
      a. Maintain aseptic technique.
      b. Observe wound color and warmth.

    c. Observe for wound healing.
    d. Monitor for signs of infection.
      (1) Fever
      (2) Tachycardia
      (3) Redness of incision area
B. Maintain proper body alignment in and out of bed.
C. Position client to relieve edema and spasms at residual limb (stump) site.
   1. Elevate residual limb (stump) for the first 24 hours postoperatively.

HESI Hint • The residual limb (stump) should be elevated on one pillow. If the residual limb (stump) is elevated too high, the elevation can cause a contracture.

2. Do not elevate residual limb (stump) after 48 hours postoperatively.
3. Keep residual limb (stump) in extended position, and turn client to prone position three times a day to prevent hip flexion contracture.
D. Be aware that phantom pain is real; it will eventually disappear, and it responds to pain medication.
E. Handle affected body part gently and with smooth movements.
F. Provide passive ROM until client is able to perform active ROM. Collaborate with rehabilitation team members for mobility improvement.
G. Encourage independence in self-care, allowing sufficient time for client to complete care and to have input into care.

Review of Musculoskeletal System

1. Differentiate between rheumatoid arthritis and osteoarthritis in terms of joint involvement.
2. Identify the categories of drugs commonly used to treat arthritis.
3. Identify pain-relief interventions for clients with arthritis.
4. What measures should the nurse encourage female clients to take to prevent osteoporosis?
5. What are the common side effects of salicylates?
6. What is the priority nursing intervention used with clients taking NSAIDs?
7. List three of the most common joints that are replaced.
8. Describe postoperative residual limb (stump) care (after amputation) for the first 48 hours.
9. Describe nursing care for the client who is experiencing phantom pain after amputation.
10. A nurse discovers that a client who is in traction for a long bone fracture has a slight fever, is short of breath, and is restless. What does the client most likely have?
11. What are the immediate nursing actions if fat embolization is suspected in a client with a fracture or other orthopedic condition?
12. List three problems associated with immobility.
13. List three nursing interventions for the prevention of thromboembolism in immobilized clients with musculoskeletal problems.

Answers to Review

1. Rheumatoid arthritis occurs bilaterally. Osteoarthritis occurs asymmetrically.
2. NSAIDs, of which salicylates are the cornerstone of treatment, and corticosteroids (used when arthritic symptoms are severe)
3. Warm, moist heat (compresses, baths, showers); diversionary activities (imaging, distraction, self-hypnosis, biofeedback); and medications
4. Possible estrogen replacement after menopause; high calcium and vitamin D intake beginning in early adulthood; calcium supplements after menopause; and weight-bearing exercise
5. GI irritation, tinnitus, thrombocytopenia, mild liver enzyme elevation
6. Administer or teach client to take drugs with food or milk.
7. Hip, knee, finger
8. Elevate residual limb (stump) for first 24 hours. Do not elevate residual limb (stump) after 48 hours. Keep residual limb (stump) in extended position, and turn client to prone position three times a day to prevent flexion contracture.
9. Be aware that phantom pain is real and will eventually disappear. Administer pain medication; phantom pain responds to medication.
10. A fat embolism, which is characterized by hypoxemia, respiratory distress, irritability, restlessness, fever, and petechiae
11. Notify physician stat, draw blood gases, administer O_2 according to blood gas results, assist with endotracheal intubation and treatment of respiratory failure.
12. Venous thrombosis, urinary calculi, skin integrity problems
13. Passive ROM exercises, elastic stockings, and elevation of foot of bed 25 degrees to increase venous return

Neurosensory System

GLAUCOMA

Chronic open-angle glaucoma is also known as simple adult primary glaucoma and as primary open-angle glaucoma.

Description: Condition characterized by increased intraocular pressure (IOP)

A. Glaucoma involves gradual, painless vision loss.

B. Glaucoma may lead to blindness if untreated.

C. Glaucoma is the second leading cause of blindness in the United States.

D. There is an increased incidence of glaucoma in older adult populations.

E. Glaucoma usually occurs bilaterally in those who have a family history of the condition.

F. Aqueous fluid is inadequately drained from the eye.

G. It is generally asymptomatic, especially in early stages.

H. It tends to be diagnosed during routine visual examinations.

I. It cannot be cured but can be treated with success pharmacologically and surgically.

Nursing Assessment

A. Early signs
1. Increase in IOP, >22 mm Hg.
2. Decreased accommodation or ability to focus

> **HESI Hint** • Glaucoma is often painless and symptom free. It is usually picked up as part of a regular eye examination.

B. Late signs include:
1. Loss of peripheral vision
2. Seeing halos around lights
3. Decreased visual acuity not correctable with glasses
4. Headache or eye pain that may be so severe as to cause nausea and vomiting (acute closed-angle glaucoma)

C. Diagnostic tests include the following:
1. Tonometer, used to measure IOP
2. Electronic tonometer, used to detect drainage of aqueous humor
3. Gonioscopy, used to obtain a direct visualization of the lens

D. Risk factors include the following:
1. Family history of glaucoma
2. Family history of diabetes
3. History of previous ocular problems
4. Medication use
   a. Glaucoma is a side effect of many medications (e.g., antihistamines, anticholinergics).
   b. Glaucoma can result from the interaction of medications.

Analysis (Nursing Diagnoses)

A. *Anxiety* related to…

B. *Disturbed sensory perception: visual* related to…

C. *Ineffective health maintenance* related to…

Nursing Plans and Interventions

A. Administer eye drops as prescribed (Table 4-30).

> **HESI Hint** • Eye drops are used to cause pupil constriction because movement of the muscles to constrict the pupil also allows aqueous humor to flow out, thereby decreasing the pressure in the eye. Pilocarpine is commonly used. Caution client that vision may be blurred for 1 to 2 hours after administration of pilocarpine and that adaptation to dark environments is difficult because of pupillary constriction (the desired effect of the drug).

B. Orient client to surroundings.

C. Avoid nonverbal communication that requires visual acuity (e.g., facial expressions).

D. Develop a teaching plan that includes the following:
1. Careful adherence to eye-drop regimen can prevent blindness.
2. Vision already lost cannot be restored.
3. Eye drops are needed for the rest of life.
4. Proper eye-drop instillation technique. Obtain a return demonstration.
   a. Wash hands and external eye.
   b. Tilt head back slightly.
   c. Instill drop into lower lid, without touching the lid with the tip of the dropper.
   d. Release the lid, and sponge excess fluid from lid and cheek.
   e. Close eye gently, and leave closed 3 to 5 minutes.
   f. Apply gentle pressure on inner canthus to decrease systemic absorption.
5. Safety measures to prevent injuries:
   a. Remove throw rugs.
   b. Adjust lighting to meet needs.

TABLE 4-30 **Treatment of Glaucoma**

Drugs	Indications	Adverse Reactions	Nursing Implications
Parasympathomimetics			
• Pilocarpine HCl (multiple brands available) 0.5% to 0.6% is the drug of choice	• Enhances papillary constriction (available in drops, gel, and time-release wafer)	• Bronchospasm • Nausea, vomiting, diarrhea • Blurred vision, twitching eyelids, eye pain with focusing	• Use cautiously with: → Pregnancy → Asthma → Hypertension • Teach proper drop instillation technique • Need for ongoing use of the drug at prescribed intervals • Blurred vision tends to decrease with regular use of this drug
Beta-Adrenergic Receptor–Blocking Agents			
• Timolol maleate optic (Timoptic Solution) • Carteolol (Ocupress)	• Inhibits formation of aqueous humor	• Side effects are insignificant. • Hypotension	• Use cautiously with → Hypersensitivity → Asthma → Second- or third-degree heart block → HF → Congenital glaucoma → Pregnancy → Teach proper drop instillation technique • Need for ongoing use of the drug at prescribed intervals • Blurred vision tends to decrease with regular use of this drug
Carbonic Anhydrase Inhibitors			
• Acetazolamide (Diamox) • Brinzolamide (Azopt) • Dorzolamide (Trusopt)	• Reduces aqueous humor production	• Numbness, tingling of hands and feet • Nausea • Malaise	• Administer orally or IV • Produces diuresis • Assess for metabolic acidosis
Prostaglandin Antagonists			
• Latanoprost (Xalatan) • Travoprost (Travatan) • Bimatoprost (Lumigan)	• Lowers intraocular pressure of glaucoma by increasing outflow of aqueous humor	• Local irritation • Foreign-body sensation • Increased brown pigmentation of iris • Increased eyelash growth	

6. Avoid activities that may increase intraocular pressure.
   a. Emotional upsets
   b. Exertion: pushing, heavy lifting, shoveling
   c. Coughing severely or excessive sneezing (Get medical attention before upper respiratory infection [URI] worsens.)
   d. Wearing constrictive clothing (tight collar or tie, tight belt or girdle)
   e. Straining at stool and constipation

HESI Hint • There is an increased incidence of glaucoma in older adult population. Older clients are prone to problems associated with constipation. Therefore, the nurse should assess these clients for constipation and postoperative complications associated with constipation and should implement a plan of care directed at prevention of and, if necessary, treatment for constipation.

Nursing Plans and Interventions: The Nonseeing (Blind) Client

A. On entering room, announce your presence clearly and identify yourself; address client by name.

B. Never touch client unless he or she knows you are there.

C. On admission, orient client thoroughly to surroundings.
   1. Demonstrate use of the call bell.
   2. Walk client around the room and acquaint him or her with all objects: chairs, bed, TV, telephone, etc.

D. Guide client when walking:
   1. Walk ahead of client, and place his or her hand in the bend of your elbow.
   2. Describe where you are walking. Note whether passageway is narrowing or you are approaching stairs, curb, or an incline.

E. Always raise side rails for newly sightless persons (e.g., clients wearing postoperative eye patches).

F. Assist with meal enjoyment by describing food and its placement in terms of the face of a clock (e.g., "meat at 6 o'clock").

G. When administering medications, inform client of number of pills, and give only a half glass of water (to avoid spills).

CATARACT

Description: Condition characterized by opacity of the lens

A. Aging accounts for 95% of cataracts (senile).

B. The remaining 5% result from trauma, toxic substances, or systemic diseases or are congenital.

C. Safety precautions may reduce the incidence of traumatic cataracts.

D. Surgical removal is done when vision impairment interferes with daily activities. Intraocular lens implants may be used.

E. Most operations are performed under local anesthesia on an outpatient basis.

HESI Hint • The lens of the eye is responsible for projecting light onto the retina so that images can be discerned. Without the lens, which becomes opaque with cataracts, light cannot be filtered and vision is blurred.

Nursing Assessment

A. Early signs include
   1. Blurred vision
   2. Decreased color perception

B. Late signs include
   1. Diplopia
   2. Reduced visual acuity, progressing to blindness
   3. Clouded pupil, progressing to a milky-white appearance

C. Diagnostic tests include use of the following:
   1. Ophthalmoscope
   2. Slit-lamp biomicroscope

Analysis (Nursing Diagnoses)

A. *Disturbed sensory perception: visual* related to…

B. *Anxiety* related to…

Nursing Plans and Interventions

A. Preoperative: Demonstrate and request a return demonstration of eye medication instillation from client or family member.

B. Develop a postoperative teaching plan that includes:
   1. Warning not to rub or put pressure on eye
   2. Teaching that glasses or shaded lens should be worn during waking hours. An eye shield should be worn during sleeping hours.
   3. Teaching to avoid lifting objects over 5 pounds, bending, straining, coughing, or any other activity that can increase IOP
   4. Teaching to use a stool softener to prevent straining at stool
   5. Teaching to avoid lying on operative side
   6. Teaching the need to keep water from getting into eye while showering or washing hair
   7. Teaching to observe and report signs of increased IOP and infection (e.g., pain, changes in vital signs)

HESI Hint • When the cataract is removed, the lens is gone, making prevention of falls important. When the lens is replaced with an implant, vision is better.

EYE TRAUMA

Description: Injury to the eye sustained as the result of sharp or blunt trauma, chemicals, or heat

A. Permanent visual impairment can occur.

B. Every eye injury should be considered an emergency.

C. Protective eye shields in hazardous work environments and during athletic sports may prevent injuries.

Nursing Assessment

A. Determine type of injury and symptoms.

B. Diagnostic tests include:
   1. Slit-lamp examination

2. Instillation of fluorescein to detect corneal injury
3. Testing of visual acuity for medical documentation and legal protection

Analysis (Nursing Diagnoses)

A. *Disturbed sensory perception: visual* related to…
B. *Acute pain* related to…

Nursing Plans and Interventions

A. Position the client according to the type of injury; a sitting position decreases intraocular pressure.
B. Remove conjunctival foreign bodies unless embedded.
C. Never attempt to remove a penetrating or embedded object. Do not apply pressure.
D. Apply cold compresses to eye contusion.
E. After chemical injuries, irrigate the eye with copious amounts of water.
F. Administer eye medications as prescribed.
G. Explain that an eye patch may be applied to rest the eye. Reading and watching TV may be restricted for 3 to 5 days.
H. Explain that a sudden increase in eye pain should be reported.

DETACHED RETINA

Description: Hole or tear in, or separation of the sensory retina from, the pigmented epithelium

A. It can be result of increasing age, severe myopia, eye trauma, retinopathy (diabetic), cataract or glaucoma surgery, family or personal history.
B. Resealing is done by surgery.
   1. Cryotherapy (freezing)
   2. Photocoagulation (laser)
   3. Diathermy (heat)
   4. Scleral buckling (most often used)

Nursing Plans and Interventions

A. The client may be on bed rest.
B. Place eye patch over affected eye.
C. Administer medication to inhibit accommodation and constriction; cycloplegics (mydriatics and homatropine) are given to dilate pupil before surgery.
D. Administer medication for postoperative pain: acetaminophen (Tylenol), meperidine (Demerol), oxycodone.
E. If gas bubble is used (inserted in vitreous), position client so bubble can rise against area to be reattached.

HEARING LOSS

Conductive Hearing Loss

Description: Hearing loss in which sound does not travel well to the sound organs of the inner ear. The volume of sound is less, but the sound remains clear. If volume is raised, hearing is normal.

A. Hearing loss is the most common disability in the United States.
B. It usually results from cerumen (wax) impaction or middle ear disorders.

> **HESI Hint** • The ear consists of three parts: the external ear, the middle ear, and the inner ear. Inner ear disorders, or disorders of the sensory fibers going to the CNS, often are neurogenic in nature and may not be helped with a hearing aid. External and middle ear problems (conductive) may result from infection, trauma, or wax buildup. These types of disorders are treated more successfully with hearing aids.

Sensorineural Hearing Loss

Description: Form of hearing loss in which sound passes properly through the outer and middle ear but is distorted by a defect in the inner ear

A. It involves perceptual loss, usually progressive and bilateral.
B. It involves damage to the eighth cranial nerve.
C. It is detected easily by the use of a tuning fork.
D. Common causes
   1. Infections
   2. Ototoxic drugs
   3. Trauma
   4. Neuromas
   5. Noise
   6. Aging process

Nursing Assessment

A. Inability to hear a whisper from 1 to 2 feet away
B. Inability to respond if nurse covers mouth when talking, indicating that client is lip reading
C. Inability to hear a watch tick 5 inches from ear
D. Shouting in conversation
E. Straining to hear
F. Turning head to favor one ear
G. Answering questions incorrectly or inappropriately
H. Raising volume of radio or TV

Analysis (Nursing Diagnoses)

A. *Disturbed sensory perception (auditory)* related to…
B. *Impaired verbal communication* related to…

Nursing Plans and Interventions

A. The nurse should do the following to enhance therapeutic communication with the hearing impaired:
1. Prior to starting conversation, reduce distraction as much as possible.
2. Turn the TV or radio down or off, close the door, or move to a quieter location.
3. Devote full attention to the conversation; do not try to do two things at once.
4. Look and listen during the conversation.
5. Begin with casual topics, and progress to more critical issues slowly.
6. Do not switch topics abruptly.
7. If you do not understand, let the client know.
8. If the client is a lip reader, face him or her directly.
9. Speak slowly and distinctly; determine whether you are being understood.
10. Allow adequate time for the conversation to take place; try to avoid hurried conversations.
11. Use active listening techniques.

HESI Hint • NCLEX-RN questions often focus on communicating with older adults who are hearing impaired.
- Speak in a low-pitched voice, slowly and distinctly.
- Stand in front of the person, with the light source behind the client.
- Use visual aids if available.

B. Be sure to inform the health care staff of the client's hearing loss.
C. Helpful aids may include a telephone amplifier, earphone attachments for the radio and TV, and lights or buzzers that indicate the doorbell is ringing, located in the most commonly used rooms of the house.

Neurologic System

ALTERED STATE OF CONSCIOUSNESS

Nursing Assessment

A. Use agency's neurologic vital signs assessment tool. It will sometimes contain a scale for scoring, such as the Glasgow Coma Scale, which objectively documents the client's level of consciousness (Table 4-31).
1. Maximum total is 15; minimum is 3.
2. A score of 7 or less indicates coma.
3. Clients with low scores (i.e., 3 to 4) have high mortality rates and poor prognosis.
4. Clients with scores greater than 8 have a good prognosis for recovery.

TABLE 4-31 Glasgow Coma Scale

Variable	Response	Score
Eye opening	Spontaneously	4
	To verbal command	3
	To pain	2
	No response	1
Motor response	To verbal command	6
	To painful stimuli	
	• Localizes pain	5
	• Flexes/withdraws	4
	• Flexor posturing (decorticate)	3
		2
	• Extensor posturing (decerebrate)	2
	• No response	1
Verbal response	Oriented and converses	5
	Disoriented, converses	4
	Uses inappropriate words	3
	Incomprehensible sounds	2
	No response	1

HESI Hint • Use of the Glasgow Coma Scale eliminates ambiguous terms to describe neurologic status, such as *lethargic, stuporous,* or *obtunded.*

B. Neurologic vital signs sheet will also address pupil size (with sizing scale), limb movement (with scale), and vital signs (blood pressure, temperature, pulse, respirations).
C. Assess skin integrity and corneal integrity.
D. Check bladder for fullness, auscultate lungs, and monitor cardiac status.
E. Family members and significant others should be assessed for knowledge of client status, coping skills, need for extra support, and the ability to assist or provide care on an ongoing basis.

Analysis (Nursing Diagnoses)

HESI Hint • Almost every diagnosis in the NANDA format is applicable because severely neurologically impaired persons require total care.

A. *Ineffective breathing pattern* related to …
B. *Ineffective airway clearance* related to …
C. *Impaired gas exchange* related to …
D. *Decreased cardiac output* related to …

E. *Risk for imbalanced body temperature (especially if hypothalamus is involved)* related to…

F. *Risk for injury* related to…

G. *Impaired physical mobility* related to…

H. *Risk for impaired skin integrity* related to…

I. *Anxiety* related to…

J. *Self-care deficit: (specify) eating, toileting, dressing, grooming* related to…

K. *Imbalanced nutrition: less than body requirements* related to…

L. *Impaired urinary elimination: incontinence* related to…

M. *Risk for constipation* related to…

HESI Hint • A client with an altered state of consciousness is fed via enteral routes because the likelihood of aspiration is high with oral feedings. Residual feeding is the amount of previous feeding still in the stomach. The presence of 100 ml of residual in an adult usually indicates poor gastric emptying, and the feeding should be withheld.

HESI Hint • Paralytic ileus is common in comatose clients. A gastric tube aids in gastric decompression.

HESI Hint • Any client on bed rest or immobilized must have ROM exercises often and very frequent position changes. Do not leave the client in any one position for longer than 2 hours. Any position that decreases venous return, such as sitting with dependent extremities for long periods, is dangerous.

Nursing Plans and Interventions

A. Maintain adequate respirations, airway, oxygenation.
  1. Document and report breathing pattern changes.
  2. Position client for maximum ventilation: three-quarters prone position or semiprone position to prevent tongue from obstructing airway and slightly to one side with arms away from chest wall.
  3. Insert airway if tongue is obstructing or if client is paralyzed.
  4. Prepare for insertion of cuffed endotracheal tube.
  5. Keep airway free of secretions with suctioning (see Table 4-3).
  6. Monitor arterial Po_2 and Pco_2.
  7. Prepare for tracheostomy if ventilator support is needed.
  8. Provide chest physiotherapy as prescribed by physician.
  9. Hyperventilate with 100% O_2 before and after suctioning.

B. Provide nutritional and fluid and electrolyte support.
  1. Keep client NPO until responsive, and provide mouth care every 4 hours.
  2. Maintain calorie count.
  3. Administer feedings as prescribed (Box 4-1).
  4. Monitor I&O.
  5. Record client's weight (weigh at same time each day).

C. Prevent complications of immobility.
  1. Monitor impairment in skin integrity.
    a. Turn client every 2 hours, and assess bony prominences.
    b. Use egg-crate or alternating-pressure mattress or waterbed.
    c. Use minimal amount of linens and underpads.,

BOX 4-1 *Unconscious Client*

Gastric Gavage

- Check bowel sounds, and begin feeding when GI peristalsis returns.
- Place client in high-Fowler position.
- Place towel over chest.
- Connect gastrostomy tube to funnel or large syringe.
- Check gastric residual to assess absorption and client tolerance; return residual.
- Pour feeding into tilted funnel, and unclamp tubing to allow feeding to flow by gravity.
- Regulate flow by raising or lowering container. Feeding too quickly causes diarrhea, gastric distention, pain. Feeding too slowly causes possible obstruction of flow.
- After feeding, irrigate tube with (tepid) water and clamp tube.
- Apply small dressing over tube opening; coil tube and attach to dressing. May cover with an abdominal binder.

Bowel Management Program

- Get bowel history from reliable source.
- Establish specific time for evacuation. Regularity is essential.
- An unconscious client can evacuate the bowel after the last tube feeding of day, because the gastrocolic and duodenocolic reflexes are active after "meal."
- Stimulate anorectal reflex by insertion of glycerin suppository 15 to 30 minutes before scheduled evacuation time. May need stronger suppository, such as bisacodyl (Dulcolax).
- Ensure adequate fiber in tube feedings and adequate fluid intake of 2 to 4 L/day.
- May apply a rectal pouch to contain fecal material (ostomy bag with seal over anal opening)

2. Potential for thrombus formation
   a. Perform passive ROM exercises to lower extremities every 4 hours.
   b. Apply sequential compression device (SCD) or elastic hose (remove and reapply every 8 hours).
   c. Avoid positions that decrease venous return.
   d. Avoid pillows under knees and Gatched bed.
3. Urinary calculi
   a. Increase fluid intake PO or via gastric tube.
   b. Assess urine for high specific gravity (dehydration) and balance between I&O.
4. Contractures and joint immobility
   a. Perform passive ROM every 4 hours.
   b. Sit client up in bed or chair, if possible, or use neuro chair if necessary.
   c. Reposition every 2 hours, maintaining proper body alignment.
   d. Apply splints or other assistive devices to prevent foot drop, wrist drop, or other improper alignment.
D. Monitor and evaluate the vital-sign changes indicating changes in condition.
   1. Pulse: a pulse rate change to <60 or >100 bpm can indicate increased ICP. A fast rate (>100 bpm) can indicate infection, thrombus formation, or dehydration.
   2. Blood pressure: rising BP or widening pulse pressure can indicate increased ICP.
   3. Temperature: report any abnormalities; temperature elevation can indicate worsening condition, damage to temperature-regulating area of brain, or infection.
   4. Level-of-consciousness changes: they may range from active to somnolent.
   5. Pupillary changes: they may range from prompt to sluggish or may increase in size.

HESI Hint • If temperature elevates, take quick measures to decrease it, because fever increases cerebral metabolism and can increase cerebral edema.

HESI Hint • Safety Features for Immobilized Clients:
• Prevent skin breakdown by frequent turning.
• Maintain adequate nutrition.
• Prevent aspiration with slow, small feedings or NG feedings.
• Monitor neurologic signs to detect the first signs that intracranial pressure may be increasing.
• Provide ROM exercises to prevent deformities.
• Prevent respiratory complications; frequent turning and positioning provide optimal drainage.

E. Prevent injury and promote safety.
   1. Place bed in low position, and keep side rails up at all times.
   2. Pad side rails if client is agitated or if there is a history of seizure activity.
   3. Restrain client if client is trying to remove tubes or attempting to get out of bed.
   4. Touch gently, and talk softly and calmly to the client, remembering that hearing is commonly intact.

HESI Hint • Restlessness may indicate a return to consciousness but can also indicate anoxia, distended bladder, covert bleeding, or increasing cerebral anoxia. Do not oversedate, and report any symptoms of restlessness.

   5. Avoid oversedating the client because sedatives and narcotics depress responsiveness and affect pupillary reaction (an important assessment in neurologic vital signs).
   6. During all activities, tell the client what you are doing, regardless of the level of consciousness.
F. Maintain hygiene and cleanliness.
   1. Provide bathing, grooming, and dressing.
   2. Provide oral hygiene.
   3. Wash hair weekly.
   4. Provide nail care within agency guidelines.
G. Observe for bladder elimination problems.
   1. Insert indwelling catheter if prescribed.
   2. Remove indwelling catheter as soon as possible; use adult brief or condom catheter.
H. Document and record bowel movements, and report abnormal patterns of constipation or diarrhea.
   1. Rapid infusion of tube feedings may cause diarrhea; lack of fiber and inadequate fluids may cause constipation.
   2. Initiate bowel program (see Box 4-1).
I. Prevent corneal injury and drying:
   1. Remove contact lenses if present.
   2. Irrigate eyes with sterile prescribed solution, and instill ophthalmic ointment in each eye every 8 hours to prevent corneal ulceration.
   3. Close eyelids if blink reflex is absent.

HEAD INJURY

Description: Any traumatic damage to the head

A. Open head injury occurs when there is a fracture of the skull or penetration of the skull by an object.
B. Closed head injury (CHI) is the result of blunt trauma (more serious because of chance of increased intracranial pressure in closed vault).

C. Increased ICP is the main concern in head injury; it is related to edema, hemorrhage, impaired cerebral autoregulation, and hydrocephalus.

> **HESI Hint** • The forces of impact influence the type of head injury. They include acceleration injury, which is caused by the head being in motion, and deceleration injury, which occurs when the head stops suddenly. Helmets are a great preventive measure for motorcyclists and bicyclists (Fig. 4-8).

Nursing Assessment

A. Unconsciousness or disturbances in consciousness
B. Vertigo
C. Confusion, delirium, or disorientation
D. Symptoms of increased ICP

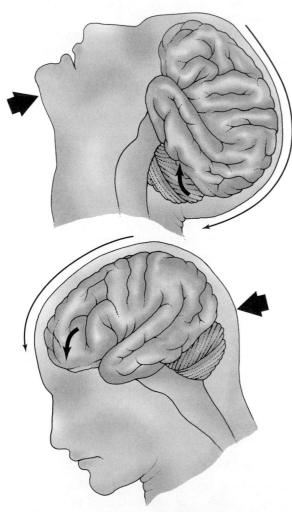

FIGURE 4-8 Head movement during acceleration-deceleration injury, which is typically seen in motor vehicle accidents. (From Ignatavicius DD, Workman ML: *Medical-surgical nursing: Patient-centered collaborative care*, ed 6. St. Louis, 2010, Saunders.)

1. Change in level of responsiveness is the most important indicator of increased ICP.

> **HESI Hint** • Even subtle behavior changes, such as restlessness, irritability, or confusion, may indicate increased ICP.

2. Changes in vital signs
   a. Slowing of respirations or respiratory irregularities
   b. Increase or decrease in pulse
   c. Rising BP or widening pulse pressure
   d. Temperature rise
3. Headache
4. Vomiting (projectile)
5. Pupillary changes reflecting pressure on optic or oculomotor nerves
   a. Decrease or increase in size or unequal size of pupils
   b. Lack of conjugate eye movement
   c. Papilledema

E. Seizures
F. Ataxia
G. Abnormal posturing (decerebrate or decorticate)
H. CSF leakage through nose (rhinorrhea) or through ear (otorrhea)

> **HESI Hint** • CSF leakage carries the risk for meningitis and indicates a deteriorating condition. Because of CSF leakage, the usual signs of increased ICP may not occur.

I. CT scan or MRI will show a lesion, such as an epidural or subdural hematoma, requiring surgery.
J. Electroencephalograph (EEG) determines presence of seizure activity.

Analysis (Nursing Diagnoses)

A. *Ineffective tissue perfusion* related to...
B. *Disturbed sensory perception* related to...
C. *Risk for injury* related to...
D. *Ineffective family coping* related to...

Nursing Plans and Interventions

A. Maintain adequate ventilation and airway.
   1. Monitor Po_2 and Pco_2 for the development of hypoxia and hypercapnia.
   2. Position client semiprone or lateral recumbent to prevent aspiration.
   3. Turn from side to side to prevent lung secretion stasis.

B. Keep head of bed elevated 30 to 45 degrees to aid venous return from the neck and to decrease cerebral volume.

C. Obtain neurologic vital signs as prescribed (at least every 1 to 2 hours), and maintain a continuous record of observations and Glasgow Coma Scale ratings.

D. Notify physician at first sign of deterioration or improvement in condition.

E. Avoid activities that increase intracranial pressure such as:
1. Change in bed position for caregiving and extreme hip flexion
2. Endotracheal suctioning
3. Compression of jugular veins (keep head straight and not to one side)
4. Coughing, vomiting, or straining of any type (no Valsalva: increased intrathoracic pressure increases ICP)

F. If temperature increases, take immediate measures to reduce it (aspirin, acetaminophen, cooling blanket) because increased temperature increases cerebral blood flow drastically; avoid shivering.

G. Use intracranial monitoring system when available:
1. A catheter is inserted into the lateral ventricle, a sensor placed on the dura, or a screw into the subarachnoid space attached to a pressure transducer.
2. Elevations of intracranial pressure over 20 mm Hg should be reported stat.

H. Administer medications prescribed by physician to reduce ICP.
1. Hyperosmotic agents and diuretics to dehydrate brain and reduce cerebral edema
   a. Mannitol (Table 4-32)
   b. Urea
2. Steroids
   a. Dexamethasone (Decadron)
   b. Methylprednisolone sodium succinate (Solu-Medrol) to reduce brain edema

3. Barbiturates
   a. To reduce brain metabolism and systemic blood pressure

I. Insert indwelling Foley catheter to prevent restlessness caused by distended bladder and to monitor balance between restricted fluid intake and output, especially if placed on osmotic diuretics.

HESI Hint • Try not to use restraints; they only increase restlessness. Avoid narcotics because they mask the level of responsiveness.

J. Physician may order passive hyperventilation on ventilator: leads to respiratory alkalosis, which causes cerebral vasoconstriction and decreased cerebral blood flow, and therefore decreased ICP.

K. Continue seizure precautions. Health care provider may order prophylactic phenytoin (Dilantin).

L. Prevent complications of immobility (see Nursing Plans and Interventions for the Unconscious/Immobilized Client, p. 144).

M. Inform at discharge of possible aftereffects of head injury.
1. Posttraumatic syndrome: headache, vertigo, emotional instability, inability to concentrate, impaired memory
2. Posttraumatic epilepsy
3. Posttraumatic neuroses or psychoses

SPINAL CORD INJURY

Description: Disruption in nervous system function, which may result in complete or incomplete loss of motor and sensory function. Changes occur in the function of all physiologic systems.

A. Injuries are described by location in the spinal cord. The most common sites are the fifth, sixth, and seventh cervical vertebrae (C-5, C-6, C-7), the twelfth thoracic (T-12), and the first lumbar (L-1).

TABLE 4-32 Osmotic Diuretic

Drug	Indications	Adverse Reactions	Nursing Implications
• Mannitol (Osmitrol)	• Acts on renal tubules by osmosis to prevent water reabsorption • In bloodstream, draws fluid from the extravascular spaces into the plasma	• Disorientation, confusion, and headache • Nausea and vomiting • Convulsions and anaphylactic reactions	• Use for short-term therapy *only* • Never give to clients with cerebral hemorrhage • IV infusion is usually adjusted to urine output; filter and watch for crystals • Never give to clients with no urine output (anuria); if output is <30 ml/hr, accumulation can cause pulmonary edema and water intoxication

B. Damage can range from contusion to complete transection.

C. Permanent impairment cannot be determined until spinal cord edema has subsided, usually by 1 week.

Nursing Assessment

A. Assess breathing pattern, and auscultate lungs.

> **HESI Hint** • Physical assessment should concentrate on respiratory status, especially in clients with injury at C-3 to C-5, because the cervical plexus innervates the diaphragm.

B. Check neurologic vital signs frequently, especially sensory and motor functions. Assess cardiovascular status.

C. Assess abdomen: girth, bowel sounds; assess lower abdomen for bladder distention.

D. Assess temperature, remembering that hyperthermia occurs commonly.

E. Assess psychosocial status.

F. Hypotension and bradycardia occur with any injury above T-6 because sympathetic outflow is affected.

Analysis (Nursing Diagnoses)

A. *Ineffective breathing pattern* related to…

B. *Ineffective tissue perfusion* related to…

C. *Impaired skin integrity* related to…

D. *Self-care deficit* (specify) related to…

E. *Urinary retention* related to…

F. *Ineffective coping* related to…

Nursing Plans and Interventions

A. In acute phase of spinal cord injury:
  1. See Nursing Plans and Interventions for the Unconscious/Immobilized Client, p. 144.
  2. Maintain client in an extended position with cervical collar on during any transfer.
  3. Stabilize the client when transferring between the accident scene and the emergency department. The client will be realigned and stabilized in the emergency room.
  4. Maintain a patent airway (most important).
  5. In cervical injuries, skeletal traction is maintained by use of skull tongs or a halo ring (Crutchfield tongs or a Gardner-Wells fixation device).
  6. High-dose corticosteroids are often given to help control edema during the first 8 to 24 hours.
  7. Use a kinetic therapy treatment table (Rotorest bed), which provides continuous side-to-side motion.

  8. Use Stryker frame or very firm mattress with board underneath.
  9. Assess for respiratory failure, especially in clients with high cervical injuries.
  10. Further loss of sensory or motor function below injury can indicate additional damage to cord due to edema and should be reported immediately.
  11. Evaluate for presence of spinal shock (a complete loss of all reflex, motor, sensory, and autonomic activity below the lesion). This is a medical emergency that occurs immediately after the injury.
     a. Hypotension, bradycardia
     b. Complete paralysis and lack of sensation below lesion
     c. Bladder and bowel distention

> **HESI Hint** • It is imperative to reverse spinal shock as quickly as possible. Permanent paralysis can occur if a spinal cord is compressed for 12 to 24 hours.

  12. Evaluate for autonomic dysreflexia (exaggerated autonomic responses to stimuli), which occurs in clients with lesions at or above T-6. This is a medical emergency that usually occurs after the period of spinal shock has finished and is usually triggered by a noxious stimulus such as bowel or bladder distention. It may also be triggered by a vaginal examination.
     a. Elevated BP
     b. Pounding headache, sweating, nasal congestion, goose bumps, bradycardia
     c. Bladder and bowel distention
  13. Watch for acute paralytic ileus, lack of gastric activity.
     a. Assess bowel sounds frequently.
     b. Initiate gastric suction to reduce distention, prevent vomiting and aspiration.
     c. Use rectal tube to relieve gaseous distention.
  14. Suction with caution to prevent vagus nerve stimulation, which can cause cardiac arrest.
  15. Administer high-dose corticosteroids to decrease edema and reduce cord damage.

B. In rehabilitative phase of spinal cord injury:
  1. Encourage deep-breathing exercises.
  2. Administer chest physiotherapy.
  3. Provide kinetic bed to promote blood flow to extremities.
  4. Apply antiembolic stockings or SCDs.
  5. Facilitate ROM exercises.
  6. Mobilize client to chair as soon as possible.
  7. Turn client frequently.

8. Keep client clean and dry.
9. Observe for impending skin breakdown.
10. Teach client importance of impeccable skin care.
11. Perform intermittent catheterization every 4 hours.
    a. Begin teaching client catheterization technique.
    b. Teach family member if client is unable.
12. Teach bladder-emptying techniques according to level of injury and bladder muscle response.
    a. UMN (spastic) bladder
    b. LMN (flaccid) bladder
13. Instruct client in monitoring I&O.
14. Encourage the client to drink fluids that promote acidic urine, including cranberry juice, prune juice, bouillon, tomato juice, and water.

HESI Hint • A common cause of death after spinal cord injury is urinary tract infection. Bacteria grow best in alkaline media, so keeping urine dilute and acidic is prophylactic against infection. Also, keeping the bladder emptied assists in avoiding bacterial growth in urine that has stagnated in the bladder.

15. Begin bowel-training program.
16. Talk with client and family about permanence of disability.
17. Encourage rehabilitation facility staff to visit client.
18. Encourage client and family to visit rehabilitation facility.
19. Assist family in finding support group, and refer to community resources after dismissal from rehabilitation facility.

BRAIN TUMOR

Description: Neoplasm occurring in the brain

A. Primary tumors can arise in any tissue of the brain.
B. Secondary tumors are a result of metastasis from other areas (most often from the lungs, followed by breast).
C. Without treatment, benign as well as malignant tumors lead to death.

HESI Hint • Benign tumors continue to grow and take up space in the confined area of the cranium, causing neural and vascular compromise in the brain, increased ICP, and necrosis of brain tissue. Even benign tumors must be treated because they may have malignant effects.

Nursing Assessment

A. Headache that is more severe on awakening
B. Vomiting not associated with nausea
C. Papilledema with visual changes

D. Behavioral and personality changes
E. Seizures
F. Aphasia, hemiplegia, ataxia
G. Cranial nerve dysfunction
H. Abnormal CT scan/MRI

Analysis (Nursing Diagnoses)

A. *Ineffective tissue perfusion* related to…
B. *Acute pain* related to…
C. *Risk for injury* related to…
D. *Anxiety* related to…

Nursing Plans and Interventions

A. Institute nursing plans and interventions that are similar to those implemented for the client with a head injury and increased ICP.
B. Elevate the head of the bed 30 to 40 degrees; maintain head in neutral position.
C. Facilitate radiation therapy.
    1. Provide skin care with non-oil-based soap and water. Avoid putting alcohol, powder, or oils on the skin.
    2. Explain that alopecia is temporary.
    3. Instruct client not to wash off the lines drawn by the radiologist.
D. Administer chemotherapy: medications may be injected intraventricularly or intravenously.
E. Facilitate surgical removal of tumor (craniotomy).
    1. Preoperative
        a. Shave head.
    2. Postoperative
        a. Perform frequent neurologic and vital sign assessment.
        b. Position client with head of bed elevated for supratentorial lesions and flat for infratentorial lesions. Position client on side opposite the operative site.
        c. Monitor dressings for signs of drainage (excess amount of CSF).
        d. Monitor respiratory status to prevent hypoventilation.
        e. Avoid activities that cause increased ICP.
        f. Monitor for seizure activity.
        g. Administer medications (see Head Injuries, p. 145).

HESI Hint • Craniotomy preoperative medications:
• Corticosteroids to reduce swelling
• Agents and osmotic diuretics to reduce secretions (atropine, glycopyrrolate [Robinul])
• Agents to reduce seizures (phenytoin)
• Prophylactic antibiotics

MULTIPLE SCLEROSIS (MS)

Description: Demyelinating disease resulting in the destruction of CNS myelin and consequent disruption in the transmission of nerve impulses

A. Onset is insidious, with 50% of clients still ambulatory 25 years after diagnosis.

B. Diagnosis determined by a combination of data:
1. Presenting symptoms
2. Increased white matter density seen on CT scan
3. Presence of plaques seen on MRI
4. CSF electrophoresis shows presence of oligoclonal (IgG) bands.

C. Current thinking is that MS is autoimmune in origin.

HESI Hint • Symptoms involving motor function usually begin in the upper extremities with weakness progressing to spastic paralysis. Bowel and bladder dysfunction occurs in 90% of cases. MS is more common in women. Progression is not "orderly."

Nursing Assessment

A. Nursing history of client to include:
1. History of symptoms
2. Progression of illness
3. Types of treatment received and the responses
4. Additional health problems
5. Current medications
6. Client's and family's perception of illness
7. Community resources used by the client

B. Physical assessment to include:
1. Optic neuritis (loss of vision or blind spots)
2. Visual or swallowing difficulties
3. Gait disturbances; intention tremors
4. Unusual fatigue, weakness, and clumsiness
5. Numbness, particularly on one side of face
6. Impaired bladder and bowel control
7. Speech disturbances
8. Scotomas (white spots in visual field, diplopia)

Analysis (Nursing Diagnoses)

A. *Impaired physical mobility* related to...
B. *Disturbed sensory perception* related to...
C. *Fatigue* related to...
D. *Impaired urinary elimination* related to...
E. *Impaired home maintenance* related to...

Nursing Plans and Interventions

A. Allow hospitalized client to keep own routine.
B. Orient client to environment, and teach strategies to maximize vision.

C. Encourage self-care and frequent rest periods.

D. With exercise programs, encourage client to work up to the point just short of fatigue.

E. Teach client that for muscle spasticity, stretch-hold-relax exercises are helpful, as are riding a stationary bicycle and swimming; take precautions against falls.

F. Initially, work with client on a voiding schedule.

G. Teach client that as incontinence worsens, the female may need to learn clean self-catheterization; the male may need a condom catheter.

H. Encourage adequate fluid intake, high-fiber foods, and a bowel regimen for constipation problems.

I. Encourage the client and the family to verbalize their concerns about ongoing care issues.

J. Encourage client to maintain contact with a support group.

K. Refer client for home health care services.

L. Encourage client to contact the local MS society for emotional support and direct services.

M. Administer steroid therapy and chemotherapeutic drugs in acute exacerbations to shorten length of attack.

HESI Hint • Drug therapy for MS clients: ACTH, cortisone, cyclophosphamide (Cytoxan), and other immunosuppressive drugs. Nursing implications for administration of these drugs should focus on the prevention of infection.

N. Remember that biologic response modifiers such as interferon-beta products have shown recent success for MS relapses.

MYASTHENIA GRAVIS

Description: Disorder affecting the neuromuscular transmission of impulses in the voluntary muscles of the body

A. It is considered an autoimmune disease characterized by the presence of acetylcholine receptor antibodies (AChRs), which interfere with neuronal transmission.

B. It usually affects females between ages 10 and 40 and men between ages 50 and 70.

Nursing Assessment

A. Diplopia (double vision), ptosis (eyelid drooping)
B. Masklike affect: sleepy appearance due to facial muscle involvement
C. Weakness of laryngeal and pharyngeal muscles: dysphagia, choking, food aspiration, difficulty speaking

D. Muscle weakness improved by rest, worsened by activity

E. Advanced cases: respiratory failure, bladder and bowel incontinence

F. Myasthenic crisis symptoms (attributed to disease worsening) associated with undermedication

G. Cholinergic crisis (attributed to anticholinesterase overdosage): diaphoresis, diarrhea, fasciculations, cramps, marked worsening of symptoms resulting from overmedication

HESI Hint • In clients with myasthenia gravis, be alert for changes in respiratory status; the most severe involvement may result in respiratory failure.

Analysis (Nursing Diagnoses)

A. *Ineffective airway clearance* related to…

B. *Risk for injury* related to…

C. *Impaired physical mobility* related to…

D. *Risk for imbalanced nutrition: less than body requirements* related to…

Nursing Plans and Interventions

A. If client is hospitalized, have tracheostomy kit available at bedside for possible myasthenic crisis.

B. Teach client the importance of wearing a Medic-Alert bracelet.

C. Administer cholinergic drugs as prescribed (Table 4-33).

D. Schedule nursing activities to conserve energy (e.g., complete daily hygiene activities, administration of medications, and treatments all at once), and allow rest periods. Plan activities during high-energy times, often in the early morning.

E. Instruct client to avoid situations that produce fatigue or physical or emotional stress (any type of stress can exacerbate symptoms).

HESI Hint • Bed rest often relieves symptoms. Bladder and respiratory infections are often a recurring problem. There is a need for health-promotion teachings.

F. Encourage coughing and deep breathing every 4 to 6 hours. (Muscle weakness limits ability to cough up secretions, promotes URI.)

G. If symptoms worsen, identify type of crisis: myasthenic or cholinergic.

HESI Hint • Myasthenic crisis is associated with a positive edrophonium (Tensilon) test, whereas a cholinergic crisis is associated with a negative test.

PARKINSON DISEASE

Description: Chronic, progressive, debilitating neurologic, disease of the basal ganglia and substantia nigra, affecting motor ability and characterized by tremor at rest, increased muscle tone (rigidity), slowness in the initiation and execution of movement (bradykinesia), and postural instability (difficulties with gait and balance).

TABLE 4-33   Treatment of Myasthenia Gravis

Drug	Indications	Adverse Reactions	Nursing Implications
• Pyridostigmine bromide (Mestinon)	• Inhibits the action of cholinesterase at the cholinergic nerve endings • To promote accumulation of acetylcholine at zcholinergic receptor sites	• Cholinergic crisis can occur with overdose	• Atropine is antidote for drug-induced bradycardia • Take drug with milk or food to decrease GI side effects • Dosage regulation required; record keeping, re: side effects, drug response • Observe for symptoms of cholinergic crisis → Fasciculations → Abdominal cramps, diarrhea, incontinence of stool or urine → Hypotension, bradycardia, respiratory depression → Lacrimation, blurred vision • Drug therapy is lifelong and requires family teaching and support

Nursing Assessment

A. Rigidity of extremities

B. Masklike facial expressions with associated difficulty in chewing, swallowing, and speaking

C. Drooling

D. Stooped posture and slow, shuffling gait

E. Tremors at rest, "pill-rolling" movement

F. Emotional lability

HESI Hint • NCLEX-RN questions often focus on the features of Parkinson disease: tremors (a coarse tremor of fingers and thumb on one hand that disappears during sleep and purposeful activity; also called "pill rolling"), rigidity, hypertonicity, and stooped posture. Focus: *safety!*

Analysis (Nursing Diagnoses)

A. *Self-care deficit* (specify) related to…

B. *Impaired physical mobility* related to…

C. *Imbalanced nutrition: less than body requirements* related to…

D. *Impaired verbal communication* related to…

E. *Disturbed body image* related to…

Nursing Plans and Interventions

A. Schedule activities later in the day to allow sufficient time for client to perform self-care activities without rushing.

B. Encourage activities and exercise. A cane or walker may be needed.

C. Eliminate environmental noise, and encourage the client to speak slowly and clearly, pausing at intervals.

D. Serve a soft diet, which is easy to swallow.

E. Administer antiparkinsonian drugs as prescribed (Table 4-34).

TABLE 4-34 Antiparkinsonian Drugs

Drugs	Indications	Adverse Reactions	Nursing Implications
Anticholinergics (parasympatholytics [older drugs])			
• Atropine sulfate (Atropisol) • Benztropine mesylate (Cogentin) • Trihexyphenidyl (Artane)	• Reduces cholinergic activity	• Increased heart rate • Postural hypotension • Dry mouth • Constipation • Urinary retention	• Review client's history for glaucoma, urinary obstruction • Warn to avoid rapid position changes • Avoid extreme heat • Provide gum, hard candy, and frequent mouth care
Dopamine Replacements			
• Levodopa (Dopar) • Levodopa-carbidopa (Sinemet) **Dopamine-Releasing Agents** • Amantadine HCl (Symmetrel) **Dopamine-Releasing Agonists** • Bromocriptine mesylate (Parlodel) • Pramipexole (Mirapex) • Pergolide (Permax)	• Stimulates dopamine production or increases sensitivity of dopamine receptors • Newer drugs require lower dosage	• Involuntary movements • Nausea • Vomiting	• Explain drugs may take months to achieve desired effects • Warn to avoid sudden position changes • Avoid foods high in vitamin B_6 (meats, liver, i.e., high-protein foods) • If insomnia occurs, suggest taking last dose earlier in day • May initially cause drowsiness; teach to avoid driving until response is determined
Monoamine Oxidase Type B Inhibitor			
• Selegiline (Eldepryl)	• Used with dopamine agonist when client symptoms do not respond	• Confusion, dizziness • Nausea, dry mouth • Insomnia	• Review drug-drug interaction carefully • Not an option if client on antidepressants (SSRIs or tricyclics)

HESI Hint • An important aspect of treatment for Parkinson disease is drug therapy. The pathophysiology involves an imbalance between acetylcholine and dopamine, so symptoms can be controlled by administering a dopamine precursor (levodopa).

GUILLAIN-BARRÉ SYNDROME

Description: Clinical syndrome of unknown origin involving peripheral and cranial nerves

A. Is usually preceded by a respiratory or GI infection 1 to 4 weeks prior to the onset of neurologic deficits.

B. Constant monitoring of these clients is required to prevent the life-threatening problem of acute respiratory failure.

C. Full recovery usually occurs within several months to a year after onset of symptoms.

D. About 10% of those diagnosed with Guillain-Barré syndrome are left with a residual disability.

Nursing Assessment

A. Paresthesia (tingling and numbness)

B. Muscle weakness of legs progressing to the upper extremities, trunk, and face

C. Paralysis of the ocular, facial, and oropharyngeal muscles, causing marked difficulty in talking, chewing, and swallowing. Assess for:
1. Breathlessness while talking
2. Shallow and irregular breathing
3. Use of accessory muscles while breathing
4. Any change in respiratory pattern
5. Paradoxical inward movement of the upper abdominal wall while in a supine position, indicating weakness and impending paralysis of the diaphragm.

D. Increasing pulse rate and disturbances in rhythm

E. Transient hypertension, orthostatic hypotension

F. Possible pain in the back and in calves of legs

G. Weakness or paralysis of the intercostal and diaphragm muscles; may develop quickly

Analysis (Nursing Diagnoses)

A. *Ineffective breathing pattern* related to…

B. *Imbalanced nutrition: less than body requirements* related to…

C. *Impaired verbal communication* related to…

Nursing Plans and Interventions

A. Monitor for respiratory distress, and initiate mechanical ventilation if necessary.

B. See Nursing Plans and Interventions for the Unconscious/Immobilized Client, p. 144.

STROKE/BRAIN ATTACK: CEREBRAL VASCULAR ACCIDENT (CVA)

Description: Sudden loss of brain function resulting from a disruption in the blood supply to a part of the brain; classified as thrombotic or hemorrhagic

HESI Hint • CNS involvement related to cause of stroke:
• Hemorrhagic: caused by a slow or fast hemorrhage into the brain tissue; often related to hypertension
• Embolytic: caused by a clot that has broken away from a vessel and has lodged in one of the arteries of the brain, blocking the blood supply. It is often related to atherosclerosis (so it may occur again).

A. Risk factors include:
1. Hypertension
2. Previous transient ischemic attacks (TIAs)
3. Cardiac disease: atherosclerosis, valve disease, history of dysrhythmias (particularly atrial flutter or fibrillation)
4. Advanced age
5. Diabetes
6. Oral contraceptives
7. Smoking

HESI Hint • Atrial flutter and fibrillation produce a high incidence of thrombus formation following dysrhythmia caused by turbulence of blood flow through all valves and heart chambers.

B. Diagnosis is made by observation of clinical signs and is confirmed by:
1. Cranial CT scan
2. MRI
3. Doppler flow studies
4. Ultrasound imaging

C. Presenting symptoms relate to the specific area of the brain that has been damaged (Table 4-35).

D. Generally there is:
1. Motor loss, usually exhibited as hemiparesis or hemiplegia
2. Communication loss, exhibited as dysarthria, dysphasia, aphasia, or apraxia
3. Perceptual disturbance that can be visual, spatial, and sensory
4. Impaired mental acuity or psychological changes, such as decreased attention span, memory loss, depression, lability, and hostility

E. Bladder dysfunction may be either incontinence or retention.

F. Rehabilitation is begun as soon as the client is stable.

TABLE 4-35 Location of Disruption in the Brain

Feature	Left Hemisphere	Right Hemisphere
• Language	• Aphasia • Agraphia	• May be alert and oriented
• Memory	• No deficit	• Disoriented • Cannot recognize faces
• Vision	• Unable to discriminate words and letters • Reading problems • Deficits in right visual field	• Visual/spatial deficits • Neglect of left visual fields • Loss of depth perception
• Behavior	• Slow • Cautious • Anxious when attempting a new task • Depression or catastrophic response to illness • Sense of guilt • Feeling of worthlessness • Worries over future • Quick anger and frustration	• Impulsive • Unaware of neurologic deficits • Confabulates • Euphoric • Constantly smiles • Denies illness • Poor judgment • Overestimates abilities • Impaired sense of humor
• Hearing	• No deficit	• Loses ability to hear tonal variations

HESI Hint • A woman who had a stroke 2 days earlier has left-sided paralysis. She has begun to regain some movement in her left side. What can the nurse tell the family about the client's recovery period?

"The quicker movement is recovered, the better the prognosis is for full or improved recovery. She will need patience and understanding from her family as she tries to cope with the stroke. Mood swings can be expected during the recovery period, and bouts of depression and tearfulness are likely."

Nursing Assessment

A. Change in level of consciousness

B. Paresthesia, paralysis

C. Aphasia, agraphia

D. Memory loss

E. Vision impairment

F. Bladder and bowel dysfunction

G. Behavioral changes

H. Assessment of client's functional abilities, including:
1. Mobility
2. Activities of daily living (ADLs)
3. Elimination
4. Communication

I. Ability to swallow, eat, and drink without aspiration

Analysis (Nursing Diagnoses)

A. *Impaired physical mobility* related to...

B. *Self-care deficit* (specify) related to...

C. *Impaired urinary elimination* related to...

D. *Impaired verbal communication* related to...

E. *Ineffective coping* related to...

F. *Ineffective family coping* related to...

G. *Disturbed body image* related to...

HESI Hint • Words that describe losses in strokes:
1. *Apraxia:* inability to perform purposeful movements in the absence of motor problems
2. *Dysarthria:* difficulty articulating
3. *Dysphasia:* impairment of speech and verbal comprehension
4. *Aphasia:* loss of the ability to speak
5. *Agraphia:* loss of the ability to write
6. *Alexia:* loss of the ability to read
7. *Dysphagia:* dysfunctional swallowing

Nursing Plans and Interventions

A. Control hypertension to help prevent future stroke.

B. Maintain proper body alignment while client is in bed. Use splints or other assistive devices (including bed rolls and pillows) to maintain functional position.

C. Position client to minimize edema, prevent contractures, and maintain skin integrity.

D. Perform full ROM exercises four times a day. Follow up with program initiated by other team members.

E. Encourage client to participate in or manage own personal care.

F. Set realistic goals; add new tasks daily.

G. Teach client that appropriate self-care activities for the hemiparetic person include:
   1. Bathing
   2. Brushing teeth
   3. Shaving with electric razor
   4. Eating
   5. Combing hair

H. Encourage client to assist with dressing activities, and modify them as necessary (client will wear street clothes during waking hours).

I. Analyze bladder elimination pattern.
   1. Offer bedpan or urinal according to client's particular pattern of elimination.
   2. Reassure client that bladder control tends to be regained quickly.

J. Follow-up speech program is initiated by the speech and language therapist.
   1. Ensure consistency with this program.

2. Reassure the client that regaining speech is a very slow process.

K. Do not place client in sensory overload; give only one set of instructions at a time.

L. Encourage total family involvement in rehabilitation.

M. Encourage client and family to join a support group.

N. Encourage family members to allow the client to perform self-care activities as outlined by the rehabilitation team.

O. Refer for outpatient follow-up or for home health care.

P. Teach that swallowing modifications may include a soft diet (pureed foods, thickened liquids) and head positioning.

> **HESI Hint** • Steroids are administered after a stroke to decrease cerebral edema and retard permanent disability. H_2 inhibitors are administered to prevent peptic ulcers.

Review of Neurologic System

1. What are the classifications of the commonly prescribed eye drops for glaucoma?
2. Identify two types of hearing loss.
3. Write four nursing interventions for the care of the blind person and four nursing interventions for the care of the deaf person.
4. In your own words, describe the Glasgow Coma Scale.
5. List four nursing diagnoses for the comatose client in order of priority. (Remember Maslow's Hierarchy of Needs to help determine priorities.)
6. State four independent nursing interventions to maintain adequate respiration, airway, and oxygenation in the unconscious client.
7. Who is at risk for stroke?
8. Complications of immobility include the potential for thrombus development. State three nursing interventions to prevent thrombi.
9. List four rationales for the appearance of restlessness in the unconscious client.
10. What nursing interventions prevent corneal drying in a comatose client?
11. When can a comatose client on IV hyperalimentation begin to receive tube feedings instead?
12. What is the most important principle in a bowel management program for a client with neurologic deficits?
13. Define stroke.
14. A client with a diagnosis of stroke presents with symptoms of aphasia and right hemiparesis but no memory or hearing deficit. In what hemisphere has the client suffered a lesion?
15. What are the symptoms of spinal shock?
16. What are the symptoms of autonomic dysreflexia?
17. What is the most important indicator of increased ICP?
18. What vital sign changes are indicative of increased ICP?
19. A neighbor calls the neighborhood nurse stating that he was knocked hard to the floor by his very hyperactive dog. He is wondering what symptoms would indicate the need to visit an emergency department. What should the nurse tell him to do?
20. What activities and situations that increase ICP should be avoided?
21. What is the action of hyperosmotic agents (osmotic diuretics) used to treat intracranial pressure?
22. Why should narcotics be avoided in clients with neurologic impairment?
23. Headache and vomiting are symptoms of many disorders. What characteristics of these symptoms would alert the nurse to refer a client to a neurologist?
24. How should the head of the bed be positioned for postcraniotomy clients with infratentorial lesions?
25. Is multiple sclerosis thought to occur because of an autoimmune process?
26. Is paralysis always a consequence of spinal cord injury?
27. What types of drugs are used in the treatment of myasthenia gravis?

Answers to Review

1. Parasympathomimetic for pupillary constriction; beta-adrenergic receptor–blocking agents to inhibit formation of aqueous humor; carbonic anhydrase inhibitors to reduce aqueous humor production; and prostaglandin agonists to increase aqueous humor outflow
2. Conductive (transmission of sound to inner ear is blocked) and sensorineural (damage to eighth cranial nerve)
3. Care of blind: announce presence clearly, call by name, orient carefully to surroundings, guide by walking in front of client with his or her hand in your elbow. Care of deaf: reduce distraction before beginning conversation, look and listen to client, give client full attention if he or she is a lip reader, face client directly.
4. An objective assessment of the level of consciousness based on a score of 3 to 15, with scores of 7 or less indicative of coma
5. Ineffective breathing pattern, ineffective airway clearance, impaired gas exchange, and decreased cardiac output
6. Position for maximum ventilation (prone or semiprone and slightly to one side); insert airway if tongue is obstructing; suction airway efficiently; monitor arterial Po_2 and Pco_2; and hyperventilate with 100% O_2 before suctioning.
7. Persons with histories of hypertension, previous TIAs, cardiac disease (atrial flutter or fibrillation), diabetes, or oral contraceptive use; and older adults.
8. Frequent range-of-motion exercises, frequent (every 2 hours) position changes, and avoidance of positions that decrease venous return.
9. Anoxia, distended bladder, covert bleeding, or a return to consciousness
10. Irrigation of eyes PRN with sterile prescribed solution, application of ophthalmic ointment every 8 hours, close assessment for corneal ulceration or drying
11. When peristalsis resumes as evidenced by active bowel sounds, passage of flatus or bowel movement
12. Establishment of regularity
13. A disruption of blood supply to a part of the brain, which results in sudden loss of brain function
14. Left
15. Hypotension, bladder and bowel distention, total paralysis, lack of sensation below lesion
16. Hypertension, bladder and bowel distention, exaggerated autonomic responses, headache, sweating, goose bumps, and bradycardia
17. A change in the level of responsiveness
18. Increased BP, widening pulse pressure, increased or decreased pulse, respiratory irregularities, and temperature increase
19. Call his physician now and inform him or her of the fall. Symptoms needing medical attention would include vertigo, confusion or any subtle behavioral change, headache, vomiting, ataxia (imbalance), or seizure.
20. Change in bed position, extreme hip flexion, endotracheal suctioning, compression of jugular veins, coughing, vomiting, and straining of any kind
21. They dehydrate the brain and reduce cerebral edema by holding water in the renal tubules to prevent reabsorption, and by drawing fluid from the extravascular spaces into the plasma.
22. Narcotics mask the level of responsiveness as well as masking pupillary responses.
23. Headache that is more severe upon awakening and vomiting not associated with nausea are symptoms of a brain tumor.
24. Supratentorial: elevated; infratentorial: flat
25. Yes
26. No
27. Anticholinesterase drugs, which inhibit the action of cholinesterase at the nerve endings to promote the accumulation of acetylcholine at receptor sites; this should improve neuronal transmission to muscles.

Hematology and Oncology

ANEMIA

Description: Deficiency of erythrocytes (RBCs) reflected as decreased Hct, Hgb, and RBCs

Nursing Assessment

A. Pallor, especially of the ears and nail beds; palmar crease; conjunctiva
B. Fatigue, exercise intolerance, lethargy, orthostatic hypotension
C. Tachycardia, heart murmurs, heart failure
D. Signs of bleeding, such as hematuria, melena, menorrhagia
E. Dyspnea
F. Irritability, difficulty concentrating
G. Cool skin, cold intolerance
H. Risk factors
   1. Diet lacking in iron, folate, and/or vitamin B_{12}
   2. Family history of genetic diseases such as sickle cell or congenital hemolytic anemia
   3. Medication history of anemia-producing drugs, such as salicylates, thiazides, and diuretics
   4. Exposure to toxic agents, such as lead or insecticides
I. Diagnostic tests indicate abnormally low results:
   1. Hgb <10 g/dl
   2. Hct <36%
   3. RBCs $<4 \times 10^{12}$
   4. Bone marrow aspiration positive for anemia

J. Blood loss either acute or chronic

K. Medical history of kidney disorders

> **HESI Hint** • Physical symptoms occur as a compensatory mechanism when the body is trying to make up for a deficit somewhere in the system. For instance, cardiac output increases when Hgb levels drop below 7 g/dl.

Analysis (Nursing Diagnoses)

A. *Activity intolerance* related to…

B. *Anxiety* related to…

C. *Ineffective tissue perfusion* related to…

Nursing Plans and Interventions

A. Administer blood products as prescribed (see Table 3-4).

B. Alternate periods of activity with periods of rest.

C. Teach about diet.
   1. Instruct in food selection and preparation to maximize intake of:
      a. Iron (red meats, organ meats, whole wheat products, spinach, carrots)
      b. Folic acid (green vegetables, liver, citrus fruits)
      c. Vitamin B_{12} (glandular meats, yeast, green leafy vegetables, milk, and cheese)
   2. Instruct in need for vitamin supplements.
      a. Give iron preparations with meals to decrease gastric irritation.
      b. Administer B_{12} and folic acid orally except to clients with pernicious anemia who should receive B_{12} parenterally.

D. If parenteral iron is required, use Z-track method for administration to prevent staining the skin (Table 4-36).

E. Provide genetic information if client has sickle cell or congenital hemolytic anemia.

F. Teach that sickle cell crisis is precipitated by hypoxia (see Chapter 5, p. 224).
   1. Provide pain relief.
   2. Provide adequate hydration.

TABLE 4-36 Administration of Iron

Do's	Don'ts
• Use Z-track method of administration • Use air bubble to avoid withdrawing medication into subcutaneous tissue	• Do *not* use deltoid muscle • Do *not* massage injection site

3. Teach client to avoid activities that cause hypoxia.

G. Teach the client to report any unusual bleeding to health care professional.

> **HESI Hint** • Use only normal saline to flush IV tubing or to run with blood. Never add medications to blood products. Two registered nurses should simultaneously check the physician's prescription, the client's identity, and the blood bag label.

LEUKEMIA

Description: Malignant neoplasm of the blood-forming organs

A. Leukemia is characterized by an abnormal overproduction of immature forms of any of the leukocytes. There is an interference with normal blood production that results in decreased numbers of erythrocytes and platelets.
   1. Anemia results from decreased RBC production and blood loss.
   2. Immunosuppression occurs because of the large number of immature white blood cells or profound neutropenia.
   3. Hemorrhage occurs because of thrombocytopenia.
   4. There may be leukemic invasion of other organ systems, such as the liver, spleen, lymph nodes, kidneys, lungs, and brain.

B. The exact cause of leukemia is unknown, but identified precipitating factors include:
   1. Genetic abnormalities.
   2. Ionizing radiation (therapeutic or atomic).
   3. Viral infections (human T cells, leukemia virus).
   4. Exposure to certain chemicals or drugs (Box 4-2)
      a. Benzene
      b. Alkylating chemotherapeutic agents
      c. Immunosuppressants
      d. Chloramphenicol
      e. Phenylbutazone

C. Incidence is highest in children 3 to 4 years of age; declines until age 35, then a steady increase occurs.

D. Diagnosis of leukemia is made by biopsy, bone marrow aspiration, lumbar puncture, and frequent blood counts.

E. Leukemia is treated with antineoplastic chemotherapy (Table 4-37).

Types of Leukemia

A. Acute myelogenous leukemia
   1. It involves the inability of leukocytes to mature; those that do are abnormal.
   2. It can occur at any time during the life cycle.

BOX 4-2 *Administration of Antineoplastic Chemotherapeutic Agents*

- Follow OSHA guidelines for administration as well as for decontamination of nondisposable areas and equipment and of self.
- Obtain complete and detailed instructions about administration (routine knowledge of procedures for IV administration is not sufficient).
- These drugs are toxic to cancer cells and normal cells in both the client and the caregivers who are infusing the drugs.
- Nurses who are pregnant or are considering becoming pregnant should notify supervisor (many agencies discourage or prohibit such caregivers from administering these drugs).
- Wear gloves when handling drugs.
- Check the drug with another nurse against the health care provider's prescription and the client's record to ensure that it is the correct medication.
- If IV catheter line is used for infusion, verify line placement and patency with another nurse and aspirate a blood return.
- If a vesicant (caustic) drug is administered peripherally, stay with the client throughout administration and check IV placement and patency frequently by aspirating a blood return.
- If a peripheral site is used for infusion, use a new site daily.
- Dispose of all IV equipment in the specially provided waste receptacle so that personnel handling trash do not come into contact with vesicant drugs.

HESI Hint • Many health care delivery systems require the nurse to be credentialed in order to administer parental chemotherapy. The practical nurse (PN) should recognize complications of chemotherapy related to administration, safety, side effects, and nursing assessment parameters and should report these to the registered nurse and health care provider.

3. Onset is insidious.
4. Prognosis is poor: 5-year survival of 20%; overall, 50% for children.
5. Cause of death tends to be overwhelming infection.
B. Chronic myelogenous leukemia
   1. It results from abnormal production of granulocytic cells.
   2. It is a biphasic disease.
   3. The chronic stage lasts approximately 3 years.
   4. The acute phase tends to last 2 to 3 months.
   5. It occurs in young to middle-aged adults.
   6. Known causes include:
      a. Ionizing radiation
      b. Chemical exposure
   7. Prognosis is poor: 5-year survival rate of 37%.
   8. Treatment is conservative, involving oral antineoplastic agents.
      a. Hydroxyurea (Hydrea, an inhibitor of DNA synthesis)
      b. Interferon (mechanism of action not known)
      c. Imatinib mesylate (Gleevec) targeted therapy that is Philadelphia chromosome positive
C. Acute lymphocytic leukemia
   1. Abnormal leukocytes are found in blood-forming tissue.
   2. It occurs in children (is the most common childhood cancer).

3. The prognosis is favorable: 80% of children treated live 5 years or longer.
D. Chronic lymphocytic leukemia
   1. It involves increased production of leukocytes and lymphocytes and proliferation of cells within the bone marrow, spleen, and liver.
   2. It occurs after the age of 35, often in older adults.
   3. The 5-year survival rate is 73% overall.
   4. Most clients are asymptomatic and are not treated.

HESI Hint • A 24-year-old is admitted with large areas of ecchymosis on both upper and lower extremities. She is diagnosed with acute myelogenous leukemia. What are the expected laboratory findings for this client, and what is the expected treatment?
   Lab: Decreased Hgb, decreased Hct, decreased platelet count, altered WBC (usually quite high)
   Treatment: Prevention of infection; prevention and control of bleeding; high-protein, high-calorie diet; assistance with ADL; drug therapy

Nursing Assessment

A. Tendency to bleed
   1. Petechiae
   2. Nosebleeds
   3. Bleeding gums
   4. Ecchymoses
   5. Nonhealing skin abrasions

TABLE 4-37   Antineoplastic Chemotherapeutic Agent

Drugs	Indications	Adverse Reactions	Nursing Implications
Alkylating Agents			
• Cyclophosphamide (Cytoxan, Neosar) • Mechlorethamine HCl (nitrogen mustard) • Cisplatin (Platinol) • Busulfan (Myleran) • Procarbazine (Matulane) • Imidazole carboxamide (Dacarbazine)	• Hodgkin • Leukemia • Neuroblastoma • Retinoblastoma • Multiple myeloma	• Bone marrow suppression • Nausea and vomiting • Cystitis • Stomatitis • Alopecia • Gonadal suppression • Toxic effects occur slowly with high dosage • Toxic to kidneys and ears • Pleural effusion • Seizures	• Use immediately after reconstitution • Avoid vapors in eyes • Vesicant; if comes in contact with skin, flush with water • Check placement of infusing system • Hydrate well before and during treatment with IV fluids and mannitol • Monitor renal functioning and watch for signs of cystitis • Force fluids • Monitor hearing and vision
Antimetabolites			

• Fluorouracil (Adrucil, 5-FU)
• Methotrexate sodium (Mexate); requires Leucovorin rescue to prevent toxic effects
• Mercaptopurine/6-MP (Purinethol)
• Cytarabine (Cytosar-U, ARA-C)
• Gemcitabine (Gemzar)
	• Acute lymphocytic leukemia
	• Acute myelocytic leukemia
	• Brain tumors
	• Ovarian, breast, prostatic, testicular cancers
		• Nausea and vomiting
		• Diarrhea
		• Myelosuppression (bone marrow depression)
		• Proctitis
		• Stomatitis
		• Dermatitis
		• Renal toxicity
		• Hepatotoxicity
		• Anaphylaxis
			• Administer antiemetics as needed
			• Teach to wear sunscreen when outdoors
			• Toxic to liver and kidney; avoid:
			  • Aspirin
			  • Sulfonamide
			  • Tetracycline
			  • Vitamins containing folic acid
			• Leucovorin is used with methotrexate as antidote for high doses; called "leucovorin rescue"
			• Give allopurinol concurrently with 6-MP to inhibit uric acid production by cell destruction; it increases drug's potency
			• Monitor liver function

Antitumor Antibiotics			
• Dactinomycin (actinomycin) • Bleomycin sulfate (Blenoxane) • Daunorubicin I (Cerubidine) • Mitomycin (Mutamycin) • Doxorubicin HCl (Adriamycin) • Idarubicin (Idamycin)	• Sarcoma • Neuroblastoma • Head and neck tumors • Testicular, ovarian, breast cancer • Hodgkin • Lymphocytic leukemia • Acute myelocytic leukemia	• Bone marrow suppression • Anorexia • Nausea and vomiting • Alopecia • Cardiac toxicity • Vesicant	• Monitor placement and patency of infusing system • Monitor for cardiac dysrhythmia • Inform client that urine turns red • Administer antiemetics as needed
Miscellaneous Antineoplastics			
• Hydroxyurea (Hydrea) • Asparaginase (Elspar)	• Urea-derived antineoplastic agent against solid tumors and CML • Anticancer enzyme against ALL	• Drowsiness • Renal dysfunction • Nausea and vomiting, diarrhea • Hepatitis • Myelosuppression	• Comfort measures for stomatitis, GI discomforts • Monitor for complications • Maintain adequate hydration

(Continued)

TABLE 4-37   Antineoplastic Chemotherapeutic Agent—cont'd

Drugs	Indications	Adverse Reactions	Nursing Implications
Plant Alkaloids			
• Vincristine sulfate (Oncovin) • Vinblastine sulfate (Velban)	• Acute lymphocytic leukemia • Hodgkin • Wilms tumor • Sarcoma • Breast cancer • Testicular cancer	• Bone marrow suppression • Neurotoxicity • Weakness • Paresthesia • Jaw pain • Constipation • Stomatitis • Alopecia • Headaches • Minimal nausea and vomiting	• Administer antiemetics as needed • Monitor for neurotoxicity • Check placement and patency of infusing system
Mitotic Inhibitors			
• Paclitaxel (Taxol) • Docetaxel (Taxotere)	• Breast cancer • Ovarian cancer • Non-small-cell lung cancer • Kaposi sarcoma	• Decreased WBCs and RBCs • Alopecia • Nausea and vomiting, diarrhea • Joint, muscle pain	• Monitor for signs and symptoms of infection • Administer antiemetics and antidiarrheals as needed
Hormonal Agents (Corticosteroids)			
• Prednisone (Cortalone) • Dexamethasone (Decadron)	• Leukemia • Hodgkin • Breast cancer • Lymphoma • Multiple myeloma • Cerebral edema (due to brain metastasis)	• See Endocrine	• See Endocrine.
Male-Specific Hormonal Agents			
• Flutamide (Eulexin) • Leuprolide (Lupron) • Goserelin (Zoladex)	• Prostate cancers • Testicular cancers	• Headache, paresthesias, cardiac dysrhythmias, nausea and vomiting, hypoglycemia, Neuropathies	• Bone pain and voiding problems • Safety with neuropathies
Female-Specific Hormonal Agents			
• Tamoxifen citrate (Nolvadex) • Megestrol (Megace) • Medroxyprogesterone (Provera)	• Breast cancer	• Hot flashes • Mild nausea	• Administer antiemetics as needed
Androgens			
• Testosterone (Oreton) • Fluoxymesterone (Halotestin)	• Breast cancer (postmenopausal women)	• Fluid retention • Nausea • Masculinization	• Low-salt diet
Topoisomerase-I Inhibitors			
• Irinotecan (Camptosar) • Topotecan (Hycamtin)	• Used after failure of initial treatment of ovarian, small-cell lung, and colorectal cancers	• Myelosuppression • Moderate nausea and vomiting • Diarrhea	• Camptosar diarrhea treated with atropine due to physiologic cause • Give antiemetics per protocol

TABLE 4-37   Antineoplastic Chemotherapeutic Agent—cont'd

Drugs	Indications	Adverse Reactions	Nursing Implications
Monoclonal Antibodies			
• Trastuzumab (Herceptin) • Rituximab (Rituxan)	• Targets specific malignant cells with less damage to healthy cells in non-Hodgkin lymphoma, breast cancer	• Fever, chills, infection • Nausea and vomiting, diarrhea • Bronchospasm, dyspnea, ARDS • Hypotension • Ventricular dysfunction, HF	• Premedicate with antiemetics • Monitor for identified side effects
BIOLOGIC RESPONSE MODIFIERS			
Antianemic			
• Epoetin (Procrit, Epogen)	• Anemia due to chronic renal failure, chemotherapy, HIV-related treatments	• Seizures • Hypertension • Pain at injection site	• Do not shake vial; may cause inactivation of medication • Monitor Hct levels • Pain at injection site; give slowly SC
Granulocyte-Stimulating Factor			
• Filgrastim (Neupogen)	• Improves immune competence by increasing neutrophils	• Medullary bone pain during initial treatment • Pain at injection site	• Monitor WBC/differential; absolute neutrophil count (ANC) • Give SC slowly due to local pain at site • Assess bone pain and medicate with analgesics
Thrombotic Growth Factor			
• Oprelvekin (Neumega)	• Stimulates production of megakaryocytes and platelets	• Dizziness, headache, insomnia, blurred vision, nervousness • Pleural effusion • Vasodilation, cardiac dysrhythmias • Bone pain, myalgia • GI upsets • Fluid retention	• Give slowly to reduce pain at injection site • Assess for complications related to fluid retention • Start within 6 to 24 hours of chemotherapy start and continue for 10 to 21 days • Monitor CBC: H&H may decrease; monitor platelets
Interferon-beta Products			
• Interferon beta-1a (Avonex) • Interferon beta-1b (Betaseron)	• Relapsing multiple sclerosis • AIDS • Kaposi sarcoma • Malignant melanoma • Hepatitis C	• Seizures, H/A, weakness, insomnia, depression, suicidal ideation • Hypertension, chest pain, vasodilation, edema, palpitations • Dyspnea • Nausea and vomiting, elevated liver function studies, GI disorders • Myalgia, flulike symptoms	• Anticipate discomfort from side effects and initiate relief measures early • Notify physician if evidence of depression • Sunscreen and protective clothing are needed because of photosensitivity • Do not shake or swirl solution; use soon after reconstitution • Monitor CBC and blood chemistries

(Continued)

TABLE 4-37   Antineoplastic Chemotherapeutic Agent—cont'd

Drugs	Indications	Adverse Reactions	Nursing Implications
Interleukins			
• Aldesleukin (Proleukin, Interleukin-2)	• Metastatic renal cell carcinoma	• Respiratory failure; pulmonary edema • HF, MI, dysrhythmias, stroke • Bowel perforation, hepatomegaly, GI disturbances • Serious electrolyte imbalances • Coagulation disorders • Pancytopenia	• Vigilance in monitoring for serious side effects with stat response
Interferon-alfa Products			
• Interferon-alfa-2a (Roferon-A) • Interferon-alfa-2b (Intron A)	• 2a: hairy cell leukemia, Kaposi sarcoma • 2b: chronic hepatitis B and C; Kaposi sarcoma; hairy cell leukemia	• Similar to those of interferon-beta products	• Similar to those of interferon-beta products
ANTIEMETICS			
• Prochlorperazine (Compazine) • Promethazine HCl (Phenergan)	• Nausea and vomiting	• Drowsiness • Dizziness • Extrapyramidal symptoms • Orthostatic hypotension • Blurred vision • Dry mouth	• Dilute oral solution with juice, etc. • Determine baseline BP prior to administration • Give deep IM • Monitor BP carefully
• Metoclopramide HCl (Reglan) • Haloperidol (Haldol)	• Nausea and vomiting	• Drowsiness • Restlessness • Fatigue • Extrapyramidal symptoms	• Caution client of decreased alertness • Avoid alcohol • Discontinue if extrapyramidal symptoms occur
• Diphenhydramine HCl (Benadryl)	• Given with Reglan and Haldol to reduce extrapyramidal symptoms	• Sedation • Dizziness • Hypotension • Dry mouth	• Same as above
• Ondansetron HCl (Zofran)	• Prevention of nausea and vomiting associated with cancer • Postoperative nausea and vomiting	• Headache often requiring analgesic for relief	• Administer tablets 30 minutes prior to chemotherapy and 1 to 2 hours prior to radiation therapy • Dilute IV injection in 50 ml of 5% dextrose or 0.9% NaCl
• Granisetron (Kytril)	• Nausea and vomiting associated with chemotherapy and abdominal radiation	• Hypertension • CNS stimulation • Elevated liver enzymes	• Assess for extrapyramidal symptoms • Monitor liver enzymes • Give only on day of chemotherapy or radiation treatment and 1 hour before

ALL, acute lymphoblastic anemia; CML, cell-mediated lympholysis.

B. Anemia
   1. Fatigue
   2. Pallor
   3. Headache
   4. Bone and joint pain
   5. Hepatosplenomegaly

C. Infection
   1. Fever
   2. Tachycardia
   3. Lymphadenopathy (swollen lymph nodes)
   4. Night sweats
   5. Skin infection, poor healing

D. GI distress
   1. Anorexia
   2. Weight loss
   3. Sore throat
   4. Abdominal pain
   5. Diarrhea
   6. Oral lesions, typically thrush

> **HESI Hint** • Infection in the immunosuppressed person may not be manifested with an elevated temperature. Therefore, it is imperative that the nurse perform a total and thorough assessment of the client frequently.

Analysis (Nursing Diagnoses)

A. *Risk for infection* related to…

B. *Risk for bleeding* related to…

C. *Fatigue* related to…

D. *Anxiety* related to…

Nursing Plans and Interventions for Immunosuppressed Clients and Clients with Bone Marrow Suppression

A. Monitor WBC count daily, and inform physician of count.

B. Routinely assess oral cavity and genital area for signs of infection.

C. Monitor vital signs frequently.
   1. Note baseline.
   2. Report fever to physician as requested.
      a. Be aware that parameters for reporting tend to be lower than those in postoperative clients.
      b. Usually report temperature elevations of 100.5°F.

D. Administer antibiotics as prescribed, maintaining a strict schedule.

E. Notify physician if delay in administration occurs.
   1. Obtain trough and peak blood levels of antibiotics.
      a. Trough: draw blood sample shortly before administration of antibiotic.
      b. Peak: draw blood sample 30 minutes to 1 hour after administration of drug.
   2. Monitor blood levels of antibiotics for therapeutic dose range.

F. Teach client and family the importance of infection control:
   1. Wash hands using good handwashing technique.
   2. Avoid contact with any infected person.
   3. Avoid crowds.
   4. Maintain daily hygiene to prevent spread of microorganisms.
   5. Avoid eating uncooked foods; they contain bacteria.
   6. Avoid water standing in cups, vases, etc., because they are excellent sources of growth for microorganisms.

G. Institute an oral hygiene regimen.
   1. Use soft-bristle toothbrush to avoid bleeding.
   2. Use salt and soda mouth rinse.
   3. Perform oral hygiene after each meal and at bedtime.
   4. Lubricate lips with water-soluble gel.
   5. Avoid lemon-glycerin swabs; they dry oral mucosa.

H. Encourage coughing and deep breathing to prevent stasis of secretions in lungs.

I. Avoid rectal thermometers and suppositories to prevent further bleeding.

J. Monitor fluid status and balance; febrile clients dehydrate rapidly.
   1. Monitor I&O.
   2. Encourage fluid intake of at least 3 L per day.

K. Encourage mobility to decrease pulmonary stasis.

L. Provide care for invasive catheters and lines (Box 4-3).
   1. Use strict aseptic technique for all invasive procedures.

> **HESI Hint** • Most oncologic drugs cause immunosuppression. Prevention of secondary infections is vital! Advise client to stay away from persons with known infections such as colds. In the hospital, place client in a private room, and maintain an environment as sterile and as clean as possible. These persons should not eat raw vegetables or fruits—only cooked foods—so as to destroy any bacteria.

   2. Change dressings two or three times per week and when soiled.
   3. Use catheter line for piggybacking medication, depending on the purpose of the line and the fluid being infused; no medications can be piggybacked with an infusion of chemotherapeutic agents.
   4. Lines can often be used for collecting blood samples, thereby avoiding "sticking" the client.

M. Protect the client from bleeding and injury.
   1. Handle the client gently.
   2. Avoid needle sticks. Use smallest gauge needle possible, and apply pressure for 10 minutes after needle sticks.

BOX 4-3 *Care of Intravenous Lines and Catheters*

Types of IV Lines and Catheters	Use and Care of IV Lines and Catheters
• CVC (nontunneled percutaneous central venous catheter) • Hickman (tunneled catheter) • Broviac (tunneled catheter) • CVC, Hickman, and Broviac type catheters; • Port-A-Cath (implanted reservoir; must • PICC (peripherally inserted central catheter)	• Stays in place for extended periods of time • Used for clients who require immunosuppressive therapy or are receiving long-term IV therapy • Exit sites include: At the upper chest Femoral area Antecubital area • To prevent an air embolus when a central line is open to air, position client in Trendelenburg position or have client perform a Valsalva maneuver if there is no slide clamp on the line. • Maintain a patent IV site by flushing with heparin or saline. (The amount of heparin used depends on size of lumen, length of tubing, whether reservoir exists [e.g., Port-A-Cath].) • Immediately after insertion of a central line, the nurse should auscultate breath sounds. • After insertion of a central line, a chest radiograph must be taken to determine correct placement and detect pneumothorax (observe for unequal expansion of chest wall).

---

3. Encourage use of electric razor only for shaving.
4. Instruct client to avoid blowing or picking nose.
5. Assess for signs of bleeding.
6. Avoid use of salicylates.

HODGKIN DISEASE

Description: Malignancy of the lymphoid system

A. Hodgkin disease is characterized by a generalized painless lymphadenopathy.

B. Incidence is higher in males and young adults.

C. Cause is unknown.

D. Prognosis is good: 5-year survival rate of 90%; however, late recurrences after 5 to 10 years are not uncommon.

E. Diagnosis is made by excision of node for biopsy; characteristic cell is called Reed-Sternberg.

F. Determination of stage of disease is done by surgical laparotomy.
   1. Stage I: Involvement of single lymph node region or a single extralymphatic organ or site.
   2. Stage II: Involvement of two or more lymph nodes on the same side of the diaphragm or localized involvement of an extralymphatic organ or site.
   3. Stage III: Involvement of lymph node areas on both sides of the diaphragm to localized involvement of one extralymphatic organ, the spleen, or both.
   4. Stage IV: Diffuse involvement of one or more extralymphatic organs, with or without lymph node involvement.

G. Treatment
   1. Radiotherapy
   2. Chemotherapy: nitrogen mustard, Adriamycin, vincristine, prednisone
   3. Splenectomy

Nursing Assessment

A. Enlarged lymph nodes (one or more)

B. Anemia, thrombocytopenia, elevated leukocytes, decreased platelets

C. Fever, increased susceptibility to infections

D. Anorexia, weight loss

E. Malaise, bone pain

F. Night sweats

Analysis (Nursing Diagnoses)

A. *Risk for infection* related to...

B. *Anxiety* related to...

C. *Imbalanced nutrition: less than body requirements* related to...

D. *Ineffective tissue perfusion* related to...

Nursing Plans and Interventions

A. Protect client from infection; monitor temperature carefully.

B. Observe for signs of anemia.

C. Provide adequate rest.

D. Provide preoperative and postoperative care for laparotomy or splenectomy.

E. Encourage high-nutrient foods.

F. Provide emotional support to client and family.

HESI Hint • Hodgkin disease is one of the most curable of all adult malignancies. Emotional support is vital. Career development is often interrupted for treatment. Chemotherapy renders many male clients sterile. May bank sperm prior to treatment, if desired.

GENERAL ONCOLOGY CONTENT

A. Oncology terms
   1. Cancer: a disease characterized by uncontrolled growth of abnormal cells
   2. Neoplasm: a new formation
   3. Carcinoma: a malignant tumor arising from epithelial tissue
   4. Sarcoma: a malignant tumor arising from non-epithelial tissue
   5. Differentiation: degree to which neoplastic tissue is different from parent tissue
   6. Metastasis: spread of cancer from the original site to other parts of the body.
   7. Adjuvant therapy: therapy supplemental to the primary therapy
   8. Palliative procedure: relieves symptoms without curing the cause

B. Tumors identified by tissue of origin.
   1. Adeno: glandular tissue
   2. Angio: blood vessels
   3. Basal cell: epithelium (sun-exposed areas)
   4. Embryonal: gonads
   5. Fibro: fibrous tissue
   6. Lympho: lymphoid tissue
   7. Melano: pigmented cells of epithelium
   8. Myo: muscle tissue
   9. Osteo: bone
   10. Squamous cell: epithelium

C. Seven warning signs of cancer
   1. Change in usual bowel and bladder function
   2. A sore that does not heal
   3. Unusual bleeding or discharge, hematuria, tarry stools, ecchymosis, bleeding mole
   4. Thickening or a lump in the breast or elsewhere
   5. Indigestion or dysphagia
   6. Obvious changes in a wart or mole
   7. Nagging cough or hoarseness

Review of Hematology and Oncology

1. List three potential causes of anemia.
2. Write two nursing diagnoses for the client suffering from anemia.
3. What is the only IV fluid compatible with blood products?
4. What actions should the nurse take if a hemolytic transfusion reaction occurs?
5. List three interventions for clients with a tendency to bleed.
6. Identify two sites that should be assessed for infection in immunosuppressed clients.
7. Name three food sources of vitamin B_{12}.
8. Describe care of invasive catheters and lines.
9. List three safety precautions for the administration of antineoplastic chemotherapy.
10. Describe the use of leucovorin.
11. Describe the method of collecting the trough and peak blood levels of antibiotics.
12. What is the characteristic cell found in Hodgkin disease?
13. List four nursing interventions for care of the client with Hodgkin disease.
14. List four topics you would cover when teaching an immunosuppressed client about infection control.

Answers to Review

1. Diet lacking in iron, folate, or vitamin B_{12}; use of salicylates, thiazides, diuretics; exposure to toxic agents, such as lead or insecticides
2. Activity intolerance and ineffective tissue perfusion
3. Normal saline
4. Turn off transfusion. Take temperature. Send blood being transfused to lab. Obtain urine sample. Keep vein patent with normal saline.
5. Use a soft toothbrush, avoid salicylates, do not use suppositories.
6. Oral cavity and genital area
7. Glandular meats (liver), milk, green leafy vegetables
8. Use strict aseptic technique. Change dressings two or three times per week or when soiled. Use caution when piggybacking drugs; check purpose of line and drug to be infused. When possible, use lines to obtain blood samples to avoid "sticking" client.
9. Double-check order with another nurse. Check for blood return prior to administration to ensure that medication does not go into tissue. Use a new IV site daily for peripheral chemotherapy. Wear gloves when handling the drugs, and dispose of waste in special containers to avoid contact with toxic substances.
10. Leucovorin is used as an antidote with methotrexate to prevent toxic reactions.
11. Collection of trough: draw blood 30 minutes prior to administration of antibiotic. Collection of peak: draw blood 30 minutes after administration of antibiotic.
12. Reed-Sternberg
13. Protect from infection. Observe for anemia. Encourage high-nutrient foods. Provide emotional support to client and family.
14. Handwashing technique. Avoid infected persons. Avoid crowds. Maintain daily hygiene to prevent spread of microorganisms.

Reproductive System

BENIGN TUMORS OF THE UTERUS (LEIOMYOMAS FIBROIDS, MYOMAS, FIBROMYOMAS, FIBROMAS)

Description: Benign tumors arising from the muscle tissue of the uterus

A. Benign tumors are more common in black women than in white women.

B. Benign tumors are more common in women who have never been pregnant.

C. The most common symptom is abnormal uterine bleeding.

D. They tend to disappear after menopause.

E. They rarely become malignant.

F. Treatment for abnormal uterine bleeding (menorrhagia)
   1. Dilation and curettage (D&C)
      a. Used only in extreme cases of bleeding
      b. For older women when endometrial biopsy and ultrasonography have not provided the necessary diagnostic information
   2. Endometrial ablation
      a. Laser or electrosurgical technique
      b. Successful with many clients with menorrhagia

G. Treatment of uterine fibroids with menorrhagia
   1. Myomectomy (removal of fibroids without removal of the uterus) via laparotomy, laparoscopy, or hysteroscopy
   2. Abdominal or vaginal hysterectomy (See Nursing Plans and Interventions for Hysterectomy, p. 168.)
   3. Hormonal regimens (e.g., synthetic analog of gonadotropin-releasing hormone [GnRH], Nafarelin [Synarel], leuprolide [Lupron] to shrink the tumor)
   4. Uterine artery embolization (UAE) of the blood vessels supplying the fibroid tumor
   5. Cryosurgery

Nursing Assessment

A. Menorrhagia (hypermenorrhea: profuse or prolonged menstrual bleeding)

B. Dysmenorrhea (extremely painful menstrual periods)

C. Uterine enlargement

D. Low back pain and pelvic pain

HESI Hint • Menorrhagia (profuse or prolonged menstrual bleeding) is the most important factor relating to benign uterine tumors. Assess for signs of anemia.

Nursing Plans and Interventions

A. GnRH
1. Explain regrowth will occur after the treatment is stopped.
2. A small loss in bone mass and changes in lipid levels can occur.
3. Amenorrhea may occur.
4. Adding raloxifene to GnRH administration has been effective in preventing these effects in premenopausal women.
5. Women who wish to avoid pregnancy should use a nonhormonal or barrier method of contraception.
6. Discuss administration methods for GnRH agonists (subcutaneous and intramuscular injections, intranasal administration, and subcutaneous implantation).

B. UAE
1. Preoperative teaching: do not to drink alcohol, smoke, take aspirin or anticoagulant medications 24 hours before the procedure.
2. During procedure: expect cramping during injection of the polyvinyl alcohol pellets (PVA) pellets into selected blood vessels.
3. Postoperatively: pelvic pain, fever, malaise, and nausea and vomiting may be caused by acute fibroid degeneration.
4. Pain may be controlled with a patient-controlled analgesia (PCA) pump
5. Postoperative nursing assessments: check for bleeding in the groin and vital signs, assess pain level, check pedal pulse and neurovascular condition of affected leg.
6. Discharge teaching
   a. Take prescribed medications as ordered.
   b. Call your physician if you have any of the following symptoms: bleeding, pain, swelling or hematoma at the puncture site, fever of 101.1°F (38°C), urinary retention, or abnormal vaginal drainage (foul odor, brown color, tissue)
   c. Eat a normal diet including fluids and fiber.
   d. Do not use tampons or douche, or have vaginal intercourse for at least 4 weeks.
   e. Avoid straining during bowel movements.
   f. Keep your follow-up appointment.
7. An ultrasound or MRI examination may be done after the UAE to determine the effectiveness of the procedure.

UTERINE PROLAPSE, CYSTOCELE, AND RECTOCELE

Description: Uterine prolapse is downward displacement of the uterus. Cystocele is the relaxation of the anterior vaginal wall with prolapse of the bladder.

Rectocele is the relaxation of the posterior vaginal wall with prolapse of the rectum.

A. Preventive measures
1. Postpartum perineal exercises
2. Spaced pregnancies
3. Weight control

B. Surgical intervention
1. Hysterectomy
2. Anterior and posterior vaginal repair (A&P repair)

C. Nonsurgical intervention (for uterine prolapse)
1. Kegel exercises
2. Knee-chest position
3. Pessary use

HESI Hint • What is the anatomic significance of a prolapsed uterus? When the uterus is displaced, it impinges on other structures in the lower abdomen. The bladder, rectum, and small intestine can protrude through the vaginal wall.

Nursing Assessment

A. Predisposing conditions
1. Multiparity
2. Pelvic tearing during childbirth
3. Vaginal muscle weakness associated with aging
4. Obesity

B. Symptoms associated with uterine prolapse
1. Dysmenorrhea
2. Pulling and dragging sensations in pelvis and back
3. Dyspareunia
4. Pressure, protrusions
5. Fatigue
6. Low backache
7. Symptoms may be worse after prolonged standing or deep penile penetration during intercourse

C. Symptoms associated with cystocele
1. Incontinence or stress incontinence (dribbling with coughing or sneezing or any activity that increases intraabdominal pressure)
2. Urinary retention
3. Bladder infections (cystitis)

D. Symptoms associated with rectocele
1. Constipation
2. Hemorrhoids
3. Sense of pressure or need to defecate

Analysis (Nursing Diagnoses)

A. *Chronic pain* related to…

B. *Deficient knowledge* related to…

C. *Disturbed body image* related to…

Nursing Plans and Interventions for Hysterectomy

A. Provide preoperative and postoperative care (see Advanced Clinical Concepts: Perioperative Care, p. 49).

B. Administer enema and douche as prescribed preoperatively.

C. Note amount and character of vaginal discharge. Postoperatively, there should be less than one saturated pad in 4 hours.

D. Avoid rectal thermometers or tubes, especially when A&P repair has been performed.

E. Check extremities for warmth and tenderness as indicators of thrombophlebitis.

F. Pain management postoperatively
   1. Assess character of pain, and determine appropriate analgesic.
   2. Administer analgesics as needed, and determine effectiveness.

G. Encourage ambulation as soon as possible.

H. Monitor urinary output (Foley catheter is usually inserted in surgery).

I. After catheter removal, assess voiding patterns; catheterize every 6 to 8 hours to void.

J. Observe incision for bleeding.

K. Note abdominal distention; it may be a sign of gas (flatus) or internal bleeding.

L. Gradually increase diet from liquids to general.

M. Provide stool softeners prior to first bowel movement and thereafter as needed.

N. Instructions to client regarding follow-up care:
   1. Limit tampon use.
   2. Avoid douching.
   3. Refrain from intercourse until approved by physician (usually 3 to 6 weeks).
   4. Avoid heavy lifting (6 to 8 lb) or heavy housework for 4 to 6 weeks postoperatively.

O. Maintain adequate fluid intake (3 L/day).

P. Notify physician of complications:
   1. Elevated temperature above 101°F
   2. Redness, pain, or swelling of suture line
   3. Foul-smelling vaginal drainage

Q. Encourage verbalization of feelings.

CANCER OF THE CERVIX

Description: Of cancers occurring in the cervix, 95% are squamous cell in origin. Some cervical cancers are directly linked to the human papillomavirus (HPV). Young women between the ages of 9 and 30 years of age are encouraged to be immunized with an intramuscular (IM) injection of quadrivalent HPV (types 6, 11, 16, 18) recombinant vaccine (Gardasil). All women should be tested for HPV, and women over 21 years of age and those who have engaged in sexual intercourse for at least 3 years should continue to have yearly Papanicolaou (Pap) tests.

A. Cancer of the cervix is easily detected early by the Pap test.

B. The precursor to cancer of the cervix is dysplasia.

C. Cancer of the cervix is subdivided into three stages.
   1. Early dysplasia can be treated in a variety of ways, including:
      a. Cryosurgery
      b. Electrocautery
      c. Laser
      d. Conization
      e. Hysterectomy

HESI Hint • Laser therapy or cryosurgery is used to treat cervical cancer when the lesion is small and localized. Invasive cancer is treated with radiation, conization, hysterectomy, or pelvic exenteration (a drastic surgical procedure where the uterus, ovaries, fallopian tubes, vagina, rectum, and bladder are removed in an attempt to stop metastasis). Chemotherapy is not useful for this type of cancer.

   2. Early carcinoma can be treated by:
      a. Hysterectomy
      b. Intracavity radiation
   3. Late carcinoma (the tumor size and stage of invasion of surrounding tissues are greater) can be treated by:
      a. External beam radiation along with hysterectomy
      b. Antineoplastic chemotherapy; this is of limited use for cancers arising from squamous cells
      c. Pelvic exenteration

HESI Hint • American College of Obstetricians and Gynecologists (ACOG) 2009 recommendations: Pap smears should begin at age 21 and women younger than 30 should be screened every 2 years; Women 30 and older may be screened every 3 years after they have had three consecutive negative cervical cytology tests. Women ages 65 to 70 may stop Pap smears if they have three consecutive normal in a row and no abnormal Pap smears in the last 10 years. Women with high risk factors may need more frequent screenings.

Care of the Client with Radiation Implants

A. Radiation implants are used to treat disease by delivering high-dose radiation directly to the affected tissue.

B. The nurse must take certain precautions for protection of self as well as the client and visitors.

C. Follow specific guidelines provided by the agency. General care guidelines include:
   1. Remind the client that she is not radioactive; only the implants contain radioactivity.
   2. Remind the client that her isolation time is limited; isolation is not necessary indefinitely.

D. Assign client to a private room, and place a "Caution: Radioactive Material" sign on the door.

E. Do not permit pregnant caretakers or pregnant visitors into the room.

F. Discourage visits by small children.

G. Keep a lead-lined container in the room for disposal of the implant, should it become dislodged.

H. Client should remain in bed with as little movement as possible.

I. Be aware that all client secretions have the potential of being radioactive.

J. Wear latex gloves when handling potentially contaminated secretions.

K. Wear a dosimeter when providing care to clients with radiation implants.
   1. Badge is not to be worn out-of-doors.
   2. Badge is checked at regular intervals by health officials.

L. Provide nursing care in an efficient but caring manner.
   1. Plan care to limit overall time in the client's room. Time at the bedside is limited—each contact should last no more than 30 minutes. Staff is rotated to limit their exposure.
   2. Staff members should wear a dosimeter during every patient contact to monitor radiation exposure.
   3. When in the room, stand at the greatest possible distance away from the client to minimize exposure.
   4. Stop by frequently to check on the client from the door.

M. Keep all supplies and equipment the client might need within reach.

OVARIAN CANCER

Description: Cancer of the ovaries can occur at all ages, including infancy and childhood. Early diagnosis is difficult because no useful screening test exists at present. Malignant germ cell tumors most common in women between 20 and 40 years of age and epithelial cancers occur most often in the perimenopausal age groups.

Nursing Assessment

A. It is asymptomatic in early stages.

B. Laparotomy is the primary tool for diagnosis and staging of the disease; ovarian cancer is surgically staged rather than clinically staged.

C. Advanced clinical manifestations include:
   1. Pelvic discomfort
   2. Low back pain
   3. Weight change
   4. Abdominal pain
   5. Increased abdominal girth
   6. Nausea and vomiting
   7. Constipation
   8. Urinary frequency

HESI Hint • Ovarian cancer is the leading cause of death from gynecologic cancers in the United States. Growth is insidious, so it is not recognized until it is at an advanced stage.

Analysis (Nursing Diagnoses)

A. *Anticipatory grieving* related to…

B. *Chronic pain* related to…

C. *Self-care deficit* (specify) related to…

Nursing Plans and Interventions

A. Provide the care required after any major abdominal surgery following laparotomy (see Nursing Plans and Interventions for Hysterectomy, p. 168).

B. Provide the care required for a client on chemotherapy (see Nursing Plans and Interventions for Immunosuppressed Clients, p. 163).

C. Teach client and family about disease and follow-up treatment.

D. Offer supportive care to client and family throughout diagnosis and treatment.

HESI Hint • The major emphasis in nursing management of cancers of the reproductive tract is early detection.

BREAST CANCER

Description: Cancer originating in the breast

A. Breast cancer is the leading cancer in women in the United States.

B. One in eight women will develop breast cancer in her lifetime.

C. Early detection is important to successful treatment.

D. Men can develop breast cancer. They account for <1% of reported cases.

E. Of all breast cancers, 90% to 95% are discovered through breast self-examination.

F. Risk factors include:
1. Positive family history
2. Menarche before 12 years of age and menopause after age 50
3. Nulliparous and those bearing first child after age 30
4. History of uterine cancer
5. Daily alcohol intake
6. Highest incidence: those age 40 to 49 and over 65

G. Breast cancer is generally adenocarcinoma, originating in epithelial cells, and it occurs in the ducts or lobes.

H. Tumors tend to be located in the upper outer quadrant of the breast and more often in the left breast than the right.

I. Early detection is important.
1. Every woman should perform a breast self-examination monthly, preferably as soon as menstrual bleeding ceases or if postmenopausal the same date every month.

HESI Hint • The importance of teaching female clients how to conduct a breast self-examination cannot be overemphasized. Early detection is related to positive outcomes.

2. Mammography is very helpful in early detection of cancer of the breast.
   a. Baseline mammogram at approximately 35 to 40 years of age
   b. Mammogram every 1 to 2 years for women in their 40s
   c. Annual mammogram for women over 50 years of age
   d. No use of lotions, talc powder, or deodorant under arms prior to procedure (may mimic calcium deposits on radiograph)
3. Physical examination by a professional skilled in examination of the breast should be done annually.

J. Tumors less than 4 cm are deemed curable.

K. Larger tumors require much more aggressive treatment (cure is difficult).

L. Definitive diagnosis of cancer of the breast is made by biopsy.

M. Common sites of metastasis (spread) are the axillary, supraclavicular, and mediastinal lymph nodes, followed by metastases to the lungs, liver, brain, and spine.

N. Bone metastasis is extremely painful.

O. Treatment is dependent on the stage of disease.
1. Mastectomy is commonly performed.
2. Adjuvant treatment consists of radiation (either external beam or implants), antineoplastic chemotherapy, and hormonal therapy.

HESI Hint • The presence or absence of hormone receptors is paramount in selecting clients for adjuvant therapy.

Nursing Assessment

A. Hard lump (not freely movable and not painful)
B. Dimpling of skin
C. Retraction of nipple
D. Alterations in contour of breast
E. Change in skin color
F. Change in skin texture (peau d'orange)
G. Discharge from nipple
H. Pain and ulcerations (late signs)
I. Diagnostic tests include:
1. Mammogram
2. Biopsy and frozen section

Analysis (Nursing Diagnoses)

A. *Disturbed body image* related to...
B. *Anticipatory grieving* related to...
C. *Acute or chronic pain* related to...
D. *Self-care deficit* (specify) related to...

Nursing Plans and Interventions

A. Assess lesion.
1. Location
2. Size
3. Shape
4. Consistency
5. Fixation to surrounding tissues
6. Lymph node involvement

B. Preoperative
1. Explore client's expectations of surgery and what the surgical site will look like postoperatively.

2. Discuss skin graft if one is possible and cosmetic reconstruction that might be implemented with mastectomy or at a later time.

C. Postoperative
1. Monitor bleeding; check under dressing, Hemo-Vac, and under client's back (bleeding will run to back).
2. Position arm on operative side on a pillow, slightly elevated.
3. Avoid BP measurements, injections, and venipuncture in affected arm.
4. Instruct client to avoid injury such as burns or scrapes to affected arm.
5. Encourage hand activity by squeezing a small rubber ball.
6. Encourage client to perform activities that will use arm, like brushing hair.
7. Teach postmastectomy exercises (wall climbing with affected arm and rope turning).

D. Encourage client to verbalize concerns.
1. Cancer
2. Death
3. Loss of breast

E. Encourage client to discuss operation, diagnosis, feelings, concerns, and fears.

F. Be with client when she first looks at the operative site; offer emotional support.

G. Arrange for Reach-to-Recovery (American Cancer Society) visit, Y-me National Breast Cancer Organization (physician prescription required).

H. Recognize the grief process.
1. Allow client to cry, withdraw, etc.
2. Help client to focus on the future while allowing discussions of loss.

I. If reconstruction was not discussed preoperatively, encourage client to discuss or explore these options postoperatively.

J. Discuss use of temporary and permanent prostheses.

TESTICULAR CANCER

Description: Cancer of the testes is the leading cause of death from cancer in males 15 to 35 years of age. If untreated, death usually occurs within 2 to 3 years. If detected and treated early, there is a 90% to 100% chance of cure.

Nursing Assessment

A. Early signs are subtle and usually go unnoticed.

B. There is a feeling of heaviness or dragging sensation in lower abdomen and groin.

C. There is a lump or swelling (painless) on the testicle. Late signs include:

1. Low back pain
2. Weight loss
3. Fatigue

Analysis (Nursing Diagnoses)

A. *Deficient knowledge* (specify) related to…

B. *Disturbed body image* related to…

C. *Anticipatory grieving* related to…

> **HESI Hint** • Men whose testes have not descended into the scrotum or whose testes descended after age 6 are at high risk for developing testicular cancer. The most common symptom is the appearance of a small, hard lump about the size of a pea on the front or side of the testicle. Testicular self-examination (TSE) should be done regularly at the same time every month by all males after age 14. It should be done after a shower by gently palpating the testes and cord to look for a small lump. Swelling may also be a sign of testicular cancer.

Nursing Plans and Interventions

A. Postoperative care following orchidectomy:
1. Observe for hemorrhage.
2. Active movement may be contraindicated.

B. Care for clients receiving radiation therapy.

C. Encourage genetic counseling (sperm banking is often recommended prior to surgery).

D. Counsel that sexual functioning is usually not affected because the remaining testis undergoes hyperplasia, producing sufficient testosterone to maintain sexual functioning. Although ejaculatory ability may be decreased, orgasm is still possible.

CANCER OF THE PROSTATE

Description: Prostate cancer rarely occurs before 40 years of age, but it is the second leading cause of death from cancer in American men. High-risk groups include those with a history of multiple sexual partners, sexually transmitted diseases (STDs), and certain viral infections.

Nursing Assessment

A. Asymptomatic if confined to gland

B. Symptoms of urinary obstruction

C. With metastasis: low back pain, fatigue, aching in legs, and hip pain

D. Elevated prostate-specific antigen (PSA)
1. PSA test should be conducted prior to a digital rectal examination so that manipulation of the prostate does not give a false-positive reading.

2. Serial blood screening should be done to observe trends. A rise in PSA or consistently high PSA is more reliable than a single assay.
3. PSA levels can rise with inflammation, benign hypertrophy, or irritation, as well as in response to cancer.

E. Elevated prostatic acid phosphatase (PAP)

F. Digital rectal examination (DRE) revealing palpable nodule

G. Transrectal ultrasound (TRUS) visualizing nonpalpable tumors

H. Definitive diagnosis by biopsy

Analysis (Nursing Diagnoses)

A. *Deficient knowledge* (specify) related to…

B. *Altered body image* related to…

C. *Bowel incontinence* related to…

D. *Anticipatory grieving* related to…

Nursing Plans and Interventions

A. Teach the importance of early detection.

B. Suggest resources: local and national prostate cancer support groups; information is also available from the American Cancer Society (Man to Man program), the American Foundation for Urologic Disease.

C. Prepare client for radiation therapy
1. External beam radiation irradiates the prostate and pelvic region, and conformal techniques allow the delivery of a higher radiation dose without increasing the risk of complications by focusing the radiation and limiting the exposure of adjacent structures.
   a. Explain how treatments help cancer.
      (1) Need for repetitive treatments
      (2) Attend all sessions for successful outcome.
   b. Expected outcomes
   c. Side effects
      (1) Radiation-induced cystitis or proctitis
      (2) Dysuria (discomfort with voiding): subsides within 4 to 6 weeks; reduce intake of foods or beverages likely to irritate the bowel or bladder, including caffeine and heavily spiced or fatty foods
      (3) Daytime voiding frequency
      (4) Increase in the number of times he awakens to void
      (5) Suprapubic discomfort—may irritate the perineal skin; teach him to cleanse the perineal skin with a mild cleanser and lukewarm water, pay special attention to skin folds, and pat dry, wearing loose cotton clothing to help relieve skin irritation.
      (6) Fatigue and loss of appetite: six small meals per day, foods that are high in protein and carbohydrates; a multivitamin should be taken daily throughout radiation therapy
2. Proton beam radiotherapy combines conformal imaging and charged protons to target more specifically prostate cancer cells while limiting damage to the overlying skin or adjacent structures including the bladder and rectum. (See Interventions for External Beam Radiation.)
3. Brachytherapy is the implantation of radioactive iodine-125 or pallidium-103 seeds directly into the prostate, which emit highly localized radiation energy to kill localized cancer cells without excessive harm to nearby healthy cells.
   a. Preparation includes bowel cleansing and administration of prophylactic antibiotics
   b. A clear liquid diet 12 to 24 hours before the procedure
   c. Rectal pressure or mild discomfort is felt when the ultrasound probe is placed, but pain is not associated with implantation of radioactive seeds
   d. A catheter is left in place that may be removed on the day of the procedure. Complete a voiding trial with removal of the catheter.
   e. Seed implantation will cause inflammation of the prostate and may cause symptoms including daytime voiding frequency, an increase in nocturia, and difficulty initiating a urinary stream. These manifestations are typically transient and subside as prostatic inflammation diminishes.
   f. Semen may have a brownish color over the first 1 to 2 months following implantation, and intercourse should be avoided during this period and childbearing is contraindicated
   g. Monitor his stool for passage of large volumes of bright red blood (rare), and advise him about how to manage radiation cystitis and proctitis
   h. Teach the client and partner the principles of radiation safety
   i. Refrain from having children (or adults) sit in their lap for a prolonged period of time during the first 2 months following therapy.

D. Provide preoperative bowel preparation to prevent fecal contamination of operative site.
1. Enemas and cathartics

2. Sulfasalazine (Azulfidine) or neomycin
3. Clear fluids only the day before surgery to prevent fecal contamination of operative site

E. Provide postoperative care.
1. Monitor for urine leaks, hemorrhage, and signs of infection.
2. Provide support dressing or supportive underwear to perineal incision.
3. Use donut cushion to relieve pressure on incision site while sitting.
4. Avoid rectal manipulation (rectal thermometers, rectal tubes, and hard suppositories).
5. Provide low-residue diet until wound healing is advanced.
6. Institute measures to prevent bowel action in the first postoperative week to prevent contamination of incision.

SEXUALLY TRANSMITTED DISEASES (STDs)

Description: STDs are diseases that can be transmitted during intimate sexual contact

A. STDs are the most prevalent communicable diseases in the United States.

B. Most cases of STDs occur in adolescents and young adults.

> **HESI Hint** • STDs in infants and children usually indicate sexual abuse and should be reported. The nurse is legally responsible to report suspected cases of child abuse.

Nursing Assessment

See Table 4-38.

Analysis (Nursing Diagnoses)

A. *Deficient knowledge* (specify) related to…

B. *Anxiety* related to…

C. *Anticipatory grieving* related to…

> **HESI Hint** • Chlamydia is the most commonly reported communicable disease in the United States.

Nursing Plans and Interventions

A. Use a nonjudgmental approach; be straightforward when taking history.

B. Reassure client that all information is strictly confidential. Obtain a complete sexual history, which should include:

1. The client's sexual orientation.
2. Sexual practices
   a. Penile-vaginal
   b. Penile-anal
   c. Penile-oral
   d. Oral-vaginal
   e. Anal-oral
3. Type of protection (barrier) used
4. Contraceptive practices
5. Previous history of STDs

C. Develop teaching plan and include:
1. Signs and symptoms of STDs
2. Mode of transmission of STDs.
3. Reminder that sexual contact should be avoided with anyone while infected.
4. Assess literacy level of client and if appropriate provide written instructions about treatment; request a return verbalization of these instructions to ensure the client has heard the instructions and understands them.

D. Encourage client to provide information regarding all sexual contacts.

E. Report incidents of STDs to appropriate health agencies and departments.

F. Instruct women of childbearing age about risks to a newborn:
1. Gonorrheal conjunctivitis
2. Neonatal herpes
3. Congenital syphilis
4. Oral candidiasis

> **HESI Hint** • Pelvic inflammatory disease (PID) involves one or more of the pelvic structures. The infection can cause adhesions and eventually result in sterility. Manage the pain associated with PID with analgesics and warm sitz baths. Bed rest in a semi-Fowler position may increase comfort and promote drainage. Antibiotic treatment is necessary to reduce inflammation and pain.

G. Teach safer sex.
1. Reduce the number of sexual contacts.
2. Avoid sex with those who have multiple partners.
3. Examine genital area, and avoid sexual contact if anything abnormal is present.
4. Wash hands and genital area before and after sexual contact.
5. Use a latex condom as a barrier.
6. Use water-based lubricants rather than oil-based lubricants.
7. Use a vaginal spermicidal gel.

TABLE 4-38 Sexually Transmitted Diseases

STD	Symptoms	Treatment
Treponema pallidum, Syphilis		
Laboratory diagnosis: VDRL, FTA-ABS	**Primary (local):** up to 90 days postexposure • Chancre (red, painless lesions with indurated border) • Highly infectious **Secondary (systemic):** 6 weeks to 6 months postexposure • Influenza-type symptoms • Generalized rash that affects palms of hands and soles of feet • Lesions contagious **Tertiary:** 10 to 30 years postexposure • Cardiac and Neurologic destruction	• Penicillin G IM (usually 2.4 to 4.8 million units)
Neisseria gonorrhoeae, Gonorrhea		
Laboratory diagnosis: smears, cultures	• Females: majority are asymptomatic • Males: dysuria, yellowish-green urethral discharge, urinary frequency	• Ceftriaxone sodium plus Doxycycline hyclate • Spectinomycin HCl plus Doxycycline hyclate
Chalmydia trachomatis, Chlamydia		
Laboratory diagnosis: tissue culture; Chlamydiazyme; MicroTrak	• Females: many asymptomatic, but may exhibit dysuria, urgency, vaginal discharge • Males: leading cause of nongonococcal urethritis	• Doxycycline hyclate or Tetracycline HCl
Trichomanas vaginalis, Trichomoniasis		
Laboratory diagnosis: wet slide	• Females: green, yellow, or white frothy foul-smelling vaginal discharge with itching. • Males: asymptomatic	• Metronidazole (Flagyl) (male partners to be treated to prevent reinfection)
Candida albicans, Candidiasis		
Laboratory diagnosis: viral culture	• Females: odorless, white or yellow, cheesy discharge with itching • Males: asymptomatic	• Miconazole nitrate (Monistat) • Clotrimazole (Gyne-Lotrimin) • Nystatin (Mycostatin)
Herpes Simplex Virus 2, Herpes		
	• Vesicles in clusters that rupture and leave painful erosions that cause painful urination • Characterized by remissions and exacerbations • May be contagious even when asymptomatic	• Acyclovir (Zovirax) partially controls symptoms. • Palliative care → Viscous lidocaine topically to ease pain → Keep lesions clean and dry.
Human Papillomavirus (HPV)		
	• Multiple strains (>70), some of which are implicated in cervical cancer • Alarming rate increase in adolescent population • Lesions may be small, wartlike or clustered. • May be flat or raised	• Applied medications such as podophyllum resin (contraindicated in pregnancy) • Trichloracetic acid (TCA) • Laser • Cryotherapy (freezing)
Human Immunodeficiency Virus (HIV), AIDS		
	(See Advanced Clinical Concepts, p. 53)	

FTA-ABS, fluorescent treponemal antibody absorption; VDRL, Venereal Disease Research Laboratory.

8. Avoid douching before and after sexual contact; douching increases risk for infections because the body's normal defenses are reduced or destroyed.
9. Seek attention from health care provider immediately if symptoms occur.

> **HESI Hint** • A client comes into the clinic with a chancre on his penis. What is the usual treatment? IM dose of penicillin (such as benzathine penicillin G, 2.4 million units). Obtain a sexual history, including the names of his sex partners, so that they can receive treatment.

Review of Reproductive System

1. What are the indications for a hysterectomy in a client who has fibromas?
2. List the symptoms and conditions associated with a cystocele.
3. What are the most important nursing interventions for the postoperative client who has had a hysterectomy with an A&P repair?
4. Describe the priority nursing care for a client who has had radiation implants.
5. What screening tool is used to detect cervical cancer? What are the American Cancer Society's recommendations for women ages 30 to 70 with three consecutive normal results?
6. Cite two nursing diagnoses for a client undergoing a hysterectomy for cervical cancer.
7. What are the three most important tools for early detection of breast cancer? How often should these tools be used?
8. Describe three nursing interventions to help decrease edema postmastectomy.
9. Name three priorities to include in a discharge plan for a client who has had a mastectomy.
10. What is the most common cause of nongonococcal urethritis?
11. What is the causative organism of syphilis?
12. Malodorous, frothy, greenish-yellow vaginal discharge is characteristic of which STD?
13. Which STD is characterized by remissions and exacerbations in both males and females?
14. Outline a teaching plan for a client with an STD.

Answers to Review

1. Severe menorrhagia leading to anemia, severe dysmenorrhea requiring narcotic analgesics, severe uterine enlargement causing pressure on other organs, severe low back and pelvic pain
2. Symptoms include incontinence or stress incontinence, urinary retention, and recurrent bladder infections. Conditions associated with cystocele include multiparity, trauma in childbirth, and aging.
3. Avoid taking rectal temperatures and rectal manipulation; manage pain; and encourage early ambulation.
4. Do not permit pregnant visitors or pregnant caretakers in room. Discourage visits by small children. Confine client to room. Nurse must wear radiation badge. Nurse limits time in room. Keep supplies and equipment within client's reach.
5. Pap smear. Women ages 30 to 70 with three consecutive normal results may have Pap smears every 2 to 3 years (screening for HPV).
6. Altered body image related to uterine removal; pain related to postoperative incision
7. Breast self-examination monthly; mammogram baseline at age 35, followed by exams every 1 to 2 years in 40s and every year after age 50; physical examination by a professional skilled in examination of the breast
8. Position arm on operative side on pillow. Avoid BP measurements, injections, and venipunctures in operative arm. Encourage hand activity and use.
9. Arrange for Reach-to-Recovery visit. Discuss the grief process with the client. Have physician discuss with client the reconstruction options.
10. *Chlamydia trachomatis*
11. *Treponema pallidum* (spirochete bacteria)
12. *Trichomonas vaginalis*
13. Herpes simplex type II
14. Signs and symptoms of STD; mode of transmission; avoiding sex while infected; providing concise written instructions regarding treatment, and requesting a return verbalization to ensure that the client understands; teaching safer sex practices

Burns

Description: Tissue injury or necrosis caused by transfer of energy from a heat source to the body

A. Categories
   1. Thermal
   2. Radiation
   3. Electrical
   4. Chemical

B. Tissue destruction results from:
   1. Coagulation
   2. Protein denaturation
   3. Ionization of cellular contents

C. Critical systems affected include:
   1. Respiratory
   2. Integumentary
   3. Cardiovascular
   4. Renal
   5. GI
   6. Neurologic

D. Severity is determined by burn depth (Fig. 4-9).
   1. First degree
      a. Superficial partial-thickness (e.g., sunburn)
      b. Leaves skin pink or red
      c. Dry
      d. Painful (relieved by cooling)
      e. Slight edema
   2. Second degree
      a. Deep partial-thickness destruction of epidermis and upper layers of dermis
      b. Injury to deeper portions of the dermis
      c. Painful (sensitive to touch and cold air)
      d. Appears red or white, weeps fluid, blisters present
      e. Hair follicles intact (i.e., hair does not pull out easily)
      f. Very edematous
      g. Blanching followed by capillary refill
      h. Heals without surgical intervention, usually does not scar
   3. Third degree
      a. Full-thickness; involves total destruction of dermis and epidermis
      b. Skin cannot regenerate
      c. Requires skin grafting
      d. Underlying tissue (fat, fascia, tendon, bone) may be involved
      e. Wound appears dry and leathery as eschar develops
      f. Painless

E. Severity is determined by extent of surface area burned.
   1. Rules of nines: head and neck 9%, upper extremities 9% each, lower extremities 18% each, front trunk 18%, back trunk 18%, perineal area 1% for adults (Fig. 4-10)
   2. Lund and Browder chart: critical body areas are face, hands, feet, and perineum (Table 4-39)

F. Three stages of burn care
   1. Stage I: Emergent phase
      a. Begins at the time of injury and concludes with the restoration of capillary permeability, which typically reverses 48 to 72 hours following the injury.

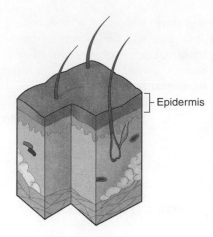

Epidermis — Superficial burns damage only the top layer of the skin—the epidermis. Healing occurs in 3-6 days.

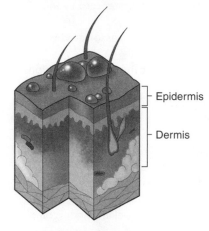

Epidermis

Dermis

Superficial partial-thickness burns are those in which the entire epidermis and variable portions of the dermis layer of skin are destroyed. Uncomplicated healing occurs in 10-21 days.

Deep partial-thickness burns extend into the deeper layers of the dermis. Healing occurs in 2-6 weeks.

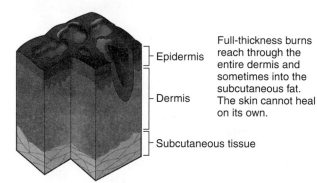

Epidermis

Dermis

Subcutaneous tissue

Full-thickness burns reach through the entire dermis and sometimes into the subcutaneous fat. The skin cannot heal on its own.

FIGURE 4-9 The tissues involved in burns of various depths. (From Ignatavicius DD, Workman ML: *Medical-surgical nursing: Patient-centered collaborative care*, ed 6. St. Louis, 2010, Saunders.)

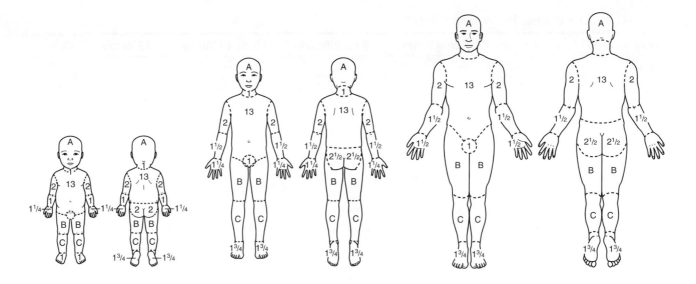

Relative percentages of areas affected by growth
(age in years)

	0	1	5	10	15	Adult
A: Half of head	$9^{1}/2$	$8^{1}/2$	$6^{1}/2$	$5^{1}/2$	$4^{1}/2$	$3^{1}/2$
B: Half of thigh	$2^{3}/4$	$3^{1}/4$	4	$4^{1}/4$	$4^{1}/2$	$4^{3}/4$
C: Half of leg	$2^{1}/2$	$2^{1}/2$	$2^{3}/4$	3	$3^{1}/4$	$3^{1}/2$

Second degree _____ and
Third degree _____ =
Total percent burned ____

FIGURE 4-10 Estimation of burn injury in children and adults. (From Hockenberry M, Wilson D: *Wong's nursing care of infants and children*, ed 8. St. Louis, 2007, Mosby.)

b. Is characterized by fluid shift from intravascular to interstitial and shock; focus of care is to preserve vital organ functioning.
  c. Expect to administer large volumes of fluid in this phase.
2. Stage II: Acute phase
  a. Occurs from beginning of diuresis to near completion of wound closure.
  b. Is characterized by fluid shift from interstitial to intravascular.
3. Stage III: Rehabilitation phase
  a. Occurs from major wound closure to return to optimal level of physical and psychosocial adjustment (approximately 5 years).
  b. Is characterized by grafting and rehabilitation specific to the client's needs.

Nursing Assessment

A. Absence of bowel sounds indicating paralytic ileus
B. Radically decreased urinary output in the first 72 hours after injury, with increased specific gravity

C. Radically increased urinary output (diuresis) 72 hours to 2 weeks after initial injury
D. Signs of inadequate hydration
  1. Restlessness
  2. Disorientation
  3. Decreased urinary volume and urinary sodium, and increased urine specific gravity
E. Signs of inhalation burn
  1. Singed nasal hairs
  2. Circumoral burns
  3. Conjunctivitis
  4. Sooty or bloody sputum
  5. Hoarseness
  6. Asymmetry of chest movements with respirations and use of accessory muscles indicative of pneumonia
  7. Rales, wheezing, and rhonchi denoting smoke inhalation
F. Description of physiologic responses to burns (Fig. 4-11)
G. Preexisting conditions or illnesses that may influence recovery

TABLE 4-39 Lund and Browder Chart

Area	1 Year	1 to 4 Years	5 to 9 Years	10 to 14 Years	15 Years	Adult
Head	19	17	13	11	9	7
Neck	2	2	2	2	2	2
Anterior trunk	13	13	13	13	13	13
Posterior trunk	13	13	13	13	13	13
Right buttock	2½	2½	2½	2½	2½	2½
Left buttock	2½	2½	2½	2½	2½	2½
Genitalia	1	1	1	1	1	1
Right upper arm	4	4	4	4	4	4
Left upper arm	4	4	4	4	4	4
Right lower arm	3	3	3	3	3	3
Left lower arm	3	3	3	3	3	3
Right hand	2½	2½	2½	2½	2½	2½
Left hand	2½	2½	2½	2½	2½	2½
Right thigh	5½	6½	8	8½	9	9½
Left thigh	5½	6½	8	8½	9	9½
Right leg	5	5	5½	6	6½	7
Left leg	5	5	5½	6	6½	7
Right foot	½	3½	3½	3½	3½	3½
Left foot	3½	3½	3½	3½	3½	3½

HESI Hint • ABCs of Assessment
- Airway
- Breathing
- Circulation

Analysis (Nursing Diagnoses)

A. *Ineffective airway clearance* related to…
B. *Impaired gas exchange* related to…
C. *Decreased cardiac output* related to…
D. *Deficient fluid volume* related to…
E. *Ineffective tissue perfusion* (specify) related to…
F. *Impaired skin integrity* related to…
G. *Acute pain* related to…
H. *Disturbed body image* related to…
I. *Imbalanced nutrition: less than body requirements* related to…
J. *Risk for infection* related to…
K. *Impaired physical mobility* related to…

Nursing Plans and Interventions

A. Emergent phase: Efforts are directed toward stabilization with ongoing assessment.
   1. Assist with admission care.
      a. Extinguish source of burn (burning may continue with clothing attached to skin).
         (1) Thermal: remove clothing, cool burns by immersion in tepid water, apply dry sterile dressings.
         (2) Chemical: flush with water or normal saline.
         (3) Electrical: separate client from electrical source.
      b. Provide an open airway; intubation may be necessary if laryngeal edema is a risk.
      c. Determine baseline data: vital signs, blood gases, weight.
      d. Determine depth and extent of burn.
      e. Administer tetanus toxoid.
      f. Initiate fluid and electrolyte therapy: lactated Ringer's solution with electrolytes and colloids adjusted according to lab results and fluid resuscitation formula used.

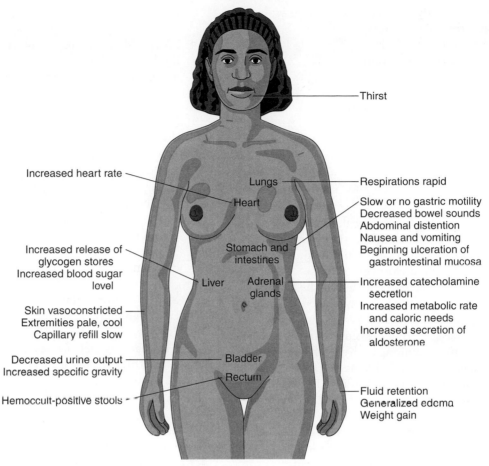

Thirst

Increased heart rate

Lungs

Heart

Respirations rapid

Slow or no gastric motility
Decreased bowel sounds
Abdominal distention
Nausea and vomiting
Beginning ulceration of
gastrointestinal mucosa

Increased release of
glycogen stores
Increased blood sugar
level

Stomach and
intestines

Liver

Adrenal
glands

Increased catecholamine
secretion
Increased metabolic rate
and caloric needs
Increased secretion of
aldosterone

Skin vasoconstricted
Extremities pale, cool
Capillary refill slow

Decreased urine output
Increased specific gravity

Bladder

Rectum

Fluid retention
Generalized edema
Weight gain

Hemoccult-positive stools

FIGURE 4-11   The physiologic actions of the sympathetic nervous system's compensatory responses to burn injury (early phase). (From Ignatavicius DD, Workman ML: *Medical-surgical nursing: Patient-centered collaborative care,* ed 6. St. Louis, 2010, Saunders.)

> **HESI Hint** • Massive volumes of IV fluids are given. It is not uncommon to give over 1000 ml/hr during various phases of burn care. Hemodynamic monitoring must be closely observed to be sure the client is supported with fluids but is not overloaded.

 g. Insert NG tube to prevent vomiting, abdominal distention, and gastric aspiration.
 h. Administer IV pain medication as prescribed.
2. Monitor hydration status.
 a. Record urinary output hourly (30 to 100 ml/hr is normal range).
 b. Maintain IV fluids titrated to keep urine output at 30 to 100 ml/hr.
 c. Accurately record I&O.
 d. Weigh daily.
 e. Observe for signs of inadequate hydration:
  (1) Restlessness
  (2) Disorientation
  (3) Hypothermia
  (4) Decreased urine output

3. Monitor respiratory functioning.
 a. Provide care for the intubated client.
 b. Suction endotracheal or nasotracheal tube.
 c. Monitor ABGs.
 d. Observe for cyanosis, disorientation.
 e. Administer O_2.
 f. Encourage use of incentive spirometer, coughing, and deep breathing.
4. Provide wound care.
 a. Use strict aseptic technique.

> **HESI Hint** • Infection is a life-threatening risk for those with burns.

 b. Perform débridement and dressing changes according to client's condition.
 c. Change dressings in minimum time (very painful); premedicate client; maintain sterile technique.
 d. Maintain room temperature above 90°F, humidified and free of drafts.

e. Monitor body temperature frequently; have hyperthermia blankets available.

5. Assess for paralytic ileus.
   a. Absence of bowel sounds
   b. Nausea and vomiting
   c. Abdominal distention
6. Assist with management of pain.
   a. Administer analgesics intravenously.
   b. Teach distraction and relaxation techniques.
   c. Teach use of guided imagery.
7. Assess for circulatory compromise in burns that constrict body parts. Prepare client for escharotomy.

B. Acute phase: Characterized by fluid shift from interstitial to intravascular (diuresis begins); occurs from 72 hours to 2 weeks after initial injury to near completion of wound closure
   1. Provide infection control, including the following:
      a. Maintain protective isolation of entire burn unit.
      b. Cover hair at all times.
      c. Wear masks during dressing changes.
      d. Use sterile technique for hydrotherapy, dressing change, and débridement.
      e. Administer IV antibiotics if indicated.
      f. Be sure any live plants and flowers are removed; they are prohibited.
   2. Splint and position client to prevent contractures. Avoid use of pillows in cases of neck burns.
   3. Perform ROM exercises; they are painful.
      a. Administer pain medication immediately prior to performing ROM exercises.
      b. Perform active ROM exercises for 3 to 5 minutes frequently during day.
      c. Mobilize as soon as possible using splints designed for the client.

d. Encourage active ROM exercises when up and about.
4. Provide fluid therapy; may use colloids to keep fluid in vascular space.
   a. Monitor serum chemistries at all times.
   b. Keep an IV site available; a saline lock is helpful.
   c. Maintain strict I&O.
   d. Encourage oral intake of fluids.
5. Provide adequate nutrition.
   a. Provide high-calorie (up to 5000 calories/day), high-protein, high-carbohydrate diet.
   b. Give nutritional supplements via NG tube feeding at night if caloric intake is inadequate.
   c. Keep accurate calorie counts.
   d. Administer all medications with either milk or juice.
   e. May require total parenteral nutrition (TPN)
   f. Weigh daily.
6. Provide burn and wound care.
   a. Cleansing per agency routine (daily or up to three times a day) in hydrotherapy or shower.
   b. Wet to dry dressing changes two to three times a day to remove necrotic tissue and debris.

> **HESI Hint** • Dressing changes are very painful! Medicate client prior to procedure!

   c. Apply silver sulfadiazine (Silvadene) or mafenide acetate (Sulfamylon) to burn as prescribed (Table 4-40).

TABLE 4-40 Topical Antimicrobial Agents

Drugs	Indications	Adverse Reactions	Nursing Implications
• Mafenide acetate (Sulfamylon)	• Treatment of burns • Usually used with open method of wound care	• Painful • Causes mild acidosis	• Administer pain medication *prior* to dressing change • Penetrates wound rapidly
• Silver sulfadiazine (Silvadene)	• Treatment of burns • Usually used with open method of wound care • Used to avoid acid-base complications • Keeps eschar soft, making débridement easier	• Penetrates wound slowly	• Administer pain medication *prior* to dressing change
• Nitrofurazone (Furacin)	• Treatment of burns • Used to prevent infections • Interferes with bacterial enzymes	• Allergic contact dermatitis • May see superinfections	• Administer pain medication *prior* to dressing change • Monitor for signs of infection

d. Cover (closed method) or leave open (open method), according to agency policy or physician's prescription.

e. Prepare client for grafting when eschar has been removed.

f. Prepare client for autografts (use of client's own skin for grafting).

g. Use heat lamp to donor site following graft to allow the area to reepithelialize.

HESI Hint • Preexisting conditions that might influence burn recovery are age, chronic illness (diabetes, cardiac problems, etc.), physical disabilities, disease, medications used routinely, and drug or alcohol abuse.

C. Rehabilitation phase: Characterized by the absence of infection risk

1. Ongoing discharge planning occurs.
2. Client may return home when the danger of infection has been eliminated.
3. High-protein fluids with vitamin supplements are recommended.
4. Pressure dressings such as Jobst garments may be worn continuously to prevent hypertrophic scarring and contractures.

Review of Burns

1. List four categories of burns.
2. Burn depth is a measure of severity. Describe the characteristics of superficial partial-thickness, deep partial-thickness, and full-thickness burns.
3. Describe fluid management in the emergent phase, acute phase, and rehabilitation phase of the burned client.
4. Describe pain management of the burned client.
5. Outline admission care of the burned client.
6. Nutritional status is a major concern when caring for a burned client. List three specific dietary interventions used with burned clients.
7. Describe the method of extinguishing each of the following burns: thermal, chemical, and electrical.
8. List four signs of an inhalation burn.
9. Why is the burned client allowed no "free" water?
10. Describe an autograft.

Answers to Review

1. Thermal, radiation, chemical, electrical
2. Superficial partial-thickness, first degree: pink to red skin (e.g., sunburn), slight edema, and pain relieved by cooling.

   Deep partial-thickness, second degree: destruction of epidermis and upper layers of dermis; white or red, very edematous, sensitive to touch and cold air, hair does not pull out easily.

   Full-thickness, third degree: total destruction of dermis and epidermis; reddened areas do not blanch with pressure; not painful; inelastic; waxy white skin to brown, leathery eschar.
3. Stage I (emergent phase): Replacement of fluids is titrated to urine output.

   Stage II (acute phase): Patent infusion site is maintained in case supplemental IV fluids are needed; saline lock is helpful; colloids may be used.

   Stage III (rehabilitation phase): No extra fluids are needed, but high-protein drinks are recommended.
4. Administer pain medication, especially prior to dressing wound. Teach distraction and relaxation techniques. Teach use of guided imagery.
5. Provide a patent airway because intubation may be necessary. Determine baseline data. Initiate fluid and electrolyte therapy. Administer pain medication. Determine depth and extent of burn. Administer tetanus toxoid. Insert NG tube.
6. High-calorie, high-protein, high-carbohydrate diet; medications with juice or milk; no "free" water; tube feeding at night. Maintain accurate, daily calorie counts. Weigh client daily.
7. Thermal: remove clothing, immerse in tepid water. Chemical: flush with water or saline. Electrical: separate client from electrical source.
8. Singed nasal hairs, circumoral burns; sooty or bloody sputum, hoarseness, and pulmonary signs, including asymmetry of respirations, rales, or wheezing.
9. Water may interfere with electrolyte balance. Client needs to ingest food products with highest biologic value.
10. Use of client's own skin for grafting.

PEDIATRIC NURSING 5

Growth and Development

Description: Growth and development follow an orderly yet individual pattern. Nurses should assess growth and the emergence of developmental skills in all pediatric clients. Knowledge of cognitive abilities allows a nurse to adapt teaching to the level of the child. Knowledge of appropriate toys and interests of children at different ages enables the nurse to use play to facilitate the child's development and minimize problems caused by the hospitalization.

INFANT (BIRTH TO 1 YEAR)

A. Developmental milestones
1. Birth weight doubles by 6 months, triples by 12 months.
2. Birth length increases by 50% at 12 months.
3. Posterior fontanel closes by 8 weeks.
4. Social smile occurs at 2 months.
5. Head turns to locate sounds at 3 months.
6. Moro reflex disappears around 4 months.
7. Steady head control is achieved at 4 months.
8. Rolls from abdomen to back and back to abdomen at 5 to 6 months.
9. Plays peek-a-boo after 6 months.
10. Transfers objects from hand to hand at 7 months.
11. Develops stranger anxiety at 7 to 9 months.
12. Sits unsupported at 8 months.
13. Crawls at 10 months.
14. Fine pincer grasp appears at 10 to 12 months.
15. Waves bye-bye at 10 months.
16. Walks with assistance at 10 to 12 months.
17. Says a few words in addition to "mama" or "dada" at 12 months.
18. Explores environment by motor and oral means.

B. Erickson's theory: Developing a sense of trust (trust versus mistrust)

C. Nursing implications
1. During hospitalization, the infant's emerging skills may disappear.
2. If the parents are not able to be with the infant, the baby may be inconsolable due to separation anxiety.
3. The nurse should plan to have the parents be part of the infant's care and should encourage them to do so.
4. Respect the infant's schedule at home by assessing and implementing components as possible.
5. Preparation and teaching should be directed to the family. However, the nurse should always speak to the infant and console the infant, especially while performing painful or stressful procedures.
6. Toys for hospitalized infants include mobiles, rattles, squeaking toys, picture books, balls, colored blocks, and activity boxes.

HESI Hint • Questions on the NCLEX-RN® examination are the only ones tested. However, these are frequently tested content areas:
- When does birth length double? Answer: by 4 years.
- When does the child sit unsupported? Answer: 8 months.
- When does a child achieve 50% of adult height? Answer: 2 years.
- When does a child throw a ball overhand? Answer: 18 months.
- When does a child speak two- to three-word sentences? Answer: 2 years.
- When does a child use scissors? Answer: 4 years.
- When does a child tie his or her shoes? Answer: 5 years.
- Be aware that a girl's growth spurt during adolescence begins earlier than a boy's (as early as 10 years of age).
- Temper tantrums are common in the toddler (i.e., they are considered normal or average behavior).
- Be aware that adolescence is a time when the child forms his or her identity and that rebellion against family values is common for this age group.

HESI Hint • Knowledge of normal growth and development is used to evaluate interventions and therapy. For example, what behavior would indicate that thyroid hormone therapy for a 4-month-old is effective? You must know which milestones are accomplished by a 4-month-old. One correct answer would be: Has steady head control, which is an expected milestone for a 4-month-old and indicates that replacement therapy is adequate for growth.

TODDLER (1 TO 3 YEARS)

A. Developmental milestones
   1. Birth weight quadruples by 30 months.
   2. Achieves 50% of adult height by 2 years.
   3. Growth velocity slows.
   4. Appears to be bowlegged and potbellied.
   5. All primary teeth (20) are present.
   6. Anterior fontanel closes by 12 to 18 months.
   7. Throws a ball overhand at 18 months.
   8. Kicks a ball at 24 months.
   9. Feeds self with spoon and cup at 2 years.
   10. Daytime toilet training can usually be started around 2 years.
   11. Two- to three-word sentences are spoken by 2 years.
   12. Three- to four-word sentences are spoken by 3 years.
   13. Own first and last name can be stated by 2½ to 3 years.
   14. Temper tantrums are common.

B. Erikson's theory: Developing a sense of autonomy (autonomy versus doubt and shame)

C. Nursing implications
   1. Give simple, brief explanations before procedures, keeping in mind that a 1-year-old does not benefit from the same explanation as that given to a 3-year-old.
   2. During hospitalization, enforced separation from parents is the greatest threat to the toddler's psychological and emotional integrity.
   3. Security objects or favorite toys from home should be provided for a toddler.
   4. Teach parents to explain their plans to the child (e.g., "I will be back after your nap").
   5. Respect the child's routine and implement when possible.
   6. Expect regression (e.g., bed-wetting).
   7. Toys for the hospitalized toddler include board and mallet, push-pull toys, toy telephones, stuffed animals, and storybooks with pictures, depending on the reason for hospitalization. Toddlers benefit from being taken to the hospital playroom when able, because mobility is very important to their development.
   8. Toddlers are learning to name body parts and are concerned about their bodies.
   9. Very basic explanations should be given to toddlers about procedures.
   10. Autonomy should be supported by providing guided choices when appropriate.

PRESCHOOL CHILD (3 TO 6 YEARS)

A. Developmental milestones
   1. Each year, a child gains about 5 pounds and grows 2½ to 3 inches.
   2. A child stands erect with more slender posture.
   3. A child learns to run, jump, skip, and hop.
   4. A 3-year-old can ride a tricycle.
   5. Handedness is established.
   6. A child uses scissors at 4 years.
   7. A child ties shoelaces at 5 years.
   8. A child learns colors, shapes.
   9. Visual acuity approaches 20/20.
   10. Thinking is egocentric and concrete.
   11. A child uses sentences of five to eight words.
   12. A child learns sexual identity (curiosity and masturbation are common).
   13. Imaginary playmates and fears are common.
   14. Aggressiveness at 4 years is replaced by more independence at 5 years.

B. Erikson's theory: Developing a sense of initiative (initiative versus guilt)

C. Nursing implications
   1. Nursing care for hospitalized preschoolers should emphasize understanding of the child's egocentricity. Explain that he or she did not cause the illness and that painful procedures are not a punishment for misdeeds.
   2. The child's questions should be answered at the child's level. Use simple words that will be understood by the child.
   3. Therapeutic play or medical play that allows the child to act out his or her experiences is helpful.
   4. Fear of mutilation by procedures is common. A Band-Aid may be quite helpful in restoring body integrity.
   5. Toys and play for the hospitalized preschooler include coloring books, puzzles, cutting and pasting, dolls, building blocks, clay, and toys that allow the preschooler to work out hospitalization experiences, depending on the reason for hospitalization.
   6. The preschooler needs preparation for procedures. He or she should understand what is and what is not going to be "fixed." Simple explanations and basic pictures are helpful. Let the child handle equipment or models of the equipment.

HESI Hint • Use facts and principles related to growth and development in planning teaching interventions. For example: What task could a 5-year-old diabetic boy be expected to accomplish by himself? One correct answer would be to let him choose the injection sites. This is possible for a preschooler to do and gives the child some sense of control.

SCHOOL-AGE CHILD (6 TO 12 YEARS)

A. Developmental milestones
   1. Each year, a child gains 4 to 6 pounds and about 2 inches in height.
   2. Girls may experience menarche.
   3. Loss of primary teeth and eruption of most permanent teeth occurs.
   4. Fine and gross motor skills mature.
   5. A child is able to write script at 8 years of age.
   6. A child can dress self completely.
   7. Egocentric thinking is replaced by social awareness of others.
   8. A child learns to tell time and understands past, present, and future.
   9. A child learns cause-and-effect relationships.
   10. Socialization with peers becomes important.
   11. Molars (6-year) erupt.

B. Erikson's theory: Developing a sense of industry (industry versus inferiority)

C. Nursing implications
   1. The hospitalized school-age child may need more support from parents than they wish to admit.
   2. Maintaining contact with peers and school activities is important during hospitalization.
   3. Explanation of all procedures is important. They can learn from verbal explanations, pictures, and books and by handling equipment.
   4. Privacy and modesty are important and should be respected during hospitalization (e.g., close curtains during procedures, allow privacy during baths).
   5. Participation in care and planning with staff fosters a sense of involvement and accomplishment.
   6. Toys for the school-age child include board games, card games, and hobbies, such as stamp collecting, puzzles, and video games.

HESI Hint • School-age children are in Erikson's stage of industry, meaning they like to do and accomplish things. Peers are also becoming important for children of this age.

ADOLESCENT (12 TO 19 YEARS)

A. Developmental milestones
   1. Girls' growth spurts during adolescence begin earlier than boys' (may begin as early as 10 for girls).
   2. Boys catch up at around 14 and continue to grow.
   3. Girls finish growth at around 15, boys at around 17.
   4. Secondary sex characteristics develop.
   5. Adult-like thinking begins around 15. They can problem-solve and use abstract thinking.
   6. Family conflicts develop.

B. Erikson's theory: Developing a sense of identity (identity versus role confusion)

C. Nursing implications
   1. Hospitalization of adolescents disrupts school and peer activities; they need to maintain contact with both.
   2. They should share a room with other adolescents.
   3. Illnesses, treatments, and procedures that alter the adolescent's body image can be viewed by the adolescent as being devastating.
   4. Teaching about procedures should include time without the parents being present. When parents are present, direct questions to the adolescent, not the parents.
   5. The age of assent for making medical decisions in children and adolescents ranges from 7 to 14 years. Parental consent is also needed for treatment.
   6. For prolonged hospitalizations, adolescents need to maintain identity (e.g., have their own clothing, posters, and visitors). A teen room or teen night is very helpful. Parents rooming in is discouraged.
   7. Some assessment questions should be asked without parents' presence.
   8. When teaching adolescents, the focus should be on the here and now—"How will this affect me today?"

HESI Hint • Age groups' concepts of bodily injury:
- Infants: After 6 months, their cognitive development allows them to remember pain.
- Toddlers: They fear intrusive procedures.
- Preschoolers: They fear body mutilation.
- School-age children: They fear loss of control of their bodies.
- Adolescents: Their major concern is change in body image.

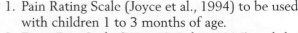

HESI Hint • Accidents are a major cause of death in children and adolescents. Teach parents and children developmentally appropriate safety and accident-prevention techniques.

Pain Assessment and Management in the Pediatric Client

Description: Historically, pain in the pediatric population has been unrecognized or undertreated. Research has shown that children, including neonates and infants, experience pain. Untreated pain may lead to complications, such as delayed recovery, alterations in sleep patterns, and alterations in nutrition.

Pain assessment is often referred to as the fifth vital sign.

Nursing Assessment

A. Verbal report by the child. Children as young as 3 years of age are able to report the location and degree of pain they are experiencing.

B. Observe for nonverbal signs of pain, such as grimacing, irritability, restlessness, and difficulty in sleeping or feeding.

C. Include the child's parents in the assessment.

D. Observe for physiologic responses to pain, such as increased heart rate, increased respiratory rate, diaphoresis, and decreased oxygen levels.

E. Physiologic responses to pain are most often seen in response to acute pain rather than in response to chronic pain.

Analysis (Nursing Diagnoses)

A. *Acute pain* related to…

B. *Anxiety* related to…

C. *Disturbed sleep pattern* related to…

D. *Ineffective infant feeding pattern* related to…

Nursing Plans And Interventions

A. A pain rating scale appropriate for the child's age and developmental level should be used.

1. Pain Rating Scale (Joyce et al., 1994) to be used with children 1 to 3 months of age.
2. Faces Pain Scale (Wong & Baker, 1996) and the Poker Chip Scale (Hester & Barcus, 1986) can be used by children of preschool age and older (Figure 5-1).
3. Numeric Pain Scale can be used by children 9 years of age and older.
4. Documentation of a child's self-report of pain is essential to effectively treating the child's pain.
5. A nonverbal child can be assessed using the FLACC pain assessment tool (Merkel et al., 1997). This tool has the nurse evaluate the child's facial expression, leg movement, activity, cry, and consolability.

B. Nonpharmacologic interventions
1. They should be used according to the child's age and developmental level.
2. Infants may respond best to pacifiers, holding, and rocking.
3. Toddlers and preschoolers may respond best to distraction. Distraction may be provided through books, music, television, bubble blowing.
4. School-aged children and adolescents may use guided imagery.
5. Other interventions may include massage, application of heat or cold, and deep-breathing exercises.

C. Pharmacologic interventions
1. Prior to administering a pain medication to a pediatric client, verify that the prescribed dose is safe for the child on the basis of the child's weight.
2. Monitor the child's vital signs following administration of opioid medications.
3. Children as young as 5 years of age may be taught to use a patient-controlled analgesia (PCA) pump.
4. Children may deny pain if they fear receiving an IM injection.

Child Health Promotion

Description: Immunization of children against communicable diseases is one of the greatest accomplishments of modern medicine. Childhood mortality and morbidity rates have greatly decreased. Protection against disease should begin in infancy according to the recommendations of the American Academy of Pediatrics and the U. S. Public Health Service (Figure 5-2; Table 5-1).

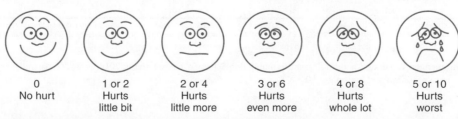

| 0 | 1 or 2 | 2 or 4 | 3 or 6 | 4 or 8 | 5 or 10 |
| No hurt | Hurts little bit | Hurts little more | Hurts even more | Hurts whole lot | Hurts worst |

FIGURE 5-1 Wong-Baker Faces Pain Rating Scale. (From Hockenberry MJ, Wilson D: *Wong's nursing care of infants and children*, ed 8. St. Louis, 2007, Mosby.)

Recommended Immunization Schedule for Persons Aged 0 Through 6 Years—United States • 2010

For those who fall behind or start late, see the catch-up schedule

Vaccine ▼ Age ►	Birth	1 month	2 months	4 months	6 months	12 months	15 months	18 months	19–23 months	2–3 years	4–6 years	
Hepatitis B[1]	HepB	HepB				HepB						Range of recommended ages for all children except certain high-risk groups
Rotavirus[2]			RV	RV	RV[2]							
Diphtheria, Tetanus, Pertussis[3]			DTaP	DTaP	DTaP	see footnote[3]	DTaP				DTaP	
Haemophilus influenzae type b[4]			Hib	Hib	Hib[4]	Hib						
Pneumococcal[5]			PCV	PCV	PCV	PCV				PPSV		
Inactivated Poliovirus[6]			IPV	IPV		IPV					IPV	
Influenza[7]						Influenza (Yearly)						Range of recommended ages for certain high-risk groups
Measles, Mumps, Rubella[8]						MMR		see footnote[8]			MMR	
Varicella[9]						Varicella		see footnote[9]			Varicella	
Hepatitis A[10]						HepA (2 doses)				HepA Series		
Meningococcal[11]										MCV		

This schedule includes recommendations in effect as of December 15, 2009. Any dose not administered at the recommended age should be administered at a subsequent visit, when indicated and feasible. The use of a combination vaccine generally is preferred over separate injections of its equivalent component vaccines. Considerations should include provider assessment, patient preference, and the potential for adverse events. Providers should consult the relevant Advisory Committee on Immunization Practices statement for detailed recommendations: **http://www.cdc.gov/vaccines/pubs/acip-list.htm**. Clinically significant adverse events that follow immunization should be reported to the Vaccine Adverse Event Reporting System (VAERS) at **http://www.vaers.hhs.gov** or by telephone, **800-822-7967**.

1. **Hepatitis B vaccine (HepB).** (Minimum age: birth)
   At birth:
   • Administer monovalent HepB to all newborns before hospital discharge.
   • If mother is hepatitis B surface antigen (HBsAg)-positive, administer HepB and 0.5 mL of hepatitis B immune globulin (HBIG) within 12 hours of birth.
   • If mother's HBsAg status is unknown, administer HepB within 12 hours of birth. Determine mother's HBsAg status as soon as possible and, if HBsAg-positive, administer HBIG (no later than age 1 week).
   After the birth dose:
   • The HepB series should be completed with either monovalent HepB or a combination vaccine containing HepB. The second dose should be administered at age 1 or 2 months. Monovalent HepB vaccine should be used for doses administered before age 6 weeks. The final dose should be administered no earlier than age 24 weeks.
   • Infants born to HBsAg-positive mothers should be tested for HBsAg and antibody to HBsAg 1 to 2 months after completion of at least 3 doses of the HepB series, at age 9 through 18 months (generally at the next well-child visit).
   • Administration of 4 doses of HepB to infants is permissible when a combination vaccine containing HepB is administered after the birth dose. The fourth dose should be administered no earlier than age 24 weeks.
2. **Rotavirus vaccine (RV).** (Minimum age: 6 weeks)
   • Administer the first dose at age 6 through 14 weeks (maximum age: 14 weeks 6 days). Vaccination should not be initiated for infants aged 15 weeks 0 days or older.
   • The maximum age for the final dose in the series is 8 months 0 days
   • If Rotarix is administered at ages 2 and 4 months, a dose at 6 months is not indicated.
3. **Diphtheria and tetanus toxoids and acellular pertussis vaccine (DTaP).** (Minimum age: 6 weeks)
   • The fourth dose may be administered as early as age 12 months, provided at least 6 months have elapsed since the third dose.
   • Administer the final dose in the series at age 4 through 6 years.
4. ***Haemophilus influenzae* type b conjugate vaccine (Hib).**
   (Minimum age: 6 weeks)
   • If PRP-OMP (PedvaxHIB or Comvax [HepB-Hib]) is administered at ages 2 and 4 months, a dose at age 6 months is not indicated.
   • TriHiBit (DTaP/Hib) and Hiberix (PRP-T) should not be used for doses at ages 2, 4, or 6 months for the primary series but can be used as the final dose in children aged 12 months through 4 years.
5. **Pneumococcal vaccine.** (Minimum age: 6 weeks for pneumococcal conjugate vaccine [PCV]; 2 years for pneumococcal polysaccharide vaccine [PPSV])
   • PCV is recommended for all children aged younger than 5 years. Administer 1 dose of PCV to all healthy children aged 24 through 59 months who are not completely vaccinated for their age.
   • Administer PPSV 2 or more months after last dose of PCV to children aged 2 years or older with certain underlying medical conditions, including a cochlear implant. See *MMWR* 1997;46(No. RR-8).

6. **Inactivated poliovirus vaccine (IPV)** (Minimum age: 6 weeks)
   • The final dose in the series should be administered on or after the fourth birthday and at least 6 months following the previous dose.
   • If 4 doses are administered prior to age 4 years a fifth dose should be administered at age 4 through 6 years. See *MMWR* 2009;58(30):829–30.
7. **Influenza vaccine (seasonal).** (Minimum age: 6 months for trivalent inactivated influenza vaccine [TIV]; 2 years for live, attenuated influenza vaccine [LAIV])
   • Administer annually to children aged 6 months through 18 years.
   • For healthy children aged 2 through 6 years (i.e., those who do not have underlying medical conditions that predispose them to influenza complications), either LAIV or TIV may be used, except LAIV should not be given to children aged 2 through 4 years who have had wheezing in the past 12 months.
   • Children receiving TIV should receive 0.25 mL if aged 6 through 35 months or 0.5 mL if aged 3 years or older.
   • Administer 2 doses (separated by at least 4 weeks) to children aged younger than 9 years who are receiving influenza vaccine for the first time or who were vaccinated for the first time during the previous influenza season but only received 1 dose.
   • For recommendations for use of influenza A (H1N1) 2009 monovalent vaccine see *MMWR* 2009;58(No. RR-10).
8. **Measles, mumps, and rubella vaccine (MMR).** (Minimum age: 12 months)
   • Administer the second dose routinely at age 4 through 6 years. However, the second dose may be administered before age 4, provided at least 28 days have elapsed since the first dose.
9. **Varicella vaccine.** (Minimum age: 12 months)
   • Administer the second dose routinely at age 4 through 6 years. However, the second dose may be administered before age 4, provided at least 3 months have elapsed since the first dose.
   • For children aged 12 months through 12 years the minimum interval between doses is 3 months. However, if the second dose was administered at least 28 days after the first dose, it can be accepted as valid.
10. **Hepatitis A vaccine (HepA).** (Minimum age: 12 months)
    • Administer to all children aged 1 year (i.e., aged 12 through 23 months). Administer 2 doses at least 6 months apart.
    • Children not fully vaccinated by age 2 years can be vaccinated at subsequent visits
    • HepA also is recommended for older children who live in areas where vaccination programs target older children, who are at increased risk for infection, or for whom immunity against hepatitis A is desired.
11. **Meningococcal vaccine.** (Minimum age: 2 years for meningococcal conjugate vaccine [MCV4] and for meningococcal polysaccharide vaccine [MPSV4])
    • Administer MCV4 to children aged 2 through 10 years with persistent complement component deficiency, anatomic or functional asplenia, and certain other conditions placing tham at high risk.
    • Administer MCV4 to children previously vaccinated with MCV4 or MPSV4 after 3 years if first dose administered at age 2 through 6 years. See *MMWR* 2009;58:1042–3.

The Recommended Immunization Schedules for Persons Aged 0 through 18 Years are approved by the Advisory Committee on Immunization Practices (**http://www.cdc.gov/vaccines/recs/acip**), the American Academy of Pediatrics (**http://www.aap.org**), and the American Academy of Family Physicians (**http://www.aafp.org**).
Department of Health and Human Services • Centers for Disease Control and Prevention

FIGURE 5-2 Recommended Childhood and Adolescent Immunization Schedule, United States, 2010. (From Department of Health and Human Services, Centers for Disease Control and Prevention, 2010.)

Recommended Immunization Schedule for Persons Aged 7 Through 18 Years—United States • 2010
For those who fall behind or start late, see the schedule below and the catch-up schedule

Vaccine ▼ Age ►	7–10 years	11–12 years	13–18 years
Tetanus, Diphtheria, Pertussis[1]		Tdap	Tdap
Human Papillomavirus[2]	see footnote 2	HPV (3 doses)	HPV series
Meningococcal[3]	MCV	MCV	MCV
Influenza[4]	Influenza (Yearly)		
Pneumococcal[5]	PPSV		
Hepatitis A[6]	HepA Series		
Hepatitis B[7]	Hep B Series		
Inactivated Poliovirus[8]	IPV Series		
Measles, Mumps, Rubella[9]	MMR Series		
Varicella[10]	Varicella Series		

Range of recommended ages for all children except certain high-risk groups

Range of recommended ages for catch-up immunization

Range of recommended ages for certain high-risk groups

This schedule includes recommendations in effect as of December 15, 2009. Any dose not administered at the recommended age should be administered at a subsequent visit, when indicated and feasible. The use of a combination vaccine generally is preferred over separate injections of its equivalent component vaccines. Considerations should include provider assessment, patient preference, and the potential for adverse events. Providers should consult the relevant Advisory Committee on Immunization Practices statement for detailed recommendations: http://www.cdc.gov/vaccines/pubs/acip-list.htm. Clinically significant adverse events that follow immunization should be reported to the Vaccine Adverse Event Reporting System (VAERS) at http://www.vaers.hhs.gov or by telephone, 800-822-7967.

1. **Tetanus and diphtheria toxoids and acellular pertussis vaccine (Tdap).** (Minimum age: 10 years for Boostrix and 11 years for Adacel)
   • Administer at age 11 or 12 years for those who have completed the recommended childhood DTP/DTaP vaccination series and have not received a tetanus and diphtheria toxoid (Td) booster dose.
   • Persons aged 13 through 18 years who have not received Tdap should receive a dose.
   • A 5-year interval from the last Td dose is encouraged when Tdap is used as a booster dose; however, a shorter interval may be used if pertussis immunity is needed.
2. **Human papillomavirus vaccine (HPV).** (Minimum age: 9 years)
   • Two HPV vaccines are licensed: a quadrivalent vaccine (HPV4) for the prevention of cervical, vaginal and vulvar cancers (in females) and genital warts (in females and males), and a bivalent vaccine (HPV2) for the prevention of cervical cancers in females.
   • HPV vaccines are most effective for both males and females when given before exposure to HPV through sexual contact.
   • HPV4 or HPV2 is recommended for the prevention of cervical precancers and cancers in females.
   • HPV4 is recommended for the prevention of cervical, vaginal and vulvar precancers and cancers and genital warts in females.
   • Administer the first dose to females at age 11 or 12 years.
   • Administer the second dose 1 to 2 months after the first dose and the third dose 6 months after the first dose (at least 24 weeks after the first dose).
   • Administer the series to females at age 13 through 18 years if not previously vaccinated.
   • HPV4 may be administered in a 3-dose series to males aged 9 through 18 years to reduce their likelihood of acquiring genital warts.
3. **Meningococcal conjugate vaccine (MCV4).**
   • Administer at age 11 or 12 years, or at age 13 through 18 years if not previously vaccinated.
   • Administer to previously unvaccinated college freshmen living in a dormitory.
   • Administer MCV4 to children aged 2 through 10 years with persistent complement component deficiency, anatomic or functional asplenia, or certain other conditions placing them at high risk.
   • Administer to children previously vaccinated with MCV4 or MPSV4 who remain at increased risk after 3 years (if first dose administered at age 2 through 6 years) or after 5 years (if first dose administered at age 7 years or older). Persons whose only risk factor is living in on-campus housing are not recommended to receive an additional dose. See MMWR 2009;58:1042–3.

4. **Influenza vaccine (seasonal).**
   • Administer annually to children aged 6 months through 18 years.
   • For healthy nonpregnant persons aged 7 through 18 years (i.e., those who do not have underlying medical conditions that predispose them to influenza complications), either LAIV or TIV may be used.
   • Administer 2 doses (separated by at least 4 weeks) to children aged younger than 9 years who are receiving influenza vaccine for the first time or who were vaccinated for the first time during the previous influenza season but only received 1 dose.
   • For recommendations for use of influenza A (H1N1) 2009 monovalent vaccine. See MMWR 2009;58(No. RR-10).
5. **Pneumococcal polysaccharide vaccine (PPSV).**
   • Administer to children with certain underlying medical conditions, including a cochlear implant. A single revaccination should be administered after 5 years to children with functional or anatomic asplenia or an immunocompromising condition. See MMWR 1997;46(No. RR-8).
6. **Hepatitis A vaccine (HepA).**
   • Administer 2 doses at least 6 months apart.
   • HepA is recommended for children aged older than 23 months who live in areas where vaccination programs target older children, who are at increased risk for infection, or for whom immunity against hepatitis A is desired.
7. **Hepatitis B vaccine (HepB).**
   • Administer the 3-dose series to those not previously vaccinated.
   • A 2-dose series (separated by at least 4 months) of adult formulation Recombivax HB is licensed for children aged 11 through 15 years.
8. **Inactivated poliovirus vaccine (IPV).**
   • The final dose in the series should be administered on or after the fourth birthday and at least 6 months following the previous dose.
   • If both OPV and IPV were administered as part of a series, a total of 4 doses should be administered, regardless of the child's current age.
9. **Measles, mumps, and rubella vaccine (MMR).**
   • If not previously vaccinated, administer 2 doses or the second dose for those who have received only 1 dose, with at least 28 days between doses.
10. **Varicella vaccine.**
   • For persons aged 7 through 18 years without evidence of immunity (see MMWR 2007;56[No. RR-4]), administer 2 doses if not previously vaccinated or the second dose if only 1 dose has been administered.
   • For persons aged 7 through 12 years, the minimum interval between doses is 3 months. However, if the second dose was administered at least 28 days after the first dose, it can be accepted as valid.
   • For persons aged 13 years and older, the minimum interval between doses is 28 days.

The Recommended Immunization Schedules for Persons Aged 0 through 18 Years are approved by the Advisory Committee on Immunization Practices (http://www.cdc.gov/vaccines/recs/acip), the American Academy of Pediatrics (http://www.aap.org), and the American Academy of Family Physicians (http://www.aafp.org). Department of Health and Human Services • Centers for Disease Control and Prevention

FIGURE 5-2, CONT'D.

TABLE 5-1 Vaccines

Type of Vaccine	Description
MMR Vaccine	
• Measles, mumps, rubella (MMR) • Offers protection against these three diseases	• It is generally administered at 12 to 15 months of age and repeated at 4 to 6 years or by 11 to 12 years. • In times of measles epidemics, it is possible to give measles protection at 6 months and repeat the MMR at 15 months. • Measles vaccine is contraindicated for persons with history of anaphylactic reaction to neomycin or eggs, those with known altered immunodeficiency, and pregnant women. It may be given to those with HIV and to breastfeeding women. • Administer subcutaneously at separate sites. • Child may have a light, transient rash 2 weeks after administration of vaccine.

HESI Hint • Pertinent history should be obtained prior to administering certain immunizations because reactions to previous immunizations or current health conditions may contraindicate current immunizations:
- DPAT: History of reactions, seizures, neurologic symptoms after previous vaccine, or systematic allergic reactions
- MMR: History of anaphylactic reaction to eggs or neomycin

Type of Vaccine	Description
DTaP Vaccine	
• Diphtheria, pertussis, tetanus • Offers protection against these diseases	• Beginning at age 2 months, administer three doses at 2-month intervals. • Booster doses given at 15 to 18 months and at 4 to 6 years. • Administer intramuscularly (separate site from other vaccine). • Not given to children past the seventh birthday; they receive Td, which contains full-strength protection against tetanus and lesser strength diphtheria protection. • When pertussis vaccine is contraindicated, give DT, full-strength diphtheria and tetanus without pertussis vaccine, until seventh birthday. • Contraindications to pertussis vaccine include: → Encephalopathy within 7 days of previous dose of DTaP. → History of seizures. → Neurologic symptoms after receiving the vaccine. → Systemic allergic reactions to the vaccine. • Systemic allergic reactions to the vaccine. • Parents should be instructed to begin acetaminophen (Tylenol) administration after the immunization (normal dosage is 10 to 15 mg/kg). • Instruct parents to report immediately any side effects of the immunization to the primary caregiver.

HESI Hint • Pertussis fatalities continue to occur in nonimmunized infants in the United States

Type of Vaccine	Description
Polio Vaccine	
• Inactive polio vaccine (IPV)	• Recommended for all persons under 18 years. • Administer at 2 months of age and again at 4 months of age. Boosters are given at 6 to 18 months and at 4 to 6 years. • Administer IPV subcutaneously or IM at separate site. • IPV is contraindicated for those with history of anaphylactic reaction to neomycin or streptomycin. • May give with all other vaccines.

TABLE 5-1 Vaccines—cont'd

Type of Vaccine	Description
Hib (Haemophilus influenzae type B) Vaccine	
• Offers protection against bacteria that cause serious illness (epiglottitis, bacterial meningitis, septic arthritis) in small children and those with chronic illnesses such as sickle cell anemia.	• Three conjugate vaccines have been recommended for administration to infants: PRP-OPMs can be given beginning as early as 2 months of age. DTaP/Hib combinations should not be used as primary immunizations at ages 2, 4, or 6 months. • Vaccines have different series administration schedules; the schedules cover children through 5 years of age. • Children at high risk who were not immunized previously should be immunized after the age of 5. • Administer intramuscularly. • There are no contraindications.
Hepatitis B	
• Offers protection against hepatitis B. • May be given to newborns prior to hospital discharge. • All children up to 18 years of age should be vaccinated.	• Is contraindicated for persons with anaphylactic reaction to common baker's yeast. • See note at bottom of Recommended Childhood Immunization Schedule, Figure 5-2.
Varicella	
• Offers protection against chickenpox. • Is a school entry requirement in 33 states. • Is safe for children with asymptomatic HIV infection.	• Administer at 12 to 18 months of age (must be at least 12 months). • Give MMR and varicella on same day or > 30 days apart (separate site). • See note at bottom of Recommended Childhood Immunization Schedule, Figure 5-2.
Tuberculosis (TB) Skin Testing	

• Offers screening for exposure to TB	• Screening is usually done using one of the following:
	  → Mantoux test with PPD (tuberculin purified protein derivative) injected intradermally on the forearm; standard method for identifying infection with *Mycobacterium tuberculosis*.
	  → Tine test (OT, old tuberculin), which consists of four prongs pressed into the forearm. These multiple puncture tests are unreliable and should not be used to determine the presence of a TB infection.
	• A positive reaction represents exposure to *M. tuberculosis*.
	• Screening can be initiated at 12 months.

HESI Hint • Subcutaneous injection, rather than intradermal injection, invalidates the Mantoux test.

HESI Hint • The common cold is not a contraindication for immunization.

HESI Hint • Following immunization, what teaching should the nurse provide to the parents?
• Irritability, fever (<102°F), redness, and soreness at injection site for 2 to 3 days are normal side effects of DTaP and IPV administration.
• Call health care provider if seizures, high fever, or high-pitched crying occurs.
• A warm washcloth on the thigh injection site and "bicycling" the legs with each diaper change decreases soreness.
• Acetaminophen (Tylenol) is administered orally every 4 to 6 hours (10 to 15 mg/kg).

COMMON COMMUNICABLE DISEASES OF CHILDHOOD

The nursing care of children with communicable diseases is virtually the same for all, regardless of the particular disease.

A. Rubeola (measles)
   1. A highly contagious viral disease that can lead to neurologic problems or death
   2. Transmitted by direct contact with droplets from infected persons
   3. Contagious mainly during the prodromal period, which is characterized by fever and upper respiratory symptoms
   4. Classic symptoms include the following:
      a. Photophobia
      b. Koplik spots on the buccal mucosa
      c. Confluent rash that begins on the face and spreads downward
B. Varicella (chickenpox)
   1. Viral disease characterized by skin lesions
   2. Lesions that begin on the trunk and spread to the face and proximal extremities
   3. Progresses through macular, papular, vesicular, and pustular stages
   4. Transmitted by direct contact, droplet spread, or freshly contaminated objects
   5. Communicable prodromal period to the time all lesions have crusted
C. Rubella (German measles)
   1. Common viral disease that has teratogenic effects on fetus during the first trimester of pregnancy
   2. Transmitted by droplet and direct contact with infected person
   3. Discrete red maculopapular rash that starts on face and rapidly spreads to entire body
   4. Rash disappears within 3 days
D. Pertussis (whooping cough)
   1. Acute infectious respiratory disease usually occurring in infancy
   2. Caused by a gram-negative bacillus
   3. Begins with upper respiratory symptoms
   4. Paroxysmal stage characterized by prolonged coughing, and crowing or whooping upon inspiration; lasts from 4 to 6 weeks
   5. Transmitted by direct contact, droplet spread, or freshly contaminated objects
   6. Treated by administering erythromycin
   7. Complications: pneumonia, hemorrhage, and seizures
E. Paramyxovirus (mumps)
   1. Incubation: 14 to 21 days
   2. Symptoms: fever, headache, malaise, parotid gland swelling and tenderness; manifestations include submaxillary and sublingual infection, orchitis, and meningoencephalitis
   3. Transmitted by direct contact or droplet spread
   4. Analgesics used for pain and antiseptics for fever
   5. Bed rest maintained until swelling subsides

Nursing Care for Children with Communicable Diseases

A. Isolate child during period of communicability.
B. Treat fever with *nonaspirin* product.
C. Report occurrence to the health department.
D. Prevent child from scratching skin (e.g., cut nails, apply mittens, and provide soothing baths).
E. Administer diphenhydramine HCl (Benadryl) as prescribed, for itching.
F. *Wash hands* after caring for child and handling secretions or child's articles.

> **HESI Hint** • Children with German measles pose a serious threat to their unborn siblings. The nurse should counsel all expectant mothers, especially those with young children, to be aware of the serious consequences of exposure to German measles during pregnancy.

> **HESI Hint** • Common childhood problems are encountered by nurses caring for children in the community or hospital settings. The child's age directly influences the severity and management of these problems.

NUTRITIONAL ASSESSMENT

Description: Profile of the child's and family's eating habits

A. Iron deficiency occurs most commonly in children 12 to 36 months old, in adolescent females, and in females during their childbearing years.
B. The vitamins most often consumed in less than appropriate amounts by preschool and school-age children are:
   1. Vitamin A
   2. Vitamin C
   3. Vitamin B_6
   4. Vitamin B_{12}

Nursing Plans and Interventions

A. Determine dietary history.
   1. The 24-hour recall: ask the family to recall all food and liquid intake during the past 24 hours.
   2. Food diary: ask the family to keep a 3-day record (2 weekdays and 1 weekend day) of all food and liquid intake.

3. Food frequency record: provide a questionnaire and ask family to record information regarding the number of times per day, week, or month a child consumes items from the four food groups.

B. Perform a clinical examination.
1. Assess skin, hair, teeth, gums, lips, tongue, and eyes.
2. Use anthropometry: measurement of height, weight, body mass index (BMI), head circumference in young children, proportion, skinfold thickness, and arm circumference.
   a. Height and head circumference reflect past nutrition.
   b. Weight, skinfold thickness, and arm circumference reflect present nutritional status (especially protein and fat reserves).
   c. Skinfold thickness provides a measurement of the body's fat content (one-half of the body's total fat stores are directly beneath the skin).
3. Obtain biochemical analysis.
   a. Plasma, blood cells, urine, or tissues from liver, bone, hair, or fingernails can be used to determine nutritional status.
   b. Laboratory testing of Hgb, Hct, albumin, creatinine, and nitrogen is commonly used to determine nutritional status.

C. Implement appropriate nursing interventions, including client and family teaching to correct identified nutritional deficits (Table 5-2).

DIARRHEA

Description: Increased number or decreased consistency of stools

A. Diarrhea can be a serious or fatal illness, especially in infancy.
B. Causes include but are not limited to:
1. Infections: bacterial, viral
2. Malabsorption problems
3. Inflammatory diseases
4. Dietary factors
C. Conditions associated with diarrhea are:
1. Dehydration
2. Metabolic acidosis
3. Shock

Nursing Assessment

A. Usually occurs in infants
B. History of exposure to pathogens, contaminated food, dietary changes
C. Signs of dehydration
1. Poor skin turgor
2. Absence of tears
3. Dry mucous membranes
4. Weight loss (5% to 15%)
5. Depressed fontanel
6. Decreased urinary output, increased specific gravity
D. Laboratory signs of acidosis:
1. Loss of bicarbonate (serum pH <7.35)
2. Loss of sodium and potassium through stools
3. Elevated hematocrit (Hct)
4. Elevated blood urea nitrogen (BUN)
E. Signs of shock
1. Decreased blood pressure
2. Rapid, weak pulse
3. Mottled to gray skin color
4. Changes in mental status

Analysis (Nursing Diagnoses)

A. *Diarrhea* related to...
B. *Risk for deficient fluid volume* related to...

Nursing Plans and Interventions

A. Assess hydration status and vital signs frequently.
B. Monitor intake and output.
C. Do *not* take temperature rectally.
D. Rehydrate as prescribed with fluids and electrolytes.
E. Calculate intravenous (IV) hydration to include maintenance and replacement fluids.
F. Collect specimens to aid in diagnosis of cause.
G. Check stools for pH, glucose, and blood.
H. Administer antibiotics as prescribed.
I. Check urine for specific gravity.
J. Institute careful isolation precautions; *wash hands*.
K. Teach home care of child with diarrhea:
1. Provide child with oral rehydration solution such as Pedialyte or Lytren.
2. Child may temporarily need lactose-free diet.
3. Children should not receive antidiarrheals (e.g., Imodium A-D).
4. Do not give child grape juice, orange juice, apple juice, cola, or ginger ale. These solutions have high osmolality.

HESI Hint • Add potassium to IV fluids *only* with adequate urine output.

BURNS

Description: Tissue injuries caused by heat, electricity, chemicals, or radiation

A. Burns are the second leading cause of accidental death in children under 15 (after automobile accidents).
B. It is estimated that 75% of burns are preventable.

TABLE 5-2   Nutritional Assessment

Nutrient	Signs of Deficiency	Food Sources
• Iron	• Anemia • Pale conjunctiva • Pale skin color • Atrophy of papillae on tongue • Brittle, ridged, spoon-shaped nails • Thyroid edema	• Iron-fortified formula • Infant high-protein cereal • Infant rice cereal • Liver • Beef • Pork • Eggs
• Vitamin B_2 (riboflavin)	• Redness and fissuring of eyelid corners; burning, itching, tearing eyes; photophobia • Magenta–colored tongue, glossitis • Seborrheic dermatitis, delayed wound healing	• Prepared infant formula • Liver • Cow's milk • Cheddar cheese • Some green leafy vegetables (broccoli, green beans, spinach) • Enriched cereals
• Vitamin A (Retinol)	• Dry, rough skin • Dull cornea; soft cornea; Bitot spots • Night blindness • Defective tooth enamel • Retarded growth; impaired bone formation • Decreased thyroxine formation	• Liver • Sweet potatoes • Carrots • Spinach • Peaches • Apricots
• Vitamin C (ascorbic acid)	• Scurvy • Receding gums that are spongy and prone to bleeding • Dry, rough skin; petechiae • Decreased wound healing • Increased susceptibility to infection • Irritability, anorexia, apprehension	• Strawberries • Oranges and orange juice • Tomatoes • Broccoli • Cabbage • Cauliflower • Spinach
• Vitamin B_6 (pyridoxine)	• Scaly dermatitis • Weight loss • Anemia • Irritability • Convulsions • Peripheral neuritis	• Meats, especially liver • Cereals (wheat and corn) • Yeast • Soybeans • Peanuts • Tuna • Chicken • Bananas

HESI Hint •
• Teach proper cooking and storage methods to preserve potency (i.e., cook vegetables in small amounts of liquid).
• Store milk in opaque container.

C. Children under age 2 have a higher mortality rate due to:
  1. Greater central body surface area. In a child under 2, a greater part of their body surface area is concentrated in the head and trunk compared to an older child or an adult; therefore the younger child is more likely to have serious effects from burns to the trunk and head (see Figure 4-10).
  2. Greater fluid volume (proportionate to body size)
  3. Less effective cardiovascular responses to fluid volume shifts

D. In childhood, a partial-thickness burn is considered a major burn if it involves more than 25% of body surface.

E. A full-thickness burn is considered major if it involves more than 10% of body surface.

F. Because of the changing proportions of the child, especially the infant, the rule of nines cannot be used to assess the percent of burn (see Figure 4-10).

G. An assessment tool such as the Lund-Browder chart, which takes into account the changing proportions of the child, should be used.

H. Fluid needs should be calculated from the time of the burn.

I. The formula for calculating fluid replacement and maintenance is based on child's body surface area and should include volume for burn losses and maintenance.

J. Adequacy of fluid replacement is determined by evaluating urinary output.

> **HESI Hint** • Urinary output for infants and children should be 1 to 2 ml/kg/hr.

K. Specific gravity should be less than 1.025.
L. See Medical Surgical Nursing, Burns, p. 176.

CHILD ABUSE

Description: Physical and mental injury, sexual abuse, and emotional and physical neglect; a national problem from which 3000 to 5000 children die each year (See Abuse in Chapter 7, Psychiatric Nursing).

POISONINGS

Description: Ingesting, inhaling, or absorbing a toxic substance

A. Poisoning, particularly by ingestion, is a common cause of childhood injury and illness.

B. Most poisonings occur in children under the age of 6, with a peak at age 2.

C. The exploratory behavior, curiosity, and oral-motor activity of early childhood place the child at risk for poisonings.

D. About 90% of poisonings occur in the home.

Nursing Assessment

A. Child found near source of poison
B. Gastrointestinal (GI) disturbance: nausea, abdominal pain, diarrhea, vomiting
C. Burns of mouth, pharynx
D. Respiratory distress
E. Seizures, changes in level of consciousness
F. Cyanosis
G. Shock

Analysis (Nursing Diagnoses)

A. *Risk for poisoning* related to…
B. *Deficient knowledge (home safety)* related to…

Nursing Plans and Interventions

A. Identify the poisonous agent quickly!
B. Assess the child's respiratory, cardiac, and neurologic status.
C. Instruct parent to bring any emesis, stool, etc., to the emergency department.
D. Determine the child's age and weight.

> **HESI Hint** • Use of syrup of ipecac is no longer recommended by the American Academy of Pediatrics. Teach parents that it is *not* recommended to induce vomiting in any way because it may cause more damage.

E. Poison removal and care may require gastric lavage, activated charcoal, or naloxone HCl (Narcan).
F. Teach home safety.
   1. Poison-proof and child proof the home.
      a. Identify location of poisons: under the sink (cleaning supplies, drain cleaners, bug poisons); medicine cabinets; storage rooms (paints, varnishes); garages (antifreeze, gasoline); poisonous plants (philodendron, dieffenbachia).
      b. Put locks on cabinets.
      c. Use safety containers: do *not* place poisonous materials in other nonsafe containers.
      d. Discard unused medications.
      e. Make sure child is always under adult supervision.
   2. Post telephone number for local poison control center next to telephone.
   3. Examine the environment from the child's viewpoint (the height to which a 2- to 5-year-old can reach).
G. Contact community health nurse or child welfare agency if necessary.

LEAD POISONING

Description: It is estimated that 2.2% of children under 6 years of age living in the United States have blood levels greater than 10 mcg/dl.

A. Children 6 years of age and younger are most vulnerable to the effects of lead.

B. Although numerous sources of lead can result in exposure in young children, the major cause of lead poisoning is deteriorating lead-based paint.

C. Lead enters the body through ingestion, inhalation, or, in the case of an unborn child, placental transfer when the mother is exposed. The most common route is ingestion either from hand-to-mouth behavior via contaminated hands, fingers, toys, or pacifiers or, less often, from eating sweet-tasting loose paint chips found in a home built before 1950s or in a play area.

D. Lead can affect any part of the body, but the renal, neurologic, and hematologic systems are the most seriously affected.

E. The blood lead level (BLL) test is currently used for screening and diagnosis.

F. Erythrocyte protoporphyrin (EP) test (a good indicator of early toxic effects of lead) remains useful as a clinical tool, along with the BLL test, to help estimate the potential body burden of lead in a child.

Nursing Assessment

A. Screen for lead poisoning using CDC guidelines of blood lead surveillance and other risk factor data collected over time to establish the status and risk of children throughout the state.

B. In areas without available data, universal screening is recommended.
1. All children should have a BLL test at the ages of 1 and 2 years.
   a. Collect blood in a capillary tube, and send to the laboratory.
   b. During collection, avoid contamination of blood specimen and lead on the skin.
2. Any child between 3 and 6 years of age who has not been screened should also be tested.

C. Obtain a history of possible sources of lead in the child's environment.

D. Physical assessment
1. General signs
   a. Anemia
   b. Acute crampy abdominal pain
   c. Vomiting
   d. Constipation
   e. Anorexia
   f. Headache
   g. Lethargy
   h. Impaired growth
2. Central nervous system (CNS) signs (early)
   a. Hyperactivity
   b. Aggression
   c. Impulsiveness
   d. Decreased interest in play
   e. Irritability
   f. Short attention span
3. CNS signs (late)
   a. Mental retardation
   b. Paralysis
   c. Blindness
   d. Convulsions
   e. Coma
   f. Death

Analysis (Nursing Diagnoses)

A. *Risk for poisoning* related to sources of lead in the environment

B. *Interrupted family processes* related to child's access to lead in the environment

C. *Risk for injury* related to ingested or inhaled lead

Nursing Plans and Interventions

A. Identify sources of lead in the environment.

B. Administer prescribed chelating agents to reduce high BLLs.
1. Ask family if child is allergic to peanuts; if so, client should not be given chelating agents such as dimercaprol (also called BAL [British anti-Lewisite]) or D-penicillamine.
2. Rotate injection sites if chelating agent is given intramuscularly.
   a. Reassure child that injections are a treatment, not a punishment.
   b. Administer the local anesthetic procaine with IM injection of $CaNa_2$ EDTA to reduce discomfort.
   c. Apply EMLA cream over puncture site 2½ hours before the injection to reduce discomfort.
3. Avoid giving iron during chelation because of possible interactive effects.
4. If home oral chelation therapy is used, teach family proper administration of medication.

C. Administer prescribed cleansing enemas or cathartic for acute lead ingestion.

D. Assist family to obtain sources of help for removing lead from the environment.
1. Do not vacuum hard-surfaced floors or windowsills or window wells in homes built before 1960, since this spreads dust.
2. Wash and dry child's hands and face frequently, especially before eating.
3. Wash toys and pacifiers frequently.
4. Make sure that home exposure is not occurring from parental occupations or hobbies.

HESI Hint • More lead is absorbed on an empty stomach. Hot water can contain higher levels of lead because it dissolves lead more quickly than cold water, so use only cold water for consumption (drinking, cooking, and especially for making infant formula).

Review of Child Health Promotion

1. List two contraindications to live virus immunization.
2. List three classic signs and symptoms of measles.
3. List the signs and symptoms of iron deficiency.
4. Identify food sources of vitamin A.
5. What disease occurs with vitamin C deficiency?
6. What measurements reflect present nutritional status?
7. List the signs and symptoms of dehydration in an infant.
8. List the laboratory findings that can be expected in a dehydrated child.
9. How should burns in children be assessed?
10. How can the nurse best evaluate the adequacy of fluid replacement in children?
11. How should a parent be instructed to childproof a house?
12. What interventions should the nurse perform *first* in caring for a child who has ingested a poison?
13. What early signs should the nurse assess for if lead poisoning is suspected?

Answers to Review

1. Immunocompromised child or a child in a household with an immunocompromised individual
2. Photophobia, confluent rash that begins on the face and spreads downward, and Koplik spots on the buccal mucosa
3. Anemia; pale conjunctiva; pale skin color; atrophy of papillae on tongue; brittle, ridged, or spoon-shaped nails; and thyroid edema
4. Liver, sweet potatoes, carrots, spinach, peaches, and apricots
5. Scurvy
6. Weight, skinfold thickness, and arm circumference
7. Poor skin turgor, absence of tears, dry mucous membranes, weight loss, depressed fontanel, and decreased urinary output
8. Loss of bicarbonate/decreased serum pH, loss of sodium (hyponatremia), loss of potassium (hypokalemia), elevated Hct, and elevated BUN
9. By using the Lund-Browder chart, which takes into account the changing proportions of the child's body
10. By monitoring urine output
11. By being taught to lock all cabinets, to safely store all toxic household items in locked cabinets, and to examine the house from the child's point of view
12. Assessment of the child's respiratory, cardiac, and neurologic status
13. Anemia, acute cramping, abdominal pain, vomiting, constipation, anorexia, headache, lethargy, hyperactivity, aggression, impulsiveness, decreased interest in play, irritability, short attention span

Respiratory Disorders

IMPORTANT SIGNS IN CHILDREN

A. Normal pulse and respiratory rates (Table 5-3)
B. Signs of respiratory distress in children
    1. Cardinal signs of respiratory distress
        a. Restlessness
        b. Increased respiratory rate
        c. Increased pulse rate
        d. Diaphoresis
    2. Other signs of respiratory distress
        a. Flaring nostrils
        b. Retractions
        c. Grunting
        d. Adventitious breath sounds (or absent breath sounds)
        e. Use of accessory muscles, head bobbing
        f. Alterations in blood gases: decreased Po_2, elevated Pco_2
        g. Cyanosis and pallor

TABLE 5-3 Normal Pulse and Respiratory Rates for Children

Age	Pulse	Respirations	Nursing Implications
Newborn	100 to 160	30 to 60	These ranges are averages only and vary with the sex, age, and condition of child. Always note whether the child is crying, febrile, or in some distress.
1 to 11 months	100 to 150	25 to 35	
1 to 3 years (toddler)	80 to 130	20 to 30	
3 to 5 years (preschooler)	80 to 120	20 to 25	
6 to 10 years (school age)	70 to 110	18 to 22	
10 to 16 years (adolescent)	60 to 90	16 to 20	

C. Nursing implications
  1. A pediatric client often goes into respiratory failure before cardiac failure.
  2. The nurse should know the signs of respiratory distress.

ASTHMA

Description: Inflammatory reactive airway disease that is commonly chronic

A. The airways become edematous.
B. The airways become congested with mucus.
C. The smooth muscles of the bronchi and bronchioles constrict.
D. Air trapping occurs in the alveoli.

Nursing Assessment

A. History of asthma in the family
B. History of allergies
C. Home environment containing pets or other allergens
D. Tight cough (nonproductive cough)
E. Breath sounds: coarse expiratory wheezing; rales; crackles
F. Chest diameter enlarges (late sign and symptom)
G. Increased number of school days missed during past 6 months
H. Signs of respiratory distress (see Important Signs in Children)

Analysis (Nursing Diagnoses)

A. *Impaired gas exchange* related to…
B. *Ineffective breathing pattern* related to…

Nursing Plans and Interventions

A. Monitor carefully for increasing respiratory distress.
B. Administer rapid-acting bronchodilators and steroids for acute attacks.
C. Maintain hydration (oral fluids or IV).

D. Monitor blood gas values for signs of respiratory acidosis (see Advanced Clinical Concepts, Fluid, and Electrolyte Balance, p. 38).
E. Administer oxygen or nebulizer therapy as prescribed.
F. Monitor pulse oximetry as prescribed (usually >95% is normal).
G. Monitor theophylline levels (10 to 20 mcg/ml is desired level). Beta-adrenergic agonists (second-generation sympathomimetic agents, such as albuterol, cromolyn sodium [Intal], levalbuteral [Xopenex], and budesonide [Pulmicort]) are the most commonly used medications (Table 5-4; and see Table 4-4).
H. Administer cromolyn sodium prophylactically to prevent inflammatory response.
I. Teach home care program, including
  1. Identifying precipitating factors
  2. Reducing allergens in the home
  3. Using metered-dose inhaler
  4. Monitoring peak expiratory flow rate at home
  5. Doing breathing exercises
  6. Monitoring drug actions, dosages, and side effects
  7. Managing acute episode and when to seek emergency care
J. Refer child and family for emotional and psychological counseling

CYSTIC FIBROSIS

Description: Autosomal-recessive disease that causes dysfunction of the exocrine glands

A. Tenacious mucus production obstructs vital structures.
B. Multiple problems result from the exocrine dysfunction
  1. Lung insufficiency (most critical problem)
  2. Pancreatic insufficiency
  3. Increased loss of sodium and chloride in sweat

TABLE 5-4 Adrenergics

Drugs/Route	Indications	Adverse Reactions	Nursing Implications
• Epinephrine HCl (Sus-Phrine)/INH, SUBCUT, IM, IV	• Rapid-acting bronchodilator • Drug of choice for acute asthma attack	• Tachycardia • Hypertension • Tremors • Nausea	• Give subcutaneously, intravenously, via nebulizer • May be repeated in 20 minutes
• Theophylline (Theo-Dur)/PO, IV	• Bronchodilator, used in asthma to reverse bronchospasm	• Tachycardia • Irritability • Palpitations • Hypotension • Nausea, vomiting	• Auscultate lungs before and after administration • Monitor blood levels

HESI Hint • When calculating a pediatric dosage, the nurse must often change the child's weight from pounds to kilograms.

2.2 lb = 1 kg (divide pounds by 2.2).

a. If the child's weight is in pounds, convert the pounds directly to kilograms.

b. If the child's weight is in pounds and ounces, convert the ounces to the nearest tenth of a pound and add this to the total pounds. Then convert the total pounds to kilograms to the nearest tenth.

HESI Hint • Weight expressed in kilograms should always be a smaller number than the weight expressed in pounds.

Nursing Assessment

A. Usually found in a white infant or child

B. Meconium ileus at birth (10% to 20% of cases)

C. Recurrent respiratory infection

D. Pulmonary congestion

E. Steatorrhea (excessive fat, greasy stools)

F. Foul-smelling bulky stools

G. Delayed growth and poor weight gain

H. Skin that tastes salty when kissed (caused by excessive secretions from sweat glands)

I. Later: cyanosis, nail-bed clubbing, congestive heart failure (CHF)

Analysis (Nursing Diagnoses)

A. *Ineffective airway clearance* related to…

B. *Imbalanced nutrition: less than body requirements* related to…

Nursing Plans and Interventions

A. Monitor respiratory status.

B. Assess for signs of respiratory infection.

C. Administer IV antibiotics as prescribed; manage vascular access.

D. Administer pancreatic enzymes (Cotazym-S, Pancrease: for infants, with applesauce, rice, or cereal; for an older child, with food).

E. Administer fat-soluble vitamins (A, D, E, K) in water-soluble form.

F. Administer oxygen (Box 5-1) and nebulizer treatments (recombinant human deoxyribonuclease [DNase] or dornase alfa [Pulmozyme]) as prescribed.

BOX 5-1 *Respiratory Client*

Administration of Oxygen

• Oxygen hood: Used for infants.

• Nasal prongs: Provide low to moderate concentrations of oxygen.

• Tents: Provide mist and oxygen. Monitor child's temperature. Keep edges tucked in. Keep child dry.

Measurement of Oxygenation

• Pulse oximetry measures oxygen saturation (SaO_2) of arterial hemoglobin noninvasively via a sensor that is usually attached to the finger or toe or, in an infant, to sole of foot.

• Nurse should be aware of the alarm parameters signaling decreased SaO_2 (usually <95%).

• Blood gas evaluation is usually monitored in respiratory clients through arterial sampling.

• Norms: Po_2: 80 to 100 mm Hg; Pco_2: 35 to 45 mm Hg for children (not infants and newborns).

G. Evaluate effectiveness of respiratory treatments.

H. Teach family percussion and postural-drainage techniques.

I. Teach dietary recommendations: high in calories, high in protein, moderate to high in fat (more calories per volume), and moderate to low in carbohydrates (to avoid an increase in CO_2 drive).

> **HESI Hint** • A child needs 150% of the usual calorie intake for normal growth and development.

J. Provide age-appropriate activities.

K. Refer family for genetic counseling.

EPIGLOTTITIS

Description: Severe life-threatening infection of the epiglottis

A. Epiglottitis progresses rapidly, causing acute airway obstruction.

B. The organism usually responsible for epiglottitis is *Haemophilus influenzae* (*H. influenzae*, primarily type B).

Nursing Assessment

A. Sudden onset

B. Restlessness

C. High fever

D. Sore throat, dysphagia

E. Drooling

F. Muffled voice

G. Child assuming upright sitting position with chin out and tongue protruding ("tripod position")

Analysis (Nursing Diagnoses)

A. *Ineffective breathing pattern* related to…

B. *Anxiety* related to…

Nursing Plans and Interventions

A. Encourage prevention with Hib vaccine (see Figure 5-2).

B. Maintain child in upright sitting position.

C. Prepare for intubation or tracheostomy.

D. Administer IV antibiotics as prescribed.

E. Prepare for hospitalization in ICU.

F. Restrain as needed to prevent extubation.

G. Employ measures to decrease agitation and crying.

> **HESI Hint** • Do not examine the throat of a child with epiglottitis (i.e., do not put a tongue blade or any object into the throat) because of the risk of obstructing the airway completely.

BRONCHIOLITIS

Description: Viral infection of the bronchioles that is characterized by thick secretions

A. Bronchiolitis is usually caused by respiratory syncytial virus (RSV) and is found to be readily transmitted by close contact with hospital personnel, families, and other children.

B. Bronchiolitis occurs primarily in young infants.

Nursing Assessment

A. History of upper respiratory symptoms

B. Irritable, distressed infant

C. Paroxysmal coughing

D. Poor eating

E. Nasal congestion

F. Nasal flaring

G. Prolonged expiratory phase of respiration

H. Wheezing, rales can be auscultated

I. Deteriorating condition that is often indicated by shallow, rapid respirations

Analysis (Nursing Diagnoses)

A. *Impaired gas exchange* related to…

B. *Ineffective airway clearance* related to…

Nursing Plans and Interventions

A. Isolate child (isolation of choice for RSV is contact isolation).

B. Assign nurses to clients with RSV who have no responsibility for any other children (to prevent transmission of the virus).

C. Monitor respiratory status; observe for hypoxia.

D. Clear airway of secretions using a bulb syringe for suctioning.

E. Provide care in mist tent; administer oxygen as prescribed.

F. Maintain hydration (oral and IV fluids).

G. Monitor antiviral agent, ribavirin aerosol, if prescribed.

H. Evaluate response to respiratory therapy treatments.

I. Administer palivizumab (Synagis) to provide passive immunity against RSV in high-risk children (less than 2 years of age with a history of prematurity, lung disease, or congenital heart disease).

> **HESI Hint** • In planning and providing nursing care, a patent airway is always the priority of care, regardless of age!

OTITIS MEDIA

Description: Inflammatory disorder of the middle ear

A. Otitis media may be suppurative or serous.
B. Anatomic structure of the ear predisposes young child to ear infections.
C. There is a risk for conductive hearing loss if untreated or incompletely treated.

Nursing Assessment

A. Fever, pain; infant may pull at ear
B. Enlarged lymph nodes
C. Discharge from ear (if drum is ruptured)
D. Upper respiratory symptoms
E. Vomiting, diarrhea

Analysis (Nursing Diagnoses)

A. *Risk for infection* related to…
B. *Acute pain* related to…

Nursing Plans and Interventions

A. Administer antibiotics if prescribed.
B. Reduce body temperature (can be very high, with risk for seizures).
   1. Tepid baths
   2. Acetaminophen (Tylenol) if prescribed
C. Position child on affected side.
D. Provide comfort measure: warm compress on affected ear.
E. Teach home care.
   1. Teach to finish all prescribed antibiotics.
   2. Encourage follow-up visit.
   3. Monitor for hearing loss.
   4. Teach preventive care (smoking and bottle feeding when child is in supine position are predisposing factors).

> **HESI Hint** • Respiratory disorders are the primary reason most children and their families seek medical care. Therefore, these disorders are frequently tested on the NCLEX-RN. Knowing the normal parameters of respiratory rates and the key signs of respiratory distress in children is essential!

TONSILLITIS

Description: Inflammation of the tonsils

A. Tonsillitis may be viral or bacterial.
B. Tonsillitis may be related to infection by a *Streptococcus* species.
C. If related to strep, treatment is *very important* because of the risk for developing acute glomerulonephritis or rheumatic heart disease.

Nursing Assessment

A. Sore throat
B. Fever
C. Enlarged tonsils (may have purulent discharge on tonsils)
D. Breathing may be obstructed (tonsils touching, called "kissing tonsils")
E. Throat culture to determine viral or bacterial cause

> **HESI Hint** • The nurse should be sure PT and PTT have been determined prior to a tonsillectomy. More important, the nurse should ask whether there has been a history of bleeding, prolonged or excessive, and whether there is a history of any bleeding disorders in the family.

Analysis (Nursing Diagnoses)

A. *Impaired swallowing* related to…
B. *Risk for injury* related to…

Nursing Plans and Interventions

A. Collect throat culture if prescribed.
B. Instruct parents in home care.
   1. Encourage warm saline gargles.
   2. Provide ice chips.
   3. Administer antibiotics if prescribed.
   4. Manage fever with acetaminophen.
C. Provide surgical care if indicated.
   1. Provide preoperative teaching and assessment.
   2. Monitor for signs of postoperative bleeding.
      a. Frequent swallowing
      b. Vomiting fresh blood
      c. Clearing throat
   3. Encourage soft foods and oral fluids (avoid red fluids, which mimic signs of bleeding); do not use straws.
   4. Provide comfort measures: ice collar helps with pain and with vasoconstriction.
   5. Teach that the highest risk for hemorrhage is during the first 24 hours and 5 to 10 days *after* surgery.

Review of Respiratory Disorders

1. Describe the purpose of bronchodilators.
2. What are the physical assessment findings for a child with asthma?
3. What nutritional support should be provided for a child with cystic fibrosis?
4. Why is genetic counseling important for the family of a child with cystic fibrosis?
5. List seven signs of respiratory distress in a pediatric client.
6. Describe the care of a child in a mist tent.

7. What position does a child with epiglottitis assume?
8. Why are IV fluids important for a child with an increased respiratory rate?
9. Children with chronic otitis media are at risk for developing what problem?
10. What is the most common postoperative complication following a tonsillectomy? Describe the signs and symptoms of this complication.

Answers to Review

1. To reverse bronchospasm
2. Expiratory wheezing, rales, tight cough, and signs of altered blood gases
3. Pancreatic enzyme replacement, fat-soluble vitamins, and a moderate- to low-carbohydrate, high-protein, moderate- to high-fat diet
4. Because the disease is autosomal recessive in its genetic pattern
5. Restlessness, tachycardia, tachypnea, diaphoresis, flaring nostrils, retractions, and grunting

6. Monitor child's temperature; keep tent edges tucked in; keep clothing dry; assess respiratory status; look at child inside tent.
7. Upright sitting, with chin out and tongue protruding ("tripod position")
8. The child is at risk for dehydration and acid-base imbalance.
9. Hearing loss
10. Hemorrhage; frequent swallowing, vomiting fresh blood, and clearing throat.

Cardiovascular Disorders

CONGENITAL HEART DISORDERS

Description: Heart anomalies that develop in utero and manifest at birth or shortly thereafter

A. Congenital heart disorders occur in 4 to 10 children per 1000 live births.
B. They may be categorized as:
   1. Acyanotic (ventricular septal defect [VSD], atrial septal defect [ASD], patent ductus arteriosus [PDA], coarctation of aorta, aortic stenosis [AS])
      a. Left-to-right shunts or increased pulmonary blood flow
      b. Obstructive defects
   2. Cyanotic (tetralogy of Fallot, truncus arteriosus [TA], transposition of the great vessels [TGV])
      a. Right-to-left shunts or decreased pulmonary blood flow
      b. Mixed blood flow
C. Hemodynamic classification may be used.
   1. Increased pulmonary blood flow defects (ASD, VSD, PDA)
   2. Obstructive defects (coarctation of aorta, AS)
   3. Decreased pulmonary blood flow defects (tetralogy of Fallot)
   4. Mixed defects (TGV, TA)

ACYANOTIC HEART DEFECTS

Ventricular Septal Defect (VSD; Increased Pulmonary Blood Flow)

A. There is a hole between the ventricles.
B. Oxygenated blood from left ventricle is shunted to right ventricle and recirculated to the lungs.
C. Small defects may close spontaneously.
D. Large defects cause Eisenmenger syndrome or congestive heart failure and require surgical closures (Fig. 5-3).

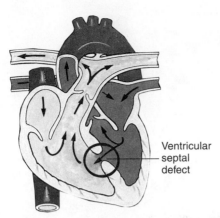

FIGURE 5-3   Ventricular septal defect. (From Hockenberry MJ, Wilson D: *Wong's nursing care of infants and children*, ed 8. St. Louis, 2007, Mosby.)

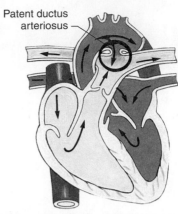

FIGURE 5-5   Patent ductus arteriosus. (From Hockenberry MJ, Wilson D: *Wong's nursing care of infants and children*, ed 8. St. Louis, 2007, Mosby.)

Atrial Septal Defect (ASD; Increased Pulmonary Blood Flow)

A. There is a hole between the atria.

B. Oxygenated blood from the left atrium is shunted to the right atrium and lungs.

C. Most defects do not compromise children seriously.

D. Surgical closure is recommended before school age. It can lead to significant problems, such as congestive heart failure or atrial dysrhythmias later in life if not corrected (Fig. 5-4).

Patent Ductus Arteriosus (PDA; Increased Pulmonary Blood Flow)

A. There is an abnormal opening between the aorta and the pulmonary artery.

B. It usually closes within 72 hours after birth.

C. If it remains patent, oxygenated blood from the aorta returns to the pulmonary artery.

D. Increased blood flow to the lungs causes pulmonary hypertension.

E. It may require medical intervention with indomethacin (Indocin) administration or surgical closure (Fig. 5-5).

Coarctation of the Aorta (Obstruction of Blood Flow from Ventricles)

A. There is an obstructive narrowing of the aorta.

B. The most common sites are the aortic valve and the aorta near the ductus arteriosus.

C. A common finding is hypertension in the upper extremities and decreased or absent pulses in the lower extremities.

D. It may require surgical correction (Fig. 5-6).

Aortic Stenosis (AS; Obstruction of Blood Flow from Ventricles)

A. It is an obstructive narrowing immediately before, at, or after the aortic valve. (It is most commonly valvular.)

B. Oxygenated blood flow from the left ventricle into systemic circulation is diminished.

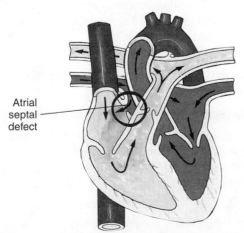

FIGURE 5-4   Atrial septal defect. (From Hockenberry MJ, Wilson D: *Wong's nursing care of infants and children*, ed 8. St. Louis, 2007, Mosby.)

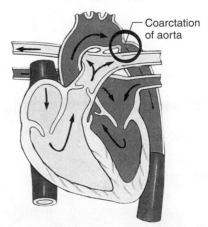

FIGURE 5-6   Coarctation of the aorta. (From Hockenberry MJ, Wilson D: *Wong's nursing care of infants and children*, ed 8. St. Louis, 2007, Mosby.)

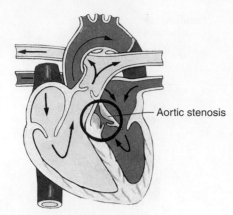

FIGURE 5-7 Aortic stenosis. (From Hockenberry MJ, Wilson D: *Wong's nursing care of infants and children*, ed 8. St. Louis, 2007, Mosby.)

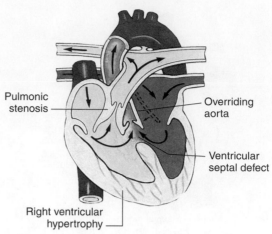

FIGURE 5-8 Tetralogy of Fallot. (From Hockenberry MJ, Wilson D: *Wong's nursing care of infants and children*, ed 8. St. Louis, 2007, Mosby.)

C. Symptoms are caused by low cardiac output.

D. It may require surgical correction (Fig. 5-7).

TRADITIONAL THREE T'S OF CYANOTIC HEART DISEASE

A. Tetralogy of Fallot is a combination of four defects:
 1. VSD
 2. Aorta placed over and above the VSD (overriding aorta)
 3. Pulmonary stenosis (PS) that obstructs right ventricular outflow
 4. Right ventricular hypertrophy (The severity of the pulmonary stenosis is related to the degree of right ventricular hypertrophy and the extent of shunting.)

B. TA, in which one artery (truncus), rather than two arteries (aorta and pulmonary artery), arises from both ventricles

C. TGA, in which the pulmonary artery leaves the left ventricle, and the aorta exits from the right ventricle

Tetralogy of Fallot (Decreased Pulmonary Blood Flow)

A. Tetralogy of Fallot consists of four defects:
 1. PS
 2. VSD
 3. Overriding aorta
 4. Right ventricular hypertrophy

B. Cyanosis occurs because unoxygenated blood is pumped into the systemic circulation.

C. Decreased pulmonary circulation occurs because of the PS.

D. The child experiences "tet" spells, or hypoxic episodes; they are relieved by the child's squatting or being placed in the knee-chest position.

E. Tetralogy of Fallot requires staged surgery for correction (Fig. 5-8).

> **HESI Hint** • Polycythemia is common in children with cyanotic defects.

Truncus Arteriosus

A. Pulmonary artery and aorta do not separate.

B. One main vessel receives blood from the left and right ventricles together.

C. Blood mixes in right and left ventricles through a large VSD, resulting in cyanosis.

D. Increased pulmonary resistance results in increased cyanosis.

E. This congenital defect requires surgical correction; only the presence of the large VSD allows for survival at birth (Fig. 5-9).

Transposition of the Great Vessels (Mixed Blood Flow)

A. The great vessels are reversed.

B. The pulmonary circulation arises from the left ventricle, and the systemic circulation arises from the right ventricle.

C. This is incompatible with life unless coexisting VSD, ASD, and/or PDA is present.

D. The diagnosis is a *medical emergency*. The child is given prostaglandin E (PGE) to keep the ductus open (Fig. 5-10).

3. Blood pressure (upper and lower extremities)
4. History of maternal infection during pregnancy

Analysis (Nursing Diagnoses)

A. *Decreased cardiac output* related to…

B. *Activity intolerance* related to…

C. *Delayed growth and development* related to…

Nursing Plans and Interventions

A. Provide care for the child with cardiovascular dysfunction.
   1. Maintain nutritional status; feed small, frequent feedings; provide high-calorie formula.

> **HESI Hint** • Infants may require tube feeding to conserve energy. Infants being tube fed need to continue to satisfy sucking needs.

   2. Maintain hydration (polycythemia increases risk for thrombus formation).
   3. Maintain neutral thermal environment.
   4. Plan frequent rest periods.
   5. Organize activities so as to disturb child only as indicated.
   6. Administer digoxin and diuretics as prescribed.
   7. Monitor for signs of deteriorating condition or CHF.
   8. Teach family the need for prophylactic antibiotics prior to any dental or invasive procedures due to risk for endocarditis.
B. Assist with diagnostic tests, and support family during diagnosis.
   1. ECG
   2. Echocardiography
C. Prepare family and child for cardiac catheterization (conducted when surgery is probable or as an intervention for certain procedures).
   1. Risks of catheterization are similar to those for a child undergoing cardiac surgery:
      a. Arrhythmias
      b. Bleeding
      c. Perforation
      d. Phlebitis
      e. Arterial obstruction at the entry site
   2. Child requires reassurance and close monitoring postcatheterization:
      a. Vital signs
      b. Pulses
      c. Incision site
      d. Cardiac rhythm
   3. Prepare family and child (as able) for surgical intervention if necessary.

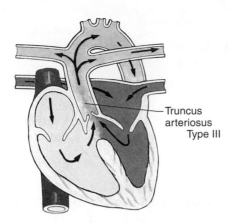

FIGURE 5-9 Truncus arteriosus. (From Hockenberry MJ, Wilson D: *Wong's nursing care of infants and children*, ed 8. St. Louis, 2007, Mosby.)

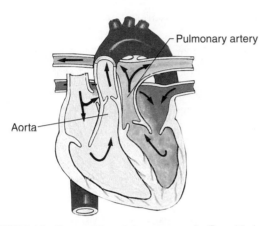

FIGURE 5-10 Transposition of the great vessels. (From Hockenberry MJ, Wilson D: *Wong's nursing care of infants and children*, ed 8. St. Louis, 2007, Mosby.)

CARE OF CHILDREN WITH CONGENITAL HEART DISEASE (CHD)

Nursing Assessment

A. Manifestations of CHD
   1. Murmur (present or absent; thrill or rub)
   2. Cyanosis, clubbing of digits (usually after age 2)
   3. Poor feeding, poor weight gain, failure to thrive (FTT)
   4. Frequent regurgitation
   5. Frequent respiratory infections
   6. Activity intolerance, fatigue
B. The following are assessed:
   1. Heart rate and rhythm and heart sounds
   2. Pulses (quality and symmetry)

> **HESI Hint** • For normal cardiac rates in children, see Respiratory Disorders, Table 5-3, in this chapter. The heart rate of a child increases with crying or fever.

D. Prepare child as appropriate for age.
  1. Show to ICU.
  2. Explain chest tubes, IV lines, monitors, dressings, and ventilator.
  3. Show family and child waiting area for families.
  4. Use a doll or a drawing for explanations.
  5. Provide emotional support.

> **HESI Hint** • Basic differences between cyanotic and acyanotic defects:
> - Acyanotic: Has abnormal circulation; however, all blood entering the systemic circulation is oxygenated.
> - Cyanotic: Has abnormal circulation with unoxygenated blood entering the systemic circulation
>
> **CHF** • Congestive heart failure is more often associated with acyanotic defects

CONGESTIVE HEART FAILURE (CHF)

Description: Condition in which the heart is unable to pump effectively the volume of blood that is presented to it

> **HESI Hint** • CHF is a common complication of congenital heart disease. It reflects the increased workload of the heart caused by shunts or obstructions. The two objectives in treating CHF are to reduce the workload of the heart and increase cardiac output.

Nursing Assessment

A. Tachypnea, shortness of breath
B. Tachycardia
C. Difficulty feeding
D. Cyanosis
E. Grunting, wheezing, pulmonary congestion
F. Edema (face, eyes of infants), weight gain
G. Diaphoresis (especially head)
H. Hepatomegaly

Analysis (Nursing Diagnoses)

A. *Decreased cardiac output* related to…
B. *Impaired gas exchange* related to…

Nursing Plans and Interventions

A. Monitor vital signs frequently, and report signs of increasing distress.
B. Assess respiratory functioning frequently.
C. Elevate head of bed, or use infant seat.
D. Administer oxygen therapy as prescribed.
E. Administer digoxin and diuretics as prescribed (Box 5-2).
F. Weigh frequently (may be every shift for infants).
G. Maintain strict input and output (I&O); weigh diapers (1 g = 1 ml).
H. Report any unusual weight gains.
I. Provide low-sodium diet or formula.
J. Gavage-feed infants if unable to get adequate nutrition by mouth.
K. Continue care for infant or child with a congenital defect as indicated.
L. See Nursing Plans and Interventions, Cyanotic Heart Defects, p. 202.

BOX 5-2 *Managing Digoxin*	
Administration	**Toxicity**
• Prior to administering digoxin, nurse *must* take child's apical pulse for 1 minute to assess for bradycardia. Hold dose if pulse is below normal heart rate for child's age.	• Nurse must be acutely aware of the signs of digoxin toxicity. A small child or infant cannot describe feeling bad or nauseated.
• Therapeutic blood levels of digoxin are 0.8 to 2.0 ng/ml (nanograms per milliliter).	• Vomiting is a common early sign of toxicity. This symptom is often overlooked because infants commonly "spit up."
• Families should be taught safe home administration of digoxin:	• Other GI symptoms include anorexia, diarrhea, and abdominal pain.
→ Administer on a regular basis; do *not* skip or make up for missed doses.	• Neurologic signs include fatigue, muscle weakness, and drowsiness.
→ Give 1 hour before or 2 hours after meals. Do *not* mix with formula or food.	• Hypokalemia can increase digoxin toxicity.
→ Take child's pulse prior to administration, and know when to call the caregiver.	
→ Keep in safe place (e.g., a locked cabinet).	

TABLE 5-5 Antiinfective

Drug/Route	Indications	Adverse Reactions	Nursing Implications
• Penicillin G (Bicillin) IM	• Prophylaxis for recurrence of rheumatic fever	• Allergic reactions ranging from rashes to anaphylactic shock and death	• Penicillin G is released very slowly over several weeks, giving sustained levels of concentration • Have emergency equipment available wherever medication is administered • *Always* determine existence of allergies to penicillin and cephalosporins; check chart and record and inquire of client and family

> **HESI Hint** • When frequent weighings are required, weigh client on the same scale at the same time of day so that accurate comparisons can be made.

RHEUMATIC FEVER

Description: Inflammatory disease

A. Rheumatic fever is the most common cause of *acquired* heart disease in children. It usually affects the aortic and mitral valves of the heart.

B. Rheumatic fever is associated with an antecedent beta-hemolytic streptococcal infection.

C. Rheumatic fever is a collagen disease that injures the heart, blood vessels, joints, and subcutaneous tissue.

Nursing Assessment

A. Chest pain, shortness of breath (carditis)

B. Tachycardia, even during sleep

C. Migratory large-joint pain

D. Chorea (irregular involuntary movements)

E. Rash (erythema marginatum)

F. Subcutaneous nodules over bony prominences

G. Fever

H. Lab findings:

1. Elevated erythrocyte sedimentation rate (ESR)
2. Elevated ASO (antistreptolysin O) titer

Analysis (Nursing Diagnoses)

A. *Decreased cardiac output* related to…

B. *Risk for injury* related to…

Nursing Plans and Interventions

A. Monitor vital signs.

B. Assess for increasing signs of cardiac distress.

C. Encourage bed rest (as needed during febrile illness).

D. Assist with ambulation.

E. Reassure child and family that chorea is temporary.

F. Administer prescribed medications.
1. Penicillin or erythromycin
2. Aspirin for antiinflammatory and anticoagulant actions

G. Teach home care program.
1. Explain the necessity for prophylactics.
   a. Antibiotics taken either orally or IM; oral penicillin BID
   b. IM penicillin G each month (Table 5-5)
2. Inform dentist and other health care providers of diagnosis so they can evaluate the necessity for prophylactic antibiotics.

Review of Cardiovascular Disorders

1. Differentiate between a right-to-left and a left-to-right shunt in cardiac disease.

2. List the four defects associated with tetralogy of Fallot.

3. List the common signs of cardiac problems in an infant.

4. What are the two objectives in treating congestive heart failure?

5. Describe nursing interventions to reduce the workload of the heart.

6. What position would best relieve the child experiencing a tet spell?

7. What are common signs of digoxin toxicity?

8. List five risks in cardiac catheterization.

9. What cardiac complications are associated with rheumatic fever?

10. What medications are used to treat rheumatic fever?

Answers to Review

1. A right-to-left shunt bypasses the lungs and delivers unoxygenated blood to the systemic circulation, causing cyanosis. A left-to-right shunt moves oxygenated blood back through the pulmonary circulation.
2. VSD, overriding aorta, pulmonary stenosis, and right ventricular hypertrophy
3. Poor feeding, poor weight gain, respiratory distress and infections, edema, and cyanosis
4. Reduce the workload of the heart, and increase cardiac output.
5. Give small, frequent feedings or gavage feedings. Plan frequent rest periods. Maintain a neutral thermal environment. Organize activities to disturb child only as indicated.
6. Knee-chest position or squatting
7. Diarrhea, fatigue, weakness, nausea, and vomiting; the nurse should check for bradycardia prior to administration.
8. Arrhythmia, bleeding, perforation, phlebitis, and obstruction of the arterial entry site
9. Aortic valve stenosis and mitral valve stenosis
10. Penicillin, erythromycin, and aspirin

Neuromuscular Disorders

DOWN SYNDROME

Description: Most common chromosomal abnormality in children

A. Down syndrome is evidenced by various physical characteristics and by mental retardation.

B. Down syndrome results from a trisomy of chromosome 21 and, in less than 5% of cases, a translocation of chromosome 21.

C. Down syndrome is associated with maternal age over 35.

Nursing Assessment

A. Common physical characteristics (Fig. 5-11)
   1. Flat, broad nasal bridge
   2. Inner epicanthal eye folds
   3. Upward, outward slant of eyes
   4. Protruding tongue
   5. Short neck
   6. Transverse palmar crease (simian)
   7. Hyperextensible and lax joints (hypotonia)

B. Common associated problems
   1. Cardiac defects
   2. Respiratory infections
   3. Feeding difficulties
   4. Delayed developmental skills
   5. Mental retardation
   6. Skeletal defects
   7. Altered immune function
   8. Endocrine dysfunctions

Analysis (Nursing Diagnoses)

A. *Delayed growth and development* related to…

B. *Risk for impaired parenting* related to…

Nursing Plans and Interventions

A. Assist and support parents during the diagnostic process and management of child's associated problems.

B. Assess and monitor growth and development.

C. Teach use of bulb syringe for suctioning nares.

D. Teach signs of respiratory infection.

E. Assist family with feeding problems.

F. Feed to back and side of mouth.

G. Monitor for signs of cardiac difficulty or respiratory infection.

H. Refer family to early intervention program.

I. Refer to other specialists as indicated: nutritionist, speech therapist, physical therapist, and occupational therapist.

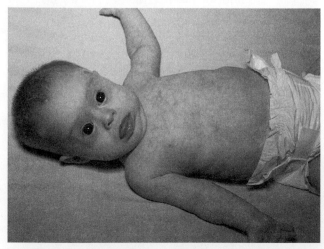

FIGURE 5-11   Down syndrome in an infant. Note small, square head with upward slant to eyes, flat nasal bridge, protruding tongue, mottled skin, and hypotonia. (From Hockenberry MJ, Wilson D: *Wong's nursing care of infants and children,* ed 8. St. Louis, 2007, Mosby.)

HESI Hint • The nursing goal in caring for a child with Down syndrome is to help the child reach his or her optimal level of functioning.

CEREBRAL PALSY (CP)

Description: Nonprogressive injury to the motor centers of the brain causing neuromuscular problems of spasticity or dyskinesia (involuntary movements)

A. Associated problems may include mental retardation and seizures.
B. Causes include
1. Anoxic injury before, during, or after birth
2. Maternal infections
3. Kernicterus
4. Low birth weight (major risk factor)

Nursing Assessment

A. Persistent neonatal reflexes (Moro, tonic neck) after 6 months
B. Delayed developmental milestones
C. Apparent early preference for one hand
D. Poor suck, tongue thrust
E. Spasticity (may be described as "difficulty with diapering" by mother or caregiver)
F. Scissoring of legs (legs are extended and crossed over each other, feet are plantarflexed; a common characteristic of spastic CP.)
G. Involuntary movements
H. Seizures

Analysis (Nursing Diagnoses)

A. *Delayed growth and development* related to…
B. *Risk for imbalanced nutrition: less than body requirements* related to…

Nursing Plans and Interventions

A. Identify CP through follow-up of high-risk infants such as premature infants.
B. Refer to community-based agencies.
C. Coordinate with physical therapist, occupational therapist, speech therapist, nutritionist, orthopedic surgeon, and neurologist.

> **HESI Hint** • Feed infant or child with cerebral palsy using nursing interventions aimed at preventing aspiration. Position child upright, and support the lower jaw.

D. Support family through grief process at diagnosis and throughout the child's life. Caring for severely affected children is very challenging.
E. Administer anticonvulsant medications such as phenytoin (Dilantin) if prescribed (Table 5-6).

F. Administer diazepam (Valium) for muscle spasms if prescribed (Table 7-4).

ATTENTION-DEFICIT DISORDER, ATTENTION-DEFICIT/HYPERACTIVITY DISORDER

Description: It is classified under DSM-IV. However, recent studies indicate that these disorders are neurologic (see Psychiatric Nursing, p. 355).

SPINA BIFIDA

Description: Malformation of the vertebrae and spinal cord resulting in varying degrees of disability and deformity (Fig. 5-12)

A. Spina bifida occulta is a defect of vertebrae only. No sac is present, and it is usually a benign condition, although bowel and bladder problems may occur.
B. With meningocele and myelomeningocele, a sac is present at some point along the spine.
C. Meningocele contains only meninges and spinal fluid and has less neurologic involvement than a myelomeningocele.
D. Myelomeningocele is more severe than meningocele because the sac contains spinal fluid, meninges, and nerves.
E. The severity of neurologic impairment is determined by the anatomic level of the defect.
F. Every child with a history of spina bifida should be screened for latex allergies.
G. Prevention: folic acid 0.4 mg is taken daily at least 3 months prior to pregnancy. The dosage is increased to 0.6 mg/day when pregnant.

Nursing Assessment

A. Spina bifida occulta: dimple with or without hair tuft at base of spine
B. Presence of sac in myelomeningocele is usually lumbar or lumbosacral
C. Flaccid paralysis and limited or no feeling below the defect
D. Head circumference at variance with norms on growth grids
E. Associated problems
1. Hydrocephalus (90% with myelomeningocele)
2. Neurogenic bladder, poor anal sphincter tone
3. Congenital dislocated hips
4. Club feet
5. Skin problems associated with anesthesia below the defect
6. Scoliosis

TABLE 5-6 Anticonvulsants

Drugs/Routes	Indications	Adverse Reactions	Nursing Implications
• Phenobarbital (Luminal)/PO, IM, IV	• Tonic-clonic and partial seizures • Is the longest acting of common barbiturates • Usually combined with other drugs	• Drowsiness • Nystagmus • Ataxia • Paradoxic excitement	• Therapeutic levels: 15 to 40 mcg/ml • Avoid rapid IV infusion • Monitor blood pressure during IV infusion
• Phenytoin (Dilantin)/PO, IV	• Tonic-clonic and partial seizures	• Gingival hyperplasia • Dermatitis • Ataxia • Nausea, anorexia • Bone marrow depression • Nystagmus	• Therapeutic levels: 10 to 20 mcg/ml • Monitor any drug interactions • Ensure meticulous oral hygiene • Monitor CBC • Report to physician if any rash develops • For IV administration, flush IV line before and after with normal saline *only* • Do not administer with milk
• Fosphenytoin sodium (Cerebyx)/ IM, IV	• Generalized convulsive status epilepticus • Prevention and treatment of seizures during neurosurgery • Short-term parenteral replacement for phenytoin oral (Dilantin)	• Rapid IV infusion (> rate of 15 mg PE/min) can cause hypotension • Severe: ataxia, CNS toxicity, confusion, gingival hyperplasia, irritability, lupus erythematosus, nervousness, nystagmus, paradoxic excitement, Stevens-Johnson syndrome, toxic epidural necrosis	• Use for short-term parenteral use (IV infusion or IM injection) only • Should always be prescribed and dispensed in phenytoin sodium equivalents (PEs) • Prior to IV infusion, dilute in D_5W or NS to administer solution of 1.5 to 25 mg PE/ml • Infuse at IV rate of no more than 150 mg PE/min
• Valproic acid (Depakene)/ PO	• Absence seizures • Myoclonic seizures	• Hepatotoxicity, especially in children less than 2 years old • Prolonged bleeding times • GI disturbances	• Monitor liver function • Potentiates phenobarbital and Dilantin, altering blood levels • Therapeutic levels: 50 to 100 mEg/ml
• Carbamazepine (Tegretol)/PO	• Tonic-clonic, mixed seizures • Drowsiness • Ataxia	• Hepatitis • Agranulocytosis	• Monitor liver function while on therapy • Therapeutic levels: 6 to 12 mcg/ml
• Lamotrigine (Lamictal)/PO	• Partial seizures • Tonic-clonic seizures • Absence seizures	• Dizziness • Headache • Nausea • Rash	• Withhold drug if rash develops • Do not discontinue abruptly
• Clonazepam (Klonopin)/PO	• Absence seizures • Myoclonic seizures	• Drowsiness • Hyperactivity • Agitation • Increased salivation	• Therapeutic levels: 20 to 80 mcg/ml • Do not abruptly discontinue drug • Monitor liver function, CBC, and renal function periodically

Nursing Plans and Interventions

A. Preoperative: place infant in prone position.
   1. Keep sac free of stool and urine.
   2. Cover sac with moist sterile dressing.
   3. Elevate foot of bed, and position child on his or her abdomen, with legs abducted.
   4. Measure head circumference at least every 8 hours or every shift; check fontanel.
   5. Assess neurologic function.
   6. Monitor for signs of infection.
   7. Empty bladder using Credé method, or catheterize if needed.
   8. Promote parent-infant bonding.

B. Postoperative: place infant in prone position.
   1. Make same assessments as preoperatively.
   2. Assess incision for drainage and infection.
   3. Assess neurologic function.

C. Long-term care
   1. Teach family catheterization program when child is young.
   2. Help older children to learn self-catheterization.
   3. Administer Pro-Banthine or urecholine as prescribed to improve continence.
   4. Develop bowel program.
      a. High-fiber diet
      b. Increased fluids
      c. Regular fluids
      d. Suppositories as needed
   5. Assess skin condition frequently.
   6. Assist with range-of-motion (ROM) exercises, ambulation, and bracing, if client is able.
   7. Coordinate with team members: neurologist, orthopedist, urologist, physical therapist, and nutritionist.

D. Support independent functioning of child.

E. Assist family to make realistic developmental expectations of child.

HYDROCEPHALUS

Description: Condition characterized by an abnormal accumulation of cerebrospinal fluid (CSF) within the ventricles of the brain

A. It is usually caused by an obstruction in the flow of CSF between the ventricles.

B. Hydrocephalus is most often associated with spina bifida; it can be a complication of meningitis.

> **HESI Hint** • The signs of increased intracranial pressure (ICP) are the opposite of those of shock:
> • Shock: increased pulse, decreased blood pressure
> • Increased ICP: decreased pulse, increased blood pressure

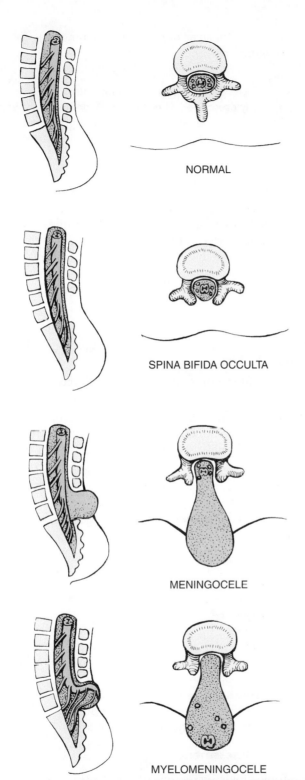

FIGURE 5-12 Midline defects of osseous spine with varying degrees of neural herniations. *A*, Normal. *B*, Spina bifida occulta. *C*, Meningocele. *D*, Myelomeningocele. (From Hockenberry MJ, *Wilson D: Wong's nursing care of infants and children*, ed 8. St. Louis, 2007, Mosby.)

NORMAL

SPINA BIFIDA OCCULTA

MENINGOCELE

MYELOMENINGOCELE

Analysis (Nursing Diagnoses)

A. *Risk for infection* related to ...

B. *Impaired urinary elimination patterns* related to ...

C. *Impaired physical mobility* related to ...

Nursing Assessment

A. Older children show classic signs of ICP
1. Change in level of consciousness (LOC)
2. Irritability
3. Vomiting
4. Headache on awakening
5. Motor dysfunction
6. Unequal pupil response
7. Seizures
8. Decline in academics
9. Change in personality

B. Signs of increased ICP in infants
1. Irritability, lethargy
2. Increasing head circumference
3. Bulging fontanels
4. Widening suture lines
5. "Sunset" eyes
6. High-pitched cry

HESI Hint • Baseline data on the child's usual behavior and level of development are essential so changes associated with increased ICP can be detected early.

Analysis (Nursing Diagnoses)

A. *Delayed growth and development* related to...
B. *Risk for injury* related to...

Nursing Plans and Interventions

A. Prepare infant and family for diagnostic procedures.
B. Monitor for signs of increased ICP.
C. Maintain seizure precautions.
D. Elevate head of bed.
E. Prepare parents for surgical procedure.
1. Shunt is inserted into ventricle.
2. Tubing is tunneled through skin to peritoneum where it drains excess CSF.
F. Postoperative care
1. Assess for signs of shunt malfunction.
a. Infant
(1) Changes in size, signs of bulging, tenseness, and separation in fontanels and suture lines.
(2) Irritability, lethargy, or seizure activity
(3) Altered vital signs and feeding behavior
b. Older child: Increase in ICP
(1) Change in LOC
(2) Complaint of headache
(3) Changes in customary behavior (sleep patterns, developmental capabilities)

2. Assess for signs of infection (meningitis).
3. Monitor I&O closely.

HESI Hint • Do not pump shunt unless specifically prescribed. The shunt is made up of delicate valves, and pumping changes the pressures within the ventricles.

G. Teach home care program.
1. Teach to watch for signs of increased ICP or infection.
2. Note that child will eventually outgrow shunt and show symptoms of difficulty.
3. Note that child will need shunt revision.
4. Provide anticipatory guidance for potential problems with growth and development.

SEIZURES

Description: Uncontrolled electrical discharges of neurons in the brain

A. Seizures are more common in children under the age of 2 years.

B. Seizures can be associated with immaturity of the CNS, fever, infection, neoplasms, cerebral anoxia, and metabolic disorders.

C. Seizures are categorized as generalized or partial.
1. Generalized seizures are:
a. Tonic-clonic (grand mal): consciousness is lost.
(1) Tonic phase: generalized stiffness of entire body
(2) Clonic phase: spasm followed by relaxation
b. Absence (petit mal): momentary loss of consciousness, posture is maintained; has minor face, eye, hand movements
c. Myoclonic: sudden, brief contractures of a muscle or group of muscles, no postictal state, may or may not be symmetrical or include loss of consciousness
2. Partial seizures arise from a specific area in the brain and cause limited symptoms. Examples are focal and psychomotor seizures.

Nursing Assessment

A. Tonic-clonic (grand mal)
1. Aura (a warning sign of impending seizure)
2. Loss of consciousness
3. Tonic phase: generalized stiffness of entire body
4. Apnea, cyanosis
5. Clonic phase: spasms followed by relaxation
6. Pupils dilated and nonreactive to light
7. Incontinence
8. Postseizure: disoriented, sleepy

B. Absence seizures (petit mal)
  1. Usually occur between 4 and 12 years of age
  2. Last 5 to 10 seconds
  3. Child appears to be inattentive, daydreaming
  4. Poor performance in school

HESI Hint • Medication noncompliance is the most common cause of increased seizure activity.

Analysis (Nursing Diagnoses)

A. *Risk for injury: trauma* related to…
B. *Noncompliance* related to…

Nursing Plans and Interventions

A. Maintain airway during seizure: turn client on side to aid ventilation.
B. Do not restrain client.
C. Protect client from injury during seizure, and support head (avoid neck flexion).
D. Document seizure, noting all data in assessment.
E. Maintain seizure precautions.
  1. Reduce environmental stimuli as much as possible.
  2. Pad side rails or crib rails.
  3. Have suction equipment and oxygen quickly accessible.
  4. Tape oral airway to the head of the bed.

HESI Hint • Do *not* use tongue blade, padded or not, during a seizure. It can cause traumatic damage to oral cavity.

F. Support during diagnostic tests: EEG, CT scan
G. Support during workup for infections such as meningitis
H. Administer anticonvulsant medications as prescribed (see Table 5-6).
  1. For tonic-clonic seizures: phenytoin (Dilantin), carbamazepine (Tegretol), phenobarbital (Luminal), and fosphenytoin (Cerebyx)
  2. For absence seizures: ethosuximide (Zarontin), valproic acid (Depakene)
I. Monitor therapeutic drug levels.
J. Teach family about drug administration: dosage, action, and side effects.

BACTERIAL MENINGITIS

Description: Bacterial inflammatory disorder of the meninges that cover the brain and spinal cord

A. Meningitis is usually caused by *Haemophilus influenzae* type B (less prevalent), *Streptococcus pneumoniae*, or *Neisseria meningitidis*.
B. The usual source of bacterial invasion is the middle ear or the nasopharynx.
C. Other sources of bacteria from wounds include fractures of the skull, lumbar punctures, and shunts.
D. Exudate covers brain, and cerebral edema occurs.
E. Lumbar puncture shows
  1. Increased WBC
  2. Decreased glucose
  3. Elevated protein
  4. Increased ICP
  5. Positive culture for meningitis

Nursing Assessment

A. Older children
  1. Classic signs of increased ICP (see Hydrocephalus, p. 209.)
  2. Fever, chills
  3. Neck stiffness, opisthotonos
  4. Photophobia
  5. Positive Kernig sign (inability to extend leg when thigh is flexed anteriorly at hip)
  6. Positive Brudzinski sign (neck flexion causing adduction and flexion movements of lower extremities)
B. Infants
  1. Absence of classic signs
  2. Ill, with generalized symptoms
  3. Poor feeding
  4. Vomiting, irritability
  5. Bulging fontanel (an important sign)
  6. Seizures

Analysis (Nursing Diagnoses)

A. *Disturbed sensory perception* (specify) related to…
B. *Risk for trauma* related to…

Nursing Plans and Interventions

A. Administer antibiotics (usually ampicillin, penicillin, or chloramphenicol) and antipyretics as prescribed.
B. Isolate for at least 24 hours.
C. Monitor vital signs and neurologic signs.
D. Keep environment quiet and darkened to prevent overstimulation.
E. Implement seizure precautions.
F. Position for comfort: head of the bed slightly elevated, with client on side if prescribed.
G. Measure head circumference daily in infants.
H. Monitor I&O closely.

I. Administer Hib vaccine to protect against *H. influenzae* infection (see Table 5-1).

> **HESI Hint** • Monitor hydration status and IV therapy carefully. With meningitis, there may be inappropriate ADH secretions causing fluid retention (cerebral edema) and dilutional hyponatremia.

REYE SYNDROME

Description: Acute, rapidly progressing encephalopathy and hepatic dysfunction

A. Causes include antecedent viral infections, such as influenza or chickenpox.

B. Occurrence is often associated with aspirin use.

C. Disease is staged according to the clinical manifestations to reflect the severity of the condition.

Nursing Assessment

A. Usually occurs in school-age children

B. Lethargy, rapidly progressing to deep coma (marked cerebral edema)

C. Vomiting

D. Elevated SGOT/AST, SGPT/ALT, lactate dehydrogenase, serum ammonia, decreased PT

E. Hypoglycemia

Analysis (Nursing Diagnoses)

A. *Excess fluid volume* related to…

B. *Ineffective breathing pattern* related to…

Nursing Plans and Interventions

A. Provide critical care early in syndrome.

B. Monitor neurologic status: frequent noninvasive assessments and invasive ICP monitoring.

C. Maintain ventilation.

D. Monitor cardiac parameters (i.e., invasive cardiac monitoring system).

E. Administer mannitol, if prescribed, to increase blood osmolality (Table 5-7).

F. Monitor I&O accurately:

G. Care for Foley catheter.

H. Provide family with emotional support.

BRAIN TUMORS

Description: Second most common cancer in children

A. Most pediatric brain tumors are infratentorial, making them difficult to excise surgically.

B. Tumors usually occur close to vital structures.

C. Gliomas are the most common childhood brain tumors.

Nursing Assessment

A. Headache

> **HESI Hint** • Headache on awakening is the most common presenting symptom of brain tumors.

B. Vomiting (usually in the morning), often without nausea

C. Loss of concentration

D. Change in behavior or personality

E. Vision problems, tilting of head

F. In infants: widening sutures, increasing frontal occipital circumference, tense fontanel

Analysis (Nursing Diagnoses)

A. *Ineffective tissue perfusion (cerebral)* related to…

B. *Risk for trauma* related to…

C. *Risk for infection (postoperative)* related to…

Nursing Plans and Interventions

A. Identify baseline neurologic functioning.

B. Support child and family during diagnostic workup and treatment.

C. If surgery is treatment of choice, provide preoperative teaching:
   1. Explain that head will be shaved.
   2. Describe ICU, dressings, IV lines, etc.
   3. Identify child's developmental level, and plan teaching accordingly.

TABLE 5-7 **Diuretic**

Drug/Route	Indications	Adverse Reactions	Nursing Implications
• Mannitol (Osmitrol)/ IV	Osmotic diuretic used to reduce: • Cerebral edema • Postoperative swelling or trauma	• Circulatory overload • Confusion • Hypokalemia • Hyponatremia	• Use in-line filter for IV administration, and avoid extravasation • Monitor I&O • Lasix may also be prescribed

D. Assess family's response to the diagnosis, and treat family appropriately.

E. After surgery, position client as prescribed by the health care provider.

> **HESI Hint** • Most postoperative clients with infratentorial tumors are prescribed to lie flat or turn to either side. A large tumor may require that the child *not* be turned to the operative side.

A. Monitor IV fluids and output carefully. Overhydration can cause cerebral edema and increased ICP.

B. Administer steroids and osmotic diuretics as prescribed (see Table 5-7).

C. Support child and family to promote optimum functioning postoperatively.

> **HESI Hint** • Suctioning, coughing, straining, and turning cause increased ICP.

MUSCULAR DYSTROPHY

Description: Inherited disease of the muscles, causing muscle atrophy and weakness

A. The most serious and most common of the dystrophies is Duchenne muscular dystrophy, an X-linked recessive disease affecting primarily males.

B. Duchenne muscular dystrophy appears in early childhood (ages 3 to 5 years). It rapidly progresses, causing respiratory or cardiac complications and death, usually by 25 years of age.

Nursing Assessment

A. Waddling gait, lordosis

B. Increasing clumsiness, muscle weakness

C. Gowers sign: difficulty rising to standing position; has to "walk" up legs, using hands

D. Pseudohypertrophy of muscles (especially noted in calves) due to fat deposits

E. Muscle degeneration, especially the thighs, and fatty infiltrates (detected by muscle biopsy); cardiac muscle also involved

F. Delayed cognitive development

G. Elevated CPK and SGOT/AST

H. Later in disease: scoliosis, respiratory difficulty, and cardiac difficulties

I. Eventual wheelchair dependency, confinement to bed

Analysis (Nursing Diagnoses)

A. *Impaired physical mobility* related to...

B. *Chronic low self-esteem* related to...

Nursing Plans and Interventions

A. Provide supportive care.

B. Provide exercises (active and passive).

C. Prevent exposure to respiratory infection.

D. Encourage a balanced diet to avoid obesity.

E. Support family's grieving process.

F. Support participation in the Muscular Dystrophy Association.

G. Coordinate with health care team: physical therapist, occupational therapist, nutritionist, neurologist, orthopedist, and geneticist.

Review of Neuromuscular Disorders

1. What are the physical features of a child with Down syndrome?
2. Describe scissoring.
3. What are two nursing priorities for a newborn with myelomeningocele?
4. List the signs and symptoms of increased ICP in older children.
5. What teaching should parents of a newly shunted child receive?
6. State the three main goals in providing nursing care for a child experiencing a seizure.
7. What are the side effects of Dilantin?
8. Describe the signs and symptoms of a child with meningitis.
9. What antibiotics are usually prescribed for bacterial meningitis?
10. How is a child usually positioned after brain tumor surgery?
11. Describe the function of an osmotic diuretic.
12. What nursing interventions increase intracranial pressure?
13. Describe the mechanism of inheritance of Duchenne muscular dystrophy.
14. What is the Gowers sign?

Answers to Review

1. Simian creases in palms, hypotonia, protruding tongue, and upward-outward slant of eyes
2. A common characteristic of spastic cerebral palsy in infants; legs are extended and crossed over each other, feet are plantarflexed
3. Prevention of infection of the sac and monitoring for hydrocephalus (measure head circumference; check fontanel; assess neurologic functioning).
4. Irritability, change in LOC, motor dysfunction, headache, vomiting, unequal pupil response, and seizures
5. Information about signs of infection and increased ICP (see Signs of Increased ICP and Meningitis, p. 209); understanding that shunt should not be pumped and that child will need revisions with growth; guidance concerning growth and development
6. Maintain patent airway, protect from injury, and observe carefully.
7. Gingival hyperplasia, dermatitis, ataxia, GI distress
8. Fever, irritability, vomiting, neck stiffness, opisthotonos, positive Kernig sign, positive Brudzinski sign; infant may not show all classic signs even though very ill
9. Ampicillin, penicillin, or chloramphenicol
10. Flat or on either side
11. Osmotic diuretics remove water from the CNS to reduce cerebral edema.
12. Suctioning and positioning, turning
13. Duchenne muscular dystrophy is inherited as an X-linked recessive trait.
14. Gowers sign is an indicator of muscular dystrophy; to stand, the child has to "walk" hands up legs.

Renal Disorders

ACUTE GLOMERULONEPHRITIS (AGN)

Description: Immune complex response to an antecedent beta-hemolytic streptococcal infection of skin or pharynx; antigen-antibody complexes become trapped in the membrane of the glomeruli, causing inflammation and decreased glomerular filtration.

Nursing Assessment

A. Recent streptococcal infection
B. Mild to moderate edema (often confined to face)
C. Irritability, lethargy
D. Hypertension
E. Dark-colored urine (hematuria)
F. Slight to moderate proteinuria
G. Elevated antistreptolysin (ASO) titer, elevated BUN and creatinine

Analysis (Nursing Diagnoses)

A. *Excess fluid volume* related to...
B. *Risk for trauma* related to...

Nursing Plans and Interventions

A. Provide supportive care.
B. Monitor vital signs (especially blood pressure) frequently.
C. Monitor I&O closely.
D. Weigh daily.
E. Provide low-sodium diet with no added salt; low potassium, if oliguric.
F. Encourage bed rest during acute phase (usually 4 to 10 days).
G. Administer antihypertensives if prescribed.
H. Monitor for seizures (hypertensive encephalopathy).
I. Monitor for signs of CHF.
J. Monitor for signs of renal failure (uncommon).

> **HESI Hint** • Decreased urinary output is the first sign of renal failure.

NEPHROTIC SYNDROME

Description: A disorder in which the basement membrane of the glomeruli becomes permeable to plasma proteins; most often idiopathic in nature

A. It usually occurs between the ages of 2 and 3 years.
B. Its course may involve exacerbations and remissions over several years.
C. Refer to Table 5-8.

Nursing Assessment

A. Edema that begins insidiously, becomes severe and generalized
B. Lethargy
C. Anorexia
D. Pallor
E. Frothy-appearing urine
F. Massive proteinuria
G. Decreased serum protein (hypoproteinemia)
H. Elevated serum lipids

TABLE 5-8 Comparison of Acute Glomerulonephritis and Nephrotic Syndrome

Variable	Acute Glomerulonephritis	Nephrotic Syndrome
Causes	Follows streptococcal infection	Usually idiopathic
Edema	Mild, usually around eyes	Severe, generalized
Blood pressure	Elevated	Normal
Urine	Dark, tea-colored (hematuria) Slight or moderate proteinuria	Dark, frothy yellow Massive proteinuria
Blood	Normal serum protein Positive ASO titer	Decreased serum protein Negative ASO titer

Analysis (Nursing Diagnoses)

A. *Excess fluid volume* related to…

B. *Imbalanced nutrition: less than body requirements* related to…

Nursing Plans and Interventions

A. Provide supportive care.

B. Monitor temperature; assess for signs of infection.

C. Protect from persons with infections.

D. Provide skin care (edematous areas are vulnerable).

E. Maintain bed rest during edematous phase.

F. Administer steroids such as prednisone and cholinergics such as bethanechol (Urecholine) as prescribed (Table 5-9).

G. Monitor I&O.

H. Measure abdominal girth daily.

I. Administer Cytoxan if prescribed (used if nonresponsive to prednisone).

J. Provide small, frequent feedings of a normal-protein, low-salt diet. Client is commonly prescribed IV albumin followed by diuretic.

K. Teach home care:
   1. Instruct to weigh child daily.
   2. Describe medication side effects.
   3. Describe signs of relapse (see Nursing Assessment, p. 214).
   4. Train to prevent infection.

URINARY TRACT INFECTION (UTI)

Description: Bacterial infection anywhere along the urinary tract (most ascend)

Nursing Assessment

A. In infants
   1. Vague symptoms
   2. Fever
   3. Irritability
   4. Poor food intake
   5. Diarrhea, vomiting, jaundice
   6. Strong-smelling urine

B. In older children
   1. Urinary frequency
   2. Hematuria
   3. Enuresis
   4. Dysuria
   5. Fever

C. *Escherichia coli* in urine cultures

Analysis (Nursing Diagnoses)

A. *Impaired urinary elimination patterns* related to…

B. *Deficient knowledge (medications)* related to…

Nursing Plans and Interventions

A. Suspect and assess for UTI in infants who are ill.

B. Assess for recurrent urinary tract infections. In infants and young boys, UTI may indicate structural abnormalities of the urinary system.

C. Collect clean voided or catheterized specimen, as prescribed (Table 5-10).

D. Administer antibiotics as prescribed.

E. Teach home program:
   1. Instruct to finish all prescribed medication.
   2. Note that follow-up specimens are needed.
   3. Teach to avoid bubble baths.
   4. Teach to increase acidic oral fluids (e.g., apple juice, cranberry juice).
   5. Instruct to void frequently.
   6. Teach to clean genital area from front to back.
   7. Note symptoms of recurrence.

TABLE 5-9 Medications Used in Renal Disorders

Drugs/Route	Indications	Adverse Reactions	Nursing Implications
• Bethanechol chloride (Urecholine)/PO, IM, IV	• Cholinergic used to treat: → Urinary retention → Neurogenic bladder → Gastric reflux	• Orthostatic hypotension • Flushing • Asthmatic reaction • GI distress	• *Do not give IV or IM (may cause circulatory collapse)* • Monitor vital signs • Preferably give on empty stomach
• Prednisone (Deltasone)/PO	• Adrenocorticosteroid used to treat: → Immunosuppression (acts as an antiinflammatory) → Edema (promotes diuresis in nephritic syndrome)	• Mood changes • Increased susceptibility to infection • Cushingoid appearance (moon face and buffalo hump) • Acne • GI distress • Thrombocytopenia • Edema • Potassium loss • *Growth failure in children*	• In children, every other day administration is best to avoid growth failure when drug is taken long term • Discontinuing this drug requires tapering dose • Avoid live virus vaccines in children receiving prednisone
• Oxybutynin (Ditropan)/PO, transdermal • Tolterodine (Detrol)/PO	• Genitourinary smooth-muscle relaxants (antispasmodics) used to treat: → Uninhibited neurogenic bladder → Reflex urogenic bladder → Both are characterized by voiding symptoms of urgency, frequency, nocturia, and incontinence	• Increased susceptibility to UTI • GI distress • Dry eyes • Dry mouth • Vision changes • Dizziness • Chest pain • Drowsiness	• Administered orally; available in extended-release forms • Do not administer with other medications that have anticholinergic effects • May exacerbate reflux esophagitis • Contraindicated in clients with untreated glaucoma or any GI narrowing (GI obstruction may occur) • Safety for use with children has not been established

TABLE 5-10 Collection of Urine Specimens

Method	Description for Children and Infants
Clean catch	• Best obtained by using a urine bag to catch the specimen. • Apply from side to side or back to front. Diaper should be applied over the bag. • Check child frequently to note urination.
Catheterization	• Sterile feeding tube is often used to catheterize small children and infants.
Sterile specimen	• In small infants it is best collected by the physician performing a bladder tap. Urine is aspirated through a needle inserted directly into the bladder. The nurse is responsible for making sure infant is appropriately hydrated and restrained during the procedure.

VESICOURETERAL REFLEX

Description: Result of valvular malfunction and backflow of urine into the ureters (and higher) from the bladder (severe cases are associated with hydronephrosis)

Nursing Assessment

A. Recurrent UTI.
B. Reflux (common with neurogenic bladder)
C. Reflux noted on voiding cystourethrogram (VCUG)

Analysis (Nursing Diagnoses)

A. *Risk for infection* related to…
B. *Risk for trauma* related to…

Nursing Plans and Interventions

A. Teach home program for prevention of UTI.
B. Teach family the importance of medication compliance, which usually leads to resolution of mild cases.
C. Provide support for children and families requiring surgery.
D. Explain the goal of ureteral reimplantation: to stop reflux and prevent kidney damage.
E. Monitor postoperative urinary drainage (may be suprapubic or urethral).
   1. Measure output from both catheters.
   2. Assess dressing and incision for drainage.
   3. Restrain child's hands as necessary.
F. Maintain hydration with IV or oral fluids.
G. Manage pain relief postoperatively
   1. Surgical pain
   2. Bladder spasms

WILMS TUMOR (NEPHROBLASTOMA)

Description: Malignant renal tumor
A. A Wilms tumor is embryonic in origin.
B. This tumor is encapsulated.
C. It occurs in preschool children.
D. With early detection, surgery, adjuvant chemotherapy, as well as radiation therapy postoperatively, the prognosis is good.

Nursing Assessment

A. A mass in the flank area, confined to midline
B. Often discovered by parents when bathing child
C. Fever
D. Pallor, lethargy
E. Elevated blood pressure (excess renin secretion)
F. Hematuria (rare)

Analysis (Nursing Diagnoses)

A. *Risk for injury: trauma* related to…
B. *Fear* related to…

Nursing Plans and Interventions

A. Support family during diagnostic period.
B. Protect child from injury; place a sign on bed stating "no abdominal palpation."
C. Prepare family and child for imminent nephrectomy.
D. Provide postoperative care.
   1. Monitor for increased blood pressure.
   2. Monitor kidney function: I&O, urine specific gravity.
   3. Provide care for abdominal surgery client.
      a. Maintain nasogastric tube.
      b. Check for bowel sounds.
   4. Support child and family during chemotherapy or radiation therapy.

HYPOSPADIAS

Description: Congenital defect of urethral meatus in males; urethra opens on ventral side of penis behind the glans

> **HESI Hint** • Surgical correction for hypospadias is usually done before preschool years to allow for the achievement of sexual identity, to avoid castration anxiety, and to facilitate toilet training.

Nursing Assessment

A. Abnormal placement of meatus
B. Altered voiding stream
C. Presence of chordee
D. Undescended testes and inguinal hernia (may occur concurrently)

Analysis (Nursing Diagnoses)

A. *Impaired urinary elimination* related to…
B. *Disturbed body image* related to…

Nursing Plans and Interventions

A. Prepare child and family for surgery (no circumcision prior to surgery).
B. Assess circulation to tip of penis postoperatively.
C. Monitor urinary drainage after urethroplasty
   1. Foley catheter
   2. Suprapubic tube
   3. Urethral stent
D. Restrain child's arms and legs as necessary.

E. Maintain hydration (IV and oral fluids).
F. Teach home care.
   1. Teach care of catheters.
   2. Teach how to empty drainage bag.

3. Teach prevention of catheter displacement or blockage.
4. Instruct to increase oral fluids.
5. Describe signs of infection.

Review of Renal Disorders

1. Compare the signs and symptoms of acute glomerulonephritis (AGN) with those of nephrosis.
2. What antecedent event occurs with AGN?
3. Compare the dietary interventions for AGN and nephrosis.
4. What is the physiologic reason for the lab finding of hypoproteinemia in nephrosis?
5. Describe safe monitoring of prednisone administration and withdrawal.
6. What interventions can be taught to prevent urinary tract infections in children?
7. Describe the pathophysiology of vesicoureteral reflux.
8. What are the priorities for a client with a Wilms tumor?
9. Explain why hypospadias correction is performed before the child reaches preschool age.

Answers to Review

1. AGN: gross hematuria, recent strep infection, hypertension, and mild edema; nephrosis: severe edema, massive proteinuria, frothy-appearing urine, anorexia
2. Beta-hemolytic streptococcal infection
3. AGN: low-sodium diet with no added salt; nephrosis: high-protein, low-salt diet
4. Hypoproteinemia occurs because the glomeruli are permeable to serum proteins.
5. Long-term prednisone should be given every other day. Signs of edema, mood changes, and GI distress should be noted and reported. The drug should be tapered, not discontinued suddenly.
6. Avoid bubble baths; void frequently; drink adequate fluids, especially acidic fluids such as apple or cranberry juice; and clean genital area from front to back.
7. A malfunction of the valves at the end of the ureters, allowing urine to reflux out of the bladder into the ureters and possibly into the kidneys.
8. Protect the child from injury to the encapsulated tumor. Prepare the family and child for surgery.
9. Preschoolers fear castration, achieving sexual identity, and acquiring independent toileting skills.

Gastrointestinal Disorders

CLEFT LIP OR PALATE

Description: Malformations of the face and oral cavity that seem to be multifactorial in hereditary origin (Fig. 5-13)
A. Cleft lip is readily apparent.
B. Cleft palate may not be identified until the infant has difficulty with feeding.
C. Initial closure of cleft lip is performed when infant weighs approximately 10 pounds and has an Hgb of 10 g/dL.
D. Closure of palate defect is usually performed at 1 year of age to minimize speech impairment.

Nursing Assessment

A. Failure of fusion of the lip, palate, or both
B. Difficulty sucking and swallowing
C. Parent reaction to facial defect

Analysis (Nursing Diagnoses)

A. *Imbalanced nutrition: less than body requirements* related to...
B. *Impaired parenting* related to...

Nursing Plans and Interventions

A. Promote family bonding and grieving during newborn period.
B. Inform family that successful corrective surgery is available.
C. In newborn period, assist with feeding.
   1. Feed in upright position.
   2. Feed slowly, with frequent bubbling.

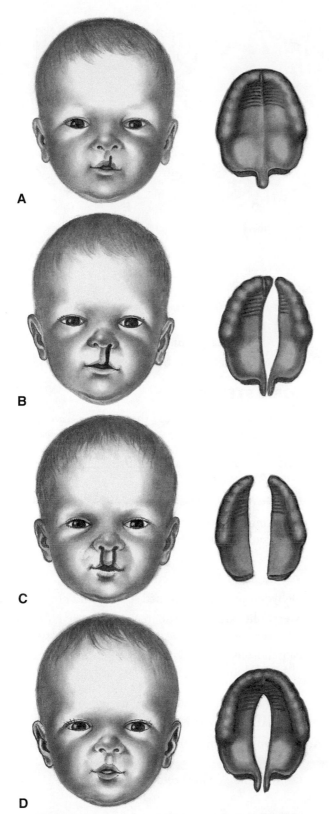

FIGURE 5-13 Variations in clefts of lip and palate at birth. *A,* Notch in vermilion border. *B,* Unilateral cleft lip and cleft palate. *C,* Bilateral cleft lip and cleft palate. *D,* Cleft palate. (From Hockenberry MJ, Wilson D: *Wong's nursing care of infants and children,* ed 8. St. Louis, 2007, Mosby.)

3. Use soft, large nipples; lamb's nipple; prosthetic palate; or rubber-tipped Asepto syringe.
4. Support mother's breast-feeding if possible.

D. Provide postoperative care:
   1. Maintain patent airway and proper positioning.
      a. Cleft lip: place client on side or upright in infant seat (not prone).
      b. Cleft palate: place client on side or abdomen.
      c. Remove oral secretions carefully with bulb syringe or Yankauer suction set.
   2. Protect surgical site.
      a. Apply elbow restraints.
      b. Minimize crying to prevent strain on lip suture line.
      c. Maintain Logan bow to lip if applied.
   3. Provide care for restrained child.
      a. Remove one restraint at a time, and perform ROM exercises.
      b. Provide age-appropriate stimulation.
   4. Resume feeding as prescribed. Cleanse suture site with sterile water after feeding; formula remaining on suture line may impede healing and lead to infection.
   5. Encourage family participation in care and feeding.
      a. Fluids are taken by a cup or an Asepto syringe with a rubber tip (gravity feeder).
      b. The diet progresses from a clear to a full liquid diet.
      c. The child may go home on a soft diet (nothing harder than mashed potatoes).

E. Usually for cleft palate: coordinate long-term care with other team members: plastic surgeon, ENT specialist, nutritionist, speech therapist, orthodontist, pediatrician, nurse.

> **HESI Hint** • Typical parent and family reactions to a child with an obvious malformation such as cleft lip or palate are guilt, disappointment, grief, sense of loss, and anger.

ESOPHAGEAL ATRESIA WITH TRACHEOESOPHAGEAL FISTULA (TEF)

Description: Congenital anomaly in which the esophagus does not fully develop (Fig. 5-14)

A. Most common: upper esophagus ends in a blind pouch, and the lower part of the esophagus is connected to the trachea.

B. This condition is a clinical and surgical *emergency.*

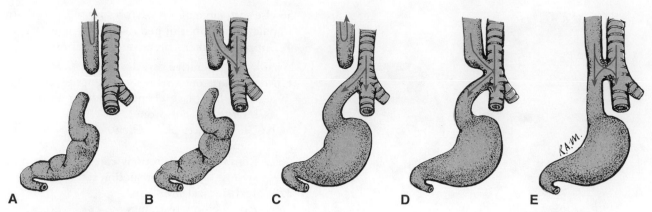

FIGURE 5-14 Five most common types of esophageal atresia and tracheoesophageal fistula. (From Hockenberry MJ, Wilson D: *Wong's nursing care of infants and children*, ed 8. St. Louis, 2007, Mosby.)

Nursing Assessment

A. Three Cs of TEF in the newborn:
1. Choking
2. Coughing
3. Cyanosis
B. Excess salivation
C. Respiratory distress
D. Aspiration pneumonia

Analysis (Nursing Diagnoses)

A. *Risk for aspiration* related to…
B. *Imbalanced nutrition: less than body requirements* related to…

Nursing Plans and Interventions

A. Provide preoperative care.
1. Monitor respiratory status.
2. Remove excess secretions (suction is usually continuous to blind pouch).
3. Elevate infant into antireflux position of 30 degrees.
4. Provide oxygen as prescribed.
5. Maintain NPO.
6. Administer IV fluids as prescribed.
B. Provide postoperative care.
1. Maintain NPO.
2. Administer IV fluids.
3. Monitor I&O.
4. Provide gastrostomy tube care and feedings as prescribed.
5. Provide pacifier to meet developmental needs.
6. Monitor child for postoperative stricture of the esophagus.
    a. Poor feeding
    b. Dysphagia

c. Drooling
d. Regurgitating undigested food
C. Promote parent-infant bonding for high-risk infant.

PYLORIC STENOSIS

Description: Narrowing of the pyloric canal; the sphincter (circular muscle of the pylorus) hypertrophies to twice the normal size.

Nursing Assessment

A. Usually occurs in first-born males
B. Vomiting (free of bile) usually begins after 14 days of life and becomes projectile.
C. Hungry, fretful infant
D. Weight loss, failure to gain weight
E. Dehydration with decreased sodium and potassium
F. Metabolic alkalosis (decreased serum chloride, increased pH and bicarbonate or CO_2 content)
G. Palpable olive-shaped mass in upper right quadrant of the abdomen
H. Visible peristaltic waves

Analysis (Nursing Diagnoses)

A. *Imbalanced nutrition: less than body requirements* related to…
B. *Deficient fluid volume* related to…

HESI Hint • Children with cleft lip or palate and those with pyloric stenosis both have a nursing diagnosis of "*Alteration in nutrition; less than body requirements.*"
• Cleft lip or palate is related to decreased ability to suck.
• Pyloric stenosis is related to frequent vomiting.

Nursing Plans and Interventions

A. Preoperative care
1. Assess for dehydration.
2. Administer IV fluids and electrolytes as prescribed.
3. Weigh daily; monitor I&O.
4. Provide small, frequent feedings if prescribed.

B. Prepare family for surgery by teaching that:
1. Hypertrophied muscle will be split
2. Prognosis is excellent

C. Postoperative care
1. Continue IV fluids as prescribed.
2. Provide small oral feedings with electrolyte solutions or glucose (usually 4 to 6 hours postoperative).
3. Position on *right* side in semi-Fowler position after feeding.
4. Burp frequently to avoid stomach becoming distended and putting pressure on surgical site.
5. Weigh daily; monitor I&O.

INTUSSUSCEPTION

Description: Telescoping of one part of the intestine into another part of the intestine, usually the ileum into the colon (called ileocolic)

A. Partial to complete bowel obstruction occurs.
B. Blood vessels become trapped in the telescoping bowel, causing necrosis.

Nursing Assessment

A. Child under 1 year of age
B. Acute, intermittent abdominal pain
C. Screaming, with legs drawn up to abdomen
D. Vomiting
E. "Currant jelly" stools (mixed with blood and mucus)
F. Sausage-shaped mass in upper right quadrant while lower right quadrant is empty

Analysis (Nursing Diagnoses)

A. *Ineffective tissue perfusion (bowel)* related to...
B. *Risk for deficient fluid volume* related to...

Nursing Plans and Interventions

A. Monitor carefully for shock and bowel perforation.
B. Administer IV fluids as prescribed.
C. Monitor I&O.
D. Prepare family for emergency intervention.
E. Prepare child for barium enema (which provides hydrostatic reduction). Two of three cases respond to this treatment; if not, surgery is necessary.

F. Provide postoperative care for infants who require abdominal surgery.

> **HESI Hint** • Nutritional needs and fluid and electrolyte balance are key problems for children with GI disorders. The younger the children, the more vulnerable they are to fluid and electrolyte imbalances and the greater is the need for the caloric intake required for growth.

CONGENITAL AGANGLIONIC MEGACOLON (HIRSCHSPRUNG DISEASE)

Description: Congenital absence of autonomic parasympathetic ganglion cells in a distal portion of the colon and rectum

A. There is a lack of peristalsis in the area of the colon where the ganglion cells are absent.
B. Fecal contents accumulate above the aganglionic area of the bowel.
C. Correction usually involves a series of surgical procedures:
1. A temporary colostomy
2. Later, a reanastomosis and closure of the colostomy

Nursing Assessment

A. Suspicion in newborn who fails to pass meconium within 24 hours
B. Distended abdomen, chronic constipation alternating with diarrhea
C. Nutritionally deficient child
D. Enterocolitis that occurs as an emergency event
E. Ribbonlike stools in the older child

Analysis (Nursing Diagnoses)

A. *Constipation* related to...
B. *Diarrhea* related to...
C. *Imbalanced nutrition: less than body requirements* related to...

Nursing Plans and Interventions

A. Provide preoperative care.
1. Begin preparation for abdominal surgery.
2. Provide bowel-cleansing program as prescribed.
3. Insert rectal tube if prescribed.
4. Observe for symptoms of bowel perforation.
   a. Abdominal distention (Measure abdominal girth.)
   b. Vomiting
   c. Increased abdominal tenderness

d. Irritability

e. Dyspnea and cyanosis

5. Initiate preoperative teaching regarding colostomy.

B. Provide postoperative care.

1. Check vital signs, axillary temperature.

> **HESI Hint** • Take axillary temperature in children with congenital megacolon.

2. Administer IV fluids as prescribed.
3. Monitor I&O.
4. Care for nasogastric tube with connection to intermittent suction.
5. Check abdominal and perineal dressings.
6. Assess bowel sounds.

C. Prepare family for home care.

1. Teach care of temporary colostomy.
2. Teach skin care.
3. Refer family to enterostomal therapist and social services.

D. Prepare child and family for closure of temporary colostomy.

E. After closure, encourage family to be patient with child when toileting.

F. Teach family to begin toilet training after age 2.

ANORECTAL MALFORMATION

Description: Congenital malformation of the anorectal section of the GI tract (imperforate anus)

A. It is often associated with a fistula.

B. It may also be associated with urinary tract anomalies.

C. Type and level of rectal anomaly determine surgical procedure and degree of bowel control possible.

Nursing Assessment

A. An unusual-appearing anal dimple

B. Newborn who does not pass meconium stool within 24 hours

C. Meconium appearing from perineal fistula or in urine

Analysis (Nursing Diagnoses)

A. *Bowel incontinence* related to…

B. *Deficient knowledge (bowel or colostomy home program)* related to…

Nursing Plans and Interventions

A. Determine newborn's first temperature, typically using a rectal thermometer, to assess for imperforate anus.

B. Assess newborn for passage of meconium.

C. Assist family's ability to cope with diagnosis.

D. Provide preoperative care to infant.

1. Assess vital signs.
2. Administer IV fluids (NPO).
3. Monitor I&O.

E. Provide postoperative care for anal reconstruction.

1. Keep perineal site clean.
2. Position infant in side-lying prone position with hips elevated (decreases pressure on perineal sutures).
3. Provide colostomy care if needed.

F. Teach home care.

1. Teach home care of colostomy if necessary.
2. Teach that with high-level defects, long-term follow-up is required.
3. Teach that toilet training is delayed and full continence may not be achieved.

Review of Gastrointestinal Disorders

1. Describe feeding techniques for a child with cleft lip or palate.
2. List the signs and symptoms of esophageal atresia with TEF.
3. What nursing actions are initiated for the newborn with suspected esophageal atresia with TEF?
4. Describe the postoperative nursing care for an infant with pyloric stenosis.
5. Describe why a barium enema is used to treat intussusception.
6. Describe the preoperative nursing care for a child with Hirschsprung disease.
7. What care is needed for a child with a temporary colostomy?
8. What are the signs of anorectal malformation?
9. What are the priorities for a child undergoing abdominal surgery?

Answers to Review

1. Use lamb's nipple or prosthesis. Feed child upright, with frequent bubbling.
2. Choking, coughing, cyanosis, and excess salivation
3. Maintain NPO immediately, and suction secretions.
4. Maintain IV hydration, and provide small, frequent oral feedings of glucose or electrolyte solutions or both within 4 to 6 hours. Gradually increase to full-strength formula. Position infant on right side in semi-Fowler position after feeding.
5. A barium enema reduces the telescoping of the intestine through hydrostatic pressure without surgical intervention.
6. Check vital signs and take axillary temperatures. Provide bowel cleansing program, and teach about colostomy.

Observe for bowel perforation; measure abdominal girth.
7. Family needs education about skin care and appliances. Referral to an enterostomal therapist is appropriate.
8. A newborn who does not pass meconium within 24 hours; meconium appearing through a fistula or in the urine; an unusual-appearing anal dimple.
9. Maintain fluid balance (I&O, nasogastric suction, monitor electrolytes); monitor vital signs; care for drains, if present; assess bowel function; prevent infection of incisional area and other postoperative complications; and support child and family with appropriate teaching.

Hematologic Disorders

IRON DEFICIENCY ANEMIA

Description: Hemoglobin levels below normal range because of the body's inadequate supply, intake, or absorption of iron

A. Iron deficiency anemia is the leading hematologic disorder in children.
B. The need for iron is greater in children than in adults because of accelerated growth.
C. Anemia may be caused by the following:
   1. Inadequate stores during fetal development
   2. Deficient dietary intake
   3. Chronic blood loss
   4. Poor utilization of iron by the body

Nursing Assessment

A. Pallor, paleness of mucous membranes
B. Tiredness, fatigue
C. Usually seen in infants 6 to 24 months old (times of growth spurt); toddlers and female adolescents most affected
D. Overweight "milk baby"
E. Dietary intake low in iron
F. Milk intake greater than 32 oz/day
G. Pica habit (eating nonfood substances)
H. Lab values:
   1. Decreased Hgb
   2. Low serum iron level
   3. Elevated total iron binding capacity (TIBC)

HESI Hint • Remember the Hgb norms:
• Newborn: 14 to 24 g/dl
• Infant: 10 to 17 g/dl
• Child: 9.5 to 15.5 g/dl

Analysis (Nursing Diagnoses)

A. *Ineffective tissue perfusion* (specify) related to...
B. *Activity intolerance* related to...

Nursing Plans and Interventions

A. Support child's need to limit activities.
B. Provide rest periods.
C. Administer oral iron (ferrous sulfate) as prescribed.

HESI Hint • Teach family about administration of oral iron:
• Give on empty stomach (as tolerated, for better absorption).
• Give with citrus juices (vitamin C) for increased absorption.
• Use dropper or straw to avoid discoloring teeth.
• Teach that stools will become tarry.
• Teach that iron can be fatal in severe overdose; keep away from other children.
• Do not give with any dairy products.

D. Teach family nutritional facts concerning iron deficiency.
   1. Limit milk intake to less than 32 oz/day.
   2. Teach about dietary sources of iron:
      a. Meat
      b. Green, leafy vegetables
      c. Fish
      d. Liver
      e. Whole grains
      f. Legumes
      g. For infants: iron-fortified cereals and formula
   3. Teach about appropriate nutrition for child's age.
E. Be aware of family's income and cultural food preferences.
F. Refer family to nutritionist.

G. Refer to Women, Infants, and Children's nutrition program, if available to family.

HEMOPHILIA

Description: Inherited bleeding disorder

A. Transmitted by an X-linked recessive chromosome (mother is the carrier; her sons may express the disease).

B. A normal individual has between 50% and 200% factor activity in blood; the hemophiliac has from 0% to 25% activity.

C. The affected individual usually is missing either factor VIII (classic, 75% of cases) or factor IX.

Nursing Assessment

A. Male child: first red flag may be prolonged bleeding at the umbilical cord or injection site (vitamin K), or following circumcision

B. Prolonged bleeding with minor trauma

C. Hemarthrosis (most frequent site of bleeding)

D. Spontaneous bleeding into muscles and tissues (less severe cases have fewer bleeds)

E. Loss of motion in joints

F. Pain

G. Lab values:
   1. PTT is prolonged.
   2. Factor assays less than 25%

Analysis (Nursing Diagnoses)

A. *Risk for trauma* related to…

B. *Deficient knowledge (home care)* related to…

Nursing Plans and Interventions

A. Administer fresh-frozen plasma, cryoprecipitate of fresh plasma, or lyophilized (freeze-dried) concentrate as prescribed.

B. Administer pain medication as prescribed (analgesics containing *no* aspirin).

C. Follow blood precautions: risk for hepatitis.

D. Teach child and family home care.
   1. Teach to recognize early signs of bleeding into joints.
   2. Teach local treatment for minor bleeds (pressure, splinting, ice).
   3. Teach administration of factor replacement.
   4. Discuss dental hygiene: use soft toothbrushes.
   5. Provide protective care: give child soft toys; use padded bed rails.
   6. Have child wear MedicAlert identification.

E. Refer family for genetic counseling.

F. Support child and family during periods of growth and development when increased risk for bleeding occurs (e.g., learning to walk, tooth loss).

HESI Hint • Inherited bleeding disorders (hemophilia and sickle cell anemia) are often used to test knowledge of genetic transmission patterns. Remember:
• Autosomal recessive: Both parents must be heterozygous, or carriers of the recessive trait, for the disease to be expressed in their offspring. With each pregnancy, there is a one in four chance that the infant will have the disease. However, all children of such parents can get the disease—not just 25% of them. This is the transmission pattern of sickle cell anemia, cystic fibrosis, and phenylketonuria (PKU).
• X-linked recessive trait: The trait is carried on the X chromosome; therefore, it usually affects male offspring, as in hemophilia. With each pregnancy of a woman who is a carrier, there is a 25% chance of having a child with hemophilia. If the child is male, he has a 50% chance of having hemophilia. If the child is female, she has a 50% chance of being a carrier.

SICKLE CELL ANEMIA

Description: Inherited autosomal recessive disorder of Hgb

A. It occurs primarily in persons of African and eastern Mediterranean descent. One in 12 persons of African ancestry is a carrier of the heterozygous gene *HgbAS*. Therefore, the risk that two parents of African ancestry will have a child with sickle cell disease is 0.7%.

B. It usually appears after 6 months of age.

C. Hemoglobin S (HgbS) replaces all or part of the normal Hgb, which causes the red blood cells to sickle when oxygen is released into the tissues.
   1. Sickled cells cannot flow through capillary beds.
   2. Dehydration promotes sickling.

HESI Hint • Hydration is very important in the treatment of sickle cell disease because it promotes hemodilution and circulation of red cells through the blood vessels.

D. HgbS has a less than normal life span (less than 40 days), which leads to chronic anemia.

E. Tissue ischemia causes widespread pathologic changes in spleen, liver, kidney, bones, and CNS.

> **HESI Hint** • Important terms
> • Heterozygous gene (*HgbAS*)—sickle cell trait
> • Homozygous gene (*HbSS*)—sickle cell disease
> • Abnormal hemoglobin (HgbS)—disease and trait

Nursing Assessment

A. Children of African descent, usually over 6 months of age

B. Parents with sickle cell trait or sickle cell anemia

C. Lab diagnosis: Hgb electrophoresis (differentiates trait from disease)

D. Frequent infections (nonfunctional spleen)

E. Tiredness

F. Chronic hemolytic anemia

G. Delayed physical growth

H. Vaso-occlusive crisis: the classic sign:
   1. Fever
   2. Severe abdominal pain
   3. Hand-foot syndrome (infants); painful edematous hands and feet
   4. Arthralgia

I. Leg ulcers (adolescents)

J. Cerebrovascular accidents (increased risk with dehydration)

Analysis (Nursing Diagnoses)

A. *Acute pain* related to…

B. *Risk for infection* related to…

C. *Deficient knowledge (crisis prevention)* related to…

Nursing Plans and Interventions

A. Teach family that to prevent crisis (hypoxia), they should:
   1. Keep child from exercising strenuously.
   2. Keep child away from high altitudes.
   3. Avoid letting child become infected, and seek care at first sign of infection.
   4. Use prophylactic penicillin if prescribed.
   5. Keep child well hydrated.
   6. Not withhold fluids at night because enuresis is a complication of both the disease and the treatment.

B. For a child hospitalized with a vaso-occlusive crisis:
   1. Administer IV fluids (one to two times maintenance levels) and electrolytes, as prescribed, to increase hydration and treat acidosis.
   2. Monitor I&O.
   3. Administer blood products as prescribed.
   4. Administer analgesics, including parenteral morphine for severe pain, as prescribed.

   5. Use warm compresses (not ice).
   6. Administer prescribed antibiotics to treat infection.

C. Administer pneumococcal vaccine, meningococcal vaccine, and Hib vaccine as prescribed.

D. Administer hepatitis B vaccine as prescribed (for child at risk because of transfusions).

E. Refer family for genetic counseling.

F. Support child and family experiencing chronic disease.

> **HESI Hint** • Supplemental iron is not given to clients with sickle cell anemia. The anemia is not caused by iron deficiency. Folic acid is given orally to stimulate RBC synthesis.

ACUTE LYMPHOCYTIC LEUKEMIA

Description: Cancer of the blood-forming organs

A. Acute lymphocytic leukemia accounts for about 80% of childhood leukemia.

B. It is noted for the presence of lymphoblasts (immature lymphocytes), which replace normal cells in the bone marrow.

C. Blast cells are also seen in the peripheral blood.

D. Acute lymphocytic leukemia is classified according to whether it involves:
   1. T lymphocytes
   2. B lymphocytes
   3. Null cells (neither T cells nor B cells)

E. More than 75% of children with acute lymphocytic leukemia have the null cell type, which has the best prognosis.

F. The signs and symptoms of leukemia result from the replacement of normal cells by leukemic cells in the bone marrow and extramedullary sites.

G. Treatment has four phases:
   1. Induction
   2. Sanctuary
   3. Consolidation
   4. Maintenance

Nursing Assessment

A. Pallor, tiredness, weakness, lethargy due to anemia

B. Petechia, bleeding, bruising due to thrombocytopenia

C. Infection, fever due to neutropenia

D. Bone joint pain due to leukemic infiltration of bone marrow

E. Enlarged lymph nodes; hepatosplenomegaly

F. Headache and vomiting (signs of CNS involvement)

G. Anorexia, weight loss

H. Lab data: bone marrow aspiration that reveals 80%–90% immature blast cells

Analysis (Nursing Diagnoses)

A. *Risk for infection* related to...

B. *Fear* related to...

C. *Deficient knowledge (disease process and chemotherapy)* related to...

Nursing Plans and Interventions

A. Recommend private room.

B. Reverse isolation if prescribed.

C. Provide child with age-appropriate explanations for diagnostic tests, treatments, and nursing care.

D. Examine child for infection of skin, needle-stick sites, dental problems.

E. Administer blood products as prescribed.

F. Administer antineoplastic chemotherapy.

G. Monitor for side effects of chemotherapeutic agents (see Table 4-37).
   1. Vincristine (induction)
   2. L-Asparaginase (induction)
   3. Methotrexate (sanctuary and maintenance)
   4. Mercaptopurine (6-MP) (maintenance)

> **HESI Hint** • Have epinephrine and oxygen readily available to treat anaphylaxis when administering L-asparaginase.

H. Provide care directed toward managing side effects and toxic effects of antineoplastic agents.
   1. Administer antiemetics as prescribed.
   2. Monitor fluid balance.
   3. Monitor for signs of infection.
   4. Monitor for signs of bleeding.
   5. Monitor for cumulative toxic effects of drugs: hepatic toxicity, cardiac toxicity, renal toxicity, and neurotoxicity.
   6. Provide oral hygiene.
   7. Provide small, appealing meals; increase calories and protein; refer to nutritionist.
   8. Promote self-esteem and positive body image if child has alopecia, severe weight loss, or other disturbance in body image.
   9. Provide care to prevent infection.

I. Provide emotional support for family in crisis.

J. Encourage family's and child's input and control in determining plans and treatment.

> **HESI Hint** • Prednisone is frequently used in combination with antineoplastic drugs to reduce the mitosis of lymphocytes. Allopurinol, a xanthine oxidase inhibitor, is also administered to prevent renal damage caused by uric acid buildup and cellular lysis.

Review of Hematologic Disorders

1. Describe the information families should be given when a child is receiving oral iron preparations.
2. List dietary sources of iron.
3. What is the genetic transmission pattern of hemophilia?
4. Describe the sequence of events in a vaso-occlusive crisis in sickle cell anemia.
5. Explain why hydration is a priority in treating sickle cell disease.
6. What should families and clients do to avoid triggering sickling episodes?
7. Nursing interventions and medical treatments for a child with leukemia are based on what three physiologic problems?

Answers to Review

1. Give oral iron on an empty stomach and with vitamin C. Use straws to avoid discoloring teeth. Tarry stools are normal. Increase dietary sources of iron.
2. Meat, green leafy vegetables, fish, liver, whole grains, legumes
3. It is an X-linked recessive chromosomal disorder transmitted by the mother and expressed in male children.
4. A vaso-occlusive crisis is caused by the clumping of red blood cells, which blocks small blood vessels; therefore, the cells cannot get through the capillaries, causing pain and tissue and organ ischemia. Lowered oxygen tension affects HgbS, which causes sickling of the cells.
5. Hydration promotes hemodilution and circulation of the red cells through the blood vessels.
6. Keep child well hydrated. Avoid known sources of infections. Avoid high altitudes. Avoid strenuous exercise.
7. Anemia (decreased erythrocytes); infection (neutropenia); bleeding thrombocytopenia (decreased platelets)

Metabolic and Endocrine Disorders

CONGENITAL HYPOTHYROIDISM

Description: Congenital condition resulting from inadequate thyroid tissue development in utero. Mental retardation and growth failure occur if it is not detected and treated in early infancy.

Nursing Assessment

A. Newborn screening reveals low T_4 (thyroxine) and high TSH (thyroid-stimulating hormone).

B. Symptoms in the newborn:
  1. Long gestation (>42 weeks)
  2. Large hypoactive infant
  3. Delayed meconium passage
  4. Feeding problems (poor suck)
  5. Prolonged physiologic jaundice
  6. Hypothermia

C. Symptoms in early infancy:
  1. Large, protruding tongue
  2. Coarse hair
  3. Lethargy, sleepiness
  4. Flat expression
  5. Constipation

> **HESI Hint** • An infant with hypothyroidism is often described as a good, quiet baby by the parents.

Analysis (Nursing Diagnoses)

A. *Delayed growth and development* related to…

B. *Deficient knowledge (medication program)* related to…

Nursing Plans and Interventions

A. Perform newborn screening programs before discharge.

B. Assess newborn for signs of congenital hypothyroidism.

C. Teach family about replacement therapy with thyroid hormone:
  1. Explain that child will have a lifelong need for the therapy.
  2. Tell parents to give child a single dose in the morning.
  3. Teach family to check child's pulse daily before giving thyroid medication.
  4. Signs of overdose include rapid pulse, irritability, fever, weight loss, and diarrhea.
  5. Signs of underdose include lethargy, fatigue, constipation, and poor feeding.
  6. Periodic thyroid testing is necessary.

PHENYLKETONURIA (PKU)

Description: Autosomal recessive disorder in which the body cannot metabolize the essential amino acid phenylalanine

A. The buildup of serum phenylalanine leads to CNS damage, most notably mental retardation.

B. Decreased melanin produces light skin and blond hair.

Nursing Assessment

A. Newborn screening using the Guthrie test; positive result: serum phenylalanine level of 4 mg/dL.

B. Frequent vomiting, failure to gain weight

C. Irritability, hyperactivity

D. Musty odor of urine

> **HESI Hint** • Early detection of hypothyroidism and phenylketonuria is essential in preventing mental retardation in infants. Knowledge of normal growth and development patterns is important because a lack of attainment can be used to detect the presence of a disease and to evaluate the treatment's effects.

Analysis (Nursing Diagnoses)

A. *Delayed growth and development* related to…

B. *Deficient knowledge (disease process and diet)* related to…

Nursing Plans and Interventions

A. Perform newborn screening at birth and again at about 3 weeks of age.

B. Teach family dietary management.
  1. Stress the importance of strict adherence to prescribed low-phenylalanine diet.
  2. Instruct family to provide special formulas for infant: Lofenalac, Phenex-1.
  3. Instruct family to provide phenyl-free milk substitute after the age of 2 years.
  4. Teach family to avoid foods high in phenylalanine, that is, high-protein foods, such as meat, milk, dairy products, and eggs.
  5. Teach family to offer foods low in phenylalanine, that is, vegetables, fruits, juices, cereals, breads, and starches.
  6. Encourage family to work with nutritionist.
  7. Teach that diet must be maintained at least until brain growth is complete (age 6 to 8 years).

C. Refer for genetic counseling.

> **HESI Hint** • NutraSweet (aspartame) contains phenylalanine and should not therefore be given to a child with phenylketonuria.

INSULIN-DEPENDENT DIABETES MELLITUS (IDDM), OR TYPE I DIABETES

Description: Metabolic disorder in which the insulin-producing cells of the pancreas are nonfunctioning as a result of some insult (see Medical-Surgical Nursing, p. 124)

A. Heredity, viral infections, and autoimmune processes are implicated in diabetes mellitus.
B. Diabetes causes altered metabolism of carbohydrates, proteins, and fats.
C. Insulin replacement, dietary management, and exercise are the treatments.

Nursing Assessment

A. Classic three P's:
   1. Polydipsia
   2. Polyphagia
   3. Polyuria, enuresis (bed-wetting) in previously continent child
B. Irritability, fatigue
C. Weight loss
D. Abdominal complaints, nausea, and vomiting
E. Usually occurs in school-age children but can occur even in infancy
F. See Table 4-27.

Analysis (Nursing Diagnoses)

1. *Imbalanced nutrition: less than body requirements* related to…
2. *Deficient knowledge (home program for diabetes)* related to…

HESI Hint • Diabetes mellitus (DM) in children was typically diagnosed as insulin-dependent diabetes (type 1) until recently. A marked increase in type 2 DM has occurred recently in the United States, particularly among Native American, African American, and Hispanic children and adolescents. Adolescence frequently causes difficulty in management because growth is rapid, and the need to be like peers makes compliance difficult. Remember to consider the child's age, cognitive level of development, and psychosocial development when answering NCLEX-RN questions.

Nursing Plans and Interventions

A. Assist with diagnosis (fasting blood sugar >120 mg/dl glucose).
B. If child is in ketoacidosis, provide care for seriously ill child (may be unconscious).
   1. Monitor vital signs and neurologic status.
   2. Monitor blood glucose, pH, serum electrolytes.

HESI Hint • When a child is in ketoacidosis, administer regular insulin IV in normal saline as prescribed.

   3. Administer IV fluids, insulin, and electrolytes as prescribed.
   4. Assess hydration status.
   5. Maintain strict I&O.
C. Initiate home teaching program as soon as possible; involve child and family.
   1. Teach insulin administration.
      a. Child usually receives two injections daily.
      b. The dose before breakfast is usually the larger dose.
      c. Use rapid-acting and intermediate-acting insulin.
   2. Teach dietary management (carbohydrate counting preferred).
      a. Meals and snacks
      b. Growth and exercise needs
      c. Four basic food groups, no concentrated sweets
      d. Advice from nutritionist
   3. Teach about exercise.
      a. Regular, planned activities
      b. Diet modification; snacks before or during exercise
   4. Teach about home glucose monitoring and urine testing.
   5. Teach the signs and symptoms of hyperglycemia and hypoglycemia.
D. Initiate program for school-age child, as appropriate.
   1. Identify issues specific to school.
      a. Physical education class and exercise
      b. Scheduled times for meals and snacks
      c. Cooperation with teachers and school nurse
      d. Need to be like peers
   2. Teach that a school-age child should be responsible for most management.
   3. Instruct the child to wear a MedicAlert ID bracelet.

HESI Hint • There has been an increase in the number of children diagnosed with type 2 diabetes. The increasing rate of obesity in children is thought to be a contributing factor. Other contributing factors include lack of physical activity and a family history of type 2 diabetes.

Review of Metabolic and Endocrine Disorders

1. How is congenital hypothyroidism diagnosed?
2. What are the symptoms of congenital hypothyroidism in early infancy?
3. What are the outcomes of untreated congenital hypothyroidism?
4. What are the metabolic effects of PKU?
5. What two formulas are prescribed for infants with PKU?
6. List foods high in phenylalanine content.
7. What are the three classic signs of diabetes?
8. Differentiate the signs of hypoglycemia and hyperglycemia.
9. Describe the nursing care of a child with ketoacidosis.
10. Describe developmental factors that would impact the school-age child with diabetes.
11. What is the relationship between hypoglycemia and exercise?

Answers to Review

1. Newborn screening revealing a low T_4 and a high TSH
2. Large, protruding tongue; coarse hair; lethargy; sleepiness; and constipation
3. Mental retardation and growth failure
4. CNS damage, mental retardation, and decreased melanin
5. Lofenalac and Phenex-1
6. Meat, milk, dairy products, and eggs
7. Polydipsia, polyphagia, and polyuria
8. Hypoglycemia: tremors, sweating, headache, hunger, nausea, lethargy, confusion, slurred speech, anxiety, tingling around mouth, nightmares. Hyperglycemia: polydipsia, polyuria, polyphagia, blurred vision, weakness, weight loss, and syncope
9. Provide care for an unconscious child, administer regular insulin IV in normal saline, monitor blood gas values, and maintain strict I&O.
10. Need to be like peers; assuming responsibility for own care; modification of diet; snacks and exercise in school
11. During exercise, insulin uptake is increased and the risk for hypoglycemia occurs.

Skeletal Disorders

FRACTURES

Description: Traumatic injury to bone
A. Fractures can be classified according to type (see Table 4-29).
1. Complete fractures: bone fragments are completely separate.
2. Incomplete fractures: bone fragments remain attached (e.g., greenstick, bends, buckles).
3. Comminuted fractures: bone fragments from the fractured shaft break free and lie in the surrounding tissue. This type of fracture is rare in children.
B. Fractures that occur in the epiphyseal plate (growth plate) may affect growth of the limb.

HESI Hint • Fractures in older children are common because they fall during play and are involved in motor vehicle accidents.
• Spiral fractures (caused by twisting) and fractures in infants may be related to child abuse.
• Fractures involving the epiphyseal plate (growth plate) can have serious consequences in terms of the growth of the affected limb.

Nursing Assessment

A. General condition
1. Visible bone fragments
2. Pain
3. Swelling
4. Contusions
5. Child guarding or protecting the extremity
B. Possibility of being able to use fractured extremity due to intact periosteum
C. The five P's (may indicate the presence of ischemia):
1. Pain
2. Pallor
3. Pulselessness
4. Paresthesia
5. Paralysis

Analysis (Nursing Diagnoses)

A. *Ineffective tissue perfusion (peripheral)* related to…
B. *Acute pain* related to…

Nursing Plans and Interventions

A. Obtain baseline data, and frequently perform neurovascular assessments.

1. Pulses: Check pulses distal to the injury to assess circulation.
2. Color: Check injured extremity for pink, brisk, capillary refill.
3. Movement and sensation: Check injured extremity for nerve impairment; compare for symmetry with uninjured extremity (child may guard injury).
4. Temperature: Check extremity for warmth.
5. Swelling: Check for an increase in swelling. Elevate extremity to prevent swelling.
6. Pain: Monitor for severe pain that is not relieved by analgesics.

B. Report abnormal assessment promptly! Compartment syndrome may occur; it results in permanent damage to the nerves and vasculature of the injured extremity due to compression.

C. Maintain traction if prescribed. Note bed position, type of traction, weights, pulleys, pins, pin sites, adhesive strips, ace wraps, splints, and casts.
   1. Skin traction: force is applied to skin.

> **HESI Hint** • Skin traction for fracture reduction should *not* be removed unless health care provider prescribes its removal.

   a. Buck extension traction: lower extremity, legs extended, no hip flexion
   b. Dunlop traction: two lines of pull on the arm
   c. Russell traction: two lines of pull on the lower extremity, one perpendicular, one longitudinal
   d. Bryant traction: both lower extremities flexed 90 degrees at hips (rarely used because extreme elevation of lower extremities causes decreased peripheral circulation)
   2. Skeletal traction: pin or wire applies pull directly to the distal bone fragment.
   a. 90-Degree traction: 90-degree flexion of hip and knee; lower extremity is in a boot cast; can also be used on upper extremities (Fig. 5-15).
   b. Dunlop traction: may be used as skeletal traction.

> **HESI Hint** • Pin sites can be source of infection. Monitor for signs of infection. Cleanse and dress pin sites as prescribed.

D. Maintain child in proper body alignment; restrain if necessary.

E. Monitor for problems of immobility.

F. Provide age-appropriate play and toys.

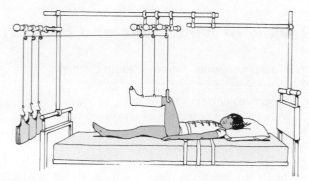

FIGURE 5-15 90-90 Traction. (From Hockenberry MJ, Wilson D: *Wong's nursing care of infants and children*, ed 8. St. Louis, 2007, Mosby.)

G. Prepare child for cast application; use age-appropriate terms when explaining procedures.

H. Provide routine cast care following application; petal cast edges.

I. Teach home cast care to family:
   1. Teach neurovascular assessment of casted extremity.
   2. Teach child not to get cast wet.
   3. Teach child not to place anything under cast.
   4. Teach child to keep small objects, toys, and food out of cast.
   5. Teach family to modify diapering and toileting to prevent cast soilage.
   6. Teach that in the presence of a hip spica, family may use a Bradford frame under a small child to help with toileting; they must *not* use abduction bar to turn child.
   7. Teach to seek follow-up care with health care provider.

> **HESI Hint** • Skeletal disorders affect the infant's or child's physical mobility, and typical NCLEX-RN questions focus on appropriate toys and activities for the child who is confined to bed rest and is immobilized.

CONGENITAL DISLOCATED HIP (DEVELOPMENTAL DYSPLASIA OF HIP)

Description: Abnormal development of the femoral head in the acetabulum

A. Conservative treatment consists of splinting.

B. Surgical intervention is necessary if splinting is not successful.

Nursing Assessment

A. Infant
   1. Positive Ortolani sign ("clicking" with abduction)
   2. Unequal folds of skin on buttocks and thigh
   3. Limited abduction of affected hip
   4. Unequal leg lengths

B. Older child
  1. Limp on affected side
  2. Trendelenburg sign

Analysis (Nursing Diagnoses)

A. *Impaired physical mobility* related to...

B. *Deficient knowledge (home care)* related to...

Nursing Plans and Interventions

A. Perform newborn assessment at birth.

B. Apply abduction device or splint (Pavlik harness; Frejka or von Rosen splint) as prescribed. Therapy involves positioning legs in flexed abducted position.

C. Teach parents home care.
  1. Teach application and removal of device (worn 24 hours a day).
  2. Teach skin care and bathing (physician may allow parents to remove device for bathing).
  3. Teach diapering.
  4. Teach that follow-up care involves frequent adjustments because of growth.

D. Teach how to provide care for an infant in Bryant traction (used if splinting is ineffective).
  1. Instruct to maintain hips in 90-degree flexion.
  2. Instruct to elevate buttocks off bed.
  3. Instruct to monitor circulation to feet.
  4. Instruct to meet developmental needs of an immobilized infant.
  5. Incorporate family in care.
  6. Prepare family for spica cast application.

E. Provide nursing care for a child requiring surgical correction.
  1. Perform preoperative teaching of child and family, including cast application.
  2. Perform postoperative care.
     a. Assess vital signs.
     b. Check cast for drainage and bleeding.

c. Perform neurovascular assessment of extremities.
d. Promote respiratory hygiene.
e. Administer narcotic analgesics (meperidine [Demerol] or morphine) either IV (preferred) or IM (Table 5-11).
f. Teach family cast care when child gets home.

> **HESI Hint** • Children do not like injections and will deny pain to avoid "shots."

SCOLIOSIS

Description: Lateral curvature of the spine (Fig. 5-16)

A. If severe, it can cause respiratory compromise.

B. Surgical correction by spinal fusion or instrumentation may be required if conservative treatment is ineffective.

Nursing Assessment

A. Occurs most commonly in adolescent females (10 to 15 years old)
  1. Elevated shoulder or hip
  2. Head and hips not aligned
  3. While child is bending forward, a rib hump is apparent. (Ask child to bend forward from the hips with arms hanging free, and examine child for a curve of the spine, rib hump, and hip asymmetry.)

Analysis (Nursing Diagnoses)

A. *Impaired physical mobility* related to...

B. *Disturbed body image* related to...

Nursing Plans and Interventions

A. Screen all adolescent children, especially females, during growth spurt.

B. Prepare child and family for conservative treatment such as the use of a brace.

TABLE 5-11   Medications Used in Skeletal Disorders

Drugs/Route	Indications	Adverse Reactions	Nursing Implications
• Infliximab (Remicade)/IV • Methocarbamol (Robaxin)/PO, IM, IV • Cyclobenzaprine (Flexeril)/PO	• Nonnarcotics to treat pain, stiffness, and discomfort	• Nausea • Vomiting • Fever • Chills • Dizziness • Drowsiness (Robaxin) • Chest pain • Allergic response: rash, difficulty breathing, etc.	• Do not give if client has increased intracranial pressure • Review history: heart disease (all); thyroid disorders; and use of MAOIs • Remicade use can worsen TB

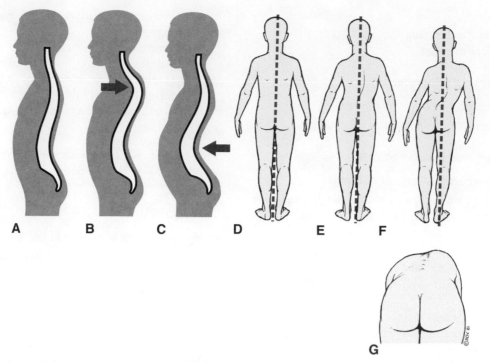

FIGURE 5-16 Defects of spinal column. *A,* Normal spine. *B,* Kyphosis. *C,* Lordosis. *D,* Normal spine in balance. *E,* Mild scoliosis in balance. *F,* Severe scoliosis not in balance. *G,* Rib hump and flank asymmetry seen in flexion caused by rotary component. (From Hockenberry MJ, Wilson D: *Wong's nursing care of infants and children,* ed 8, St. Louis, 2007, Mosby.)

1. Teach application of Milwaukee brace.
   a. Instruct to wear 23 hours a day.
   b. Instruct to wear a T-shirt under brace to decrease skin irritation.
   c. Instruct to check skin for areas of irritation or breakdown.
2. Suggest clothing modifications to camouflage brace.
3. Reinforce prescribed exercise regimen for back and abdominal muscles.
4. Plan with adolescent ways of improving self-concept.
5. Teach family that severe, untreated scoliosis can cause respiratory difficulty.

HESI Hint • A brace does not correct the spine's curve in a child with scoliosis; it only stops or slows the progression.

C. Prepare child and family for surgical correction if required.
   1. Teach child and family log-rolling technique.
   2. Teach how to practice respiratory hygiene.
   3. Orient child to ICU.
   4. Discuss postoperative tubes: Foley, nasogastric tube, and chest tube (if anterior fusion is performed).

5. Describe postoperative pain management; patient-controlled analgesic (PCA) may be used.
6. Obtain a baseline neurologic assessment.

D. Provide postoperative care.
   1. Perform frequent neurologic assessments.
   2. Log-roll for 5 days (Box 5-3).
   3. Administer IV fluids and analgesics as prescribed.
   4. Perform oral hygiene (client NPO).
   5. Monitor nasogastric tube and bowel sounds.
   6. Assist with ambulation, provide body jacket, progressively ambulate.
   7. Teach child and family that body jacket will be worn for several months until the bone fusion is stable.
   8. Determine the need for a teacher in the home.
   9. Encourage child's participation in care to promote self-esteem.

BOX 5-3 *Log Rolling*

- Usually requires two or more persons, depending on the size of the client.
- Client is carefully moved on a draw sheet to the side of the bed away from which they are to be turned (moved to the left if they are to face to the right).
- Client is then turned in a simultaneous motion (log-rolled), maintaining the spine in a straight position.
- Pillows are arranged for support and comfort, and they assist the client to maintain alignment.

JUVENILE RHEUMATOID ARTHRITIS (JRA) OR JUVENILE IDIOPATHIC ARTHRITIS (JIA)

Description: Chronic inflammatory disorder of the joint synovium

A. Single or multiple joints may be involved.

B. It may also have a systemic presentation.

C. It occurs between ages 2 and 5 and between ages 9 and 12.

Nursing Assessment

A. Joint swelling and stiffness (usually large joints)

B. Painful joints

C. Generalized symptoms: fever, malaise, and rash

D. Periods of exacerbations and remissions

E. Varying severity: mild and self-limited or severe and disabling

F. Lab data: latex fixation test (usually negative) and elevated ESR

G. Poorest prognosis:
   1. Positive rheumatoid factor
   2. Polyarticular systemic onset

Analysis (Nursing Diagnoses)

A. *Impaired physical mobility* related to…

B. *Chronic pain* related to…

Nursing Plans and Interventions

A. Plan home program of prescribed exercise, splinting, and activity.

B. Assist in identifying adaptations in routine (e.g., Velcro fasteners, frequent rest periods).

C. Support the maintaining of school schedule and activities appropriate for age.

D. Teach about medication regimen; combination drugs are used (see Medical-Surgical Nursing, p. 131).
   1. Nonsteroidal antiinflammatory drugs
      a. Aspirin
      b. Tolmetin sodium
      c. Ibuprofen
      d. Naproxen
   2. Antirheumatic drugs (gold salts; see Table 5-11)
   3. Corticosteroids (prednisone)
   4. Cytotoxic drugs (cyclophosphamide, methotrexate)

E. Teach child and family about side effects and toxic effects of prescribed drugs.

F. Inform child and family that the optimum antiinflammatory effects of drugs may take a month to achieve.

G. Encourage periodic eye exams for early detection of iridocyclitis so as to prevent vision loss.

H. Encourage family to allow child's independence.

> **HESI Hint** • Corticosteroids are used in the short term in low doses during exacerbations. Long-term use is avoided because of side effects and their adverse effects on growth.

Review of Skeletal Disorders

1. List normal findings in a neurovascular assessment.
2. What is compartment syndrome?
3. What are the signs and symptoms of compartment syndrome?
4. Why are fractures of the epiphyseal plate a special concern?
5. How is skeletal traction applied?
6. What discharge instructions should be included concerning a child with a spica cast?
7. What are the signs and symptoms of congenital dislocated hip in infants?
8. How would the nurse conduct a scoliosis screening?
9. What instructions should a child with scoliosis receive about the Milwaukee brace?
10. What care is indicated for a child with juvenile rheumatoid arthritis?

Answers to Review

1. Warm extremity, brisk capillary refill, free movement, normal sensation of the affected extremity, and equal pulses
2. Damage to nerves and vasculature of an extremity due to compression
3. Abnormal neurovascular assessment: cold extremity, severe pain, inability to move the extremity, and poor capillary refill
4. Fractures of the epiphyseal plate (growth plate) may affect the growth of the limb.
5. Skeletal traction is maintained by pins or wires applied to the distal fragment of the fracture.
6. Check child's circulation. Keep cast dry. Do not place anything under cast. Prevent cast soilage during toileting or diapering. Do not turn child using an abductor bar.

7. Unequal skin folds of the buttocks, Ortolani sign, limited abduction of the affected hip, and unequal leg lengths
8. Ask the child to bend forward from the hips, with arms hanging free. Examine the child for a curve in the spine, a rib hump, and hip asymmetry.
9. The child should be instructed to wear the brace 23 hours per day; wear a T-shirt under brace; check skin for irritation; perform back and abdominal exercises; and modify clothing. The child should be encouraged to maintain normal activities as able.
10. Prescribed exercise to maintain mobility; splinting of affected joints; and teaching about medication management and side effects of drugs.

For more review, go to **http://evolve.elsevier.com/HESI/RN** for HESI's online study exams.

MATERNITY NURSING **6**

Anatomy and Physiology of Reproduction

THE MENSTRUAL CYCLE

Description: The cycle is composed of four phases. The normal cycle is 21 to 45 days in length. The mean age for menarche (first menstruation) in the United States is 12.87 years or 1 to 3 years after breast budding. Pregnancy can occur after the very first menstrual cycle. Most women have ovulatory cycles within 24 months after menarche (Fig. 6-1).

Phases of the Menstrual Cycle

A. Menstrual phase: Days 1 to 5 of cycle
   1. Shedding of the endometrium occurs in the form of uterine bleeding.
B. Proliferation (follicular) phase: Day 5 to ovulation
   1. Endometrium is restored under primary hormone influence of estrogen
   2. In this preovulatory phase, follicle stimulating hormone (FSH) is secreted by the anterior pituitary
   3. Preovulatory surge of luteinizing hormone (LH) converts the follicle to a corpus luteum, which produces progesterone
C. Secretory (luteal) phase: Ovulation to approximately 3 days before menstrual cycle
   1. Estrogen levels level off.
   2. Progesterone levels increase.
D. Ischemic phase: Approximately 3 days before menstruation to onset of menstruation
   1. If fertilization did not occur, the corpus luteum degenerates.
   2. Estrogen and progesterone levels drop.
   3. Endometrium becomes "blood starved," leading to onset of menstruation.

> **HESI Hint** • The menstrual phase varies in length in most women.

> **HESI Hint** • Between ovulation and the beginning of the next menstrual cycle, there are usually exactly 14 days. In other words, ovulation occurs 14 days before the next menstrual period.

> **HESI Hint** • Sperm live approximately 3 days (48 to 72 hours), and eggs live about 24 hours. A couple must avoid unprotected intercourse for several days before the anticipated ovulation and for 3 days after ovulation to prevent pregnancy.

Fertilization

A. Indications of ovulation
   1. A slight drop in temperature occurs 1 day prior to ovulation; a rise of 0.5°F to 1°F in temperature occurs at ovulation; it remains elevated for approximately 10 to 12 days.
   2. Cervical mucus is abundant, watery, clear, and more alkaline.
   3. Cervical os dilates slightly, softens, and rises in the vagina.
   4. Spinnbarkeit (egg-white stretchiness of cervical mucus) is present.
   5. Ferning is seen under microscope.
B. Conditions for fertilization
   1. Postcoital test demonstrates live, motile, normal sperm present in cervical mucus.
   2. Fallopian tubes are patent.
   3. Endometrial biopsy indicates adequate progesterone and secretory endometrium.
   4. Semen is supportive to pregnancy: 2 ml semen; at least 20 million sperm per ml; >60% are normal; and >50% are motile (moving forward).
C. Implantation
   1. Fertilization takes place in ampulla (outer third) section of the fallopian tube.
   2. The zygote (fertilized ovum) takes 3 to 4 days to enter the uterus.

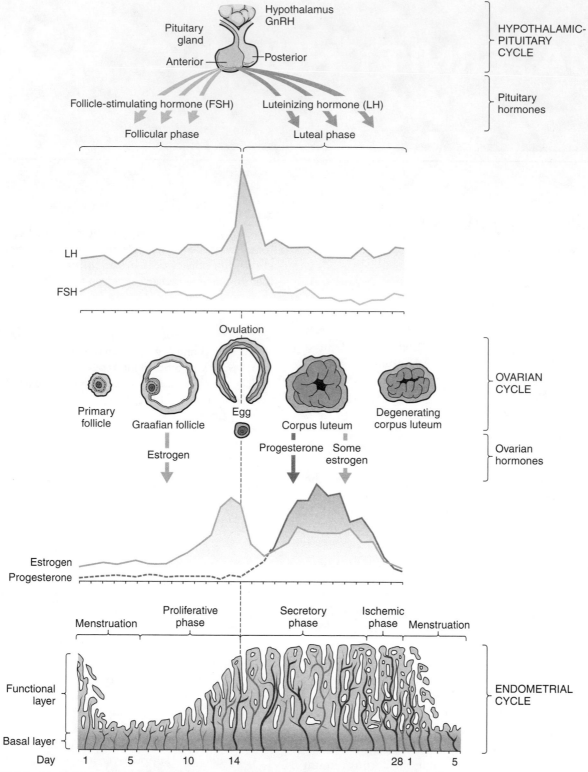

FIGURE 6-1 Menstrual cycle: hypothalamic-pituitary, ovarian, and endometrial. (From Lowdermilk DL, Perry SE: *Maternity nursing,* ed 9. St. Louis, 2010, Mosby.)

3. It takes 7 to 10 days to complete the process of nidation (implantation).
D. Fetal development
   1. Zygote
      a. 12 to 14 Days after fertilization
      b. From the time the ovum is fertilized until it is implanted in the uterus
   2. Embryo
      a. 3 to 8 Weeks after fertilization
      b. Embryo most vulnerable to teratogens (viruses, drugs, radiation, or infections), which can cause major congenital anomalies
   3. Fetus
      a. 9 Weeks after fertilization to term (38+ weeks)
      b. Fewer major anomalies (Fig. 6-2) caused by teratogens

MATERNAL PHYSIOLOGIC CHANGES DURING PREGNANCY

A. Pregnancy length: counted from the first day of last menstrual period (LMP)
   1. 280 Days (approximately)
   2. 40 Weeks
   3. 10 Lunar months (perfect 28-day months)
   4. 9 Calendar months
B. Pregnancy divided into three 13-week trimesters:
   1. First trimester: from the first day of LMP through 13 weeks
   2. Second trimester: 14 weeks through 26 weeks
   3. Third trimester: 27 weeks to 40 weeks

> **HESI Hint** • Because some women experience implantation bleeding or spotting, they do not know they are pregnant.

Fetal and Maternal Changes

8 Weeks

A. Fetal development
   1. Development is rapid.
   2. Heart begins to pump blood.
   3. Limb buds are well developed.
   4. Facial features are discernible.
   5. Major divisions of brain are discernible.
   6. Ears develop from skin folds.
   7. Tiny muscles are formed beneath this skin embryo.
   8. Weight is 2 g.
B. Maternal changes
   1. Nausea persists up to 12 weeks.
   2. Uterus changes from pear to globular shape.
   3. Hegar sign occurs (softening of the isthmus of cervix).
   4. Goodell sign occurs (softening of cervix).
   5. Cervix flexes.
   6. Leukorrhea increases.

7. Ambivalence about pregnancy may occur.
8. There is no noticeable weight gain.
9. Chadwick sign (bluing of vagina) appears as early as 4 weeks.
C. Nursing interventions
   1. Teach prevention of nausea.
      a. Suggest eating dry crackers before getting out of bed in the morning.
      b. Suggest eating small, frequent meals; avoiding fatty foods; and avoiding skipping meals.
   2. Teach safety.
      a. Avoid hot tubs, saunas, and steam rooms throughout pregnancy (increases risk for neural tube defects in first trimester; hypotension may cause fainting).
   3. Prepare client for pregnancy.
      a. Discuss attitudes toward pregnancy.
      b. Discuss value of early pregnancy classes that focus on what to expect during pregnancy.
      c. Provide information about childbirth preparation classes.
      d. Include father and family in preparation for childbirth (expectant fathers experience many of the same feelings and conflicts experienced by the expectant mother).

12 Weeks

A. Fetal development
   1. Embryo becomes a fetus.
   2. Heart is discernible by ultrasound.
   3. Lower body develops.
   4. Sex is determinable.
   5. Kidneys produce urine.
   6. Fetus weighs 19 to 28 g (<1 oz).
B. Maternal changes
   1. Uterus rises above pelvic brim.
   2. Braxton Hicks contractions are possible (continue throughout pregnancy).
   3. Potential for UTI increases (exists throughout pregnancy).
   4. Weight gain is 2 to 4 lb during the first trimester.
   5. Placenta is fully functioning and producing hormones.
C. Nursing interventions
   1. Teach prevention of urinary tract infections.
      a. Encourage adequate fluid intake (3 L/day).
      b. Instruct to void frequently (every 2 hours while awake).
      c. Encourage to void before and after intercourse.
      d. Teach to wipe from front to back.
   2. Discuss nutrition and exercise.
      a. Increase caloric intake by 300 calories per day.
      b. Stress the value of regular exercise.
   3. Discuss possible effects of pregnancy on sexual relationship. Recognize father's role as he labors to incorporate the parental role into his self-identity.

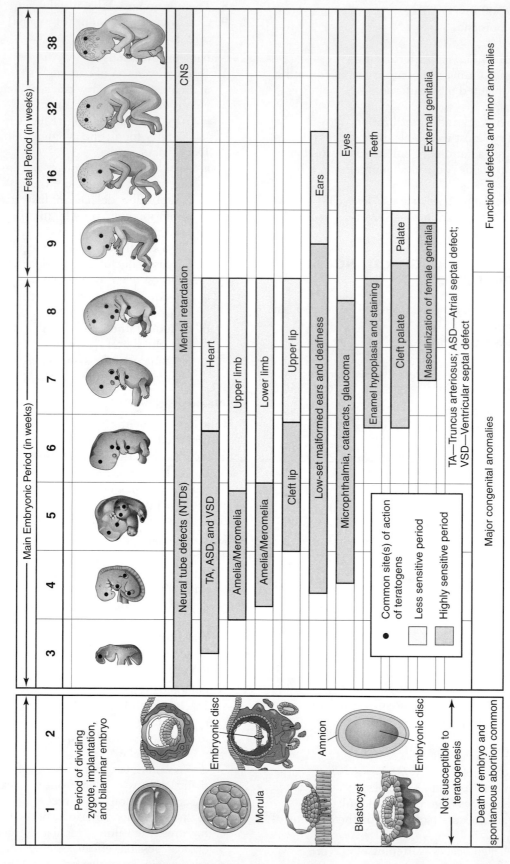

FIGURE 6-2 Sensitive, or critical, periods in human development. Dark color denotes highly sensitive periods; light color indicates stages that are less sensitive to teratogens. (From Moore K, Persaud T: *Before we are born: essentials of embryology and birth defects*, ed 7. St. Louis, 2008, Saunders.)

16 Weeks

A. Fetal development
1. Head still dominant, but face looks human and arm/leg ratio is proportionate
2. Scalp hair appears.
3. Meconium in bowel, and anus open
4. Most bones and joint cavities seen on ultrasound, and muscular movements detected
5. Heart muscle well developed, and blood formation active in spleen
6. Elastic fibers appear in lungs and terminal; respiratory bronchioles appear
7. Kidneys in position
8. Cerebral lobes delineated, and cerebellum assumes some prominence
9. General sense organs differentiated
10. Testes in position for descent into scrotum, or vagina open

B. Maternal changes
1. Quickening, the mother's first perception of fetal movement, may be noted between weeks 16 and 20.
2. Colostrum, the creamy white to yellowish premilk, may be expressed from the nipples as early as 16 weeks of gestation.
3. Serum cholesterol increases from 16 to 32 weeks of pregnancy and remains at this level until after birth.
4. By 14 to 16 weeks, the placenta is clearly defined.
5. Insulin resistance begins as early as 14 to 16 weeks of gestation and continues to rise until it stabilizes during the last few weeks of pregnancy.
6. Approximately weight gain of 1 lb per week beginning in the second trimester and continuing until delivery.

C. Nursing interventions
1. Explain the screening test, and obtain blood sample for maternal serum alpha-fetoprotein (MSAFP) between 15 and 22 weeks of gestation, ideally between 16 and 18 weeks of gestation.
   a. Elevated levels are associated with open neural tube defects and multiple gestations
   b. Low levels are associated with Down syndrome. Abnormal levels are followed by second-trimester ultrasonography for more in-depth investigation.
2. Explain the multiple-marker, or triple-screen, blood test, and obtain a specimen for screening between 16 and 18 weeks of gestation, to measure the MSAFP, human chorionic gonadotropin (hCG), and unconjugated estriol, the levels of which are combined to yield one value.
   a. Low levels may be associated with Down syndrome and other chromosomal abnormalities.

20 Weeks

A. Fetal development
1. Vernix protects the body.
2. Lanugo (fine hair) covers the body and protects body.
3. Eyebrows, eyelashes, and head hair develop.
4. Fetus sleeps, sucks, and kicks.
5. Fetus weighs 200 to 400 g (11 to 14 oz).

B. Maternal changes
1. Fundus reaches level of umbilicus.
2. Breasts begin secreting colostrum; areolae darken.
3. Amniotic sac holds approximately 400 ml of fluid.
4. Postural hypotension may occur.
5. Fetal movement felt (quickening); pregnancy becomes "real."
6. Nasal stuffiness may begin.
7. Leg cramps may begin.
8. Varicose veins may develop.
9. Constipation may develop.

C. Nursing interventions
1. Teach comfort measures.
   a. Encourage to remain active.
   b. Encourage to sit with feet elevated when possible.
   c. Teach to avoid pressure on lower thighs.
   d. Teach that use of support stockings may be helpful.
   e. Teach to dorsiflex foot to relieve leg cramps.
   f. Suggest applying heat to muscles affected by cramps.
   g. Suggest that cool-air vaporizer or saline nasal spray may help with nasal stuffiness.
2. Teach measures to avoid constipation.
   a. Encourage to eat raw fruits, vegetables, cereals with bran.
   b. Encourage to drink 3 L of fluid per day.
   c. Encourage to exercise frequently.

24 Weeks

A. Fetal development
1. Body fairly well proportioned; skin red and wrinkled; sweat glands forming
2. Blood formation increases in bone marrow and decreases in liver.
3. Alveolar ducts and sacs present, and lecithin begins to appear in amniotic fluid (weeks 26 to 27)
4. Neuronal proliferation in cerebral cortex ends
5. Can hear
6. Testes at inguinal ring in descent to scrotum

B. Maternal changes
1. Uterus rises to the level of the umbilicus.
2. Diastolic BP gradually increases at 24 to 32 weeks, after having decreased in the first trimester, and returns to prepregnancy levels by term. Systolic BP usually remains the same as the prepregnancy level.

C. Nursing interventions
1. Explain and obtain a blood sample for a glucose challenge that is usually done between 24 and 28 weeks' gestation.
2. At between 24 and 32 weeks' gestation, two or three ultrasound measurements may be taken 2 weeks apart to compare against standard fetal growth curves

28 Weeks

A. Fetal development
1. Fetus can breathe, swallow, and regulate temperature.
2. Surfactant forms in lungs.
3. Fetus can hear.
4. Fetus's eyelids open.
5. Period of greatest fetal weight gain begins.
6. Fetus weighs 1100 g (2½ lb).

B. Maternal changes
1. Fundus is halfway between umbilicus and xiphoid process.
2. Thoracic breathing replaces abdominal breathing.
3. Fetal outline is palpable.
4. Woman becomes more introspective and concentrates interest on the unborn child.
5. Heartburn may begin.
6. Hemorrhoids may develop.

C. Nursing interventions
1. Teach treatment of hemorrhoids.
   a. Suggest sitz baths.
   b. Suggest topical anesthetic agents.
   c. Suggest taking stool softeners as prescribed.
2. Teach comfort measures.
   a. Encourage woman to elevate legs when sitting.
   b. Suggest that woman assume side-lying position when resting.
3. Teach measures to avoid heartburn.
   a. Teach woman to eat small, frequent meals.
   b. Teach avoidance of fatty foods.
   c. Encourage woman to avoid lying down after meals.
   d. Teach that antacids may be prescribed.
   e. Teach woman to avoid sodium bicarbonate.
4. Prepare woman for delivery and parenthood.
   a. Discuss mother's, father's, and family's expectations of labor and delivery.
   b. Discuss mother's, father's, and family's expectations about caring for infant.
   c. Encourage woman to start childbirth-preparation classes.

32 Weeks

A. Fetal development
1. Brown fat deposits develop beneath skin to insulate baby following birth.
2. Fetus is 15 to 17 inches in length.
3. Fetus begins storing iron, calcium, and phosphorus.
4. Fetus weighs 1800 to 2200 g (4 to 5 lb).

B. Maternal changes
1. Fundus reaches xiphoid process.
2. Breasts are full and tender.
3. Urinary frequency returns.
4. Swollen ankles may occur.
5. Sleeping problems may develop.
6. Dyspnea may develop.

C. Nursing interventions
1. Teach measures to decrease edema.
   a. Encourage woman to elevate legs one or two times per day for approximately 1 hour.
2. Teach comfort measures.
   a. Encourage woman to wear well-fitting supportive bra.
   b. Encourage woman to maintain proper posture.
   c. Teach woman to use semi-Fowler position at night for dyspnea.
3. Prepare woman for childbirth.
   a. Review signs of labor.
   b. Discuss plans for other children (if any).
   c. Discuss plans for transportation to agency.
   d. Assess father's (family member's) role during childbirth.

36 to 40 Weeks

A. Fetal development
1. Fetus occupies entire uterus; activity is restricted.
2. Maternal antibodies are transferred to fetus (provide immunity for approximately 6 months, until infant's own immune system can take over).
3. L/S (lecithin/sphingomyelin) ratio is 2:1 and phosphatidylglycerol (PG) is present.
4. Fetus weighs 3200+ g (7+ lb).

B. Maternal changes
1. Lightening occurs.
2. Placenta weighs approximately 20 oz.
3. Mother is eager for birth, may have burst of energy.
4. Backaches increase.
5. Urinary frequency increases.
6. Braxton Hicks contractions intensify (cervix and lower uterine segment prepare for labor).

C. Nursing interventions
1. Teach safety measures.
   a. Teach to wear low-heeled shoes or flats.
   b. Instruct to avoid heavy lifting.
   c. Encourage sleeping on side to relieve bladder pressure and urinating frequently.
2. Encourage preparation for delivery.
   a. Teach woman to do pelvic tilt exercises.
   b. Encourage packing a suitcase.
   c. Encourage couple to tour labor and delivery area.
   d. Discuss postpartum circumstances: circumcision, rooming-in, possibility of postpartum blues, birth control, need for adequate rest, father's role.

Antepartum Nursing Care

PSYCHOSOCIAL RESPONSES TO PREGNANCY

Maternal Responses

A. First trimester
1. Ambivalence: whether pregnancy is planned or unplanned, ambivalence is normal.
2. Financial worries about increased responsibility are normal.
3. Career concerns may arise.

B. Second trimester
1. Quickening occurs and pregnancy becomes real.
2. Pregnant woman accepts pregnancy.
3. Ambivalence wanes.

C. Third trimester
1. Pregnant woman becomes introverted and self-absorbed.
2. Pregnant woman begins to ignore partner (may strain the relationship).

D. Throughout pregnancy
1. Wide mood swings (joy, anticipation, fear) occur.
2. Pregnant woman is ultrasensitive.
3. Strained relationship with partner may occur.

HESI Hint • Look for signs of maternal-fetal bonding during pregnancy; for example, talking to fetus in utero, massaging abdomen, and nicknaming fetus are all healthy psychosocial activities.

Paternal Responses

A. Announcement phase, acceptance of the biological fact of pregnancy
1. At the confirmation of pregnancy, men may react with joy or dismay, depending on whether the pregnancy is desired or unplanned or unwanted.
2. Ambivalence in the early stages of pregnancy is common.
3. Some men experience pregnancy-like symptoms, such as nausea, weight gain, and other physical symptoms, which is known as the *couvade syndrome*.
4. May last from a few hours to a few weeks

B. Moratorium phase, the period of adjustment to the reality of pregnancy
1. Accepts the pregnancy
2. May put conscious thought of the pregnancy aside for a time and become more introspective by engaging in many discussions about his philosophy of life, religion, childbearing, and childrearing practices and relationships with family members, particularly with his father.

3. This phase may be relatively short or persist until the last trimester, depending on the father's readiness for the pregnancy.

C. Focusing phase, active involvement in both the pregnancy and his relationship with his child
1. Negotiates with the mother the role he is to play in labor and to prepare for parenthood.
2. Concentrates on his experience of the pregnancy and begins to think of himself as a father.
3. Begins in the last trimester

ACTIVITIES DURING FIRST PRENATAL VISIT

A. Obtain history.
1. Medical history
2. Obstetric history
3. History of current pregnancy

HESI Hint • For many women, battering (emotional or physical abuse) begins during pregnancy. Women should be assessed for abuse in private, away from the male partner, by a nurse who is familiar with local resources and knows how to determine the safety of the client.

B. Determine gravidity and parity.
1. *Gravida* refers to the number of times a woman has been pregnant, regardless of the outcome.
2. *Para* refers to the number of deliveries (not children) that have occurred after 20 weeks of gestation.
3. When calculating parity, multiple births count as only one.
4. Pregnancy losses occurring before 20 weeks are counted as abortions (whether spontaneous or voluntary terminations) and add only to a client's gravidity count.
5. A fetal death after 20 weeks is added to the parity count.
6. TPAL (term births, preterm births, abortions [spontaneous or elective], and living children) may be calculated.

HESI Hint • Practice determining gravidity and parity. A woman who is 6 weeks pregnant has the following maternal history:
• She has a healthy 2-year-old, daughter.
• She had a miscarriage at 10 weeks.
• She had an elective abortion at 6 weeks, 5 years earlier.
• With this pregnancy, she is a gravida 4, para 1 (only 1 delivery after 20 weeks' gestation).
• GPAL is 4-1-0-2-1

C. Assist with physical examination.
D. Calculate gestational age: estimated date of birth (EDB) using the Nägele rule:
   1. Count back 3 months from the first day of the last normal menstrual period, and add 7 days.
   2. For example: if the LMP was March 23, the EDB would be December 30.

> **HESI Hint** • Practice calculating EDB. If the first day of a woman's last normal menstrual period was October 17, what is her EDB, using the Nägele rule? July 24. Count back 3 months and add 7 days (always give February 28 days).

E. Vital signs
   1. BP should rise no more than 30 points systolic and 15 points diastolic from previous baseline normal. Average BP is 90 to 140 mm Hg systolic and 60 to 90 mm Hg diastolic.
   2. Average pulse is 60 to 90 beats per minute (bpm).
   3. Average respiration is 16 to 24 breaths per minute (breaths/min).
   4. Average temperature is 97° to 100°F.
F. Future office visits
   1. Low-risk client's schedule is:
      a. Every 4 weeks until 28 weeks.
      b. Every 2 weeks from 28 weeks until 36 weeks.
      c. Every week from 36 weeks until delivery.
   2. High-risk client's schedule is determined by client's needs; visits are scheduled as necessary.
G. Obtain laboratory data (Appendix A, p. 375).
   1. Hgb: values during pregnancy >11
   2. Hct: values during pregnancy >33

> **HESI Hint** • At approximately 28 to 32 weeks' gestation, the maximum plasma volume increase of 25% to 40% occurs, resulting in normal hemodilution of pregnancy and Hct values of 32% to 42%. High Hct values may look good, but in reality they represent pregnancy-induced hypertension and a depleted vascular space.

   3. WBC and differential
   4. Hgb electrophoresis (sickle cell)
   5. Pap smear and cytology (gonorrhea and *Chlamydia*)
   6. Antibody screens
      a. HIV
      b. Hepatitis B
      c. Toxoplasmosis
      d. Rubella (>1:10 = immunity)
      e. Syphilis (RPR, VDRL)
      f. Cytomegalovirus
   7. Tuberculin skin testing (PPD)
   8. Rh and blood type
   9. Urinalysis

> **HESI Hint** • Hgb and Hct data can be used to evaluate nutritional status. Example: A 22-year-old primigravida at 12 weeks' gestation has an Hgb of 9.6 g/dL and an Hct of 31%. She has gained 3 pounds during the first trimester. A weight gain of 2 to 4 pounds during the first trimester is recommended, and this client is anemic. Supplemental iron and a diet higher in iron are needed.
>
> Foods high in iron:
> • Fish and red meats
> • Cereals and yellow vegetables
> • Green leafy vegetables and citrus fruits
> • Egg yolks and dried fruits

ACTIVITIES DURING SUBSEQUENT VISITS

A. Check urine.
   1. Albumin: no more than a trace in a normal finding (related to preeclampsia)
   2. Glucose: no more than 1+ in a normal finding (related to gestational diabetes)
   3. Protein: a trace amount of protein may be present in the urine; a higher presence may indicate contamination by vaginal secretions, kidney disease, or preeclampsia. ≥30 mg/dl (≥1+) on dipstick (mild preeclampsia); 2+ to 3+ protein on dipstick (severe preeclampsia)
B. Graph weight gain.
   1. 2 to 4 lb weight gain in the first trimester is recommended.
   2. 1 lb per week weight gain thereafter is recommended (>2 lb/week related to preeclampsia-edema).
   3. Total weight gain during the pregnancy should be between 25 and 35 pounds.
C. Check fundal height (Fig. 6-3).
   1. 12 to 13 weeks: fundus rises out of symphysis.
   2. From gestational weeks 18 to 32, the height of the fundus, measured in centimeters and with an empty bladder, is approximately the same as the number of weeks of gestation. Example: 24 weeks' gestation should be 24 cm when measured from the symphysis pubis to the top of the fundus.

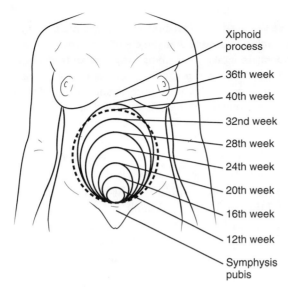

Xiphoid process

36th week
40th week
32nd week
28th week
24th week
20th week
16th week
12th week

Symphysis pubis

FIGURE 6-3 Fundal height assessment.

> **HESI Hint** • As pregnancy advances, the uterus presses on abdominal vessels (vena cava and aorta). Teach the woman that a left side-lying position relieves supine hypotension and increases perfusion to uterus, placenta, and fetus.

D. Check fetal heart rate.
1. 10 to 12 weeks: detectable by using Doppler
2. 15 to 20 weeks: detectable by using fetoscope
3. 110 to 160 bpm: normal range

> **HESI Hint** • Fetal well-being is determined by assessing fundal height, fetal heart tones and rate, fetal movement, and uterine activity (contractions). Changes in fetal heart rate are the first and most important indicators of compromised blood flow to the fetus, and these changes require action! Remember, the normal fetal heart rate is 110 to 160 bpm.

E. Teach the importance of continuing prenatal care.
F. Provide anticipatory guidance: first trimester
1. Discomforts such as nausea, fatigue, and urinary frequency subside after 13 weeks.
2. Sleep needs increase to 8 hr/day.
3. Rest periods should be planned.
4. Exercise is fine as long as woman is able to converse easily while exercising. If not, she should slow down.
5. Work is acceptable if there is no exposure to hazardous chemicals or toxins.
6. Bathing is acceptable until membranes rupture (usually within hours of delivery).

7. Travel by car is acceptable, but woman will need frequent breaks and must wear seat belt.
8. Air travel is acceptable, but policies vary with airline. Advise woman to remain well hydrated and to move about frequently to minimize the risk for thrombophlebitis
9. It is best to ingest no medications and no alcohol and to stop smoking.
G. Provide anticipatory guidance: second trimester
1. Sexual needs and desires may change for better or for worse. Encourage communication with partner regarding adjustments.
2. Encourage woman to have regular dental check-ups; to maintain dental hygiene (gum hypertrophy is common); and to delay radiographs and major dental work if possible.
H. Provide anticipatory guidance: third trimester:
1. Encourage woman to schedule childbirth classes.
2. Note that urinary frequency and dyspnea return.
3. Review interventions for leg cramps (dorsiflex foot), nasal stuffiness, varicose veins, and constipation.
4. Teach safety related to balance.
5. Teach about positioning with pillows for comfort.
6. Note that round-ligament pain will occur.
7. Instruct client to come to hospital when contractions are occurring regularly 5 minutes apart.
8. Provide information on feeding methods.
9. Encourage choosing a pediatrician and clinic.
10. Reinforce nutritional needs because third trimester is a period of rapid fetal growth.
11. Teach the risks and symptoms of preterm labor.

> **HESI Hint** • Teach clients to report immediately any of the following danger signs. Early intervention can optimize maternal and fetal outcome. Possible indications of preeclampsia and eclampsia are:
> • Visual disturbances
> • Swelling of face, fingers, or sacrum
> • Severe, continuous headache
> • Persistent vomiting
> • Infection. Signs include:
>   • Chills
>   • Temperature over 100.4°F
>   • Dysuria
>   • Pain in abdomen
> • Fluid discharge or bleeding from vagina (anything other than normal leukorrhea)
> • Change in fetal movement or increased fetal heart rate (FHR)

NUTRITION

Nursing Assessment

A. Diet
1. Ask client to recall diet for past 24 hours.
2. Use a questionnaire to determine individual deficiencies.
3. Determine body mass index (BMI).
4. Note symptoms of malnutrition:
   a. Glossitis
   b. Cracked lips
   c. Dry, brittle hair
B. Dental caries, periodontitis
C. Weight (those who weigh <100 lb or >200 lb are at risk)

Analysis (Nursing Diagnoses)

A. *Imbalanced nutrition: less than/more than body requirements* related to...
B. *Deficient knowledge* (specify) related to...

Nursing Plans and Interventions

A. Teach about minimum nutritional increases. Teach that client should:
1. Increase intake by 300 calories above basal and activity needs.
2. Increase protein by 30 g/day.
3. Increase intake of iron (30+ mg) and folic acid (800 to 1000 mcg) through diet and supplements.
4. Increase intake of vitamin A, vitamin C, and calcium through diet.

> **HESI Hint** • Most providers prescribe prenatal vitamins to ensure that the client receives an adequate intake of vitamins. However, only the health care provider can prescribe prenatal vitamins. It is the nurse's responsibility to teach about proper diet and about taking prescribed vitamins if they have been prescribed by the health care provider.

5. Drink a total of 8 to 10 glasses of fluid per day; 4 to 6 glasses should be water.
B. Relate recommended weight gain by trimester to fetal growth and fetal health.
1. Record weight at each visit, using graph.
2. Advise client to maintain steady weight gain of 1 lb/week in second and third trimesters.
C. Provide a copy of daily food guide to post on refrigerator (consider cultural food patterns in choices given). Include the following:
1. Three servings from dairy group (milk, cheese)
2. Five servings of protein (meats, eggs, legumes)
3. Five servings of vegetables (Green and deep yellow vegetables are good sources of vitamin C.)
4. Six servings of breads or cereals.
5. Four servings of fruit.
D. Advise regarding vitamin and iron supplementation.
E. Explain that poor nutrition can lead to anemia, preterm labor, obesity, and intrauterine growth restriction.

> **HESI Hint** • It is recommended that pregnant women consume the equivalent of 3 cups of milk or yogurt per day. This will ensure that the daily calcium needs are met and help to alleviate the occurrence of leg cramps.

Review of Anatomy and Physiology of Reproduction and Antepartum Nursing Care

1. State the objective signs that signify ovulation.
2. Ovulation occurs how many days before the next menstrual period?
3. State three ways to identify the chronological age of a pregnancy (gestation).
4. What maternal position provides optimum fetal and placental perfusion during pregnancy?
5. Name the major discomforts of the first trimester and one suggestion for amelioration of each.
6. If the first day of a woman's last normal menstrual period was May 28, what is the estimated date of birth (EDB) using the Nägele rule?
7. At 20 weeks' gestation, the fundal height would be_____; the fetus would weigh approximately _____ and would look like _____.
8. State the normal psychosocial responses to pregnancy in the second trimester.
9. The hemodilution of pregnancy peaks at _____ weeks and results in a/an _____ in a woman's Hct.
10. State three principles relative to the pattern of weight gain in pregnancy.
11. During pregnancy a woman should add _____ calories to her diet and drink _____ of milk per day.
12. Fetal heart rate can be auscultated by Doppler at _____ weeks' gestation.
13. Describe the schedule of prenatal visits for a low-risk pregnant woman.

Answers to Review

1. Abundant, thin, clear cervical mucus; spinnbarkeit (egg-white stretchiness) of cervical mucus; open cervical os; slight drop in basal body temperature and then 0.5° to 1°F rise; ferning under the microscope
2. 14 days
3. 10 lunar months; 9 calendar months consisting of three trimesters of 3 months each; 40 weeks; 280 days
4. The knee-chest position; but the ideal position of comfort for the mother, which supports fetal, maternal, and placental perfusion, is the side-lying position (removes pressure from the abdominal vessels [vena cava, aorta]).
5. Nausea and vomiting: crackers before rising; fatigue: rest periods and naps and 7 to 8 hours of sleep at night.
6. Count back 3 months and add 7 days: March 7 (Always give February 28 days.)
7. At the umbilicus; 300 to 400 g; a baby—with hair, lanugo, and vernix, but without any subcutaneous fat
8. Ambivalence wanes and acceptance of pregnancy occurs; pregnancy becomes "real"; signs of maternal-fetal bonding occur.
9. 28 to 32 weeks; decrease
10. Total gain should average 25 to 35 lb. Gain should be consistent throughout pregnancy. An average of 1 lb/week should be gained in the second and third trimesters.
11. 300; 3 cups
12. 10 to 12
13. Once every 4 weeks until 28 weeks; every 2 weeks from 28 to 36 weeks; then once a week until delivery

Fetal and Maternal Assessment Techniques

Description: Techniques used to obtain data regarding fetal and maternal physiologic status

A. Maternal risk factors include but are not limited to:
1. Age under 17 or over 34
2. High parity (>5)
3. Pregnancy (3 months since last delivery)
4. Hypertension, preeclampsia in current pregnancy
5. Anemia, history of hemorrhage, or current hemorrhage
6. Multiple gestations
7. Rh incompatibility
8. History of dystocia or previous operative delivery
9. A height of 60 inches (5 feet) or less
10. Malnutrition (15% under ideal weight) or extreme obesity (20% over ideal weight)
11. Medical disease during pregnancy (diabetes, hyperthyroidism, hyperemesis, clotting disorders such as thrombocytopenia)
12. Infection in pregnancy: toxoplasmosis, other agents, rubella, cytomegalovirus, herpes simplex (TORCH diseases); influenza; HIV; *Chlamydia*; human papillomavirus (HPV)
13. History of family violence, lack of social support

B. Various techniques are used to determine fetal and maternal well-being.

> **HESI Hint** • In some states, screening for neural tube defects by testing either maternal serum alpha-fetoprotein (AFP) levels or amniotic fluid AFP levels is mandated by state law. This screening test is highly associated with both false positives and false negatives.

ULTRASONOGRAPHY

Description: High-frequency sound waves are beamed onto the abdomen; echoes are returned to a machine that records the fetus's location and size.

A. Used in the first trimester to determine
1. Number of fetuses
2. Presence of fetal cardiac movement and rhythm
3. Uterine abnormalities
4. Gestational age

B. Used in the second and third trimesters to determine
1. Fetal viability and gestational age
2. Size-date discrepancies
3. Amniotic fluid volume
4. Placental location and maturity
5. Uterine anomalies and abnormalities
6. Results of amniocentesis

C. Findings
1. Fetal heart activity is apparent as early as 6 to 7 weeks' gestation.
2. Serial evaluation of biparietal diameter and limb length can differentiate between wrong dates and true intrauterine growth restriction (IUGR).

3. A biophysical profile (BPP) is made to ascertain fetal well-being.
   a. Five variables are assessed: fetal breathing movements, gross body movements, fetal tone, reactivity of fetal heart rate, and amniotic fluid volume.
   b. A score of 2 or 0 can be obtained for each variable. An overall score of 10 designates that the fetus is well on the day of the examination.
D. Nursing care
   1. Instruct the woman to drink 3 to 4 glasses of water prior to coming for examination and not to urinate. When the fetus is very small (in the first and second trimesters), the client's bladder must be full during the examination in order for the uterus to be supported for imaging. (A full bladder is not needed if ultrasound is done transvaginally instead of abdominally.)
   2. Position the woman with pillows under neck and knees to keep pressure off bladder; late in the third trimester, place wedge under right hip to displace uterus to the left.
   3. Position display so woman can watch if she wishes.
   4. Have bedpan or bathroom immediately available.
E. Complications
   1. There are no known complications.
   2. There is controversy regarding routine use of ultrasound in pregnancy.

> **HESI Hint** • Gestational age is best determined by an early sonogram rather than a later one.

CHORIONIC VILLI SAMPLING (CVS)

Description: Removal of a small piece of villi during the period between 8 and 12 weeks' gestation under ultrasound guidance (cannot replace amniocentesis completely because no sample of amniotic fluid can be obtained for AFP or Rh disease testing)

A. Findings
   1. The test determines genetic diagnosis early in the first trimester.
   2. The results are obtained in 1 week.
B. Nursing care
   1. Have informed consent signed before any procedure.
   2. Place woman in lithotomy position using stirrups.
   3. Warn of slight sharp pain upon catheter insertion.
   4. Results should not be given over the phone.

C. Complications
   1. Spontaneous abortion (5%)
   2. Controversy regarding fetal anomalies (limb)

AMNIOCENTESIS

Description: Removal of amniotic fluid sample from uterus as early as 14 to 16 weeks

A. Is used to determine:
   1. Fetal genetic diagnosis (usually in the first trimester)
   2. Fetal lung maturity (last trimester)
   3. Fetal well-being
B. Is performed when uterus rises out of symphysis at 13 weeks and amniotic fluid has formed
C. Usually takes 10 days to 2 weeks to develop cultured cell karyotype. Therefore, woman could be well into second trimester before diagnosis is made, making choice for abortion more dangerous.
D. Findings
   1. Genetic disorders
      a. Karyotype: determines Down syndrome (trisomy 21), other trisomies, and sex chromatin (sex-linked disorders)
      b. Biochemical analysis: determines more than 60 types of metabolic disorders (Tay-Sachs)
      c. AFP: elevations may be associated with neutral tube defects; low levels may indicate trisomy 21
   2. Fetal lung maturity
      a. L:S ratio: 2:1 ratio indicates fetal lung maturity unless mother is diabetic or has Rh disease, or fetus is septic.
      b. L:S ratio and presence of PG: most accurate determination of fetal maturity. PG is present after 35 weeks' gestation.
      c. Lung maturity is the best predictor of extrauterine survival.
      d. Creatinine: renal maturity indicator >1.8
      e. Orange-staining cells: lipid-containing exfoliating sebaceous gland maturity; >20% stained orange means 35 weeks or more.
   3. Fetal well-being
      a. Bilirubin delta optical density (OD) assessment should be performed in mother previously sensitized to the fetal Rh+ RBCs and having antibodies to the RH+ circulating cells. The delta OD test measures the change in optical density of the amniotic fluid caused by staining with bilirubin. Done at 24 weeks' gestation.
      b. Meconium in amniotic fluid may indicate fetal distress.
E. Nursing care
   1. Obtain baseline vital signs and FHR.

2. Place client in supine position with hands across chest.

3. If prescribed, shave area and scrub with povidone-iodine (Betadine).

4. Draw maternal blood sample for comparison with postprocedure blood sample to determine maternal bleeding.

5. Provide emotional support, explain procedure, stay with the client (do not leave her alone).

6. Label samples; if bilirubin test is prescribed, darken room and immediately cover the tubes with aluminum foil or use opaque tubes.

7. After specimen is drawn, wash abdomen; assist woman to empty bladder. A full bladder can irritate the uterus and cause contractions.

8. Monitor FHR for 1 hour after procedure, and assess for uterine contractions and irritability.

9. Instruct woman to report any contractions, change in fetal movement, or fluid leaking from vagina.

F. Complications
1. Spontaneous abortion (1%)
2. Fetal injury
3. Infection

HESI Hint • When an amniocentesis is done in early pregnancy, the bladder must be full to help support the uterus and to help push the uterus up in the abdomen for easy access. When an amniocentesis is done in late pregnancy, the bladder must be empty so it will not be punctured.

ELECTRONIC FETAL MONITORING

Variables Measured by Fetal Monitoring

A. Contractions
1. Beginning, peak (acme), and end of each contraction
2. Duration: length of each contraction from beginning to end
3. Frequency: beginning of one contraction to beginning of the next (Three to five contractions must be measured.)
4. Intensity: measured not by external monitoring but in mm Hg by internal (intrauterine) monitoring after amniotic membranes have ruptured; ranges from 30 mm Hg (mild) to 70 mm Hg (strong) at peak.

B. Baseline FHR
1. The range of FHR (average 110 to 160 bpm) between contractions, monitored over a 10-minute period
2. The balance between parasympathetic and sympathetic impulses usually produces no observable changes in the FHR during uterine contractions (with a healthy fetus, a healthy placenta, and good uteroplacental perfusion; Fig. 6-4).

Nursing Actions Based on Fetal Heart Rate

A. Baseline FHR
1. Normal rhythmicity
2. Average FHR 110 to 160 bpm

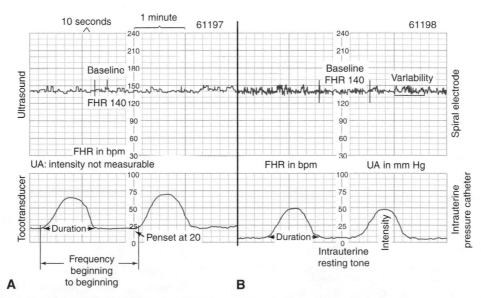

FIGURE 6-4 Fetal heart rate and uterine activity. Display of fetal heart rate and uterine activity on chart paper. *A*, External mode with ultrasound and tocotransducer as signal course. *B*, Internal mode with spiral electrode and intrauterine catheter as signal source. Frequency of contractions is measured from the beginning of one contraction to the beginning of the next. Peak-to-peak measurement is sometimes used when electronic uterine activity monitoring is done. (From Tucker SM: *Pocket guide to fetal monitoring and assessment*, ed 6. St. Louis, 2009, Mosby.)

3. Description
   a. The FHR results from the balance between the parasympathetic and the sympathetic branches of the autonomic nervous system.
   b. It is the most important indicator of the health of the fetal central nervous system (CNS).

B. Variability
   1. A characteristic of the baseline FHR and described as normal irregularity of the cardiac rhythm. (Note: The NICHD definitions no longer distinguish between long and short term variability since they occur together).
   2. There are four categories of variability:
      a. absent - amplitude range undetectable
      b. minimal - amplitude range detectable up to and including 5 beats/min
      c. moderate - amplitude range of 6 to 25 beats/min
      d. marked - amplitude range >25 beats/min.

C. Nursing actions
   1. Assess contractions using monitor strip.
   2. Assess FHR for normal baseline range and variability.

D. Periodic changes
   1. FHR changes in relation to uterine contractions (Fig. 6-5).
   2. Description:
      a. Accelerations
         (1) Caused by sympathetic fetal response
         (2) Occur in response to fetal movement
         (3) Indicative of a reactive, healthy fetus
      b. Early decelerations (Fig. 6-6)
         (1) Benign pattern caused by parasympathetic response (head compression)
         (2) Heart rate slowly and smoothly decelerates at beginning of contraction and returns to baseline at end of contraction.

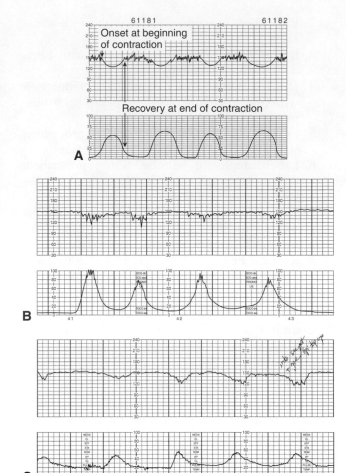

FIGURE 6-6 *A,* Early deceleration (illustration, with key points identified). *B* and *C,* Early decelerations (actual tracings). (From Tucker SM: *Pocket guide to fetal monitoring and assessment,* ed. 6, St. Louis, 2009, Mosby.)

E. Nursing actions for early decelerations
   1. No nursing interventions are required except to monitor the progress of labor.
   2. Document the processes of labor.

Nonreassuring Warning Signs

A. Variability (Fig. 6-7)
   1. FHR is absent or minimal.
   2. Causes:
      a. Hypoxia (asphyxia)
      b. Acidosis
      c. Maternal drug ingestion (narcotics, CNS depressants such as magnesium sulfate)
      d. Fetal sleep

B. Bradycardia
   1. Baseline FHR is below 110 bpm (assessed between contractions) for 10 minutes (as differentiated from a periodic change).

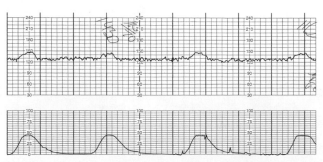

FIGURE 6-5 Periodic accelerations with uterine contractions. (From Tucker SM: *Pocket guide to fetal monitoring and assessment,* ed. 6, St. Louis, 2009, Mosby.)

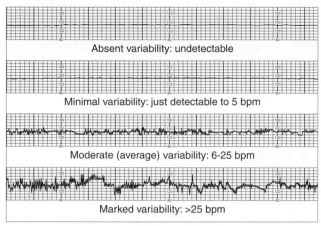

FIGURE 6-7 Classification of variability. (From Tucker SM: *Pocket guide to fetal monitoring and assessment*, ed. 6, St. Louis, 2009, Mosby.)

2. Causes:
  a. Late manifestation of fetal hypoxia
  b. Medication-induced (narcotics, MgSO₄)
  c. Maternal hypotension
  d. Fetal heart block
  e. Prolonged umbilical cord compression

C. Tachycardia
  1. Baseline FHR is above 160 bpm (assessed between contractions) for 10 minutes.
  2. Causes:
   a. Early sign of fetal hypoxia
   b. Fetal anemia
   c. Dehydration
   d. Maternal infection, maternal fever
   e. Maternal hyperthyroid disease
   f. Medication-induced (atropine, ritodrine, terbutaline, hydroxyzine)

D. Nursing actions for decreased variability, bradycardia, and tachycardia:
  a. Treatment is based on cause.

E. Variable deceleration pattern (Figure 6-8)
  1. It is the most common periodic pattern.
  2. It occurs in 40% of all labors and is caused mainly by cord compression but can also indicate rapid fetal descent. It is characterized by an abrupt transitory decrease in the FHR that is variable in duration, depth of fall, and timing relative to the contraction cycle.
  3. An occasional variable is usually benign.

F. Nursing actions for variable decelerations:
  1. Change maternal position.
  2. Stimulate fetus if indicated.
  3. Discontinue oxytocin if infusing.
  4. Administer oxygen at 10 L by tight face mask.
  5. Perform a vaginal examination to check for cord prolapse.
  6. Report findings to physician and document.

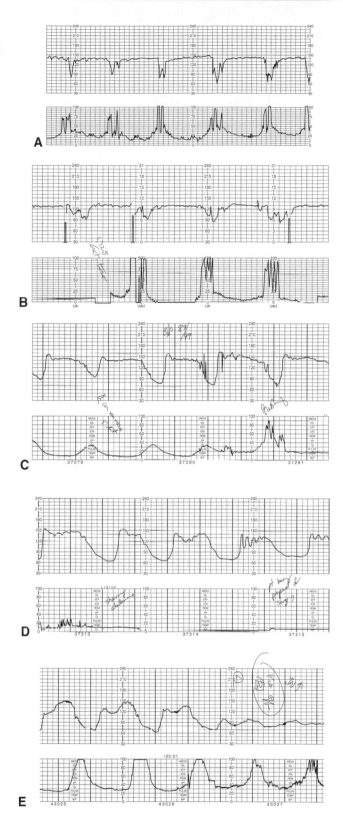

FIGURE 6-8 Variable decelerations. Note the progression in severity from panel *A* to panel *E*, with overshoots and decreasing variability and eventually a prolonged and smooth deceleration (actual tracings). (From Tucker SM: *Pocket guide to fetal monitoring and assessment*, ed. 6, St. Louis, 2009, Mosby.)

Nonreassuring (Ominous) Signs

A. Severe variable decelerations
1. FHR below 70 bpm lasting longer than 30 to 60 seconds
2. Slow return to baseline
3. Decreasing or absent variability

B. Late decelerations (Fig. 6-9)
1. An ominous and potentially disastrous nonreassuring sign
2. Indicative of uteroplacental insufficiency (UPI)
3. The shape of the deceleration is uniform, and the FHR returns to baseline after the contraction is over.
4. The depth of the deceleration does not indicate severity; rarely falls below 100 bpm.

C. Nursing actions
1. Immediately turn client onto left side.
2. Discontinue oxytocin if infusing.
3. Administer oxygen at 10 L by tight face mask.
4. Assist with fetal blood sampling if indicated.
5. Maintain intravenous line, and if possible, elevate legs to increase venous return.

6. Correct any underlying hypotension by increasing IV rate or with prescribed medications.
7. Determine presence of FHR variability.
8. Notify health care provider.
9. Document pattern and response to each nursing action.

HESI Hint • Early decelerations, caused by head compression and fetal descent, usually occur between 4 and 7 cm and in the second stage of labor. Check for labor progress if early decelerations are noted (Fig. 6-10A).

HESI Hint • If cord prolapse is detected, the examiner should position the mother to relieve pressure on the cord (i.e., knee-chest position) or push the presenting part off the cord until immediate cesarean delivery can be accomplished.

HESI Hint • Late decelerations indicate uteroplacental insufficiency and are associated with conditions such as postmaturity, preeclampsia, diabetes mellitus, cardiac disease, and abruptio placentae (Fig. 6-10B).

HESI Hint • When deceleration patterns (late or variable) are associated with decreased or absent variability and tachycardia, the situation is ominous (potentially disastrous) and requires immediate intervention and fetal assessment.

HESI Hint • A decrease in uteroplacental perfusion results in late decelerations; cord compression results in a pattern of variable decelerations (Fig. 6-10C). Nursing interventions should include changing maternal position, discontinuing Pitocin infusion, administering oxygen, and notifying the health care provider.

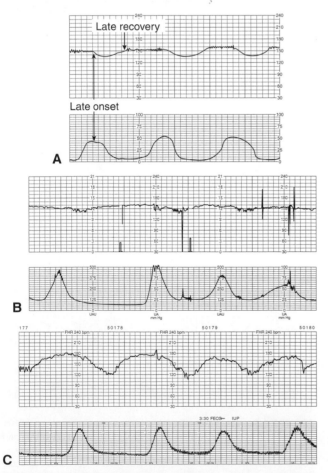

FIGURE 6-9 *A,* Late decelerations (illustration, with key points identified). *B* and *C,* Late decelerations (actual tracings). (From Tucker SM: *Pocket guide to fetal monitoring and assessment,* ed. 6, St. Louis, 2009, Mosby.)

ADDITIONAL ANTEPARTUM TESTS

A. Nonstress test
1. Description
   a. It is used to determine fetal well-being in high-risk pregnancy and especially useful in postmaturity (notes response of the fetus to its own movements).

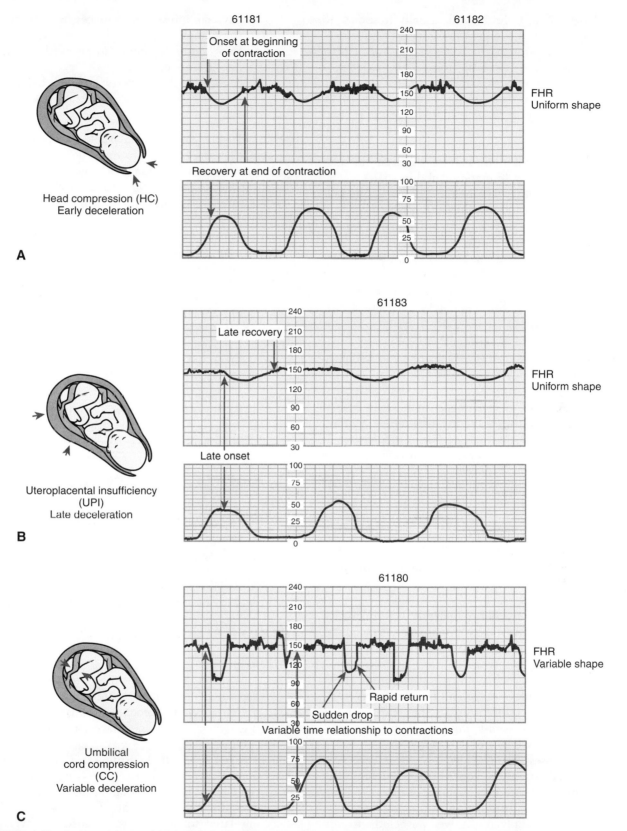

61181   61182

Onset at beginning
of contraction

FHR
Uniform shape

Recovery at end of contraction

Head compression (HC)
Early deceleration

A

Uteroplacental insufficiency
(UPI)
Late deceleration

B

61183

Late recovery

FHR
Uniform shape

Late onset

Umbilical
cord compression
(CC)
Variable deceleration

C

61180

FHR
Variable shape

Rapid return

Sudden drop

Variable time relationship to contractions

FIGURE 6-10 Review of fetal variability. *A,* Early decelerations caused by head compression. *B,* Late decelerations caused by uteroplacental insufficiency. *C,* Variable decelerations caused by cord compression. (From Tucker SM: *Pocket guide to fetal monitoring and assessment,* ed 6. St. Louis, 2009, Mosby.)

b. A healthy fetus will usually respond to its own movement by means of an FHR acceleration of 15 beats, lasting for at least 15 seconds after the movement, twice in a 20-minute period.

c. The fetus that responds with the 15/15 acceleration is considered "reactive" and healthy.

2. Nursing care

a. Apply fetal monitor, ultrasound, and tocodynamometer to maternal abdomen.

b. Give mother handheld event marker, and instruct her to push the button whenever fetal movement is felt or recorded as FM on the fetal heart rate strip.

c. Monitor client for 20 to 30 minutes, observing for reactivity.

d. Suspect fetus is sleeping if there is no fetal movement. Stimulate fetus acoustically or physically, or have mother move fetus around and begin test again.

B. Contraction stress test (CST) or oxytocin challenge test (OCT)

1. Description

a. The fetus is challenged with the stress of labor by the induction of uterine contractions, and the fetal response to physiologically decreased oxygen supply during uterine contractions is noted.

b. An unhealthy fetus will develop nonreassuring fetal heart rate patterns in response to uterine contractions; late decelerations are indicative of UPI.

c. Contractions can be induced by nipple stimulation or by infusing a dilute solution of oxytocin.

2. Nursing care

a. Assess for contraindications: prematurity, placenta previa, hydramnios, multiple gestation, and previous uterine classical scar, rupture of membranes.

b. Place external monitors on abdomen (FHR ultrasound monitor and tocodynamometer).

c. Record a 20-minute baseline strip to determine fetal well-being (reactivity) and presence or absence of contractions.

d. To assess for fetal well-being, a recording of at least three contractions in 10 minutes must be obtained.

e. If nipple stimulation is attempted, have woman apply warm, wet washcloths to nipples and roll the nipple of one breast for 10 minutes. Begin rolling both nipples if contractions do not begin in 10 minutes. Proceed with oxytocin infusion if unsuccessful with nipple stimulation.

f. Exogenous oxytocin can be used to stimulate uterine contractions.

g. A negative test suggests fetal well-being (i.e., no occurrence of late decelerations).

> **HESI Hint** • The danger of nipple stimulation lies in controlling the "dose" of oxytocin delivered by the posterior pituitary. The chance of hyperstimulation or tetany (contractions over 90 seconds or contractions with less than 30 seconds in between) is increased.

C. Biophysical profile (BPP)

1. Description

a. Ultrasonography is used to evaluate fetal health by assessing five variables:
   (1) Fetal breathing movements (FBM)
   (2) Gross body movements (FM)
   (3) Fetal tone (FT)
   (4) Reactive fetal heart rate (nonstress test)
   (5) Qualitative amniotic fluid volume (AFV)

b. Each variable receives 2 points for a normal response or 0 points for an abnormal or absent response.

2. Nursing care

a. Prepare client for procedure.

b. Inform client of purpose of examination.

c. Provide psychological support, especially if testing will continue throughout the pregnancy.

d. Advise client that a low score indicates fetal compromise that would warrant more detailed investigation.

e. A score of 8-10 indicates fetal well-being

FETAL PH BLOOD SAMPLING

A. Description

1. This technique is performed only in the intrapartum period when the fetal blood from the presenting part (breech or scalp) can be taken (i.e., when membranes have ruptured and the cervix is dilated 2 to 3 cm).

2. The test is used to determine true acidosis when nonreassuring fetal heart rate is noted (late decelerations, severe variable decelerations unresponsive to treatment, decreased variability unrelated to nonasphyxial causes, tachycardia unrelated to maternal variables).

3. Because fetal blood gas values vary rapidly with transient circulatory changes, this test is

usually done only in tertiary centers that have the capability of repetitive sampling and rapid results.

B. Nursing care
1. Place client in lithotomy position at end of labor bed, and prepare with perineal cleansing and sterile draping.
2. Assist the health care provider by gathering sterile supplies and providing ice in cup or emesis basin to carry pipette filled with blood to unit's pH machine or to lab.

> **HESI Hint** • Percutaneous umbilical blood sampling (PUBS) can be done during pregnancy under ultrasound for prenatal diagnosis and therapy. Hemoglobinopathies, clotting disorders, sepsis, and some genetic testing can be done using this method.

> **HESI Hint** • The most import determinant of fetal maturity for extrauterine survival is the lung maturity:lung surfactant (L:S) ratio (2:1 or higher).

Review of Fetal and Maternal Assessment Techniques

1. Name five maternal variables associated with diagnosis of a high-risk pregnancy.
2. Is one ultrasound examination useful in determining the presence of IUGR?
3. What does the biophysical profile (BPP) determine?
4. List three necessary nursing actions prior to an ultrasound examination for a woman in the first trimester of pregnancy.
5. State the advantage of CVS over amniocentesis.
6. Why are serum or amniotic AFP levels done prenatally?
7. What is the most important determinant of fetal maturity for extrauterine survival?
8. Name the three most common complications of amniocentesis.
9. Name the four periodic changes of the FHR, their causes, and one nursing treatment for each.
10. What is the most important indicator of fetal autonomic nervous system integrity and health?
11. Name four causes of decreased FHR variability.
12. State the most important action to take when a cord prolapse is determined.
13. What is a reactive nonstress test?
14. What are the dangers of the nipple-stimulation stress test?
15. Normal fetal scalp pH in labor is _____, and values below _____ indicate true acidosis.

Answers to Review

1. Age (under 17 or over 34 years of age); parity (over 5); <3 months between pregnancies; diagnosis of preeclampsia, diabetes mellitus, or cardiac disease
2. No. Serial measurements are needed to determine IUGR.
3. Fetal well-being
4. Have client fill bladder. Do not allow client to void. Position client supine and with uterine wedge.
5. Can be done between 8 and 12 weeks' gestation, with results returned within 1 week, which allows for decision about termination while still in first trimester.
6. To determine whether AFP levels are elevated, which may indicate the presence of neural tube defects; or whether they are low, which may indicate trisomy 21.
7. L:S ratio (lung maturity, lung surfactant development)
8. Spontaneous abortion, fetal injury, infection
9. Accelerations are caused by a burst of sympathetic activity; they are reassuring and require no treatment. Early decelerations are caused by head compression; they are benign and alert the nurse to monitor for labor progress and fetal descent. Variable decelerations are caused by cord compression; change of position should be tried first. Late decelerations are caused by UPI and should be treated by placing client on her side and administering oxygen.
10. Fetal heart rate variability
11. Hypoxia, acidosis, drugs, fetal sleep
12. Examiner should position mother to relieve pressure on the cord or push the presenting part off the cord with fingers until emergency delivery is accomplished.
13. FHR acceleration of 15 bpm for 15 seconds in response to fetal movement
14. The inability to control oxytocin "dosage" and the chance of tetany/hyperstimulation
15. 7.25 to 7.35; 7.2

Intrapartum Nursing Care

Description: Begins with true labor and consists of four stages

A. First stage of labor: From the beginning of regular contractions or rupture of membranes to 10 cm of dilatation and 100% effacement (Table 6-1)

B. Second stage of labor: 10 cm to delivery of the fetus

C. Third stage of labor: Delivery of the fetus to delivery of the placenta

D. Fourth stage of labor: arbitrarily lasts about 2 hours after delivery of the placenta (recovery)

INITIAL EXAMINATION

> **HESI Hint** • Be able differentiate true labor from false labor.
>
> **True Labor:**
> • Pain in lower back that radiates to abdomen
> • Pain accompanied by regular rhythmic contractions
> • Contractions that intensify with ambulation
> • Progressive cervical dilatation and effacement
>
> **False Labor:**
> • Discomfort localized in abdomen
> • No lower back pain
> • Contractions decrease in intensity or frequency with ambulation

Nursing Assessment

A. Prodromal labor signs include the following:
1. Lightening (fetus drops into true pelvis)
2. Braxton Hicks contractions (practice contractions)
3. Cervical softening and slight effacement
4. Bloody show or expulsion of mucous plug
5. Burst of energy, "nesting instinct"

B. Determine the following:
1. Gravidity and parity >5 (grand multiparity)
2. Gestational age 38 to 40 weeks (term gestation)
3. FHR best heard over fetal back (Fig. 6-11 and Box 6-1)
4. Maternal vital signs
5. Contraction frequency, intensity, and duration

C. Perform vaginal examination to determine
1. Fetal presentation and position
2. Cervical dilatation, effacement, position, and consistency
3. Fetal station

D. Assess the client for
1. Status of membranes (ruptured or intact)
2. Urine glucose and albumin data
3. Comfort level
4. Labor and delivery preparation
5. Presence of support person
6. Presence of true or false labor

Vaginal Examination

A. It is preceded by antiseptic cleansing, with client in modified lithotomy position.
1. Sterile gloves are worn.
2. Examinations are not done routinely. They are sharply curtailed after membranes rupture so as to prevent infection.

TABLE 6-1 First Stage of Labor

Phase	Description	Psychological and Physical Responses
• Latent	• From beginning of true labor until 3 to 4 cm cervical dilatation	• Mildly anxious, conversant • Able to continue usual activities • Contractions mild, initially 10 to 20 minutes apart, 15 to 20 seconds' duration; later 5 to 7 minutes apart, 30 to 40 seconds' duration
• Active	• From 4 to 7 cm cervical dilatation	• Increased anxiety • Increased discomfort • Unwillingness to be left alone • Contractions moderate to severe, 2 to 3 minutes apart, 30 to 60 seconds' duration
• Transition	• From 8 to 10 cm cervical dilatation	• Changed behavior • Sudden nausea, hiccups • Extreme irritability and unwillingness to be touched, although desirous of companionship • Contractions severe, 1½ minutes apart, 60 to 90 seconds' duration

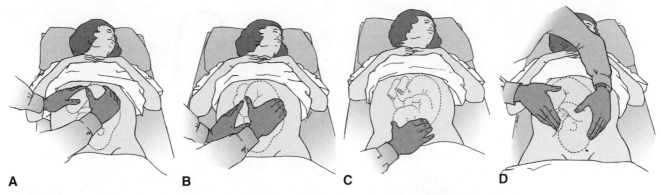

FIGURE 6-11   Leopold maneuvers. (From Lowdermilk DL, Perry SE: *Maternity nursing*, ed 9. St. Louis, 2010, Mosby.)

BOX 6-1   *Leopold Maneuvers*

Description: Abdominal palpations used to determine fetal presentation, lie, position, and engagement

A. With client in supine position, place both cupped hands over fundus and palpate to determine whether breech (soft, immovable, large) or vertex (hard, movable, small).

B. Place one hand firmly on side and palpate with other hand to determine presence of small parts or fetal back. (Fetal heart rate is heard best through fetal back.)

C. Facing client, grasp the area over the symphysis with the thumb and fingers and press to determine the degree of descent of the presenting part. (A ballotable or floating head can be rocked back and forth between the thumb and fingers.)

D. Facing the client's feet, outline the fetal presenting part with the palmar surface of both hands to determine the degree of descent and attitude of the fetus. (If cephalic prominence is located on the same side as small parts, assume the head is flexed.)

3. Examinations are performed
   a. Prior to analgesia and anesthesia
   b. To determine the progress of labor
   c. To determine whether second-stage pushing can begin

B. The purpose of a vaginal examination is to determine:
   1. Cervical dilation: cervix opens from 0 to 10 cm
   2. Cervical effacement: cervix is taken up into the upper uterine segment; expressed in percentages from 0% to 100%. Cervix is "shortened" from 3 cm to <0.5 cm in length; often called "thinning of the cervix," a misnomer
   3. Cervical position: cervix can be directly anterior and palpated easily or posterior and difficult to palpate.
   4. Cervical consistency: it is firm to soft.

C. Fetal station: location of presenting part in relation to midpelvis or ischial spines; expressed as cm above or below the spines (Fig. 6-12)
   1. Station 0 is engaged.
   2. Station −2 is 2 cm above the ischial spines.

D. Fetal presentation: the part of the fetus that presents to the inlet (Fig. 6-13):
   1. Vertex (head, cephalic)
   2. Shoulder (acromion)
   3. Breech (buttocks)
   4. Other variations include brow (sinciput) and chin (mentum)

E. Fetal position: The relationship of the point of reference (occiput, sacrum, acromion) on the fetal presenting part (vertex, breech, shoulder) to the mother's pelvis. Most common is LOA (left occiput anterior). The point of reference on the vertex (occiput) is pointed up toward the symphysis

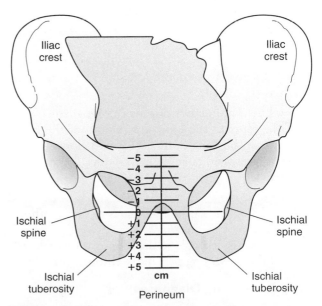

FIGURE 6-12   Fetal stations. Stations of presenting part, or degree of descent. The lowermost portion of the presenting part is at the level of the ischial spines, station 0. (From Lowdermilk DL, Perry SE: *Maternity nursing*, ed 9. St. Louis, 2010, Mosby.)

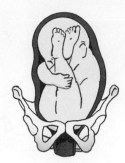

Frank breech

Lie: Longitudinal or vertical
Presentation: Breech (incomplete)
Presenting part: Sacrum
Attitude: Flexion, except for legs at knees

A

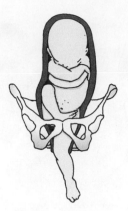

Single footling breech

Lie: Longitudinal or vertical
Presentation: Breech (incomplete)
Presenting part: Sacrum
Attitude: Flexion, except for one leg extended
at hip and knee

B

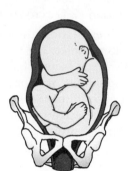

Complete breech

Lie: Longitudinal or vertical
Presentation: Breech (sacrum and feet presenting)
Presenting part: Sacrum (with feet)
Attitude: General flexion

C

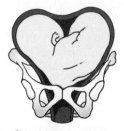

Shoulder presentation

Lie: Transverse or horizontal
Presentation: Shoulder
Presenting part: Scapula
Attitude: Flexion

D

FIGURE 6-13 Fetal presentations. *A, B, C,* Breech (sacral) presentation. *D,* Shoulder presentation. (From Lowdermilk DL, Perry SE: *Maternity nursing,* ed 9. St. Louis, 2010, Mosby.)

and directed toward the left side of the maternal pelvis (Fig. 6-14).

F. Fetal lie: The relationship of the long axis (spine) of the fetus to the long axis (spine) of the mother. It can be longitudinal (up and down), transverse (perpendicular), or oblique (slanted; see Fig. 6-13).

G. Fetal attitude
   1. Relationship of the fetal parts to one another
   2. Flexion or extension
   3. Flexion is desirable so that the smallest diameters of the presenting part move through the pelvis.

Analysis (Nursing Diagnoses)

A. *Deficient knowledge (labor/delivery)* related to…

B. *Acute pain* related to…

C. *Anxiety* related to…

HESI Hint • It is important to know the normal findings for a client in labor:
• Normal FHR in labor: 110 to 160 bpm
• Normal maternal BP: <140/90
• Normal maternal pulse: <100 bpm
• Normal maternal temperature: <100.4°F
• Slight elevation in temperature may occur because of dehydration and the work of labor. Anything higher indicates infection and must be reported immediately.

Nursing Plans and Interventions

A. Determine FHR (auscultation schedule).
   1. FHR every 30 minutes in early latent stage
   2. FHR every 15 to 30 minutes in midactive stage
   3. FHR every 15 minutes in transition stage

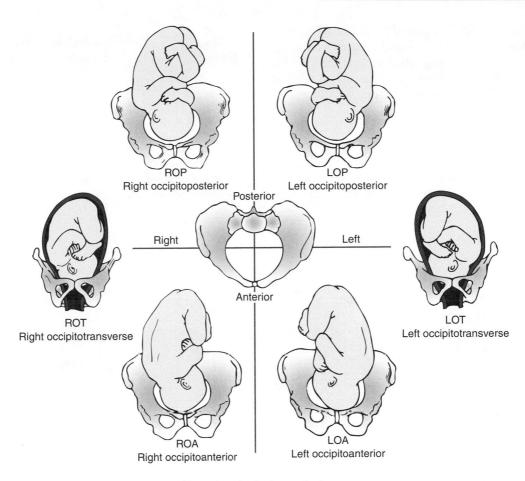

ROP
Right occipitoposterior

LOP
Left occipitoposterior

Posterior

Right   Left

Anterior

ROT
Right occipitotransverse

LOT
Left occipitotransverse

ROA
Right occipitoanterior

LOA
Left occipitoanterior

Lie: Longitudinal or vertical
Presentation: Vertex
Reference point: Occiput
Attitude: Complete flexion

FIGURE 6-14 Fetal positions. Examples of fetal vertex (occiput) presentations in relation to front, back, or side of maternal pelvis. (From Lowdermilk DL, Perry SE: *Maternity nursing,* ed 9. St. Louis, 2010, Mosby.)

B. Assess maternal vital signs.
  1. Take BP *between* contractions, in side-lying position at least every hour unless abnormal (BP increases during contractions).
  2. Take temperature every 4 hours until membranes rupture, then every hour.
C. Explain all activities and procedures to mother and support person.
D. Determine birth plan and desires for:
  1. Analgesia and anesthesia
  2. Delivery situation

HESI Hint • If infant's head is floating, watch for cord prolapse.

E. Assess urine every 8 hours unless abnormal. Normal findings:
  1. Protein (<trace)
  2. Glucose (1+ or less)

F. Assess contractions when assessing FHR.
  1. *Frequency.* Time contractions from beginning of one contraction to the beginning of the next (measured in minutes apart).
  2. *Duration.* Time the length of the entire contraction (from beginning to end).
  3. *Strength.* Assess the intensity of strongest part (peak) of contraction. It is measured by clinical estimation of the indentability of the fundus (use gentle pressure of fingertips to determine it):
    a. Very indentable (mild)
    b. Moderately indentable (moderate)
    c. Unindentable (firm)
  4. *Norms.* Contraction frequency, duration, and intensity vary with the stage of labor.
G. If membranes or bag of waters (BOW) has ruptured:
  1. Nitrazine paper turns black or dark blue.
  2. Vaginal fluid ferns under microscope.
  3. Color and amount of amniotic fluid should be noted.

4. Woman should be allowed to ambulate during labor only if the FHR is within a normal range and if the fetus is engaged (zero station). If the fetus is not engaged, there is an increased risk that a prolapsed cord will occur.

H. Begin graph of labor progress (Friedman graph; Fig. 6-15).
   1. Prolonged latent phase lasts >20 hours in primigravida, >14 hours in multipara.
   2. A primigravida dilates an average of 1.2 cm/hr in the midactive phase; a multipara, 1.5 cm/hr.

HESI Hint • Meconium-stained fluid is yellow-green or gold-yellow and may indicate fetal stress

I. Take client to bathroom or offer bedpan at least every 2 hours during labor (a full bladder can impede labor progress).

J. Assist woman with use of psychoprophylactic coping techniques, such as breathing exercises and effleurage (abdominal massage).

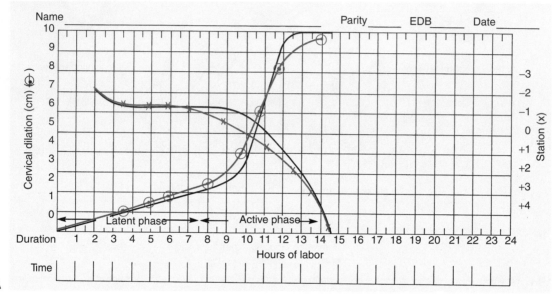

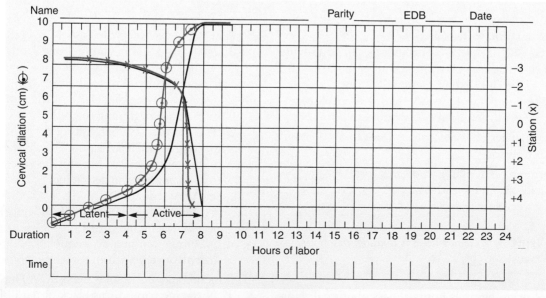

FIGURE 6-15 Labor graph. Partogram for assessment of patterns of cervical dilatation and descent. Individual woman's labor patterns (colored) are superimposed on labor graph (black) for comparison. *A*, Nulliparous labor. *B*, Multiparous labor. The rate of cervical dilatation is indicated by the symbol O. A line drawn through the symbols depicts the slope of the curve. Station is indicated by an X. A line drawn through the Xs reveals the pattern of descent. (From Lowdermilk DL, Perry SE: *Maternity nursing*, ed 9. St. Louis, 2010, Mosby.)

HESI Hint • Breathing techniques, such as deep chest, accelerated, and cued, are not prescribed by the stage and phase of labor but by the discomfort level of the laboring woman. If coping is decreasing, switch to a new technique.

K. Provide mouth care, ice chips, and hard candy as needed for dry mouth.

HESI Hint • Hyperventilation results in respiratory alkalosis that is caused by blowing off too much CO_2.
Symptoms include:
• Dizziness
• Tingling of fingers
• Stiff mouth
   Have woman breathe into her cupped hands or a paper bag in order to rebreathe CO_2.

L. Maintain asepsis in labor by means of frequent perineal care and by changing linen and underpads.
M. Allow sips of clear fluid if no general anesthesia is anticipated.

N. Offer anesthesia or analgesia in midactive phase of labor.
   1. If given too early, they will retard the progress of labor.
   2. If given too late, narcotics increase the risk of neonatal respiratory depression.
O. Monitor fetus continuously if any high-risk situation occurs.
P. Notify health care provider if any of the following occurs:
   1. Labor progress is retarded.
   2. Maternal vital signs are abnormal.
   3. Fetal distress noted.

SECOND STAGE OF LABOR

Description: Heralded by the involuntary need to push, 10 centimeters of cervical dilatation, rapid fetal descent, and birth

A. The second stage of labor averages 1 hour for a primigravida, 15 minutes for a multipara.
B. The addition of abdominal force to the uterine contraction force enhances the cardinal movements of the fetus: engagement, descent, flexion, internal rotation, extension, restitution, and external rotation (Fig. 6-16).

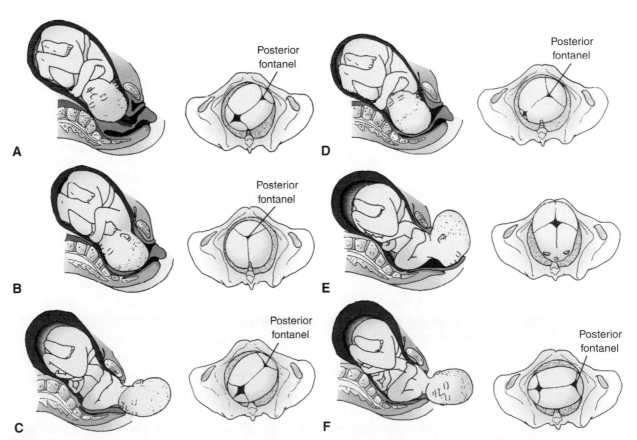

FIGURE 6-16 Cardinal movement of the mechanism of labor. Left occipitoanterior (LOA) presentation. *A,* Engagement and descent. *B,* Flexion. *C,* Internal rotation to occipitoanterior (OA) position. *D,* Extension. *E,* External rotation beginning (restitution). *F,* External rotation. (From Lowdermilk DL, Perry SE: *Maternity nursing,* ed 9. St. Louis, 2010, Mosby.)

Nursing Assessment

A. Assess BP and pulse every 5 to 15 minutes.

B. Determine FHR with every contraction.

C. Observe perineal area for the following:
   1. Increase in bloody show
   2. Bulging perineum and anus
   3. Visibility of the presenting part

D. Palpate bladder for distention.

E. Assess amniotic fluid for color and consistency.

Analysis (Nursing Diagnoses)

A. *Acute pain* related to…

B. *Risk for injury* related to…

C. *Deficient knowledge* (specify) related to…

Nursing Plans and Interventions

A. Document maternal BP and pulse every 15 minutes between contractions.

B. Check FHR with each contraction or by continuous fetal monitoring.

C. Continue comfort measures: mouth care, linen change, positioning.

D. Decrease outside distractions.

E. Teach mother positions such as squatting, side-lying, or high-Fowler/lithotomy for pushing.

F. Teach mother to hold breath for no longer than 10 seconds during pushing.

G. Teach mother to exhale when pushing or use "gentle" pushing technique (pushing down on vagina while constantly exhaling through open mouth, followed by deep breath).

> **HESI Hint** • Determine cervical dilatation before allowing client to push. Cervix should be completely dilated (10 cm) before the client begins pushing. If pushing starts too early, the cervix can become edematous and never fully dilate.

H. If delivering in another room or setting:
   1. Transfer multipara at 8 to 9 cm, +2 station.
   2. Transfer primigravida at 10 cm, with presenting part visible between contractions *and* during contractions.

I. Set up delivery table, including bulb syringe, cord clamp, and sterile supplies.

J. Perform perineal cleansing.

K. At crowning, put gentle counterpressure against the perineum. Do not allow rapid delivery over woman's perineum.

L. Make sure client and support person can visualize delivery if they so desire. If siblings are present, make sure they are closely attended to by support person explaining that their mom is all right.

M. Record *exact* delivery time (complete delivery of baby).

THIRD STAGE OF LABOR

Description: From complete expulsion of the baby to complete expulsion of the placenta

A. Average length of third stage of labor is 5 to 15 minutes.

B. The longer the third stage of labor, the greater the chance for uterine atony or hemorrhage to occur.

Nursing Assessment

A. Signs of placental separation:
   1. Lengthening of umbilical cord outside vagina.
   2. Gush of blood.
   3. Uterus changes from oval (discoid) to globular.

B. Mother describes a "full" feeling in vagina.

C. Firm uterine contractions continue.

Analysis (Nursing Diagnoses)

A. *Risk for deficient fluid volume* related to…

B. *Anxiety* related to…

Nursing Plans and Interventions

> **HESI Hint** • Give the oxytocin after the placenta is delivered because the drug will cause the uterus to contract. If the oxytocic drug is administered before the placenta is delivered, it may result in a retained placenta, which predisposes the client to hemorrhage and infection.

A. Place hand under drape and palpate fundus of uterus for firmness and placement at or below the umbilicus. At signs of placental separation, instruct mother to push gently.

B. Take maternal BP before and after placental separation.

C. Check patency and site integrity of infusing IV.

D. Administer oxytocic medication immediately after delivery of the placenta (Table 6-2).

E. Observe for blood loss and ask physician for estimate of blood loss (EBL).

F. Dry and suction infant, perform Apgar assessment, place blanket on mother's abdomen or allow skin-to-skin contact with mother after delivery.

TABLE 6-2 Uterine Stimulants

Drug	Indications	Adverse Reactions	Nursing Implications
• Oxytocin, synthetic (Pitocin, Syntocinon)	• Uterine atony	• Severe afterpains in multipara • Hypertension	• Give immediately after delivery of placenta to avoid "trapped" placenta. • Continue to monitor vaginal bleeding and uterine tone. • May stimulate let-down milk reflex and flow of milk when engorged
• Methylergonovine maleate (Methergine)	• Uterine atony	• Hypertension	• Use with caution in clients with elevated BP or preeclampsia. • Take BP prior to administration and if 140/90 or above, withhold and notify physician.
• Prostaglandin F$_2$ (Hemabate)	• Uterine atony	• Headache • Nausea and vomiting • Fever • Bronchospasm, wheezing	• Contraindicated for clients with asthma • May be given intramyometrially by provider • Check temperature every 1 to 2 hours. • Auscultate breath sounds frequently.

HESI Hint • Methergine is *not* given to clients with hypertension because of its vasoconstrictive action. Pitocin is given with caution to those with hypertension.

HESI Hint • Never give Methergine or Hemabate to a client while she is in labor or before delivery of the placenta.

G. Place stockinette cap on newborn's head or cover head to prevent heat loss.

H. Allow father or other support person to hold infant during repair of episiotomy.

I. Allow any siblings present to hold new family member.

J. Gently cleanse vulva and apply sterile perineal pad.

HESI Hint • APPLICATION OF PERINEAL PADS AFTER DELIVERY
• Place two on perineum.
• Do not touch inside of pad.
• Do apply from front to back, being careful not to drag pad across the anus.

K. Remove both legs simultaneously if legs are in stirrups.

L. Provide clean gown and warm blanket.

M. Lock bed before moving mother, and raise side rails during transfer.

FOURTH STAGE OF LABOR

Description: The fourth stage of labor is the first 1 to 4 hours after delivery of placenta.

Nursing Assessment

A. Review antepartum and labor and delivery records for possible complications.
 1. Postpartum hemorrhage
 2. Uterine hyperstimulation
 3. Uterine overdistention
 4. Dystocia
 5. Antepartum hemorrhage
 6. Magnesium sulfate therapy
 7. Bladder distention

B. Routine postpartum physical assessment

C. Mother-infant bonding

Analysis (Nursing Diagnoses)

A. *Risk for deficient fluid volume* related to…

B. *Risk for injury* related to…

C. *Risk for impaired parenting* related to…

Nursing Plans and Interventions

A. Maintain bed rest for at least 2 hours to prevent orthostatic hypotension.

B. Assess BP, pulse, and respirations every 15 minutes for 1 hour, then every 30 minutes until stable (BP < 140/90, pulse <100, and respiration <24).

C. Assess temperature at beginning of fourth stage and prior to discharge to postpartum room. If above >100.4°F, report it to physician and monitor hourly.

D. Assess fundal firmness and height, bladder, lochia, and perineum every 15 minutes for 1 hour, then every 30 minutes for 2 hours.
1. Fundus: firm, midline, at or below the umbilicus. Massage if soft or boggy. Suspect full bladder if above umbilicus and to the right side of abdomen.

> **HESI Hint** • Full bladder is one of the most common reasons for uterine atony or hemorrhage in the first 24 hours after delivery. If the nurse finds the fundus soft, boggy, and displaced above and to the right of the umbilicus, what action should be taken first? First, perform fundal massage; then have the client empty her bladder. Recheck fundus every 15 minutes for 1 hour, then every 30 minutes for 2 hours.

2. Lochia: rubra (red), moderate, and clots <2 to 3 cm. Suspect undetected laceration if fundus is firm and bright-red blood continues to trickle. Always check perineal pad *and* under buttocks.
3. Perineum: intact, clean, and slightly edematous. Suspect hematomas if very tender or discolored or if pain is disproportionate to vaginal delivery.

E. Report to health care provider:
1. Abnormal vital signs
2. Uterus not becoming firm with massage
3. Second perineal pad soaked in 15 minutes
4. Signs of hypovolemic shock: pale, clammy, tachycardic, light-headed, hypotensive

F. Monitor infusion of intravenous Pitocin. (Check health care provider's prescription and hospital policy.)

G. Change perineal pads and cleanse vulva and perineum with each change.

H. Prevent the discomfort of afterpains.
1. Keep bladder empty. Catheterize only if absolutely necessary.
2. Place warm blanket on abdomen.
3. Administer analgesics as prescribed (usually codeine, acetaminophen, or ibuprofen).

> **HESI Hint** • If narcotic analgesics (codeine, meperidine) are given, raise side rails and place call light within reach. Instruct client not to get out of bed or ambulate without assistance. Caution client about drowsiness as a side effect.

I. Offer fluids PO when woman is alert and able to swallow.

J. Apply ice pack to perineum to minimize edema, especially if a third- or fourth-degree episiotomy has been performed or if lacerations are present.

K. Apply witch hazel compresses to perineum for comfort.

> **HESI Hint** • A first-degree tear involves only the epidermis. A second-degree tear involves dermis, muscle, and fascia. A third-degree tear extends into the anal sphincter. A fourth-degree tear extends up the rectal mucosa. Tears cause pain and swelling. Avoid rectal manipulations.

L. Support parental emotional needs and promote bonding.
1. Allow extended time with newborn.
2. Openly share in the joy and excitement of childbirth; also grieve with parents experiencing loss.
3. Encourage initiation of breastfeeding.
4. Provide a warm, darkened environment so newborn will open eyes.
5. Withhold eye prophylaxis for up to 1 hour.
6. Perform newborn admission and routine procedures in room with parents.

NEWBORN CARE (DELIVERY ROOM)

Description: Care provided to newborn, usually performed by the nurse

Nursing Assessment

A. Maternal history and labor data indicating potential problems with newborn

B. Apgar scores

C. Findings of brief physical examination performed in delivery room

Analysis (Nursing Diagnoses)

A. *Risk for ineffective airway clearance* related to…

B. *Risk for injury* related to…

Nursing Plans and Interventions

A. Immediately dry infant under warmer or skin to skin with mother; suction mouth and nose with bulb syringe; keep head slightly lower than body; and assess airway status.

1. Assess for five symptoms of respiratory distress.
   a. Retractions
   b. Tachypnea (rate >60)
   c. Dusky color, circumoral cyanosis
   d. Expiratory grunt
   e. Flaring nares
2. Do not hyperextend the newborn neck at any time (may close glottis). Place infant in "sniff" position (neck slightly extended as if sniffing the air) to open airway.

HESI Hint • If it was documented that the fetus passed meconium in utero or the nurse noted *late* passage of meconium in delivery room, the neonate must be attended to by a pediatrician, neonatologist, or nurse practitioner to determine,

through endotracheal tube observation and suction, whether meconium is present below the vocal cords. Such a presence can result in pneumonitis and meconium aspiration syndrome, which necessitate a sepsis workup, including a chest radiograph early in the transitional newborn period.

B. Obtain Apgar score at 1 and 5 minutes (Table 6-3).
C. Continue to allow maternal/parent contact if newborn is stable.
D. Keep neonate's head covered.
E. Do quick gestational age assessment (Table 6-4).
   1. Sole creases
   2. Breast tissue bud

TABLE 6-3 Apgar Assessment

- Performed at exactly 1 and 5 minutes after birth
- Cannot just eyeball; must have hands-on examination
- Score:
  → 7 to 10: Good
  → 4 to 6: Needs moderate resuscitative efforts
  → 0 to 3: Severe need for resuscitation

HESI Hint • Do *not* wait until a 1-minute Apgar is assigned to begin resuscitation of the compromised neonate.

• Heart rate	Absent = 0; <100 = 1; ≥100 = 2
• Respiratory effort	No cry = 0; weak cry = 1; vigorous cry = 2
• Muscle tone	Flaccid = 0; some flexion = 1; total flexion = 2
• Reflex irritability	No response to foot tap = 0; slight response to foot tap (grimace) = 1; quick foot removal = 2
• Color	Dusky, cyanotic = 0; acrocyanotic = 1; totally pink = 2

HESI Hint • Apgar scores of 6 or lower at 5 minutes require an additional Apgar assessment at 10 minutes.

TABLE 6-4 Gestational Age Assessment

• 28 Weeks	• No nipple bud • Testes in the inguinal canal or labia majora widely separated, with labia minora prominent, open, and equal in size • Vernix (cheesy coating) over the entire body • Lanugo (fine, downy hair) over the entire body • Full extension of extremities in resting posture
• 40 Weeks	• Raised nipple with a tissue bud underneath • Descended testes with large rugae (folds) on the scrotum • Labia majora large and covering the minora • Vernix only in the creases • Lanugo perhaps only over the shoulders • Hypertonic flexion of extremities in resting posture

3. Skin, vessels, and peeling
4. Genitalia
5. Resting posture

F. Examine cord for presence of three vessels (two arteries, one vein), and document.

G. Make sure cord blood is collected for analysis and sent to lab.
   1. Rh
   2. Blood type
   3. Hct
   4. Possible cord blood gases

H. Document passage of meconium or urine after delivery.

I. Place two identity bands on neonate and one on mother.

J. Obtain newborn footprints and maternal thumb and fingerprint. Follow institutional policy regarding identification procedures.

K. Perform brief physical examination of newborn.
   1. Check for gross anomalies: spina bifida, hydrocephaly, and cleft lip or palate.
   2. Elicit reflexes: Moro (startle) and Rooting (suck).
   3. Examine cord clamp for closure, absence of blood oozing from cord; again check for presence of three vessels.

L. May instill eye prophylaxis in delivery room (Table 6-5).

M. If parents desire an open-eye bonding period, may delay eye prophylaxis for up to 1 hour. The Centers for Disease Control and Prevention (CDC) states that a delay of up to 1 hour is safe.

LABOR WITH ANALGESIA OR ANESTHESIA

A. Analgesia and anesthesia are usually withheld until the midactive phase of labor.
   1. If given in the early latent phase of the first stage of labor, it may retard the progress of labor.
   2. If given late in transition or in the second stage, it may depress the newborn (some narcotic analgesics).

B. Most drugs used for systematic pain relief and relaxation cause CNS depression, which can slow labor and harm fetus.

C. Regional blocks (epidural, caudal, and subarachnoid) cause a temporary interruption of nerve impulses (especially pain) but also cause vasodilation in area below block, causing pooling of blood and hypotension.

Nursing Assessment

A. Acute pain is experienced during active labor.

B. Birth plan includes use of analgesic and anesthetic agents.

C. Decreased coping and increased anxiety are observed.

D. Assess the client and obtain the following data:
   1. Vital signs and fetal heart rate
   2. Labor progress (e.g., cervical dilatation and effacement, fetal position and lie)
   3. Last time and amount of food or fluids ingested
   4. Lab values (Hgb, Hct, clotting time)
   5. Hydration status
   6. Signs and symptoms of infection

TABLE 6-5   Newborn Prophylactic Eye Care

Drugs	Indications	Adverse Reactions	Nursing Implications
Ointments • Erythromycin • Tetracycline	• Prevention of ophthalmia neonatorum and *Chlamydia trachomatis* conjunctivitis	• Most commonly used agents • None known, except puffy eyes resulting from manipulation	• Place a thin line of ointment along the entire lower lid in conjunctival sac • Use only one tube per baby and *discard* • Manipulate upper lids to ensure complete eye coverage • After 1 minute, may wipe excess from around eyes
• Silver nitrate (use in the United States is minimal because silver nitrate does not protect against chlamydial infection and can cause chemical conjunctivitis)	• Prevention of ophthalmia neonatorum resulting from gonorrhea exposure through the birth canal in a vaginal delivery	• Chemical conjunctivitis (red, puffy eyes) • Staining of skin if contact occurs	• Eye prophylaxis is mandatory in the United States • May not kill other organisms such as *Chlamydia* species • Instill medication in lower conjunctival sac, making sure drops spread over entire eye • Do *not* irrigate eyes following instillation

Analysis (Nursing Diagnoses)

A. *Acute pain* related to…

B. *Ineffective coping* related to…

C. *Risk for injury (mother or fetus)* related to…

Nursing Plans and Interventions

A. Administration of analgesic drugs in labor
  1. Document baseline maternal vital signs and FHR prior to administration of narcotics or sedatives (Table 6-6).
  2. Assess phase and stage of labor.
  3. Obtain physician's order for medication.
  4. Determine client's and family's desires regarding analgesics, and verbally praise informed choice.
  5. Do *not* give PO medications. Labor retards gastrointestinal activity and absorption.
  6. Administer medications IV when possible, IM if necessary.

> **HESI Hint** • IV administration of analgesics is preferred to IM administration for a client in labor because the onset and peak occur more quickly, and the duration of the drug is shorter. It is important to know the following:

IV ADMINISTRATION
- Onset: 5 minutes
- Peak: 30 minutes
- Duration: 1 hour

IM ADMINISTRATION
- Onset: within 30 minutes
- Peak: 1 to 3 hours after injection
- Duration: 4 to 6 hours

  7. Push IV bolus into line *slowly*, at the beginning of a contraction (i.e., give medication during contraction, when uterine blood vessels are constricted, so less analgesic reaches the fetus).
  8. Explain the purpose of the drug to the laboring woman, but do not promise results.

B. After drug administration
  1. Record the woman's response and level of pain relief.
  2. Monitor maternal vital signs, FHR, and characteristics of uterine contractions every 15 minutes for 1 hour after administration.
  3. Monitor bladder for distention and retention (medication can decrease perception of bladder filling).

TABLE 6-6 Analgesics

Drugs	Indications	Adverse Reactions	Nursing Implications
• Fentanyl (Sublimaze) • Morphine sulfate (MS Contin)	• Opioid agonists • Narcotic used to produce analgesia, euphoria, and sedation in labor • Analgesia during labor	• Respiratory depression • Fetal narcosis, distress • Hypotension • Itching • Urinary retention • Respiratory depression	• Store in narcotics cabinet • Record use accurately • Do *not* administer if respirations <12/min • Have narcotic antagonist available (Narcan) • Monitor respirations, pulse, BP closely • Refer to Table 6-21, p. 306
• Butorphanol tartrate (Stadol) • Nalbuphine (Nubain)	• Opioid agonist/antagonists • Provision of analgesia in labor • Narcotic analgesic	• Woman with preexisting narcotic dependency will experience withdrawal symptoms immediately (abstinence syndrome)	• Give IV or IM • Obtain drug history before administration • Monitor respirations, pulse
• Naloxone HCl (Narcan)	• Narcotic antagonist used to counteract narcotic effects on mother/fetus	• Decreased respirations rarely occur	• Monitor respirations closely because drug action is shorter than the narcotic (may need to readminister) • Pain returns after administration to mother • Can be administered to newborn after delivery (0.01 mg/kg body weight) to counteract narcotic depression

4. Decrease environmental stimuli: darken room, reduce number of visitors, turn off TV.
5. Note on delivery record the time between drug administration and birth of baby.
6. If baby delivers during peak drug absorption time, notify pediatrician or neonatologist for delivery room assistance and possible use of Narcan for neonate (see Table 6-6).

C. General anesthesia is rarely used in today's obstetric units. It might be used in emergency deliveries or when regional block anesthesia is contraindicated or refused.
1. Administer drugs to reduce gastric secretions (e.g., cimetidine [Tagamet]) or clear (nonparticulate) antacids to neutralize gastric acid. (The most common cause of maternal death is aspiration of gastric contents into the lung.)

> **HESI Hint** • Tranquilizers (ataractics and phenothiazines), such as Phenergan and Vistaril, are used in labor as analgesic-potentiating drugs to decrease the amount of narcotic needed and to decrease maternal anxiety.

> **HESI Hint** • Agonist narcotic drugs (Demerol, morphine) produce narcosis and have a higher risk for causing maternal and fetal respiratory depression. Antagonist drugs (Stadol, Nubain) have less respiratory depression but must be used with caution in a mother with preexisting narcotic dependency because withdrawal symptoms occur immediately.

2. Assist with speedy delivery. (General anesthesia may depress fetus if delivery is not accomplished quickly.)
3. Assess closely for uterine atony; check fundal firmness and uterine contraction. (General anesthesia is associated with postpartum uterine atony.)

REGIONAL BLOCK ANESTHESIA

A. Local anesthesia
1. Is used for pain relief during episiotomy and perineal repair
2. Is safe for mother and infant
B. Regional blocks
1. Used for relief of perineal and uterine pain
2. Is usually safe for mother and infant unless severe hypotension occurs
3. Types of regional blocks
   a. Pudendal block: given in second stage to deaden pudendal nerve plexus, thus deadening pain in the perineum and vagina
      (1) Has no effect on pain of uterine contractions
      (2) Is safe for mother and infant
   b. Peridural (epidural, caudal) block: given in first or second stage of labor to block nerve impulses from T10 to S5, thereby deadening pain of contractions
      (1) Used in conjunction with local or pudendal block for delivery; or given to deaden perineum for delivery.
      (2) May be given in single dose or continuously through catheter threaded into epidural space
      (3) Is moderately associated with hypotension, which can cause maternal and fetal distress
      (4) Epidural block associated with prolonged second stage due to decreased effectiveness of pushing
   c. Intradural (subarachnoid, spinal) block: given in second stage of labor to deaden uterine and perineal pain
      (1) Rapid onset, but highly associated with maternal hypotension which can cause maternal and fetal distress
      (2) Client must remain flat for 6 to 8 hours after delivery.

C. Contraindications to subarachnoid and peridural blocks
1. Client's refusal or fear
2. Anticoagulant therapy or presence of bleeding disorder
3. Presence of antepartum hemorrhage causing acute hypovolemia
4. Infection or tumor at injection site
5. Allergy to -caine drugs
6. CNS disorders, previous back surgery, or spinal anatomic abnormality

> **HESI Hint** • Pudendal block and subarachnoid (saddle) block are used only in the second stage of labor. Peridural and epidural blocks may be used during all stages of labor.

Nursing Assessment

A. No contraindications to regional block anesthesia
B. Experiencing severe pain
C. Possible need for cesarean delivery
D. BP before block >100/70 mm Hg
E. Status of maternal-fetal unit

Analysis (Nursing Diagnoses)

A. *Risk for ineffective tissue perfusion (mother and fetus)* related to…

B. *Risk for injury (fetus/client)* related to…

C. *Urinary retention* related to…

Nursing Plans and Interventions

A. Ensure that the health care provider has explained the procedures, the risks, the benefits, and the alternatives.

B. Prehydrate client to counteract possible hypotension: 500 to 1000ml IV fluid (isotonic) are infused over 20 to 30 minutes before initiation of regional block.

C. Place client in a modified Sims position or sitting on side of bed with head flexed.

D. Ask client to describe symptoms after test dose of medication is given.
   1. Metallic taste in mouth and ringing in ears denote possible injection of medication into bloodstream.
   2. Nausea and vomiting are among the first signs of hypotension.

> **HESI Hint** • The first sign of a block's effectiveness is usually warmth and tingling in the ball of foot or big toe.

E. Determine BP every 1 to 2 minutes for 15 minutes after injection of anesthetic drug, and initiate continuous fetal monitoring.

F. Determine BP every 15 minutes during continuous regional block infusion.

G. Assist client to keep bladder empty.

H. Assess level of pain relief using the sharp-dull technique, and record return of pain sensation.

I. Report return of pain sensation, incomplete anesthesia, or uneven anesthesia to anesthesiologist.

J. If hypotension occurs, do the following:
   1. Immediately turn client onto left side.
   2. Increase intravenous infusion.
   3. Begin O_2 at 10L/min by facemask.
   4. Notify health care provider stat and have ephedrine available at bedside.
   5. Assess FHR.

K. Assist client in the pushing technique once complete dilatation has been achieved.

> **HESI Hint** • Stop continuous infusion at end of stage I or during transition to increase effectiveness of pushing.

> **HESI Hint** • **REGIONAL BLOCK ANESTHESIA AND FETAL PRESENTATION**
> - Internal rotation is harder to achieve when the pelvic floor is relaxed by anesthesia; this results in a persistent occiput-posterior position of fetus.
> - Monitor fetal position. Remember, the mother cannot tell you she has back pain, which is the cardinal sign of persistent posterior fetal position.
> - Regional blocks, especially epidural and caudal blocks, commonly result in assisted (forceps or vacuum) delivery because of the inability to push effectively during the second stage.

> **HESI Hint** • Nerve block anesthesia (spinal or epidural) during labor blocks motor as well as nerve fibers. Vasodilation below the level of the block results in blood pooling in the lower extremities, causing maternal hypotension. Approximately 20 minutes prior to nerve block anesthesia, the client should be hydrated with 500 to 1000ml lactated Ringer's solution IV. Monitor maternal vital signs and FHR every 15 minutes. If hypotension occurs, turn the client onto her side, administer O_2 at 10L/min by facemask, and increase IV rate.

Review of Intrapartum Nursing Care

1. List five prodromal signs of labor the nurse might teach the client.
2. How is true labor discriminated from false labor?
3. State two ways to determine whether the membranes have truly ruptured.
4. Are psychoprophylactic breathing techniques prescribed for use according to the stage and phase of labor?
5. Identify two reasons to withhold anesthesia and analgesia until the midactive phase of stage I labor.
6. Hyperventilation often occurs in the laboring client. What results from hyperventilation, and what actions should the nurse take to relieve the condition?
7. Describe the maternal changes that characterize the transition phase of labor.
8. When should a laboring client be examined vaginally?

9. Define cervical effacement.
10. Where is the fetal heart rate best heard?
11. Normal fetal heart rate during labor is _____.
12. Normal maternal BP during labor is _____.
13. Normal maternal pulse during labor is _____.
14. Normal maternal temperature during labor is _____.
15. List four nursing actions for the second stage of labor.
16. List three signs of placental separation.
17. When should the postpartum dosage of Pitocin be administered? Why is it administered?
18. State one contraindication to the use of ergot drugs (Methergine).
19. State five symptoms of respiratory distress in the newborn.
20. If meconium was passed in utero, what action must the nurse take in the delivery room?
21. What is considered a good Apgar score?
22. What is the purpose of eye prophylaxis in the newborn?
23. What is the danger associated with regional blocks?
24. What is the major cause of maternal death when general anesthesia is administered?
25. Why are PO medications avoided in labor?
26. State the best way to administer IV drugs during labor.

27. When is it dangerous to administer butorphanol (Stadol), an agonist/antagonist narcotic?
28. Hypotension commonly occurs after the laboring client receives a regional block. What is one of the first signs the nurse might observe?
29. State three actions the nurse should take when hypotension occurs in a laboring client.
30. The fourth stage is defined as.
31. What actions can the nurse take to assist in preventing postpartum hemorrhage?
32. To promote comfort, what nursing interventions are used for a third-degree episiotomy that extends into the anal sphincter?
33. What nursing interventions are used to enhance maternal-infant bonding during the fourth stage of labor?
34. List three nursing interventions to ease the discomfort of afterpains.
35. List the symptoms of a full bladder that might occur in the fourth stage of labor.
36. What action should the nurse take first when a soft, boggy uterus is palpated?
37. What are the symptoms of hypovolemic shock?
38. How often should the nurse check the fundus during the fourth stage of labor?

Answers to Review

1. Lightening, Braxton Hicks contractions, increased bloody show, loss of mucous plug, burst of energy, and nesting behaviors.
2. True labor: regular, rhythmic contractions that intensify with ambulation, pain in the abdomen sweeping around from the back, and cervical changes
   False labor: irregular rhythm, abdominal pain (not in back) that decreases with ambulation
3. Nitrazine testing: paper turns dark blue or black
   Demonstration of fluid ferning under microscope
4. No. Clients should use these techniques according to their discomfort level and should change techniques when one is no longer working for relaxation.
5. If analgesia and anesthesia are given too early, they can retard labor; if given too late, they can cause fetal distress.
6. Respiratory alkalosis occurs; it is caused by blowing off CO_2 and is relieved by breathing into a paper bag or cupped hands.
7. Irritability and unwillingness to be touched, but does not want to be left alone; nausea, vomiting, and hiccupping
8. Vaginal examinations should be done prior to analgesia and anesthesia to rule out cord prolapse, to determine labor progress if it is questioned, and to determine when pushing can begin.
9. The taking up of the lower cervical segment into the upper segment; the shortening of the cervix expressed in percentages from 0 to 100%, or complete effacement.

10. Through the fetal back in vertex, OA positions
11. 110 to 160 bpm
12. <140/90
13. <100 bpm
14. <100.4°F
15. Make sure cervix is completely dilated before pushing is allowed. Assess FHR with each contraction. Teach woman to hold breath for no longer than 10 seconds. Teach pushing technique.
16. Gush of blood, lengthening of cord, and globular shape of uterus
17. Give immediately after placenta is delivered to prevent postpartum hemorrhage and atony.
18. Hypertension
19. Tachypnea, dusky color, flaring nares, retractions, and grunting
20. Arrange for immediate endotracheal tube observation to determine the presence of meconium below the vocal cords (prevents pneumonitis and meconium aspiration syndrome).
21. 7 to 10
22. To prevent ophthalmia neonatorum, which results from exposure to gonorrhea in the vagina
23. Hypotension resulting from vasodilatation below the block, which pools blood in the periphery, reducing venous return
24. Aspiration of gastric contents
25. Gastric activity slows or stops in labor, decreasing absorption from PO route; it may cause vomiting.

26. At beginning of contraction, push a little medication in while uterine blood vessels are constricted, thereby reducing dose to fetus.

27. When the client is an undiagnosed drug abuser of narcotics, it can cause immediate withdrawal symptoms.

28. Nausea

29. Turn client to left side.
Administer O$_2$ by mask at 10 L/min.
Increase speed of intravenous infusion (if it does not contain medication).

30. The first 1 to 4 hours after delivery of placenta

31. Massage the fundus (gently) and keep the bladder emptied.

32. Ice pack, witch hazel compresses, and no rectal manipulation

33. Withhold eye prophylaxis for up to 1 hour. Perform newborn admission and routine procedures in room with parents. Encourage early initiation of breastfeeding. Darken room to encourage newborn to open eyes.

34. Keep bladder empty. Provide a warm blanket for abdomen. Administer analgesics prescribed by health care provider.

35. Fundus above umbilicus; dextroverted (to the right side of abdomen); increased bleeding (uterine atony)

36. Perform fundal massage.

37. Pallor, clammy skin, tachycardia, lightheadedness, and hypotension

38. Every 15 minutes for 1 hour; every 30 minutes for 2 hours if normal

Normal Puerperium (Postpartum)

Description: Period after pregnancy and delivery (usually 6 weeks) when the body returns to the nonpregnant state

A. Care during this period is focused on wellness and family integrity.

B. Teaching must be initiated early to cover the physical self-care needs and the emotional needs of the mother, infant, and family.

NORMAL PUERPERIUM CHANGES

A. Reproductive system
1. Uterus
a. Myometrial contractions occur for 12 to 24 hours postdelivery due to high oxytocin levels (prominent in multiparas, breastfeeding women, and women who have experienced overdistention of the uterus).
b. Involution occurs (1 to 2 cm/day).
(1) First day: at or 1 to 2 cm above umbilicus
(2) 7 to 10 days: decreases to 12-week size, slides back under symphysis pubis
c. Placenta site contracts and heals without scarring.
2. Cervix
a. Becomes parous, with a transverse slit
b. Heals within 6 weeks
3. Vagina
a. Rugae (folds) reappear within 3 weeks.
b. Walls are thin and dry.
4. Breasts
a. Nonlactating
(1) Nodules are palpable.
(2) Engorgement may occur 2 to 3 days postpartum.
b. Lactating
(1) Milk sinuses (lumps) are palpable.
(2) Colostrum (yellowish fluid) is expressed first, then milk (bluish-white).
(3) Breasts may feel warm, firm, tender for 48 hours.

B. Cardiovascular system
1. At delivery
a. Maternal vascular bed is reduced by 15%.
b. Pulse may decrease to 50 (normal puerperal bradycardia).
c. These changes are hypothesized to result in client's "shivering."
d. BP and pulse should quickly return to prepregnant levels.
2. First 72 hours
a. 24 to 48 hours postpartum, cardiac output remains elevated (returns to nonpregnant levels in 2 to 3 weeks).
b. Plasma loss > RBC loss; reverses hemodilution of pregnancy (Hct rises)
c. Diaphoresis (especially at night) helps restore normal plasma volume.

C. Hematologic system
1. Hct rises.
2. WBC count is elevated (12,000 to 25,000).
3. It is difficult to use WBC for determination of infection.
4. Blood-clotting factors are elevated; increases risk for thromboembolism.

D. Urinary system
1. Diuresis occurs; woman excretes up to 3000 ml/day of urine.
2. Bladder distention and incomplete emptying are common.
3. Persistent dilatation of ureter and renal pelvis increase risk for UTI.
4. Urine glucose, creatinine, and BUN levels are normal after 7 days.

E. Gastrointestinal system
1. Excess analgesia and anesthesia may decrease peristalsis.
2. No bowel movements are expected for 2 to 3 days.

F. Integumentary system
1. Chloasma and hyperpigmentation areas (linea nigra, areolae) regress; some areas may remain permanently darker.
2. Palmar erythema declines quickly.
3. Spider nevi fade; some in legs may remain.

G. Musculoskeletal system
1. Pelvic muscles regain tone in 3 to 6 weeks.
2. Abdominal muscles regain tone in 6 weeks unless diastasis recti (separation of rectus abdominis muscles) occurs.

HESI Hint • Normal leukocytosis of pregnancy averages 12,000 to 15,000 mm³. During the first 10 to 12 days postdelivery, values of 25,000 mm³ are common. Elevated WBC and the normal elevated ESR may confuse interpretation of acute postpartal infections. For example, if the nurse assesses a client's temperature to be 101°F on the client's second postpartum day, what assessments should be made before notifying the physician? Assess fundal height and firmness; assess perineal integrity; check for a positive Homan sign and other symptoms of thromboembolism; assess pulse, respirations, and BP; assess client's subjective description of symptoms (e.g., burning on urination, pain in leg, excessive tenderness of uterus).

HESI Hint • Client and family teaching is a common subject of NCLEX-RN® questions. Remember that when teaching, the first step is to assess the client's (parents') level of knowledge and to identify their readiness to learn. Client teaching regarding lochia changes, perineal care, breastfeeding, and sore nipples are subjects that are commonly tested.

Nursing Assessment

A. Review prenatal, antepartum, L&D (labor and delivery), and early postpartum records for status, lab data, and possible complications.

B. Review newborn's record for Apgar scores, sex, possible complications, and relevant psychosocial information (adoption, single parent, etc.).

C. Assess postpartum status (Table 6-7): vital signs, fundal height and firmness, lochia, urination, perineum, bowel sounds, presence of thrombophlebitis.

D. Assess maternal-infant bonding and identify teaching needs of mother and family.

Analysis (Nursing Diagnoses)

A. *Acute pain* related to…

B. *Risk for infection* related to…

C. *Urinary retention* related to…

D. *Deficient knowledge* (specify) related to…

E. *Risk for situational low self-esteem* related to…

Nursing Plans and Interventions

A. Monitor vital signs every 4 hours for 24 hr, then every 8 hr.

B. Check fundal height and firmness:
1. On the first postpartum day (first day following birth), the top of the fundus is located approximately 1 cm below the umbilicus (Fig. 6-17).
2. The fundus should be midline and firm immediately after delivery.
3. Massage the fundus if it is soft or boggy by stabilizing the back of uterus before applying pressure; teach mother the procedure but advise against overstimulation, which can lead to atony.
4. Teach about the normalcy of afterpains.

C. Assess and document lochia:
1. Lochia rubra: blood-tinged discharge, including shreds of tissue and decidua; lochia rubra lasts 2 to 3 days postpartum.

TABLE 6-7 Normal Postpartal Vital Signs

Vital Sign	Description
Temperature	May rise to 100.4°F due to dehydrating effects of labor. Any higher elevation may be due to infection and must be reported.
Pulse	May decrease to 50 (normal puerperal bradycardia). Pulse >100 may indicate excessive blood loss or infection.
Blood pressure	Should be normal. Suspect hypovolemia if it decreases, preeclampsia if it increases.
Respirations	Rarely change. If respirations increase significantly, suspect pulmonary embolism, uterine atony, or hemorrhage.

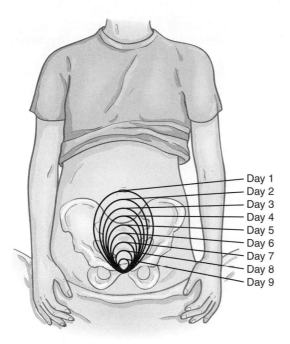

Day 1
Day 2
Day 3
Day 4
Day 5
Day 6
Day 7
Day 8
Day 9

FIGURE 6-17 Involution of the uterus. Height of the uterine fundus decreases by approximately 1 cm per day. (From Murray SS, McKinney ES: *Foundations of maternal-newborn and women's health nursing*, ed 5. St. Louis, 2010, Saunders.)

2. Lochia serosa: pale pinkish to brownish discharge lasting 1 week postpartum.
3. Lochia alba: thicker, whitish-yellowish discharge with leukocytes and degenerated cells; lochia alba lasts up to 4 weeks postpartum.

HESI Hint • After the first postpartum day, the most common cause of uterine atony is retained placental fragments. The nurse must check for the presence of fragments in lochial tissue.

4. Subinvolution: placental site does not heal; lochia persists, with brisk periods of lochia rubra; a D&C may be necessary.
5. Document amount of lochia.
   a. Scant: <1 inch stain on pad
   b. Small: <4 inch stain on pad
   c. Moderate: <6 inch stain on pad
   d. Heavy: saturated pad within 1 hour
   e. Clots: <2 to 3 cm
   f. Odor: fleshy, not foul
6. Teach client about normal lochia changes.

HESI Hint • Women can tolerate blood loss, even slightly excessive blood loss, in the postpartal period because of the 40% increase in plasma volume during pregnancy. In the postpartal period, a woman can void up to 3000 ml/day to reduce the volume increase that occurred during pregnancy.

D. Assess perineum and episiotomy site.
   1. Place woman in lateral Sims position, don gloves, and use flashlight to increase accuracy of visualization.
   2. Check for redness, edema, intactness, and presence of hematomas; teach self-inspection with mirror.
   3. Teach hygiene and comfort and healing measures.
      a. Instruct to change pad as needed and with every voiding and defecation.
      b. Instruct to wipe perineum front to back.
      c. Instruct to use good handwashing technique.
      d. Teach about use of ice packs, sitz baths, using a squeeze bottle for perineal lavage, and topical application of anesthetic spray and pads (Box 6-2).
E. Examine breasts.
   1. Assess nipples for cracks, fissures, redness, and tenderness.
   2. Assess breasts for engorgement.
   3. Palpate breasts for lumps and nodules.
   4. Determine woman's motivation to breastfeed or bottle-feed.
   5. If not breastfeeding, teach woman nonpharmacologic measures of milk suppression: supportive bra or binder, ice packs, and avoiding breast stimulation.
   6. Teach breast self-examination (see Box 6-2).

HESI Hint • Client should void within 4 hours of delivery. Monitor client closely for urine retention. Suspect retention if voiding is frequent and <100 ml per voiding.

BOX 6-2 *Postpartum Teaching*

Breast Self-examination

- Begin with inspection in a mirror. Place both hands at sides and observe; then look again with hands overhead and bending forward. Assess for:
  - Change in size and shape.
  - Dimpling, puckering, scaling, redness, swelling of any part of breast.
- Lie flat with right hand under head and pillow or towel under right shoulder.
- Use left hand to palpate using concentric circles around right breast, feeling for lumps, nodules, or thickening.
- Repeat with left breast.

Episiotomy Care

- Perineal care
- Fill a squeeze bottle with warm water and, if prescribed, an ounce of povidone-iodine solution.
- Lavage perineum with several squirts and blot dry instead of rubbing; avoid anal area

HESI Hint • Women often have a syncopal (fainting) spell on the first ambulation after delivery (usually related to vasomotor changes, orthostatic hypotension). The astute nurse will check client's Hgb and Hct for anemia and BP, sitting and lying down, to ascertain orthostatic hypotension.

F. Assist mother and infant with breastfeeding (Table 6-8).
G. Assess bladder and urine output.
   1. Palpate for spongy, full feeling over symphysis.
   2. Check urge to void when bladder is palpated.
   3. Assist client to ambulate for first void (orthostatic hypotension may occur); measure if possible.
   4. Run warm water over perineum or place spirit of peppermint in bedpan to relax urethra if necessary.

5. Catheterize only if necessary.
6. Teach symptoms of UTI: dysuria, frequency, and urgency.
7. Promote retoning of perineal muscles by Kegel exercises.

HESI Hint • Kegel exercises increase the integrity of the introitus and improve urine retention. Teach client to alternate contraction and relaxation of the pubococcygeal muscles.

H. Assess bowel and anal area:
   1. Inspect for hemorrhoids; describe size and number.
   2. Administer antihemorrhoidal cream, ointment, or suppositories as prescribed.
   3. Auscultate bowel sounds; check abdominal distention.

TABLE 6-8 Teaching Breastfeeding

Topics to Include	Data Related to Topics
• Advantages of breastfeeding	• Low cost • Distinct immunologic advantages for newborn
• Milk production	• Stimulated by the decrease in postpartum estrogen production, which allows release of prolactin from the pituitary
• Let-down reflex (milk ejection)	• Caused by action of oxytocin released from posterior pituitary, which stimulates myoepithelial cells around milk ducts and sinuses
• Breast size	• Has no relationship to successful breastfeeding
• Inverted and retracted nipples	• Women with inverted or retracted nipples can wear shields, which may help the infant latch onto the nipple
• Diet during breastfeeding and lactation	• Avoid dieting • Add 500 calories to prepregnancy intake • Drink 2 quarts (8 glasses) of noncaffeinated beverages daily
• Avoid	• Smoking and the intake of drugs, alcohol, and caffeine • Stress; it is the most common reason for decreased milk supply
• Encourage	• Rest
• Care of breasts and nipples	• Newborn should remain on first breast 10 minutes, then switch to second breast and suckle until satisfied (it is no longer recommended to limit breastfeeding time to 2 to 3 minutes first day, 5 minutes second day, etc.) • Use warm water, not drying soap, on nipples • Let nipples air-dry for 15 minutes 2 to 3 times daily • Breast creams should not be routinely used; colostrum may be expressed and rubbed on nipples
• Engorgement	• Nurse more frequently, and manually express milk to soften areola before feeding • Wear supportive bra • Take warm or hot showers (water over breasts promotes milk flow) • Watch for symptoms of mastitis (commonly occurs when breasts are not emptied)
• Incorrect positioning	• Incorrect positioning of baby on breast is most common reason for sore nipples • Make sure baby has as much of areola as possible in mouth • Break suction with insertion of little finger into the baby's mouth

4. Document flatus and bowel movement.
5. Encourage early ambulation.
6. Encourage increased fluids and use of roughage and bulk in diet.

7. Administer stool softeners (Colace), enemas, or suppositories (Dulcolax) as prescribed (Table 6-9).
8. Avoid rectal manipulation if third- or fourth-degree episiotomy was performed.

TABLE 6-9 Postpartum Drugs

Drugs	Indications	Adverse Reactions	Nursing Implications
• Bisacodyl (Dulcolax suppository)	• Constipation	• Abdominal cramping	• Insert suppository into anus past internal rectal sphincter • Because it is a contact laxative that stimulates rectal mucosa directly, there may be some burning • Usually effective in 15 minutes to 1 hour
• Docusate sodium (Colace)	• Constipation • Painful defecation due to fourth-degree tear	• Abdominal cramping	• Encourage increased fluid intake • Results usually occur within 1 to 3 days of continual use

• $Rh_o(D)$ immune globulin (RhoGAM)	• Prevention of Rh isoimmunization with next pregnancy	• None known	• Given to Rh-negative women after miscarriage, abortion, or any procedure or complication that increases the risk for maternal-fetal blood exchange (amniocentesis, PUBS, abdominal trauma)
			• Routinely given at 28 weeks' gestation to Rh-negative mothers with a negative antibody titer
			• Given postpartally to Rh-negative mother after delivery or abortion when fetus is Rh-positive
			• Never given to an infant or father
			• Must be given within 72 hours of delivery
			• Always given IM
			• Is a blood product:
			  → Must be checked by two nurses
			  → Syringe must be returned to lab with label
			  → Not given to a mother with positive indirect Coombs; she is already sensitized to fetal cells and has developed antibodies

• Rubella vaccine	• Rubella titer of ≤1:10 or enzyme immunoassay (EIA) of ≤0.10	• Transient benign arthralgia • Transient rash • Hypersensitivity if allergic to duck eggs • Slight elevation in temperature	• Given subcutaneously before hospital discharge to nonimmune women • Woman may breastfeed • Do not give if woman or other family members are immunocompromised • Requires informed consent • Teach about contraception; women should avoid pregnancy for 2 to 3 months after immunization

HESI Hint • Remember, RhoGAM is given to an Rh-negative mother who delivers an Rh-positive fetus and has a negative direct Coombs test. If the mother has a positive Coombs test, there is no need to give RhoGAM because the mother is already sensitized.

HESI Hint • Because Rh immune globulins suppress the immune system, the client who receives both RhoGAM and the rubella vaccine should be tested for rubella immunity at 3 months.

I. Prevent thrombophlebitis.
1. Encourage early ambulation.
2. Encourage foot paddling and ankle rolling after general anesthesia.
3. Check for positive Homan sign (per hospital policy).

> **HESI Hint** • Assess for thromboembolism: Examine legs of postpartum client daily for pain, warmth, and tenderness or a swollen vein that is tender to the touch. Client may or may not exhibit a positive Homan sign (dorsiflexion of foot causes compression of tibial veins and pain if thrombus is present).

J. Determine the need for RhoGAM (see Table 6-9).

K. Determine the need for a rubella vaccine.

L. Assess maternal psychological adaptation. Reva Rubin identified three distinct emotional stages after delivery:
1. Taking in: dependency behaviors for 24 to 48 hours; asking for help on the simplest of tasks.
2. Taking hold: less focus on physical discomforts, beginning confidence with infant care taking. Not uncommon for mother to feel inadequate caring for infant; the astute nurse will not take over but will praise efforts of parents. At this time, new parents are usually most receptive to teaching about infant care.
3. Letting go: total separation of newborn from self; confident in care taking activities of self and newborn.

M. Assess mother-infant bonding behaviors.
1. Eye contact between mother and neonate
2. Exploration of infant from head to toe
3. Stroking, kissing, and fondling the neonate
4. Smiling, talking, singing to the neonate
5. Use of claiming expressions (e.g., "He's got my feet")
6. Absence of negative statements such as "She just doesn't like me."
7. Naming the newborn quickly and calling the infant by name.

N. Promote mother-infant bonding.
1. Ensure mother is comfortable: provide pain relief, hygiene, and adequate rest.
2. If possible, have baby roomin; include family in teaching; praise and reinforce all positive parenting behaviors.

3. Teach about neonatal behavioral traits.
4. Assure normalcy of comparing idealized child to looks and sex of real child but prevent long-term disappointment by encouraging verbalization of those feelings now.
5. Teach responses to cues from the baby.
   a. Pick baby up when he or she is crying (reciprocity).
   b. Soothe with calm, interactive responses until baby returns to quiet, active state (synchrony).
6. Encourage verbalization of feelings; offer support in nonjudgmental manner.

> **HESI Hint** • "Postpartum blues" are usually normal, especially 5 to 7 days after delivery (unexplained tearfulness, feeling down, and having a decreased appetite). Encourage use of support persons to help with housework for first 2 postpartum weeks. Refer to community resources.

O. Instruct client to notify health care provider or clinic promptly of:
1. Heavy, vaginal bleeding with clots
2. Temperature of 100.4°F or higher lasting 24 hours or longer
3. A red, warm lump in breast
4. Pain on urination
5. Tenderness in calf

P. Teach self-care for discharge.
1. Instruct to continue perineal care and pad changes.
2. Encourage balanced diet and fluid intake.
3. Encourage client to rest or nap when newborn does.

Q. Warn about sibling rivalry, especially if there is a toddler (age 18 months to 3 years) at home.
1. Warn that sibling may regress.
2. Suggest taking a present to toddler from the newborn, and encourage mother to hug toddler.
3. Encourage client to plan time alone with siblings.
4. Teach to abstain from sexual intercourse until lochia has ceased. Warn that first sexual experience may not be pleasant because of vaginal dryness.

R. Assist client with choice of contraceptive method. Teach use, risks, and technique prior to discharge (Table 6-10).

TABLE 6-10 Methods of Contraception

Method	Use, Risk, and Technique
• Diaphragm	• Used with spermicide • Must be fitted by a nurse practitioner or doctor • Must be left in place for 6 hours after intercourse • Must be refitted if excessive weight gain or loss occurs • Must be checked for integrity • Can irritate urethra
• Cervical cap	• Used with spermicide • Contraindicated if cervical anomalies exist • Associated with cervical changes • Pap smear recommended 3 months after use
• Condom (with spermicide)	• Used with spermicide to increase effectiveness • Recommended if any suspicion of STD • Penis must be withdrawn while erect or condom may fall off • Petroleum jelly can deteriorate rubber; water-soluble jelly should be used
• Symptothermal, prothermal, or fertility awareness	• Signs of ovulation should be taught: → Cervical mucus assessment → Basal body temperature assessment → Mittelschmerz (abdominal pain in the region of an ovary during ovulation)
• IUD (intrauterine device)	• Contraindications: diabetes, anemia, abnormal Pap, history of pelvic infections • High association with dysmenorrhea and infection
• Oral contraceptives	• Estrogen in pills prevents pituitary secretion of FSH, preventing ovulation. • Woman still menstruates. • Lowest failure rate of methods • Contraindications: history of coagulation problems, thromboembolism, liver disease, reproductive cancer, coronary artery disease • Compliance is a problem because pill must be taken every day. • If one pill is missed, it should be taken as soon as remembered and the next one taken at the usual time. • If two pills are missed, two pills should be taken for 2 days and an alternative method of contraception should be used for next 7 days. • If more than two pills are missed in the third week, or three or more pills are missed at any time, pills for that cycle should not be taken; alternative method of contraception should be used. Pills should be resumed on fifth day of menstruation.
• Ethinyl estradiol/ norelgestromin (OrthoEvra) transdermal contraceptive patch	• Mechanism of action, efficacy, contraindications, and side effects are similar to those of oral contraceptives. • Delivers continuous levels of progesterone and estradiol • Can be applied to lower abdomen, upper outer arm, buttock, or upper torso (except the breasts) • To be applied on the same day once a week for 3 weeks, followed by 1 week without patch
• Norplant (levonorgestrel implant)	• Sustained-release, subdermal, progestin-only contraceptive • Consists of six thin, flexible capsules made of soft Silastic tubing • Placed in a fanlike pattern just beneath the skin of the upper arm • Effective within 24 hours after insertion; effective for approximately 5 years • Efficacy is not dependent on client compliance once inserted • Reversible with return to previous level of fertility after removal • Side effects include menstrual pattern changes, headache, nervousness • Works by suppression of ovulation as well as by thickening of cervical mucus • Efficacy challenged; not available in United States; two-rod implant approved by FDA

(Continued)

TABLE 6-10   Methods of Contraception—cont'd

Method	Use, Risk, and Technique
• Depo-Provera	• IM injection of 100 mg every 3 months for contraception • Administered during the first 5 days of menstrual cycle • New mothers may be given the injection during the postpartum period, before discharge • Efficacy of 99% • Protection from pregnancy is immediate after injection • Most women experience weight gain and irregular or unpredictable menstrual bleeding (after 1 year's use, many women stop having menstrual periods altogether) • Must monitor for signs and symptoms of thrombophlebitis • Contraindications: history of breast cancer, stroke, blood clots, liver disease • Side effects: nervousness, dizziness, GI disturbances, headaches, and fatigue; may also increase risk for osteoporosis
• Ethinyl estradiol/etonogestrel (NuvaRing)	• A 2-inch diameter ring is an ethylene vinyl acetate complex impregnated with ethinyl estradiol and etonogestrel. • Continuous slow absorption of estrogen/progestin allows for lower estrogen dosing than with oral contraceptives. • The ring is placed deep into the vagina once every 3 weeks and is removed on day 21, then, after a 7-day drug-free interval, a new ring is inserted for an additional 21 days. • Requires an additional form of contraception for the first 7 days of therapy. • The vaginal ring estrogen/progestin administration has the same risks, adverse effects, contraindications, precautions, and drug interactions as the oral contraceptives.

Review of Normal Puerperium (Postpartum)

1. A nurse discovers a postpartum client with a boggy uterus that is displaced above and to the right of the umbilicus. What nursing action is indicated?

2. Which women experience afterpains more than others?

3. Upon admission to the postpartum room, 3 hours after delivery, a client has a temperature of 99.5°F. What nursing actions are indicated?

4. A client feels faint on the way to the bathroom. What nursing assessments should be made?

5. What factor places the postpartum client at risk for thromboembolism?

6. A breastfeeding mother complains of very tender nipples. What nursing actions should be taken?

7. Three days postpartum, a lactating mother has full, warm, taut, tender breasts. What nursing actions should be taken?

8. What information should be given to a client regarding resumption of sexual intercourse after delivery?

9. A woman has decided to take birth control pills as her contraceptive method. What should she do if she misses taking the pill for 2 consecutive days?

10. A woman asks why she is urinating so much in the postpartum period. The nurse bases the response on what information?

11. A woman's white blood count is 17,000; she is afebrile and has no symptoms of infection. What nursing action is indicated?

12. What is the most common cause of uterine atony in the first 24 hours postpartum?

13. What is the purpose of giving docusate sodium (Colace) to the postpartum client?

14. What should the fundal height be at 3 days postpartum for a woman who has had a vaginal delivery?

15. List three signs of positive bonding between parents and newborn.

Answers to Review

1. Perform immediate fundal massage. Ambulate to the bathroom or use bedpan to empty bladder because cardinal signs of bladder distention are present.
2. Breastfeeding women, multiparas, and women who experienced overdistention of the uterus
3. Temperature is probably elevated due to dehydration and work of labor; force fluids and retake temperature in an hour; notify physician if above 100.4°F.
4. Assess BP sitting and lying; assess Hgb and Hct for anemia.
5. Increased clotting factors
6. Have her demonstrate infant position on breast (incorrect positioning often causes tenderness). Leave bra open to air-dry nipples for 15 minutes three times daily. Express colostrum and rub on nipples.
7. She is engorged; have newborn suckle frequently; take measures to increase milk flow: warm water, breast massage, and supportive bra.
8. Avoid until postpartum examination. Use water-soluble jelly. Expect slight discomfort due to vaginal changes.
9. Take two pills for 2 days and use an alternative form of birth control.
10. Up to 3000 ml per day can be voided because of the reduction in the 40% plasma volume increase during pregnancy.
11. Continue routine assessments; normal leukocytosis occurs during postpartal period because of placental site healing.
12. A full bladder
13. To soften the stool in mothers with third- or fourth-degree episiotomies, hemorrhoids, or cesarean section delivery.
14. Three fingerbreadths/cm below the umbilicus.
15. Calling infant by name, exploring newborn head to toe, using en face position.

The Normal Newborn

Description: During the immediate transitional period (first 6 to 8 hours of life) and the early newborn period (first few days of life), the nurse assesses, plans, and provides nursing interventions based on the outcomes of the individual newborn's examination.

Nursing Assessment

A. Review labor and delivery (L&D) report of neonatal history to determine risks during newborn transition caused by medical and obstetric complications.
   1. Cesarean delivery; missing of vaginal squeeze
   2. Prematurity or postmaturity
   3. Diabetic mother
   4. Prolonged rupture of membranes (ROM) >24 hours: sepsis workup
   5. Rh+ isoimmunization (+direct Coombs test)
   6. Traumatic (forceps or vacuum suction) delivery
B. Review L&D report of neonatal history to determine risks during newborn transition caused by drugs and anesthesia during labor and delivery.
   1. Magnesium sulfate during labor: Hypermagnesemia in neonate causes depressed respirations, hypocalcemia, and hypotonia.
   2. Narcosis (late administration of narcotic analgesics); causes decreased respirations and hypotonia.
C. Review L&D report of neonatal history to determine risks during newborn transition caused by degree of birth asphyxia.
   1. Asphyxia during labor: documented late decelerations, decreased variability, severe variable decelerations
   2. Apgar scores at 1 and 5 minutes
D. Review significant social history: mother with a sexually transmitted disease (STD), single parent, language barrier, substance abuse, and lack of support system.
E. Assess vital signs every 30 minutes for 2 hours, then every 1 hour for 5 hours (Table 6-11).
F. Measure the neonate (Table 6-12).
G. Perform a physical examination of the newborn (Table 6-13).
H. Perform neuromuscular assessment. The absence of expected reflexes requires investigation into birth trauma and asphyxia or CNS anomaly (Table 6-14 and Fig. 6-18).
I. Perform a systematic gestational age assessment (Table 6-15; and see Fig. 6-18). Plot measurements on percentile scale to determine whether neonate is small, average, or large for gestational age.
J. Perform a behavioral assessment using the Brazelton Neonate Behavioral Assessment Scale to evaluate newborn's behavioral uniqueness.
   1. Waiting 2 to 3 days to perform assessment gives neonate a chance to rid body of effects of analgesia, anesthesia, and trauma of birth.
   2. The scale measures six categories: habituation, orientation, motor activity, self-quieting ability, social behaviors, sleep and awake states.

TABLE 6-11 Newborn Vital Sign Norms

Vital Sign	Normal	Nursing Implications
• Respirations	• Rate: 30 to 60 breaths/min	• Remember the ABCs (airway, breathing, circulation) • Count 1 full minute by observing abdomen or auscultating breath sounds. • Note five symptoms of respiratory distress: → Tachypnea → Cyanosis → Flaring nares → Expiratory grunt → Retractions
• Heart rate	• 110 to 160 bpm; may fall as low as 100 during sleep, as high as 180 during crying	• Auscultate for 1 full minute at the PMI (point of maximal impulse): third to fourth intercostal space
• Temperature	• Range: 97.7°F to 99.4°F, 36.5°C to 37.5°C	• Rectal approach may perforate rectum; if taken rectally, insert only ¼ to ½ inch for 5 minutes and hold legs firmly to prevent trauma.
• Blood pressure	• Average 80/50 mm Hg	• Not usually measured unless problems in circulation have been assessed.

TABLE 6-12 Physical Measurements

Assessment	Normal	Nursing Implications
• Weight	• Average: 7 lb 8 oz • Majority weigh between 2700 and 4000 g (6 to 9 lb)	• Weigh at birth and daily, with neonate completely naked • Normally lose 5% to 15% (average 10%) of birth weight in first week of life; weight should be documented carefully
• Length	• Average range: 18 to 21 inches, 46 to 52.5 cm	• Measured from crown to rump and rump to heel, or from crown to heel at birth
• Head circumference	• Average range: 33 to 35 cm (normally, 2 cm larger than chest circumference)	• Tape measure placed above eyebrows and stretched around fullest part of occiput, at posterior fontanel (FOC, frontal-occipital circumference)
• Chest circumference	• Average range: 31 to 33 cm	• Tape measure is stretched around scapulae and over nipple line

HESI Hint • PHYSICAL ASSESSMENT
A detailed physical assessment is performed by the nurse or physician. Regardless of who performs the physical assessment, the nurse must know normal versus abnormal variations in the newborn. Observations must be recorded and the physician notified regarding abnormalities.

3. Performing test with the parents present familiarizes them with their newborn's uniqueness and may provide them with cues about the best ways to respond to newborn.

NURSING CARE OF THE NEWBORN

A. Aspiration
  1. Keep bulb syringe or suction immediately available: suction mouth, then nose.

2. Turn neonate on side or stomach and pat firmly on the back, holding head 10 to 15 degrees lower than feet.

HESI Hint • Suction the mouth first and then the nose. Stimulating the nares can initiate inspiration, which could cause aspiration of mucus in oral pharynx.

Text continues on p. 283

TABLE 6-13 Physical Examination of the Newborn

Normal	Abnormal	Rationale
General Appearance		
• Awake • Flexed extremities • Moves all extremities • Strong, lusty cry • Obvious presence of subcutaneous fat • No obvious anomalies	• Little subcutaneous fat	• Intrauterine growth problems • Fetal stress
	• Frog position	• Prematurity
	• Flaccid	• Asphyxia • Prematurity
	• Hard to arouse	• Sepsis • CNS problems • Asphyxia
	• High-pitched cry	• CNS damage or anomalies • Hypoglycemia • Drug withdrawal
Integument		
• Smooth, elastic turgor and subcutaneous fat, superficial peeling after 24 hours; veins rarely visible • Milia, vernix increases • Lanugo, mottling • Harlequin sign (pink-red skin on one side of body) • Erythema toxicum (pink papular rash is normal) • Mongolian spots • Telangiectatic nevi (stork bites)	• Extreme desquamation	• Postmaturity
	• Many visible veins	• Prematurity
	• Meconium staining	• Fetal distress
	• Cyanosis	• Heart disease • Asphyxia
	• Jaundice (within 24 hr)	• Blood incompatibilities • Sepsis • Drug reactions
	• Vesicles	• Herpes, syphilis
	• Café-au-lait spots	• Neurofibromatosis
Head		
• Round or slightly molded • Caput succedaneum (edema over occiput) • Open, flat anterior and posterior fontanels, sutures slightly separated or overlapping due to molding	• Bulging fontanel	• Increased ICP
	• Sunken fontanel	• Dehydration
	• Widely separated sutures	• Hydrocephalus
	• Premature suture closure	• Genetic disorders
	• Cephalhematoma	• Blood under periosteum due to trauma

HESI Hint • It is difficult to differentiate between caput succedaneum (edema under the scalp) and cephalhematoma (blood under the periosteum). The caput crosses suture lines and is usually present at birth, whereas the cephalhematoma does *not* cross suture lines and manifests a few hours after birth. The danger of cephalhematoma is increased hyperbilirubinemia due to excess RBC breakdown.

Normal	Abnormal	Rationale
Eyes		
• Symmetrically placed • Pseudostrabismus • Chemical conjunctivitis (from eye prophylaxis) • Clear cornea • White-blue sclera • Subconjunctival hemorrhage from pressure • Absence of tears • Doll's eye movement (slight nystagmus)	• Purulent discharge	• Gonorrhea or chlamydia
	• Brushfield spots in iris	• Down syndrome
	• Absence of red reflex	• Congenital cataracts
	• Epicanthal folds	• Down syndrome
	• Setting-sun sign	• CNS disorders
	• Absent glabellar reflex (blink)	• CNS or neuromuscular problem

(Continued)

TABLE 6-13 Physical Examination of the Newborn—cont'd

Normal	Abnormal	Rationale
Ears		
• Pinna at or above level of line drawn from outer canthus of eye • Well-formed and firm with instant recoil if folded against head	• Low-set	• Down syndrome
	• Unformed, soft	• Prematurity
	• Preauricular sinus	• Possible renal anomaly
Nose		
• In midline • Appears flattened • Is being used for breathing • Occasional sneezing	• Short, upturned small philtrum (creases under nose)	• Fetal alcohol syndrome
	• Nasal flaring	• Respiratory distress
	• Grunting	• Respiratory distress • Choanal atresia (obstruction between nares and pharynx)
	• Snuffles	• Syphilis
	• Excessive sneezing	• Drug withdrawal
Mouth and Chin		
• Symmetrical movement • Intact lip and palate • Epstein pearls • Mobile tongue • Sucking pads in cheeks • Presence of rooting, sucking, swallowing, and gagging reflexes	• Asymmetry	• Facial nerve injury (Bell palsy)
	• Cleft lip	• Genetic disorder
	• White plaques on cheeks, tongue	• Monilia infection/thrush
	• Absence of protective reflexes	• Prematurity • CNS disorders
	• Excessive drooling	• Esophageal atresia
Neck		
• Short • ROM • Nonpalpable thyroid • Ability to lift head momentarily	• Limited ROM	• Torticollis (wry neck)
	• Nuchal rigidity	• Meningitis
	• Enlarged thyroid	• Hyperthyroidism
	• Crepitus over clavicle	• Fractured clavicle
Chest		
• Symmetrical excursion • Breath sounds clear and equal • Transient rales at birth • Round • Breast engorgement (hormonal) • Transient murmurs	• Persistent murmur	• Patent ductus arteriosus
	• Visible activity over precordium	• Congenital heart anomaly • Heart failure
	• Retractions	• Respiratory distress
	• Asymmetrical chest	• Pneumothorax
Back, Hips, Buttocks, and Anus		
• Spine intact • Symmetrical gluteal folds • Equal limb lengths • Patent anus	• Pilonidal dimple or sinus (at base of sacrum)	• CNS anomaly • Covert spina bifida
	• Hip click • Unequal limb lengths • Asymmetrical gluteal folds	• Congenital hip dislocation
	• Absence of stools after 24 hours	• Imperforate anus • GI obstruction

TABLE 6-13 Physical Examination of the Newborn—cont'd

Normal	Abnormal	Rationale
Abdomen		
• Full, rounded, soft • Present bowel sounds • Palpable liver 1 to 2 cm below right costal margin • Two arteries, one vein in cord; white cord with Wharton jelly	• Scaphoid	• Diaphragmatic hernia
	• Distention	• Meconium ileus • GI obstruction • Hirschsprung disease
	• Hepatosplenomegaly	• Sepsis
	• Purulent discharge at base of cord, foul odor	• Omphalitis (cord infection)
	• One artery	• Renal or heart anomalies
	• Omphalocele	• Abdominal contents in umbilicus (anomaly)
	• Gastroschisis	• Abdominal contents outside of abdomen (anomaly)
Genitals		
Female • Slightly edematous labia covering clitoris and labia minora • Pseudomenstruation • Visible hymenal tag	• Labia minora and clitoris visible	• Prematurity
Male • Penis with foreskin intact • Meatus in middle at tip of penis • Descended testes • Slight edema of scrotum • Rugae on scrotum	• Undescended testes	• Prematurity
	• Meatus on dorsal surface penis	• Epispadias
	• Meatus on ventral surface penis	• Hypospadias
	• Fluid in testes	• Hydrocele
	• Intestine in inguinal canal	• Inguinal hernia
Extremities		
• Arms, hands, fingers, legs, feet, toes • Flexion • Symmetrical movement • Palpable brachial and radial pulses • Palmar and plantar grasp reflex present • Strong grasp reflex • Multiple palmar and plantar creases • Slightly bowed legs • Femoral pulses present • Positive Babinski reflex	• Incurving little finger	• Down syndrome
	• Simian crease	• Down syndrome
	• Flapping tremors	• Drug withdrawal
	• Polydactyly	• Extra digit (family trait)
	• Syndactyly	• Webbed digit (family trait)
	• Difference in pulses between upper and lower extremities	• Coarctation of aorta
	• Absence of plantar creases	• Prematurity
	• Rigid fixation of ankle	• Club feet (talipes)
	• Absent Babinski reflex	• CNS injury

HESI Hint • The umbilical cord should always be checked at birth. It should contain three vessels: one vein, which carries oxygenated blood to the fetus, and two arteries, which carry unoxygenated blood back to the placenta. This is the opposite of normal circulation in the adult. Cord abnormalities usually indicate cardiovascular or renal anomalies.

HESI Hint • Postnatally, the fetal structures of foramen ovale, ductus arteriosus, and ductus venosus should close. If they do not, cardiac and pulmonary compromise will develop.

TABLE 6-14 **Neuromuscular Assessment**

Reflex	Normal Response	Lasts Until
• Rooting	• Baby turns toward stimulus when cheek or corner of lip is touched.	• 3 to 4 months (possibly 1 year)
• Moro	• When startled, baby symmetrically extends and abducts all extremities. • Forefingers form a C shape.	• 3 to 4 months
• Tonic neck	• When neck is turned to side, baby assumes fencing posture.	• 3 to 4 months
• Babinski	• When sole of foot is stroked from heel to ball, toes hyperextend and fan apart from big toe.	• 1 year to 18 months
• Palmar grasp	• When examiner's finger is placed in the infant's palm, the newborn will curl his or her fingers around the examiner's finger.	• Lessens by 3 to 4 months
• Plantar	• A finger at base of toes causes them to curl downward	• 8 months
• Stepping	• When infant is held in upright position with feet touching a hard surface, walking motions are made.	• 3 to 4 months

NEUROMUSCULAR MATURITY

PHYSICAL MATURITY

Skin	sticky friable transparent	gelatinous red, translucent	smooth pink, visible veins	superficial peeling or rash, few veins	cracking pale areas rare veins	parchment deep cracking no vessels	leathery cracked wrinkled
Lanugo	none	sparse	abundant	thinning	bald areas	mostly bald	
Plantar Surface	heel-toe 40-50 mm: -1 <40 mm: -2	>50 mm no crease	faint red marks	anterior transverse crease only	creases ant. 2/3	creases over entire sole	
Breast	imperceptible	barely perceptible	flat areola no bud	stippled areola 1-2 mm bud	raised areola 3-4 mm bud	full areola 5-10 mm bud	
Eye/Ear	lids fused loosely: -1 tightly: -2	lids open pinna flat stays folded	sl. curved pinna; soft; slow recoil	well-curved pinna; soft but ready recoil	formed & firm instant recoil	thick cartilage ear stiff	
Genitals (male)	scrotum flat, smooth	scrotum empty faint rugae	testes in upper canal rare rugae	testes descending few rugae	testes down good rugae	testes pendulous deep rugae	
Genitals (female)	clitoris prominent labia flat	prominent clitoris small labia minora	prominent clitoris enlarging minora	majora & minora equally prominent	majora large minora small	majora cover clitoris & minora	

MATURITY RATING

score	weeks
-10	20
-5	22
0	24
5	26
10	28
15	30
20	32
25	34
30	36
35	38
40	40
45	42
50	44

FIGURE 6-18 Estimation of gestational age. New Ballard scale for newborn maturity rating. Expanded scale includes extremely premature infants and has been refined to improve accuracy in more mature infants. (From Ballard J et al: New Ballard score, expanded to include extremely premature infants. *J Pediatr* 119(3):4177, 1991.)

TABLE 6-15 Gestational Age Assessment

By Date	By Weight
Preterm: 20 to 37 weeks' gestation	Small for gestational age (SGA): Weight below the tenth percentile for estimated weeks of gestation
Term: 38 to 40 weeks' gestation	Average for gestational age (AGA): Weight between the tenth and ninetieth percentiles for estimated weeks of gestation
Postterm: >40 weeks' gestation	Large for gestational age (LGA): Weight above the ninetieth percentile for estimated weeks of gestation

HESI Hint • These neurologic reflexes are transient and, as such, disappear usually within the first year of life. In the pediatric client, prolonged presence of these reflexes can indicate CNS defects. Anticipate NCLEX-RN questions regarding normal newborn reflexes. Physical assessment questions focus on normal characteristics of the newborn and the differentiation of conditions such as caput succedaneum and cephalhematoma.

B. Infection
   1. *Hand washing!!* This is the most effective preventive measure.
   2. Scrupulous cord care: swab cord with alcohol at each diaper change or keep clean with mild soap and water (varies with hospital and provider).
   3. After circumcision a petrolatum gauze dressing or a generous amount of petrolatum may be applied with each diaper change for 1 or 2 days to prevent the diaper from adhering to the site.
   4. Do not allow visitors or personnel to attend to newborn if active infection is present or if newborn has diarrhea, open wounds, an infectious skin rash, or herpesvirus.
   5. Encourage breastfeeding for immunologic factors.

HESI Hint • Circumcision has become controversial because there is no real medical indication for the procedure, and it does cause trauma and pain to the newborn. It was once thought to decrease the incidence of penile and cervical cancer, but some researchers say this is unfounded.

C. Hypothermia
   1. Keep newborn dry and warm.
   2. Place stockinette cap on head (greatest heat loss is through scalp).
   3. Take newborn's temperature at admission and every 4 to 6 hours.
   4. If newborn's temperature falls below 97.6°F (36.4°C), place in radiant warmer and apply skin temperature probe to regulate isolette temperature. May also double-wrap or put skin to skin (kangaroo) with mother.

HESI Hint • Hypothermia (heat loss) leads to depletion of glucose and, therefore, to the use of brown fat (special fat deposits fetus develops in last trimester; they are important to thermoregulation) for energy. This results in ketoacidosis and possible shock. Prevent by keeping neonate warm!

D. Hypoglycemia
   1. Perform a heel-stick blood glucose assessment on all SGA or LGA babies; on infants of diabetic mothers (IDMs); on jittery babies; and on babies with high-pitched cries (Box 6-3).
   2. Report any blood glucose levels under 40 mg/dl in the full-term infant, under 30 mg/dl in the preterm infant. Normal serum glucose is 40 to 80 mg/dl.
   3. Feed the baby early (5% dextrose water, breast milk, or formula) if a low glucose level is detected.
   4. Prevent cold stress, which leads to hypoglycemia.

E. Hemorrhagic disorders: Administer vitamin K to prevent hemorrhagic disorders (Table 6-16).

F. Hyperbilirubinemia
   1. Evaluate for Rh isoimmunization (Rh+ newborn, Rh− mother; maternal Rh+ antibodies are

BOX 6-3 *Heel-Stick Procedure for Newborns*

- Wash hands and put on gloves.
- Clean heel with alcohol and dry with a gauze pad.
- Choose a site for puncture that avoids the plantar artery in the middle of the heel.
- Use only the lateral surfaces of the heel.
- Puncture deep enough to trigger a free flow of blood. Wipe away first drop with sterile gauze pad.
- Collect blood in appropriate tube, on card, or on glucose "stick."

TABLE 6-16 Vitamin K

Drug	Indications	Adverse Reactions	Nursing Implications
• Vitamin K (phytonadione) (AquaMEPHYTON)	• Prevention of hemorrhagic disorder in newborn • Infants are born with sterile gut; no enteric bacteria present for synthesis of vitamin K	• Inflammation at the injection site	• Give IM in the first hour after birth. • Use the vastus lateralis muscle of the thigh (never the gluteus until walking for at least 1 year). • Hold knee secure during procedure because neonate will try to move during injection.

passed to the fetus and cause RBC hemolysis); and for ABO incompatibility (mother blood type O, newborn blood type A or B; maternal anti-A or anti-B antibodies are passed to newborn and cause less severe hemolysis).

2. Bilirubin (byproduct of RBC destruction) binds to protein for excretion or metabolism.
3. Promote stooling by early feedings of milk (protein binds bilirubin for excretion).
4. Assess at birth and daily for presence of jaundice:
   a. Yellowish skin color, sclera, and mucous membranes
   b. Proceeds cephalocaudally (relationship between the head and the base of the spine)
5. Give adequate fluids.
6. Monitor bilirubin levels.
7. Assist with phototherapy if needed.

HESI Hint • Physiologic jaundice occurs at 2 to 3 days of life. If it occurs before 24 hours or persists beyond 7 days, it becomes pathologic. Typically, NCLEX-RN questions ask about the normal problem of physiologic jaundice, which occurs 2 to 3 days after birth due to the immature liver's normal inability to keep up with RBC destruction and to bind bilirubin. Remember, unconjugated bilirubin is the culprit.

Nursing Plans and Interventions

A. The nurse is responsible for monitoring the newborn whether the infant is rooming-in or in the nursery!
B. Facilitate parent-infant attachment.
C. Document the infant's elimination pattern daily.
   1. Stool progression: meconium (black, tarry, sticky) stool within the first 24 hours to transitional (yellowish-green) to milk stool (yellow). Report if no stool within 24 hours.
   2. Infant should void within 4 to 6 hours of birth; then should use one diaper for each

day of life, minimum, until day 6. On day 6 and beyond infant should use a minimum of six to eight diapers per day. Report if there is no urination within 24 hours. There may be brick-red "dust" in the first voidings (uric acid crystals).

HESI Hint • To evaluate exact urine output, weigh dry diaper before applying. Weigh the wet diaper after infant has voided. Calculate and record each gram of added weight as 1 ml urine.

D. Screen for phenylketonuria (PKU) after 24 hours of breast milk or formula ingestion. State laws differ regarding newborn screening. Many also screen for hypothyroidism, sickle cell, and galactosemia.
E. Document nutrition intake and calculate nutrition needs:

HESI Hint • Do *not* feed a newborn when the respiratory rate is over 60. Inform the physician and anticipate gavage feedings in order to prevent further energy utilization and possible aspiration.

   1. Demand feeding (bottle or breast) is preferred.
   2. Most bottle-fed newborns eat every 3 to 4 hours; breast-fed infants eat every 2 to 3 hours (the milk is digested more quickly).
   3. After the initial weight loss period, the infant should gain approximately 1 oz (30 g) per day.
   4. An infant needs about 50 calories/lb or 108 calories/kg of body weight for the first 6 months.

HESI Hint • A 7 lb 8 oz baby would need 50 calories × 7 lb = 350 calories plus 25 calories (½ lb or 8 oz) = 375 calories per day. Most infant formulas contain 20 calories per oz. Dividing 375 by 20 = 18.75 oz of formula needed per day.

F. Monitor lab values for anemia, infection, and poly-cythemia (Appendix A).
   1. Hct
   2. Hgb
   3. Platelets
   4. WBC
   5. Provide parent and family with teaching plan for newborn care.
      a. *Bathing.* Teach *not* to submerge infant in water until cord falls off (7 to 10 days); continue cord care and keep diaper off cord.
      b. *Diapering.* Teach to use warm water to clean infant after voiding; use soap and water with stools. (Remember, cleanse female perineum front to back); may use A&D cream or ointment for rashes.
      c. *Crying.* Teach that infant may cry 2 hours per day when hungry, wet, or bored. Encourage picking the baby up. Teach to identify fussy periods and change environment when they occur.
      d. *Comfort.* Encourage parents to enjoy swaddling, to avoid startling infant when picking up; to try to burp when fussy or crying (may be a gas bubble).
G. Recognize signs and symptoms of a sick newborn who needs medical attention.
   1. Lethargy or difficulty waking
   2. Temperature above 100°F (37.8°C)
   3. Vomiting (large emesis, not spitting up)
   4. Green, liquid stools
   5. Refusal of two feedings in a row

> **HESI Hint** • Teach parents to take infant's temperature, both axillary and rectal. Axillary is recommended, but some pediatricians request a rectal (core) temperature.
> • Axillary: Place thermometer under infant's arm and hold thermometer in place for 5 minutes.
> • Rectal: Use thermometer with *blunt* end. Insert thermometer ¼ to ½ inch and hold in place for 5 minutes. Hold feet and legs firmly.

Review of the Normal Newborn

1. The newborn transitional period consists of the first _____ of life.
2. The nurse anticipates which newborns will be at greater risk for problems in the transitional period. State three factors that predispose to respiratory depression in the newborn.
3. What is the danger to the newborn of heat loss in the first few hours of life?
4. Normal newborn temperature is _____. Normal newborn heart rate is _____. Normal newborn respiratory rate is ___. Normal newborn blood pressure is _____.
5. The nurse records a temperature below 97°F on admission of the newborn. What nursing actions should be taken?
6. True or False: The newborn's head is usually smaller than the chest.
7. During the physical examination of the newborn, the nurse notes the cry is shrill, high-pitched, and weak. What are the possible causes?
8. The nurse notes a swelling over the back part of the newborn's head. Is this a normal newborn variation?
9. What symptoms are common to most newborns with Down syndrome?
10. Identify three ways to determine the presence of congenital hip dislocation in the newborn.
11. Should the normal newborn have a positive or negative Babinski reflex?
12. A small-for-gestational-age newborn is identified as one who _____.
13. When suctioning the newborn with a bulb syringe, which should be suctioned first, the mouth or the nose?
14. A new mother asks the nurse whether circumcision is medically indicated in the newborn. How should the nurse respond?
15. Normal blood glucose in the term neonate is _____.
16. Why does the newborn need vitamin K in the first hour after birth?
17. Physiologic jaundice in the newborn occurs _____. It is caused by _____.
18. When is the screening test for phenylketonuria done?
19. A term newborn needs to take in _____ calories per pound per day. After the initial weight loss is sustained, the newborn should gain _____ per day.
20. List five signs and symptoms new parents should be taught to report immediately to a doctor or clinic.

Answers to Review

1. 6 to 8 hours
2. Cesarean section delivery; magnesium sulfate given to mother in labor; asphyxia or fetal distress during labor
3. It leads to depletion of glucose (there is very little glycogen storage in immature liver); body begins to use brown fat for energy, producing ketones and causing subsequent ketoacidosis and shock.
4. 97.7 to 99.4°F; 110 to 160 bpm; 30 to 60; 80/50
5. Place newborn in isolette or under radiant warmer and attach a temperature skin probe to regulate temperature in isolette or radiant warmer. Wrap newborn double if no isolette or warmer is available, and put cap on head. Watch for signs of hypothermia and hypoglycemia.
6. False: The head is usually 2 cm larger unless severe molding occurred.
7. CNS anomalies, brain damage, hypoglycemia, drug withdrawal
8. It depends on the finding. If it crosses suture lines and is a caput (edema), it is normal. If it does not cross suture lines, it is a cephalhematoma with bleeding between the skull and periosteum. This could cause hyperbilirubinemia. This is an abnormal variation.
9. Low-set ears, simian crease on palm, protruding tongue, Brushfield spots in iris, epicanthal folds
10. Hip click determination, asymmetric gluteal folds, unequal limb lengths

11. Positive; the transient reflex is present until 12 to 18 months of age.
12. Has a weight below the tenth percentile for estimated weeks of gestation.
13. The mouth; stimulating the nares can initiate inspiration, which could cause aspiration of mucus in oral pharynx.
14. There is controversy concerning this issue, but we do know it causes pain and trauma to the newborn, and the medical indications (prevention of penile and cervical cancer) may be unfounded.
15. 40 to 80 mg/dl
16. The sterile gut at delivery lacks intestinal bacteria necessary for the synthesis of vitamin K; vitamin K is needed in the clotting cascade to prevent hemorrhagic disorders.
17. Jaundice occurs at 2 to 3 days of life and is caused by immature liver's inability to keep up with the bilirubin production resulting from normal RBC destruction.
18. At 2 to 3 days of life, or after enough breast milk or formula, usually after 24 hours, is ingested to allow for determination of body's ability to metabolize amino acid phenylalanine.
19. 50; 1 oz, or 30 g
20. Lethargy, temperature >100°F, vomiting, green stools, refusal of two feeds in a row

High-Risk Disorders

ANTEPARTUM HEMORRHAGE: MISCARRIAGE (SPONTANEOUS ABORTION)

A. It is indicated by bleeding between conception and 20 weeks' gestation.
B. About 75% of spontaneous abortions occur between 8 and 13 weeks; they are usually related to chromosomal defects.
C. It is considered a medical emergency.

Nursing Assessment

A. Gestational age of 20 weeks or less; fetal viability absent
B. Uterine cramping, backache, and pelvic pressure
C. Bright-red vaginal bleeding
  1. Note number of perineal pads per hour.
  2. Note symptoms of shock:
    a. Rapid, thready pulse
    b. Pallor
    c. Hypotension
    d. Cool, clammy skin

3. Assess client's and family's emotional status, needs, and support systems

Analysis (Nursing Diagnoses)

A. *Deficient fluid volume* related to...
B. *Anxiety* related to...

Nursing Plans and Interventions

A. Identify type of abortion and subsequent management.
B. Monitor vital signs, level of consciousness every hour until stable.
C. Save all peripads, linens.
D. Start an IV with at least an 18-gauge over-the-needle catheter.
E. Give RhoGAM if indicated (Rh-negative mother).
F. Teach client to notify nurse if the following occur:
  1. Temperature above 100.4°F
  2. Foul-smelling vaginal discharge
  3. Bright-red bleeding accompanied by any tissue larger than a dime
G. Implement grief protocol if fetus loss occurs.

1. Provide a memory packet (footprints, bracelet).
2. Give client and family opportunity to see fetus (sex of fetus).
3. Explain the grief process and refer to community resources for grief and loss. (RESOLVE and SHARE are examples of national bereavement support groups.)

Types and Treatments of Miscarriage

A. Threatened
   1. Description: spotting without cervical changes
   2. Treatment: bed rest for 24 to 48 hours; no sexual intercourse for 2 weeks
B. Inevitable or incomplete
   1. Description: moderate to heavy bleeding with tissue and products of conception present; open cervical os
   2. Treatment: hospitalization; dilation and curettage (D&C)
C. Complete
   1. Description: all products of conception passed; cervix closed
   2. Treatment: no need for treatment
D. Septic
   1. Description: fever, abdominal pain and tenderness; foul-smelling vaginal discharge; bleeding from scant to heavy
   2. Treatment: termination of pregnancy; antibiotic therapy; monitoring for septic shock
E. Missed
   1. Description: fetus dead; placenta atrophied but passage of products of conception has *not* occurred; cervix closed
   2. Treatment: watchful waiting; check clotting factors and possibly terminate pregnancy to lessen the chances of developing disseminated intravascular coagulation (DIC).
F. Recurrent/habitual
   1. Description: loss of three or more previable pregnancies
   2. Treatment: varies based on cause; if premature cervical dilatation (incompetent cervix) is cause, prophylactic cerclage may be done.

> **HESI Hint** • Clients with prior traumatic delivery, history of D&C, and multiple abortions (spontaneous or induced) and daughters of DES mothers may experience miscarriage or preterm labor related to incompetent cervix. The cervix may be surgically repaired prior to pregnancy, or during gestation. A cerclage (a McDonald suture) is placed around the cervix to constrict the internal os. The cerclage may be removed prior to labor if labor is planned or left in place if cesarean birth is planned.

GESTATIONAL TROPHOBLASTIC DISEASE (HYDATIDIFORM MOLE)

A. Chorionic villi degenerate into a bunch of clear vesicles in grapelike clusters.
B. Hydatidiform mole is a developmental anomaly.
C. An embryo is rarely present.
D. It predisposes the client to choriocarcinoma.

Nursing Assessment

A. Vaginal bleeding usually in first trimester.
B. Size and date discrepancy (uterus larger than expected for gestational age)
C. Other common findings
   1. Anemia
   2. Excessive nausea and vomiting
   3. Abdominal cramping
   4. Early symptoms of preeclampsia

Analysis (Nursing Diagnoses)

A. *Grieving* related to...
B. *Deficient knowledge* (specify) related to...
C. *Anxiety* related to...

Nursing Plans and Interventions

A. Provide preoperative and postoperative D&C care.
B. Assess the following:
   1. Vital signs
   2. Vaginal discharge
   3. Uterine cramping
C. Provide discharge instructions.
   1. Instruct to prevent pregnancy for 1 year.
   2. Instruct to obtain monthly serum human chorionic gonadotropin (hCG) levels for 1 year.
D. Teach signs of complications to be reported immediately to health care provider or clinic:
   1. Bright-red, frank vaginal bleeding
   2. Temperature spike over 100.4°F
   3. Foul-smelling vaginal discharge

> **HESI Hint** • If hCG levels do not diminish, choriocarcinoma may develop. Pregnancy may mask the signs and symptoms of choriocarcinoma.

E. Refer to community resource for grief and loss.

ECTOPIC PREGNANCY

A. Fertilized ovum is implanted outside the uterine cavity, usually in a fallopian tube.

B. It occurs in 1 of 200 pregnancies.

C. It commonly occurs as the result of tubular obstruction or blockage that prevents normal transit of the fertilized ovum.

D. It is considered a medical emergency.

Nursing Assessment

A. Possible absence of early symptoms of pregnancy

B. Missed period; full feeling in lower abdomen, lower-quadrant tenderness

C. Positive pregnancy test

D. Signs of acute rupture:
1. Vaginal bleeding
2. Adnexal or abdominal mass
3. Sharp, unilateral or bilateral pelvic pain; abdominal pain
4. Referred shoulder pain
5. Syncope; shock

Analysis (Nursing Diagnoses)

A. *Acute pain* related to...

B. *Grieving* related to...

C. *Risk for deficient fluid volume* related to...

Nursing Plans and Interventions

A. Provide admission care.
1. Assess vital signs stat.
2. Check for vaginal bleeding.
3. Start IV to administer fluids.
4. Notify health care provider immediately.

B. Perform gentle, moderate abdominal palpation and percussion.

C. Explain procedures as interventions continue; allow family member to be present if possible.

D. Prepare client for abdominal ultrasound.

E. Prepare client for possible laparotomy; give preoperative and postoperative surgical instructions.

F. Type and crossmatch for two units packed red blood cells.

HESI Hint • Suspect ectopic pregnancy in any woman of childbearing age who presents at an emergency room, clinic, or office with unilateral or bilateral abdominal pain. Most are misdiagnosed as appendicitis.

ABRUPTIO PLACENTAE AND PLACENTA PREVIA

HESI Hint • A client who is at 32 weeks' gestation calls the health care provider because she is experiencing dark-red vaginal bleeding. She is admitted to the emergency department, where the nurse determines the FHR to be 100 bpm. The client's abdomen is rigid and boardlike, and she is complaining of severe pain. What action should the nurse take first? First, the nurse must use her or his knowledge base to differentiate between abruptio placentae (this client) and placenta previa (painless bright-red bleeding occurring in the third trimester). The nurse should immediately notify the health care provider, and no abdominal or vaginal manipulation or examinations should be done. Administer O_2 by facemask. Monitor for bleeding at IV sites and gums because of the increased risk for DIC. Emergency cesarean section is required because uteroplacental perfusion to the fetus is being compromised by early separation of the placenta from the uterus.

Comparison of Abruptio Placentae and Placenta Previa

Description

Abruptio Placentae	Placenta Previa

A. Partial or complete premature detachment of the placenta from its site of implantation in the uterus
B. Occurs in 1 of 200 pregnancies
C. Usually occurs in late third trimester or in labor
D. Is the cause of 15% of maternal deaths
E. One-third of infants born to mothers with abruptio placentae die.
F. A medical emergency!
	A. Abnormal implantation of placenta in lower uterine segment
	B. Occurs in 1 of 250 pregnancies
	C. Bleeding usually begins in the third trimester
	D. Degrees of previas:
	    1. Partial: placenta lies over part of cervical os.
	    2. Complete: placenta lies over entire cervical os.
	    3. Marginal: edge of placenta meets the rim of the cervical os.

Abruptio Placentae	Placenta Previa
G. Cause unknown but is related to: 1. Hypertensive disorders 2. High gravidity 3. Abdominal trauma (uncommon) 4. Short umbilical cord 5. Cocaine abuse	4. Low-lying: placenta implants in lower uterine segment with a placental edge lying near the cervical os. E. Associated with previous uterine scars, surgery, and fibroid tumors F. A medical emergency!

Nursing Assessment

Abruptio Placentae	Placenta Previa
A. Bleeding: concealed or overt (if overt, is dark red) B. Uterine tenderness C. Persistent abdominal pain. D. Rigid, board-like abdomen E. FHR abnormalities	A. Painless, bright-red vaginal bleeding in third trimester B. Soft uterus C. Possible signs of shock D. Placenta in lower uterine segment (indicated by ultrasound). E. FHR is usually normal.

Nursing Plans and Interventions

Abruptio Placentae	Placenta Previa

A. Institute bed rest with *no* vaginal or rectal manipulation, and notify health care provider immediately.
B. Monitor BP and pulse every 15 minutes; apply electric BP monitor if available.
C. Apply external uterine and fetal monitor.
D. Place client in side-lying position to increase uterine perfusion.
E. Closely monitor contractions and FHR.
F. Begin IV infusion with 16- to 18-gauge catheter
G. Review results for CBC, clotting studies, Rh factor, and type/crossmatch stat.
H. Watch for signs of developing DIC:
  1. Bleeding gums or nose
  2. Reduced lab values for platelets, fibrinogen, and prothrombin
  3. Bleeding from injection sites, IV sites
  4. Ecchymosis
I. Prepare for immediate emergency cesarean section.
J. Monitor blood loss; save pads and linens.
K. Provide constant nurse surveillance and allow presence of family if available.
L. Provide emotional support; teach regarding usual management and expected outcomes of abruption.
	A. Use bed rest to extend the period of gestation until fetal lung maturity is achieved (determined by an L:S ratio of at least 2:1); then delivery is accomplished.
	B. If determined during labor, institute bed rest immediately and notify physician.
	C. Monitor BP and pulse every 15 minutes.
	D. Start IV to administer fluids.
	E. Obtain blood specimen for CBC, clotting studies, Rh factor, and type/crossmatch.
	F. Monitor contractions and FHR; place external monitor on client immediately.
	G. Place in side-lying position.
	H. Continue monitoring blood loss; save pads and linen.
	I. Prepare client for ultrasound diagnosis.
	J. Prepare client and family for possible cesarean birth if placenta previa is complete.
	K. Provide emotional support and appropriate teaching regarding usual management and outcomes of placenta previa.

HESI Hint • Disseminated intravascular coagulation (DIC) is a syndrome of abnormal clotting that is systematic and pathologic. Large amounts of clotting factors, especially fibrinogen, are depleted, causing widespread external and internal bleeding. DIC is related to fetal demise, infection and sepsis, pregnancy-induced hypertension (preeclampsia), and abruptio placentae. (DIC is discussed in greater detail in Advanced Clinical Concepts, p. 33.)

HESI Hint • Clients with abruptio placentae or placenta previa (actual or suspected) should undergo *no* abdominal or vaginal manipulation.
- No Leopold maneuvers
- No vaginal examination
- No rectal examinations, enemas, or suppositories
- No internal monitoring

ANEMIA

A. A decrease in the oxygen-carrying capacity of blood; often related to iron deficiency and reduced dietary intake

B. Occurs in 20% of pregnant women

C. Associated with increased incidence of miscarriage, preterm labor, preeclampsia, infection, postpartum hemorrhage, and intrauterine growth retardation

Nursing Assessment

A. Fatigue, pallor

B. Hgb and Hct signs of anemia:
   1. Hgb <11 g/dL, Hct <37% in first trimester
   2. Hgb <10.5 g/dL, Hct <35% in second trimester
   3. Hgb <10 g/dL, Hct <32% in third trimester

C. See Chapter 5, Sickle Cell Anemia, p. 224.

D. Poor nutritional intake

E. Noncompliance with prenatal vitamin and iron supplementation

Analysis (Nursing Diagnoses)

A. *Ineffective tissue perfusion* related to...

B. *Imbalanced nutrition: less than body requirements* related to...

Nursing Plans and Interventions

A. Analyze 24-hour dietary recall.

B. Review and teach nutritional requirements for pregnancy (see Appendix B, p. 385).

C. Teach about oral administration of iron (Table 6-17).

INFECTIONS

A. Includes STDs and general infections

B. Infections can be harmful to mother and fetus during the antepartum period (Table 6-18).

C. Simple viral infections in the first trimester can cause serious fetal teratogenic effects.

D. STDs have a predilection to manifest at genital and paragenital sites.

Nursing Assessment

A. History of multiple sex partners

B. Previous history of STD or vaginal infections

C. Employment involving high exposure to infection (e.g., child care worker, health care worker)

D. Nonspecific symptoms: fever, malaise

E. General symptoms of STDs: vaginal discharge, genital lesions, dysuria, and dyspareunia

F. Specific symptoms (e.g., herpes simplex blisters)

G. Laboratory studies: antibody titers, TORCH, VDRL (may be negative if drawn too early), RPR, gonorrhea screen, vaginal wet-mount

Analysis (Nursing Diagnoses)

A. *Risk for injury (mother/fetus)* related to...

B. *Deficient knowledge* (specify) related to...

Nursing Plans and Interventions

A. See Nursing Plans and Interventions for STDs, p. 173.

B. Advise regarding immunity to rubella; if client lacks immunity, advise against working with children in terms of risk for exposure.

C. If diagnosed with infection, teach and counsel regarding maternal and fetal effects and how and why to follow the prescribed medical regimen.

PSYCHOSOCIAL CONCERNS: TEENAGE (ADOLESCENT) PREGNANCY

Definition: Pregnancy occurring at age 19 or younger

A. Teen pregnancy rates rose in the United States for the first time since 1991.

B. Teen pregnancy is associated with anemia, preeclampsia, cephalopelvic disproportion (CPD), sexually transmitted diseases (STDs), intrauterine growth retardation (IUGR), and ineffective parenting.

TABLE 6-17 Iron

Drug	Indications	Adverse Reactions	Nursing Implications
• Ferrous sulfate (Feosol)	• Iron deficiency anemia	• Constipation • Diarrhea • Gastric irritation • Nausea or vomiting	• Iron is best absorbed on an empty stomach • To be taken with vitamin C source such as orange juice to increase absorption • Should not be taken with cereal, eggs, or milk, which decrease absorption • Should be taken in the evening if problem exists with morning sickness • Stools will turn dark green to black • Lab values should be checked for increased reticulocytes and rising Hgb and Hct

TABLE 6-18 Infections: Maternal and Fetal Effects

Infections	Maternal Effects	Fetal Effects	Treatment
• *Chlamydia trachomatis*	• Mucopurulent vaginal discharge • Dysuria • Acute salpingitis • Pelvic inflammatory disease (PID) • Sterility or infertility	• Stillbirth or neonatal death • Preterm birth • Ophthalmia neonatorum • Pneumonia	• Erythromycin • May need to treat partner: azithromycin (Zithromax)

HESI Hint • Tetracycline is contraindicated in pregnancy because it darkens the teeth of the newborn.

Infections	Maternal Effects	Fetal Effects	Treatment
• Human papillomavirus (HPV) (TORCH disease)	• Small or large, dry, wartlike growth on vulva, vagina, cervix, or rectum (condyloma acuminatum)	• Possible chronic respiratory papillomatosis	• Laser ablation or cryotherapy • In a pregnant woman, lesions usually left alone, unless mild laser treatment needed • Explain need for possible abdominal delivery due to fetal effect

HESI Hint • Podophyllin, which is usually used to treat HPV, is contraindicated in pregnancy because it is associated with fetal death, preterm labor, and cervical carcinoma. Quadrivalent human papillomavirus (types 6, 11, 16, 18) recombinant vaccine (Gardasil) is available to nonpregnant females 9 years and older to prevent HPV.

Infections	Maternal Effects	Fetal Effects	Treatment
• Gonorrhea (TORCH disease)	• Dysuria • Purulent vaginal discharge • PID	• Ophthalmia neonatorum • Sepsis	• Includes both partners • Penicillin and/or Erythromycin and Ceftriaxone used in pregnancy. • Have partners use condoms until cultures negative two times
• Syphilis (TORCH disease)	• Chancre • Late abortion (syphilis is most common cause) • Positive antibody screen; will not show positive if tested too soon after exposure (usually positive 6 weeks after exposure) • Positive tests for *Treponema pallidum* (FTA-ABS)	• Stillbirth • Congenital syphilis, characterized by snuffles (rhinitis) if mother has latent or tertiary syphilis • Hydrocephaly • Congenital cataracts • Copper-colored rash • Cracks around the mouth • Hypothermia (neonate may have difficulty with thermoregulation)	• Treatment before 16 weeks prevents placental transmission to fetus • Penicillin G • Erythromycin
• Toxoplasmosis (TORCH disease)	• Effects are absent or manifest as flulike symptoms	• Stillbirth • Microcephaly • Hydrocephalus • Blindness • Deafness	• Treatment during pregnancy by sulfa drugs • May consider therapeutic abortion if discovered before 20 weeks

HESI Hint • Toxoplasmosis is usually related to exposure to cats, gardening (where cat feces may be found), or eating raw meat.

(Continued)

TABLE 6-18 **Infections: Maternal and Fetal Effects—cont'd**

Infections	Maternal Effects	Fetal Effects	Treatment
• Hepatitis (TORCH disease)	• May result in preterm birth	• Baby is HBsAg positive, IgM positive	• Carriers of hepatitis B are given a series of hepatitis immunizations that may prevent carrier status and chronic liver disease in newborn
• Rubella (TORCH disease)	• Most severe if contacted in first trimester • Therapeutic abortion offered	• Congenital heart defects • IUGR • Congenital cataracts • Hearing or vision problems may arise in later childhood	• No maternal treatment for the virus is available

HESI Hint • Rubella is teratogenic to the fetus during the *first* trimester, causing congenital heart disease, congenital cataracts, or both. All women should have their titers checked during pregnancy. If a woman's titers are low, she should receive the vaccine *after* delivery and be instructed not to get pregnant within 3 months. Breastfeeding mothers may take the vaccine.

Infections	Maternal Effects	Fetal Effects	Treatment
• Cytomegalovirus (CMV) or cytomegalic inclusion disease (CID; TORCH disease)	• Maternal effects are absent or mononucleosis-like	• Stillbirth • Congenital CMV • Microcephaly • IUGR • Cerebral palsy • Mental retardation • Rash • Jaundice • Hepatosplenomegaly	• No treatment is available for mother or infant
• Herpes simplex virus (HSV; TORCH disease)	• A primary or recurrent infection • Painful vesicular genital lesions • Cesarean delivery recommended during active lesion breakout	• Disseminated or localized skin infection • CNS abnormalities	• Safety of systematic acyclovir (Zovirax) in pregnant clients has not been established; should be used in pregnant clients only when infection is life-threatening

HESI Hint • Acyclovir (used to treat herpes simplex) is *not* recommended during pregnancy.

Infections	Maternal Effects	Fetal Effects	Treatment
• Human immunodeficiency virus (HIV) • Acquired immune deficiency syndrome (AIDS) (TORCH disease)	• Usually asymptomatic • Chronic vaginitis • Susceptible to opportunistic diseases and immunologic suppression	• Affects fetus through transplacental transfer, exposure to maternal blood and body fluids, and through breast milk	• See Advanced Clinical Concepts, HIV Infection, p. 53
• Bacterial vaginosis (vaginal infection)	• Milklike discharge with fishlike odor • Itching, burning pain • Can cause premature rupture of membranes • Postpartum endometritis	• Neonatal sepsis and death	• Treated with clindamycin or ampicillin or metronidazole (Flagyl)

TABLE 6-18 Infections: Maternal and Fetal Effects—cont'd

Infections	Maternal Effects	Fetal Effects	Treatment
• Monlial vaginitis (*Candida albicans*, yeast; vaginal infection)	• Common in diabetics and clients on long-term antibiotic therapy • Odorless thick, cheesy vaginal discharge • Severe vaginal itching • Dyspareunia	• Oral thrush or perineal rash	• Treated with Miconazole nitrate cream or Nystatin cream in pregnancy • Client to wear cotton undergarments and to abstain from intercourse until cured
• Trichomoniasis vaginalis (*Trichomonas protozoa*)	• Profuse, frothy, yellowish discharge • Irritation, itching • Dysuria • Dyspareunia	• Usually no fetal effects	• Treat with vaginal suppositories to reduce symptoms during the first and second trimesters of pregnancy

HESI Hint • Although metronidazole (Flagyl) is the treatment of choice for some vaginal infections, its use is contraindicated in the first trimester of pregnancy, and its use during the second trimester is controversial.

HESI Hint • Medications usually recommended for a nonpregnant client with an STD may be contraindicated for the pregnant client because of effects on the fetus.

Nursing Assessment

A. Determine that client's age is between 12 and 19.

B. Assess factors that influence the outcome of pregnancy.
1. Previous history of menstrual or obstetric complications
2. Nutritional status: 24-hour diet recall and analysis
3. Attitude toward pregnancy and becoming a mother
4. Social support system (i.e., family, spouse or boyfriend, friends, school)
5. Exposure to battering from boyfriend, spouse, father, or other male
6. Peer activities regarding smoking, drugs, and unsafe behaviors
7. Client's activities regarding smoking, drugs, and unsafe behaviors
8. Economic status
9. Educational level, knowledge of pregnancy, childbearing, and childrearing
10. Access to prenatal care

Analysis (Nursing Diagnoses)

A. *Deficient knowledge* (specify) related to…

B. *Imbalanced nutrition: less than/more than body requirements* related to…

Nursing Plans and Interventions

A. Establish trust and rapport through interview first, and then proceed to therapeutic relationship.

B. Avoid authoritative, punitive approach to counseling; use an information-sharing approach.

C. Provide information in private regarding options of pregnancy termination, adoption, and local agencies supporting pregnant adolescents.

D. Praise adolescent for all health-maintenance activities (e.g., coming for pregnancy testing, making prenatal visits, and well-thought-out questions).

E. Allow support person to attend prenatal visits.

F. Relate nutrition information to resumption of figure postpartum, skin health, hair integrity, and other normal adolescent concerns.

G. Teach dangers related to substance abuse during pregnancy.
1. Smoking: low-birth-weight infant
2. Alcohol: fetal alcohol syndrome
3. Cocaine: preterm labor and abruptio placentae; subtle neurologic changes in the neonate

H. Teach that teratogenic fetal effects are highest in first trimester.

I. Encourage normal activities to achieve early developmental task of identity versus role confusion and late adolescent developmental task of intimacy versus isolation.

J. Encourage to stay in school, continue identity as student.

K. Prevent social isolation by encouraging adolescent to continue normal activities (e.g., attendance at school functions, games, and family activities).

L. Provide information regarding childbirth classes, peer support groups.

M. Teach major milestones in fetal development (major fetal growth in third trimester).

N. Monitor carefully for development of preeclampsia, nutritional disorders (anemia, IUGR).

> **HESI Hint** • The outcome of adolescent pregnancy depends on prenatal care. Nutrition is a key factor because the adolescent's physiologic needs for growth are already higher, and the additional stress of pregnancy only increases those needs.

PRETERM LABOR

Description

A. Onset of labor between 20 to 37 6/7 weeks' gestation

B. Predisposing factors to preterm labor include
  1. Diabetes, cardiac disease, preeclampsia, and placenta previa.
  2. Infection, especially UTI.
  3. Overdistention of uterus due to multiple pregnancy, hydramnios, large-for-gestational-age baby.

C. Psychosocial factors
  1. Working outside home, if stressful
  2. Two or more children under age 5
  3. Financial stress
  4. No social support system
  5. Smoking >10 cigarettes per day.

D. Preterm labor is responsible for two of three neonatal deaths.

E. Neonates over 2000 g (4.5 lb) or 32 weeks' gestation have best chance of survival.

Nursing Assessment

A. True labor present: contractions with cervical change are occurring (e.g., more than 5 contractions per hour, cervix <4 cm, <50% effaced, membranes intact and not bulging).

B. FHR 110 to 160 bpm with no distress

C. No medical or obstetric disorder contraindicating continuance of pregnancy

D. Fetal fibronectin test obtained from a cervical swab indicating that preterm labor has begun

Analysis (Nursing Diagnoses)

A. *Anxiety* related to...

B. *Deficient knowledge* related to...

C. *Risk for injury (mother or fetus)* related to...

Nursing Plans and Interventions for Premature Labor

A. Antepartum
  1. Use fetal development chart to show client when baby has mature lungs (36 weeks).
  2. Teach warning signs of labor.
    a. Uterine contractions every 10 minutes or more often
    b. Menstrual-like cramps; low, dull backache; and pelvic pressure
    c. Increase or change in vaginal discharge
    d. Rupture of membranes
  3. Teach self-assessment of uterine contractions.
    a. Instruct to lie on left side, place fingers on top of uterus.
    b. Teach to note a periodic hardening or tightening, with or without pain (contraction).
    c. Teach that more than five contractions in an hour should be reported immediately to health care provider or clinic.
  4. Use follow-up teaching with written instructions about warning signs of labor.

B. Intrapartum
  1. Home management
    a. Teach need for bed rest with fetus off of the cervix (e.g., no sitting or kneeling).
    b. Teach side-lying position and elevation of foot of bed to increase uterine perfusion and decrease uterine irritability.
    c. Teach side effects and warning signs of medications. (Client may be taking oral tocolytic drugs [ritodrine or terbutaline]; Table 6-19.)
    d. Teach to avoid sexual stimulation: no sexual intercourse, nipple stimulation, or orgasm.
    e. Teach to increase oral fluid (2 to 3 L/day).
    f. Teach to empty bladder every 2 hours.
    g. Review what to do if membranes rupture or if signs of infection occur (fever, foul-smelling vaginal discharge).
  2. Hospital management
    a. Place on bed rest in side-lying position with continuous fetal monitoring (external).
    b. Notify health care provider *immediately*.
    c. Administer magnesium sulfate: decreases uterine activity through relaxation of smooth muscle secondary to magnesium's replacing calcium in the cells.
    d. Administer terbutaline (Brethine) and ritodrine (Yutopar): beta-adrenergic agent that acts on B_2 receptors, causing uterine muscle relaxation.
    e. Administer tocolytics as prescribed (see Table 6-19).
    f. Administer glucocorticoids (betamethasone) if prescribed to enhance fetal lung maturation or surfactant production if fetus is <35 weeks' gestation.
    g. Prepare for birth or low-birth-weight infant if preterm labor is not arrested.
    h. Continuously monitor fetal heart rate.

TABLE 6-19   Medications for Intrapartal Complications

Drugs	Indications	Adverse Reactions	Nursing Implications
• Ritodrine HCl (Yutopar) beta-sympathomimetic agent • Terbutaline sulfate (Brethine) beta-sympathomimetic agent, bronchodilator	• To stop preterm labor contractions	• CNS effects: → Severe nervousness → Tremulousness → Headache • CV effects → Severe palpitations → Tachycardia → Chest pain → Pulmonary edema • GI effects → Nausea → Vomiting → Diarrhea → Epigastric pain • Lab value distortions → Low K⁺ → Hyperglycemia	• Administer IV • Increase infusion rate every 15 minutes, depending on uterine response and maternal side effects • Obtain maternal ECG and lab values prior to beginning infusion • Place mother on bedside cardiac monitor • Monitor fetus continuously • Monitor vital signs every 15 min • Maternal pulse should not exceed 140 bpm • FHR should not exceed 180 bpm • I&O; weigh daily • Prepare woman for side effects • Notify health care provider of → High pulse, FHR changes, abnormal lab values → Signs of heart failure: dyspnea, jugular vein distention, dry cough, rales in lung bases → Have antidote available (e.g., a beta-blocking agent such as propranolol [Inderal])
• Magnesium sulfate	• CNS depressant administered to a preeclamptic client to prevent seizures • May be used as a tocolytic to stop preterm labor contractions	• CNS depression manifested by: → Depressed respirations → Depressed DTRs • Decreased urine output • Pulmonary edema	• Hold if respiration <12/min, urine output <100 ml/4 hr • Deep tendon reflexes absent • Monitor magnesium levels as prescribed and report values outside therapeutic range (5 to 8 mg/dl) • Remind client of warm, flushed feeling with IV administration • Keep calcium gluconate (antidote) at bedside
• Nifedipine (Procardia)	• Calcium channel blocker • Relaxes smooth muscles of uterus by blocking calcium • Used as a first-line tocolytic or to continue treatment after stabilization with magnesium sulfate	• Maternal → Hypotension → Fatigue → Overdose produces nausea, drowsiness, confusion, slurred speech → Peripheral edema → Facial flushing • Fetal/newborn (rare) → Problems related to maternal hypotension, which would affect uteroplacental perfusion	• Check BP for hypotension immediately before giving medication • Avoid use with magnesium sulfate; can cause severe hypotension • Rise slowly from laying to sitting position, then dangle feet at side of bed • Do not use sublingual route of administration
• Indomethacin (Indocin)	• Prostaglandin Synthetase Inhibitor (NSAIDS)	• Maternal → Nausea and vomiting → Dyspepsia, pyrosis → Dizziness	• Administer for 48 hours or less. • Do not use for women with bleeding potential (coagulopathy, thrombocytopenia), NSAID-

(Continued)

TABLE 6-19   Medications for Intrapartal Complications—cont'd

Drugs	Indications	Adverse Reactions	Nursing Implications
	• Relaxes uterine smooth muscle by inhibiting prostaglandins • Used when other methods fail only if gestational age is less than 32 weeks	→ Oligohydramnios → Reduced platelet aggregation increasing risk for hemorrhage • Fetal → Constriction of ductus arteriosus progressing to premature closure → Decrease in renal function with oligohydramnios • Neonate → Bronchopulmonary dysplasia, respiratory distress syndrome → Intraventricular hemorrhage → Necrotizing enterocolitis → Hyperbilirubinemia → Pulmonary hypertension	sensitive asthma, peptic ulcer disease, significant renal or hepatic impairment, oligohydramnios • Determine amniotic fluid volume and function of fetal ductus arteriosus before initiating therapy and within 48 hours of discontinuing therapy; assessment is critical if therapy continues for more than 48 hours • Administer with food or use rectal route to decrease GI distress • Monitor for signs of postpartum hemorrhage

HESI Hint • Although the toxic side effects of magnesium sulfate are well known and watched for, it is just as important to get serum blood levels of magnesium sulfate above 4 mg/dl in order to prevent convulsions and reach therapeutic range.

HESI Hint • Hold next dose of magnesium sulfate and notify health care provider if any toxic symptoms occur (<12 respirations/min, urine output <100 ml/4 hr, absent DTRs, magnesium sulfate serum levels >8 mg/dl).

HESI Hint • When administering magnesium sulfate, always have antidote available (calcium gluconate, 20 ml vial of a 10% solution).

HESI Hint • Tachycardia is the major side effect of tocolytic drugs, which are beta-adrenergic agents, such as terbutaline (Brethine) and ritodrine (Yutopar); they are used to stop preterm labor. Teach the client to take her pulse prior to administration and withhold medication if pulse is not within the prescribed parameters (usually withheld if pulse is >120 to 140). If administration is via a continuous pump, teach client to monitor pulse periodically.

DYSTOCIA

A. Difficult birth resulting from any cause

B. Can result from any one or all of the "5 Ps":
1. Powers: primary uterine contractions and secondary abdominal bearing-down efforts
2. Passage: maternal pelvis, uterus, cervix, vagina, perineum
3. Passenger: fetus and placenta
4. Psyche: response to labor by woman
5. Position: position of the laboring woman

C. Dystocia is suspected when there is:
1. A lack of progress in cervical dilatation
2. A lack of fetal descent
3. A lack of change in uterine contraction characteristics (frequency, strength, and duration)

D. Dystocia, dysfunctional labor, and uterine inertia are terms used interchangeably.

Nursing Assessment

A. Hypertonic or hypotonic uterine contractions

B. Inability to bear down or push efficiently

C. Prolonged labor patterns (Table 6-20)

TABLE 6-20 Prolonged Labor Patterns

Pattern	Nullipara	Multipara
Prolonged latent phase	>20 hr	>14 hr
Prolonged active phase	<1.2 cm/hr	<1.5 cm/hr
Secondary arrest	No change for >2 hr	No change for >2 hr
Prolonged deceleration phase	>3 hr	>1 hr
Protracted descent	Descent of fetus <1 cm/hr	Descent of fetus <2 cm/hr
Arrest of descent	>1 hr	>½ hr

Analysis (Nursing Diagnoses)

A. *Acute pain* related to…

B. *Anxiety* related to…

C. *Risk for injury (mother/fetus)* related to…

Nursing Plans and Interventions

A. Notify health care provider if prolonged labor patterns occur according to the Friedman curve.

B. Assist with diagnostic procedures (ultrasound, pelvimetry, vaginal examination) to rule out cephalopelvic disproportion (CPD).

C. Assist with amniotomy performed by health care provider: artificial rupture of membranes (AROM) may enhance labor forces.
   1. Explain procedure (it is painless).
   2. FHR is assessed *immediately* after rupture to determine if there is a cord prolapse.
   3. Assess fluid for color, odor, and consistency (blood, meconium, or vernix particles).

D. Initiate oxytocin infusion for induction (initiation) or augmentation (stimulation) of labor, and manage infusion delivery (Box 6-4).

HESI Hint • In 1978, the Food and Drug Administration banned the use of oxytocin for elective inductions. The health care provider must provide, for the record, the medical reason for oxytocin use.

HESI Hint • Dystocia frequently requires the use of oxytocin for augmentation or induction of labor. Uterine tetany is a harmful complication, and careful monitoring is required. The desired effect is contractions every 2 to 3 minutes, with duration of contractions no longer than 90 seconds. Continuously monitor FHR and uterine resting tone. If tetany occurs, turn off oxytocin (Pitocin), turn client to a side-lying position, and administer O_2 by facemask. Check output (should be at least 100 ml/4 hr). Oxytocin's most important side effect is its antidiuretic (ADH) effect, which can cause water intoxication. Using IV fluids containing electrolytes decreases the risk for water intoxication.

BOX 6-4 *Nursing Protocol for Administration of Oxytocin*

- Determine any contraindications to use of oxytocin.
  - Known cephalopelvic disproportion (CPD)
  - Fetal stress
  - Placenta previa
  - Prior classical incision into uterus
  - Active genital herpes infection
  - Floating fetus
  - Unripe cervix
- Add oxytocin (Pitocin, Syntocinon) to IV fluid.
  - Piggyback at the lowest port on the primary IV line.
  - Using the lowest port ensures that very little Pitocin will be in the primary line if an emergency requires discontinuing the drug.
  - Begin infusion slowly and increase at 20- to 30-minute increments until contractions occur every 2 to 3 minutes, are 40 to 60 seconds in duration, and firm.
- Using external or internal fetal monitoring, continuously monitor the following:
  - FHR
  - Uterine resting tone
  - Contraction frequency, duration, and strength

HESI Hint • Women with previous uterine scars are prone to uterine rupture, especially if oxytocin or forceps is used. If a woman complains of a sharp pain accompanied by the abrupt cessation of contractions, suspect uterine rupture, a *medical emergency*. Immediate surgical delivery is indicated to save the fetus and mother.

HESI Hint • The uterus is most sensitive to becoming tetanic at the beginning of the infusion. The client must *always* be attended and contractions monitored. Contractions should last no longer than 90 seconds to prevent fetal hypoxia.

HYPERTENSIVE DISORDERS OF PREGNANCY

A. Gestational hypertension
1. BP elevation occurs for the first time after midpregnancy.
2. There is no proteinuria.

B. Transient hypertension
1. Gestational hypertension, with no other signs of preeclampsia, is present at time of birth.
2. It resolves by 12 weeks after birth.

C. Preeclampsia
1. It is a pregnancy-specific syndrome that usually occurs after 20 weeks' gestation (except with gestational trophoblastic disease [hydatidiform mole]).
2. It involves gestational hypertension plus proteinuria.

D. Hemolysis, elevated liver enzymes, low platelets (HELLP) syndrome: Although not technically classified as a separate hypertensive disorder of pregnancy, HELLP syndrome is a variant of severe preeclampsia, and it can have a wide variety of risk factors and signs and symptoms.

E. Eclampsia: Seizures (with no known cause, like epilepsy) occur in a woman with preeclampsia.

F. Chronic hypertension: Hypertension has been observed before pregnancy or is diagnosed before the twentieth week of gestation (with the exception of hydatidiform mole).

G. Preeclampsia superimposed on chronic hypertension: Chronic hypertension with new-onset proteinuria and a worsening of the already present hypertension, thrombocytopenia, or increased liver enzyme values.

Preeclampsia and Eclampsia

A. This is the most common hypertensive disorder; it develops during pregnancy and is characterized by elevated BP, edema, and proteinuria.

B. Preeclampsia is characterized by an increase in BP of 30 mm Hg systolic or 15 mm Hg diastolic over previous or usual baseline, with concomitant evidence of preeclampsia.

C. It usually develops during last 10 weeks of gestation or up to 48 hours postdelivery.

D. It occurs in 6% to 7% of all pregnancies.

E. It occurs predominately in primigravida and in multigravida if had as a primigravida.

F. Preeclampsia is a major cause of maternal death and fetal hypoxia and death.

G. It is differentiated into three types:
1. Preeclampsia
2. Eclampsia: preeclampsia with seizures and coma
3. HELLP syndrome

H. There is no known cause of preeclampsia. Pathophysiology is characterized by:
1. Generalized vasospasm and vasoconstriction leading to vascular damage over time
2. Loss of plasma protein into the interstitial spaces (fluid is drawn into the extravascular spaces, which results in hypovolemia)
3. Hypovolemia, which results in decreased perfusion to major organs, including the uterus

Nursing Assessment

A. Baseline BP is obtained at first prenatal visit.

B. Risk factors associated with preeclampsia are:
1. Age below 17 years or above 35 years
2. Low socioeconomic status
3. Poor protein intake
4. Previous hypertension
5. Diabetes (gestational or preexisting)
6. Multiple gestations
7. Hydatidiform mole
8. Prior pregnancy with preeclampsia
9. Family history (mothers or sisters with preeclampsia)

C. Mild preeclampsia
1. BP rise to 30 mm Hg systolic and 15 mm Hg diastolic over previous baseline, or 140/90 or greater
2. Proteinuria of ≥0.3 g in a 24-hour specimen
3. Presence of associated conditions (outlined earlier)
4. Weight gain >2 lb/week
5. Proteinuria ≥1+
6. Edema, especially around eyes, face, and fingers
7. Reflexes may be normal or 1+
8. CNS symptoms: possible mild headache, slight irritability
9. IUGR, evidenced by size-date discrepancy

D. Severe preeclampsia: all of the above symptoms *plus* any two of the following:
1. BP of 160 mm Hg/110 mm Hg on two or more occasions
2. Proteinuria 2+ to 3+ (2 g in a 24-hour specimen)
3. Generalized edema (very puffy face and hands)
4. Deep tendon reflexes (DTRs) 3+ or greater, plus clonus
5. Oliguria (less than 100 ml/4 hr)
6. CNS symptoms: severe headache, visual disturbances (blurred vision, photophobia, blind spots), and possibly epigastric pain
7. Elevated serum creatinine, thrombocytopenia, and marked liver enzyme elevation (AST)

E. Severe IUGR; late decelerations of the FHR
1. Eclampsia
2. Presence of seizure in a woman with preeclampsia
3. Tonic-clonic seizures

F. HELLP syndrome
   1. It is characterized by hemolysis (H), elevated liver enzymes (EL), and low platelets (LP).
   2. There is increased risk for abruption, acute renal failure, hepatic rupture, preterm birth, and fetal or maternal death or both.
   3. Its causes arise from changes that occur with preeclampsia.
   4. It is most commonly seen in older, white multiparous women.
   5. Signs and symptoms include history of malaise, epigastric or right upper quadrant pain, nausea, and vomiting.
   6. Many women are normotensive and do not have proteinuria.
   7. These women should still be treated prophylactically with magnesium sulfate (because of the increased CNS irritability that is part of the disease), even if hypertension is not present.
   8. Women with HELLP are at high risk for developing the syndrome again in future pregnancies as well as for developing preeclampsia in other pregnancies not complicated by HELLP.

Analysis (Nursing Diagnoses)

A. *Risk for injury (fetus/mother)* related to…
B. *Risk for ineffective tissue perfusion* related to…
C. *Deficient knowledge* (specify) related to…

Nursing Care for the Client with Preeclampsia Antepartum

A. Home management
   1. Inform client that absolute bed rest with bathroom privileges is necessary (except for regularly scheduled prenatal visits).
   2. Have client weigh herself daily and report >2 lb/week gain.
   3. Teach client to test urine daily for protein.
   4. Provide client with list of signs to report immediately to caregiver.
      a. CNS symptoms: visual disturbances, headache, nausea and vomiting, hyperreflexia, convulsions
      b. Hepatic sign: epigastric pain
      c. Renal signs: oliguria, proteinuria
      d. Fetal distress signs: decreased or absent fetal activity, unusual or extreme fetal activity
      e. Signs of abruptio placentae: vaginal bleeding, abdominal pain
   5. Teach prescribed diet.
      a. High protein
      b. Limited salt intake (no longer completely restricted)
      c. Maintenance of minimum of 35 cal/kg of body weight

6. Teach that signs and symptoms include history of malaise, epigastric or right upper quadrant pain, nausea and vomiting.
7. Teach that many women are normotensive and do not have proteinuria.
8. Inform that the woman could be hospitalized to be treated prophylactically with magnesium sulfate (because of the increased CNS irritability that is part of the disease), even if hypertension is not present.
9. Teach that women with HELLP are at high risk for developing the syndrome again in future pregnancies as well as for developing preeclampsia in other pregnancies not complicated by HELLP.

B. Hospital management
   1. If preeclampsia progresses to severe preeclampsia, hospitalization will be necessary.
   2. Monitor level of consciousness, BP, and vital signs every 4 hours or more often if levels are elevated or abnormal.
   3. Obtain fetal assessment continuously; apply external fetal monitor.
   4. Assess for vaginal bleeding and abdominal pain.
   5. Provide bed rest in left side-lying position.
   6. Start intravenous infusion with 16- to 18-gauge veno catheter.
   7. Insert indwelling urinary catheter with urine meter.
   8. Monitor I&O hourly.
   9. Maintain quiet, slightly darkened environment and limit visitors.
   10. Administer magnesium sulfate and antihypertensive drugs (rare unless diastolic BP consistently over 100), and possibly Pitocin for initiation and augmentation of labor (see Table 6-19).
   11. Assess daily for signs of coagulopathy.
      a. Petechiae under BP cuff
      b. Platelet decrease or increase
      c. Fibrinogen increase or decrease
   12. Assess deep tendon reflexes (DTR) and assess for clonus once each shift or more often if prescribed or abnormal.
   13. Transfer to labor and delivery department if necessary.
      a. Signs of pulmonary edema occur.
      b. HELLP syndrome occurs.
      c. Late decelerations of the fetal heart rate occur.
      d. Preterm labor begins.

Nursing Care for the Client with Preeclampsia Intrapartum

A. When a client with preeclampsia begins labor, control the amount of stimulation in the labor room.

1. Keep nurse-to-client ratio at 1:1.
2. If possible, put client in darkened, quiet private room.
3. Keep client on absolute bed rest, side-lying and with side rails up.
4. Disturb client as little as possible with nursing interventions.
B. Have client choose support person to stay with her and limit other visitors.
C. Constantly explain rationale for procedures and care.
D. Maintain intravenous line with 16- to 18-gauge catheter.
E. Monitor BP every 15 to 30 minutes, keeping BP cuff on or using electronic BP monitor if available.
F. Check urine for protein every hour and report any increase.
G. Determine deep tendon reflexes every hour and report any increase.
H. Administer magnesium sulfate (see Table 6-19).
1. It is usually given IV with a loading dose of 4 g in 100 ml to 250 ml of solution; administer over 20 to 30 minutes to get the blood level up to therapeutic serum levels (5 to 8 mg/dl).
2. Serum blood levels are usually maintained by infusing up to 2 g/hr after loading dose.
I. Monitor for toxicity during magnesium sulfate administration:
1. Urinary output <30 ml/hr
2. Respirations <12/min
3. Deep tendon reflexes absent
4. Deceleration of the FHR, bradycardia
J. When magnesium sulfate is prescribed to be given IM:
1. Give 10 g (5 g in each buttock) with 1 ml 1% lidocaine to decrease pain.
2. Administer deep in dorsal gluteal site with 3-inch, 20-gauge needle; use Z-track or rotation method.
3. Expect onset within 30 minutes to 1 hour, lasting 3 to 4 hours.
K. If convulsions or seizures do occur:
1. Stay with client and use call button to summon help. Have someone get health care provider stat!
2. Turn client onto side to prevent aspiration.
3. Do *not* attempt to force objects inside mouth or put fingers into woman's mouth.
4. Administer O₂ at 10 L/min by facemask and have suction available.
5. Give magnesium sulfate as prescribed (see Table 6-19).
6. Assess labor and delivery status.
L. During the postdelivery period:
1. Assess BP, respirations, DTRs, and urine output every 4 hours for 48 hours (if still on magnesium sulfate, may assess every hour).

2. Carefully assess uterine tone and fundal height for uterine atony resulting from magnesium sulfate administration.
3. Monitor for blood loss: preexisting hypovolemia makes these women sensitive to even normal blood loss.
4. Instruct client to report headache, visual disturbances, or epigastric pain.
5. Check with the health care provider before administration of *any* ergot derivatives.

HESI Hint • The major goal of nursing care for a client with preeclampsia is to maintain uteroplacental perfusion and prevent seizures. This requires the administration of magnesium sulfate. Withhold administration of magnesium sulfate if signs of toxicity exist: respirations <12/min, absence of DTRs, or urine output <30 ml/hr.

HESI Hint • Rarely are antihypertensive drugs used in the preeclamptic client. They are given only in the event of diastolic BP above 110 mm Hg (danger of stroke). The drug of choice is hydralazine HCl (Apresoline).

HESI Hint • Although delivery is often described as the "cure" for preeclampsia, the client can convulse up to 48 hours after delivery.

MATERNAL AND INFANT CARDIAC DISEASE

A. Impaired cardiac function usually results from a congenital defect or history of rheumatic heart disease with valve prolapse or stenosis.
B. It is seen more commonly in women today because of surgical correction techniques in infancy that enable them to live to childbearing age.
C. Impaired cardiac function is dangerous because of the plasma volume increase that accompanies pregnancy.
D. Type and extent of disease
1. Class I: Unrestricted physical activity; ordinary physical activity does not cause cardiac symptomatology.
2. Class II: ordinary activity causes fatigue, palpitations, dyspnea, and angina; physical activity is limited.
3. Class III: With less than ordinary activity, cardiac decompensation symptoms ensue; moderate to marked limitation of activity.
4. Class IV: Symptoms of cardiac insufficiency occur even at rest; no activity is allowed.

Nursing Assessment

A. History of preexisting cardiac disease

B. Cardiac decompensation
  1. Subjective symptoms, determined by client
     a. Increasing fatigue
     b. Dyspnea
     c. Feeling of smothering
     d. Dry, hacky cough
     e. Racing heart
     f. Swelling of feet, legs, and fingers
  2. Objective symptoms, determined by health professional
     a. Pulse >100 bpm
     b. Crackles at lung bases even after deep breathing
     c. Orthopnea and dyspnea
     d. Respirations >25/min
  3. Anemia possible (Hct <32%, Hgb <10 mg/dl)

Analysis (Nursing Diagnoses)

A. *Deficient knowledge* (specify) related to…

B. *Anxiety* related to…

C. *Compromised family coping* related to…

D. *Ineffective tissue perfusion* (specify) related to…

Nursing Care for the Cardiac Maternity Client

A. Antepartum
  1. Teach client to report any symptoms of cardiac decompensation (listed earlier).
  2. Encourage 8 to 10 hours of sleep each night and daily rest periods.
  3. Teach self-administration of heparin if prescribed (see Medical-Surgical Nursing, p. 97).
  4. Give client diet plan, which includes high iron, high protein, and adequate calorie intake.
  5. Inform client of anticipated difficult period for control at 28 to 32 weeks, when plasma volume peaks in pregnancy.
  6. Teach client to notify health care provider at first sign of infection.

B. Intrapartum
  1. Maintain a calm atmosphere, allowing presence of support persons, and keep family informed at all times.
  2. Maintain cardiac perfusion:
     a. Put client in semi-Fowler, side-lying position.
     b. Prevent Valsalva maneuvers, even during second stage (obstructs left ventricular outflow).
     c. Avoid hypotension if epidural anesthesia is used.
     d. Avoid use of stirrups in delivery room (can cause popliteal vein compression and decreased venous return).
  3. Provide pain relief and supportive measures because pain can contribute to cardiac distress.

  4. Monitor forceps delivery and episiotomy (will likely be performed to decrease the time of the second stage).

C. Postpartum
  1. Tailor care to the woman's functional classification.
  2. Continue semi- or high-Fowler position (head of bed raised), with side-lying maintained.
  3. Progress ambulation: dangling, sitting, standing, short to long ambulation according to tolerance and absence of symptoms of cardiac decompensation.
  4. Administer stool softeners as prescribed to prevent straining during bowel movement.
  5. Watch for symptoms of urinary infection: dysuria, white cells in urine, and pus in urine.
  6. Report *any* symptoms of cardiac decompensation to health care provider immediately:
     a. Tachycardia (pulse >100)
     b. Tachypnea (respirations >25)
     c. Dry cough
     d. Rales in the lung bases
  7. Report immediately any temperature spike over 100.4°F.
  8. Plan with the mother and family for support when returning home. If necessary, refer to community resources for homemaking services.

HESI Hint • Nursing care during labor and delivery for the client with cardiac disease is focused on prevention of cardiac embarrassment, maintenance of uterine perfusion, and alleviation of anxiety.

HESI Hint • Should these clients experience preterm labor, the use of beta-adrenergic agents such as terbutaline (Brethine) and ritodrine HCl (Yutopar) is contraindicated because of the risk for myocardial ischemia.

HESI Hint • Normal diuresis, which occurs in the postpartum period, can pose serious problems to the new mother with cardiac disease because of the increased cardiac output.

CONGENITAL HEART DISEASE IN THE NEWBORN

Nursing Assessment

A. Weak cry, cyanosis worsening with crying

B. Lethargy, hypotonia, and flaccidity

C. Persistent bradycardia or tachycardia

D. Tachypnea or other signs of respiratory distress

E. Decreased or absent femoral or pedal pulses

Nursing Plans and Interventions

A. Decrease energy utilization immediately: no nippling (no pacifiers, no excessive stimulation).

B. Notify health care provider stat of findings.

C. Transfer neonate to neonatal intensive care unit (NICU) for diagnostic workup.

> **HESI Hint** • Coumadin may *not* be taken during pregnancy due to its ability to cross the placenta and affect the fetus. Heparin is the drug of choice; it does not cross the placental membrane.

HYPEREMESIS GRAVIDARUM

A. This is the inability to control nausea and vomiting during pregnancy.

B. Hyperemesis gravidarum is characterized by the inability to keep down fluids and solid foods for 24 hours.

C. It is linked to maternal hormones and possibly to psychological reactions to pregnancy.

Nursing Assessment

A. Weight loss during pregnancy

B. Signs of dehydration:
   1. Increased urine specific gravity
   2. Oliguria

C. Psychological distress (different from normal ambivalence in pregnancy)

D. Fluid and electrolyte imbalance; potential metabolic acidosis

Analysis (Nursing Diagnoses)

A. *Risk for fluid volume deficit* related to…

B. *Anxiety* related to…

C. *Imbalanced nutrition: less than body requirements* related to…

Nursing Plans and Interventions

A. Weigh daily at same time with like clothing.

B. Check urine three times daily for ketones.

C. Monitor electrolytes and hydration status. Report abnormal lab values to health care provider stat.

D. Progress diet from clear liquids to full liquids to bland diet, to full diet.

E. Check fetal heart rate (if possible, auscultate by Doppler) every 8 hours.

F. Provide psychological support to offset client's concerns.

> **HESI Hint** • Recent research has found that infection by *Helicobacter pylori* (the bacterium that causes stomach ulcers) is another possible causative factor in hyperemesis. Other pregnancy and nonpregnancy risk factors for hyperemesis gravidarum include first pregnancy, multiple fetuses, age under 24, history of this condition in other pregnancies, obesity, and high-fat diets.

> **HESI Hint** • In severe cases of hyperemesis gravidarum, the health care provider may prescribe antihistamines, vitamin B_6, or phenothiazines to relieve nausea. The provider may also prescribe metoclopramide (Reglan) to increase the rate at which the stomach moves food into the intestines or antacids to absorb stomach acid and help prevent acid reflux.

> **HESI Hint** • Women who suffer from hyperemesis gravidarum are often deficient in thiamin, riboflavin, vitamin B_6, vitamin A, and retinol-binding proteins.

DIABETES MELLITUS

A. It may manifest for the first time in pregnancy as the diabetogenic effects of pregnancy increase.

B. Hormonal changes during pregnancy act to increase maternal cell resistance to insulin so that an abundant supply of glucose is available to the fetus.

C. A preexisting reduction in insulin and the glucose-sparing effects of pregnancy compromise the health of the mother and fetus.

D. If insulin cannot move glucose into maternal cells, the mother will begin to metabolize fat and protein for energy-producing ketones and fatty acids, which result in ketoacidosis.

Nursing Assessment

A. Predisposing factors include:
   1. Family history of diabetes
   2. History of more than two spontaneous abortions
   3. Hydramnios
   4. Previous baby with a weight over 4000 g (8 lb 13.5 oz)
   5. Previous baby with unexplained congenital anomalies
   6. High parity
   7. Obesity

8. Recurrent monilial vaginitis
9. Glycosuria

B. Abnormal glucose screen: A 1-hour glucose screen is routinely done on all pregnant women between 24 and 26 weeks' gestation.

C. Elevated glycosylated hemoglobin A_C used to evaluate diabetic control by reflecting blood glucose level during the previous 6 to 8 weeks, indicates uncontrolled diabetes.

D. Types of diabetes mellitus include:
1. Type 1 (insulin dependent). Client to be scheduled for hemoglobin A_C test (glycosylated hemoglobin reflects glucose control for the life span of the red blood cell, 120 days); prone to ketosis.
2. Type 2 (non-insulin-dependent). In pregnancy, insulin is required to control maternal blood glucose levels.
3. Type 3 (gestational diabetes). Onset during pregnancy and return to normal glucose tolerance after delivery.

E. Symptoms include the three Ps: polyphagia, polydipsia, and polyuria.

F. Hypoglycemia (usually first trimester); insulin need may decrease.

G. Hyperglycemia (second and third trimesters); amount of insulin needed increases.

H. Increased incidence of preeclampsia, infection, and hydramnios

Analysis (Nursing Diagnoses)

A. *Deficient knowledge (diabetes mellitus during pregnancy)* related to…

B. *Risk for injury (fetus/mother)* related to…

Nursing Plans and Interventions

A. At diagnosis, implement the following.
1. Review pathophysiology of disease.
2. Teach home glucose monitoring (urine and blood).
3. Demonstrate insulin administration.
4. Identify signs of hypo- and hyperglycemia and the immediate actions to be taken if signs are noted (see Diabetes Mellitus in Medical-Surgical Nursing, p. 124).
5. Stress importance of regular prenatal visits.
6. Encourage verbalization of concerns regarding diagnosis.

B. Refer client to dietitian for individualized diet management:
1. Calories: 35 to 50 cal/kg of ideal body weight
2. Complex carbohydrates: 50% of diet
3. Proteins: 20% of diet
4. Fat: less than 30% of diet
5. Distribute calories among three meals and four snacks.
6. Review relationship between exercise and diet. Hyperglycemia can be prevented by consistent utilization of calories through exercise.

C. Remind client of expected increased insulin needs in second and third trimesters, related to increasing diabetogenic effects of pregnancy.

D. Review situations that will complicate diabetic control: illness, diarrhea, and vomiting.

E. Teach client to drink orange juice followed by a glass of low-fat milk for hypoglycemic reaction or insulin reaction.

F. Teach client signs and symptoms of ketoacidosis (fruity odor to breath, nausea and vomiting, exaggerated respiratory effort, altered mental state) and that she should go to hospital immediately if any of these symptoms occur.

G. Remind client of need for the possibility of a scheduled induction, between 38 and 40 weeks' gestation, when control of diabetes becomes more difficult.

H. See subsequent material: Nursing Care for the Diabetic Maternity Client, p. 304.

I. Provide care for the infant (see Nursing Care for Infant of Diabetic Mother, p. 304)

HESI Hint • GLUCOSE SCREEN
Client does not have to fast for this test; 50 g of glucose is given and blood is drawn after 1 hour. If the blood glucose is greater than 140 mg/dl, a 3-hour glucose tolerance test (GTT) is done.

HESI Hint • A high incidence of fetal anomalies occurs in pregnant diabetic women. Therefore, fetal surveillance is very important:
- Ultrasound examination
- Alpha-fetoprotein (to determine neural tube anomalies).
- Nonstress and contraction stress tests

HESI Hint • Oral hypoglycemics are not taken during pregnancy because of the potential teratogenic effects on the fetus. Insulin is used for therapeutic management.

HESI Hint • When a pregnant woman is admitted with a diagnosis of diabetes mellitus:
- She is more prone to preeclampsia, hemorrhage, and infection.
- Most diabetic pregnancies are allowed to progress to term (38 to 40 weeks' gestation) as long as metabolic control is maintained and fetal growth is within standards.

Nursing Care for the Diabetic Maternity Client

A. Predelivery period
1. Insert an intravenous line for infusion of insulin and a glucose-containing solution. Insulin does not cross the placental barrier.
2. On the day of delivery, carefully assess client for insulin administration.
3. Titrate regular insulin and glucose-containing solution to maintain blood glucose levels between 70 and 90 mg/dl during labor.
4. Determine blood glucose hourly by finger stick and maintain between 60 to 80 mg/dl.
5. Position woman on left side to avoid pressure on vena cava by large fetus or hydramnios.
6. Check urine for ketones hourly. Report any over 2+.
7. Monitor fetus continuously, using electronic fetal monitoring system.

B. Postdelivery period
1. Use a sliding-scale approach to insulin administration because of the precipitous fall in insulin requirements postdelivery.
2. Continue a 5% glucose infusion at 100 to 125 ml/hr.
3. Check urine each shift for ketones (sign of hyperglycemia, utilization of fat and protein for energy).
4. Monitor for complications:
   a. Preeclampsia
   b. Postpartum uterine atony associated with uterine overt distention
   c. Infection
5. Encourage breastfeeding, which decreases insulin requirements. Insulin does not cross into breast milk.
6. Contraception: diaphragm with spermicide.

> **HESI Hint** • It is useful to discontinue long-acting insulin administration on the day before delivery is planned because insulin requirements are less during labor and drop precipitously after delivery.

> **HESI Hint** • Estrogen-containing birth control pills affect glucose metabolism by increasing resistance to insulin. The intrauterine device may be associated with an increased risk for infection in these already vulnerable women.

Nursing Care for Infant of Diabetic Mother

A. Assessment
1. Macrosomia
2. IUGR
3. Hypoglycemia, hypocalcemia
4. Hyperbilirubinemia, polycythemia
5. Congenital anomalies
6. Infection
7. Prematurity

B. Nursing plans and interventions
1. Observe for birth trauma: clavicle fracture or cerebral trauma.
2. Perform heel sticks for glucose assessment at 30 minutes of age, 1 hour, and as prescribed.
3. Observe for hypoglycemia: jitteriness.
4. Observe for hypocalcemia: jitteriness.
5. Begin small, frequent feedings at 1 hour of age.

EMERGENCY DELIVERY

Description: Emergency delivery (rapid, uncontrolled delivery) is a nonsterile or an unassisted delivery that can be managed without complications to mother or fetus.

Nursing Assessment

A. Bulging perineum
B. Woman screaming that the baby is coming
C. Presenting part visible at introitus

Analysis (Nursing Diagnoses)

A. *Risk for injury (mother or fetus)* related to…
B. *Anxiety* related to…

Nursing Plans and Interventions

A. Do not, at any time, leave the client alone. Have another nurse or staff member bring any equipment needed.
B. If possible, get precipitous delivery basin from ER or closet if birth is occurring in labor room (précis basin includes towels, scissors, cord clamps, bulb syringe, and placenta basin).
C. Place clean towel under mother's buttocks.
D. Have client use hee-blow or blow-blow breathing technique to slow expulsion of head over perineum.
E. If amnion is still present, rupture with fingers or clean implement when head crowns.
F. Apply gentle counterpressure against presenting part (vertex) to prevent the fetus from "popping" over the perineum, which can lacerate tissue and cause fetal cerebral trauma.
G. Check for cord around neck and remove if loose; cut if tight.
H. Deliver anterior shoulder first by gently pressing downward under symphysis.

I. Apply upward pressure over perineum to deliver posterior shoulder.

J. Deliver entire body, holding baby in slightly head-down position to facilitate mucus drainage.

K. Suction baby with bulb syringe quickly (mouth and nares).

L. Dry infant and cover with blanket or towel.

M. If equipment is available, clamp cord in two places and cut in between. If sterile supplies are not available, leave cord intact.

N. Do not milk the cord.

O. When signs of placental separation are seen (gush of blood, lengthening of cord), ask woman to gently push placenta out.

P. Put baby to mother's breast to contract uterus.

CESAREAN BIRTH

A. Delivery of a fetus or fetuses through the abdomen.

B. Whether planned (elective) or unplanned (emergency), such a client is prone to complications:
   1. Anesthesia complications
   2. Usual abdominal surgery complications
   3. Sepsis
   4. Thromboembolism
   5. Injury to the urinary tract

C. The rate of cesarean section births has approached 25% in the United States and is increasing.

D. Vaginal birth after cesarean (VBAC) rate is decreasing due to the complications associated with the procedure.

Nursing Assessment

A. Elective or repeat cesarean birth scheduled.

B. Emergency cesarean birth performed to prevent harm to mother or fetus.

Analysis (Nursing Diagnoses)

A. *Anxiety* related to…

B. *Risk for injury (mother)* related to…

C. *Impaired urinary elimination* related to…

Nursing Care for a Client with Cesarean Birth

A. Before cesarean birth
   1. If surgery is planned, encourage couple to attend cesarean birth class.
      a. Tour of surgical area is usually provided.
      b. Film of cesarean birth is shown.
      c. Discussion is led by staff member.
   2. If emergency cesarean is necessary, obtain informed consent, including health care provider's explanation of risks, benefits, and alternatives to surgery.
   3. Inform anesthesiologist of need for preoperative assessment.
   4. Assist with anesthesia, usually epidural.
   5. Administer preoperative medications if prescribed.
      a. Usually, because fetus is in utero, no analgesia or sedative is prescribed preoperatively
      b. Client may receive antacid to alkalize stomach contents (if aspiration occurs, less damage will be done to lung tissue) or a drug such as a histamine receptor antagonist, which is a gastric antisecretory drug that reduces the production of gastric secretions.
   6. Shave abdomen from xiphoid to one quarter way down thigh, including pubic area (varies according to institution).
   7. Insert Foley catheter.
   8. Obtain lab studies: type and cross-match for two units packed red blood cells, CBC, and chemistry.
   9. Obtain catheterized or clean-catch urinalysis.
   10. Have client remove dentures, contact lenses, rings, and fingernail polish and give to support person.
   11. Notify nursery, neonatologist, and pediatrician of impending cesarean birth.
   12. Allow presence of support person in operative suite unless hospital policy contraindicates it.
   13. Maintain safety during transfer to operative suite.

B. Intraoperative care
   1. Prior to abdominal preparation:
      a. Place wedge under one hip to displace uterus laterally.
      b. Keep client warm with warm blankets.
      c. Monitor and document fetal heart tones continuously.
   2. Apply grounding pad to leg.
   3. Perform abdominal scrub (prep).
   4. Perform circulating nurse duties per institutional protocol.
   5. If client is awake, assess and meet psychosocial needs.

C. After cesarean birth
   1. Receive complete report, including the type of uterine incision performed.
   2. Fundal height and consistency assessment may be difficult due to abdominal bandage and pain. Note on chart if unable to determine, but gentle attempts should be made.
   3. Assess temperature every hour in recovery room, then every 4 hours for 24 hours, and every 8 hours thereafter if temperature is within normal limits.
   4. Assess heart rate, respirations, breath sounds, bowel sounds, and SaO_2 according to unit protocol.
   5. Begin I&O assessment every 8 hours.

6. Administer pain medication as prescribed. The trend is toward patient-controlled analgesia (PCA pumps) and postoperative epidural analgesia with morphine sulfate (Duramorph), fentanyl citrate (Sublimaze) or meperidine (Demerol; Table 6-21).
7. Encourage participation in infant care as soon as possible, and take mother or couple to nursery often.
8. Demonstrate splinting of abdomen, coughing, deep breathing, and use of incentive spirometer to prevent respiratory complications due to stasis of lung secretions.
9. Maintain aseptic technique to prevent sepsis.
   a. Teach hand-washing technique.
   b. Assess incisional healing every 8 hours.
   c. Perform scrupulous perineum care and pad changes.
   d. Assess lochia for foul odor (indicative of infection).

HESI Hint • If a woman is medicated, the responsible adult accompanying her must sign the necessary consent forms. State laws differ as to the acceptability of a friend signing the consent form rather than a relative.

HESI Hint • Babies delivered abdominally miss out on the vaginal squeeze and are born with more fluid in their lungs, predisposing them to transient tachypnea (TTN) and respiratory distress.

HESI Hint • The preferable low-transverse uterine incision usually results in less postoperative pain, less bleeding, and fewer incidents of ruptured uterus. The classical, vertical incision of the uterus may involve part of the fundus, resulting in more postoperative pain, more bleeding, and an increased chance for uterine rupture.

HESI Hint • Due to the exploration and cleansing of the uterus just after delivery of the placenta, the amount of lochia may be scant in the recovery room. However, pooling in the vagina and uterus while on bed rest may result in blood running down the client's leg when she first ambulates. Cesarean birth clients have the same lochial changes, placental site healing, and aseptic needs as do vaginal birth clients.

HESI Hint • A laparotomy of any kind, including cesarean birth, predisposes the client to postoperative paralytic ileus. When the bowel is manipulated during surgery, it ceases peristalsis, and this condition may persist. Symptoms include absent bowel sounds, abdominal distention, tympany on percussion, nausea and vomiting, and of course, obstipation (intractable constipation). Early ambulation is an effective nursing intervention.

TABLE 6-21 Narcotic Analgesics

Drugs	Indications	Adverse Reactions	Nursing Implications
• Fentanyl citrate (Sublimaze)	• Used as an adjunct to anesthesia	• Respiratory depression, apnea • Bradycardia, hypotension	• Have resuscitation equipment readily available • Do not mix with IV barbiturates
• Morphine sulfate (Astramorph PF, Duramorph, MS Contin) (see Table 3-16, p. 60)	• Often first choice for severe pain	• Nausea, vomiting, constipation • Respiratory depression, depression of cough reflexes • Hypotension	• Check respirations and BP prior to administration; hold administration if respirations <12 or if hypotension exists • Have antagonist, naloxone HCl (Narcan), available in case of respiratory depression

Review of High-Risk Disorders

1. What instructions should the nurse give the woman with a threatened abortion?

2. Identify the nursing plans and interventions for a woman hospitalized with hyperemesis gravidarum.

3. Describe discharge counseling for a woman after hydatidiform mole evacuation by D&C.

4. What condition should the nurse suspect if a woman of childbearing age presents to an emergency room with bilateral or unilateral abdominal pain, with or without bleeding?

5. List three symptoms of abruptio placentae and three symptoms of placenta previa.

6. What specific information should the nurse include when teaching about human papillomavirus detection and treatment?

7. State three principles pertinent to counseling and teaching a pregnant adolescent.

8. What complications are pregnant adolescents particularly prone to develop?

9. All pregnant women should be taught preterm labor recognition. Describe the warning symptoms of preterm labor.

10. List the factors predisposing a woman to preterm labor.

11. When is preterm labor able to be arrested?

12. What is the major side effect of beta-adrenergic tocolytic drugs (Terbutaline, Ritodrine)?

13. What special actions should the nurse take during the intrapartum period if preterm labor is unable to be arrested?

14. A prolonged latent phase for a multipara is _____ and for a nullipara is _____. Multiparas' average cervical dilatation is _____ cm/hr in the active phase, and nulliparas' average cervical dilatation is _____ cm/hr in the active phase.

15. What are the major goals of nursing care related to pregnancy-induced hypertension with preeclampsia?

16. Magnesium sulfate is used to treat preeclampsia.

    A. What is the purpose of administering magnesium sulfate?

    B. What is the main action of magnesium sulfate?

    C. What is the antidote for magnesium sulfate?

    D. List the three main assessment findings indicating toxic effects of magnesium sulfate.

17. What are the major symptoms of preeclampsia?

18. What is the priority nursing action after spontaneous or artificial rupture of membranes?

19. What is the most common complication of oxytocin augmentation or induction of labor? List three actions the nurse should take if such a complication occurs.

20. List the symptoms of water intoxication resulting from the effect of Pitocin (oxytocin) on the antidiuretic hormone (ADH).

21. State three nursing interventions during forceps delivery.

22. What is the cause of preeclampsia?

23. What interventions should the nurse implement to prevent further CNS irritability in the preeclampsia client?

24. A woman on Orinase (oral hypoglycemic) asks the nurse if she can continue this medication during pregnancy. How should the nurse respond?

25. Name three maternal and three fetal complications of gestational diabetes.

26. When should the nurse hold the dose of magnesium sulfate and call the physician?

27. State three priority nursing actions in the postdelivery period for the client with preeclampsia.

28. What are the two most difficult times for control in the pregnant diabetic?

29. Why is regular insulin used in labor?

30. List three conditions clients with diabetes mellitus are more prone to develop.

31. When is cardiac disease in pregnancy most dangerous?

32. Does insulin cross the placenta-breast barrier?

33. The goal for diabetic management during labor is euglycemia. How is it defined?

34. What contraceptive technique is recommended for diabetic women?

35. List the symptoms of cardiac decompensation in a laboring client with cardiac disease.

36. What interventions can the nurse implement to maintain cardiac perfusion in a laboring cardiac client?

37. Gentle counterpressure against the perineum during an emergency delivery prevents _____ and _____.

38. When may a vaginal birth after cesarean (VBAC) be considered by a woman with a previous cesarean section?

39. Prior to anesthesia for cesarean section delivery, the mother may be given an antacid or a gastric antisecretory drug (histamine receptor antagonist). State the reasons these drugs are given.

40. Clients who have had a cesarean section are prone to what postoperative complications?

Answers to Review

1. Maintain strict bed rest for 24 to 48 hours. Avoid sexual intercourse for 2 weeks.
2. Weigh daily; check urine ketone three times daily; give progressive diet; check FHR every 8 hours; monitor for electrolyte imbalances.
3. Prevent pregnancy for 1 year. Return to clinic or MD for monthly hCG levels for 1 year. Postoperative D&C instructions: call if bright-red vaginal bleeding or foul-smelling vaginal discharge occurs, or temperature spikes over 100.4°F.
4. Ectopic pregnancy
5. Abruptio placentae: fetal distress; rigid, board-like abdomen; pain; dark-red or absent bleeding
   Previa: pain-free; bright-red vaginal bleeding; normal FHR; soft uterus
6. Detection of dry, wartlike growths on vulva or rectum. Need for Pap smear in the prenatal period. Treatment with laser ablation (cannot use podophyllin during pregnancy). Associated with cervical carcinoma in mother and respiratory papillomatosis in neonate. Teach about immunization for females age 9 to 30 with Gardasil.
7. Nurse must establish trust and rapport before counseling and teaching begin. Adolescents do not respond to an authoritarian approach. Consider the developmental tasks of identity and social and individual intimacy.
8. Preeclampsia, IUGR, CPD, STDs, anemia
9. More than five contractions per hour; cramps; low, dull backache; pelvic pressure; change in vaginal discharge
10. Urinary tract infection; overdistention of uterus; diabetes; preeclampsia; cardiac disease; placenta previa, psychosocial factors such as stress.
11. Cervix is <4 cm dilated, <50% effacement, and membranes are intact and not bulging out of the cervical os.
12. Tachycardia
13. Monitor the FHR continuously and limit drugs that cross placental barriers so as to prevent fetal depression or further compromise.
14. >14 hours, >20 hours, 1.5, 1.2
15. Maintenance of uteroplacental perfusion; prevention of seizures; prevention of complications such as HELLP syndrome, DIC, and abruption
16. Answers are as follows:
    A. To prevent seizures by decreasing CNS irritability
    B. Central nervous system depression (seizure prevention)
    C. Calcium gluconate
    D. Reduced urinary output, reduced respiratory rate, and decreased reflexes
17. Increase in BP of 30 mm Hg systolic and 15 mm Hg diastolic over previous baseline; proteinuria (albuminuria); CNS disturbances
18. Assessment of the fetal heart rate
19. Tetany. Turn off Pitocin. Turn pregnant woman onto side. Administer O_2 by mask.
20. Nausea and vomiting, headache, and hypotension
21. Ensure empty bladder. Auscultate FHR before application, during process, and between traction periods. Observe for maternal lacerations and newborn cerebral or facial trauma.
22. The person who determines the exact cause will be our next Nobel Prize winner! However, the underlying pathophysiology appears to be generalized vasospasm with increased peripheral resistance and vascular damage. This decreased perfusion results in damage to numerous organs.
23. Darken room, limit visitors, maintain close 1:1 nurse:client ratio, place in private room, plan nursing interventions all at the same time so client is disturbed as little as possible.
24. No. Oral hypoglycemic medications are teratogenic to the fetus. Insulin will be used.
25. Maternal: hypoglycemia, hyperglycemia, ketoacidosis
    Fetal: macrosomia, hypoglycemia at birth, fetal anomalies
26. When the client's respirations are <12/min, DTRs are absent, or urinary output is <100 ml/4 hr
27. Monitor for signs of blood loss. Continue to assess BP and DTRs every 4 hours. Monitor for uterine atony.
28. Late in the third trimester and in the postpartum period, when insulin needs drop sharply (The diabetogenic effects of pregnancy drop precipitously.)
29. It is short-acting, predictable, can be infused intravenously, and can be discontinued quickly if necessary
30. Preeclampsia, hydramnios, infection
31. At peak plasma volume increase, between 28 and 32 weeks' gestation; and during stage II labor
32. No. Therefore, insulin-dependent women may breastfeed.
33. 70 to 90 mg/dl
34. Diaphragm with spermicide; clients should avoid birth control pills, which contain estrogen, and IUDs, which are an infection risk.
35. Tachycardia, tachypnea, dry cough, rales in lung bases, dyspnea, and orthopnea
36. Position client in a semi- or high Fowler position. Prevent Valsalva maneuvers. Position client in a side-lying position for regional anesthesia. Avoid stirrups because of possible popliteal vein compression and decreased venous return.
37. Maternal lacerations, fetal cerebral trauma
38. If a low uterine transverse incision was performed and can be documented and if the original complication does not recur, i.e., CPD
39. Antacid buffers alkalize the stomach secretions. If aspiration occurs, less lung damage ensues. An antisecretory drug reduces gastric acid, reducing the risk for gastric aspiration.
40. Paralytic ileus, infection, thromboembolism, respiratory complications, and impaired maternal-infant bonding

Postpartum High-Risk Disorders

POSTPARTUM INFECTIONS

Description: Any clinical infection of the vaginal canal and perineum that occurs within 28 days of delivery

Nursing Assessment

A. Women predisposed to infection include those with:
1. Rupture of membranes >24 hours.
2. Any lacerations or operative incisions (forceps, episiotomy, or cesarean section).
3. Hemorrhage.
4. Hematomas.
5. Lapses in aseptic technique before or after delivery (e.g., faulty perineal care).
6. Anemia or poor physical health prior to delivery.
7. Intrauterine manipulation, manual removal of placenta, retained placental fragments.

B. Women predisposed to puerperal morbidity include those:
1. With a temperature of 100.4°F or higher.
2. In whom morbidity occurs within the first 24 hours after delivery.
3. In whom temperature elevation occurs on two successive days or in two successive 4-hour assessments.

C. Signs of infection (see subsequent section, Assessment Data for Puerperal Infection)

D. Most common organisms are streptococcal and anaerobic organisms; least common organism is staphylococcus.

Assessment Data for Puerperal Infection

A. Perineal infection
1. Temperature 101° to 104°F (38.3° to 40°C)
2. Red, swollen, very tender perineum (episiotomy site)
3. Purulent drainage, induration

B. Endometritis (infection of lining of uterus)
1. Temperature 101° to 102°F (38.3° to 39.9°C)
2. Pulse >100
3. Malaise, anorexia
4. Excess fundal tenderness long after it is expected
5. Uterine subinvolution
6. Lochia returning to rubra from serosa
7. Foul-smelling lochia

C. Parametritis (pelvic cellulitis)
1. Temperature 103° to 104°F (39.4° to 40°C)
2. Tachycardia, tachypnea
3. Severe uterine and cervical tenderness
4. WBC >25,000
5. Palpable pelvic abscess

D. Peritonitis
1. Chills and temperature to 105°F
2. Rapid, thready pulse to 140 bpm
3. Decreased urinary output
4. Paralytic ileus, abdominal distention, absence of bowel sounds

E. Thrombophlebitis (deep vein)
1. Minimal fever, if any
2. Positive Homan sign (if assessed)
3. Pain in calf or dull ache in leg
4. Swelling in extremity below pain

F. Urinary tract infection or cystitis (bladder)
1. Slight or no temperature
2. Dysuria, frequency, urgency, suprapubic tenderness
3. Hematuria, bacteriuria
4. Cloudy urine

G. Pyelonephritis (kidney)
1. Temperature 102°F and higher, chills
2. Flank pain and costovertebral-angle tenderness
3. Nausea and vomiting
4. Dysuria, urgency, cloudy urine, hematuria, bacteriuria

H. Mastitis (breast)
1. Sore, cracked nipple
2. Flulike symptoms: malaise, chills, and fever
3. Red, warm lump in breast

Analysis (Nursing Diagnoses)

A. *Risk for injury* related to…

B. *Deficient knowledge* (specify) related to…

C. *Acute pain* related to…

Nursing Plans and Interventions

A. Implement general care pertinent to any client with a diagnosed infection:
1. Use and teach good hand-washing technique (HWT).
2. Assess and record vital signs, especially temperature, every 4 hours or more often if indicated.
3. Manage fever by increasing fluids, providing cool cloths, administering acetaminophen (Tylenol) PO or by suppository.
4. Assess for signs of dehydration: inelastic skin turgor, dry mucous membranes, increased urine specific gravity.
5. Maintain hydration: increase fluid intake to 2 to 3 L/day.
6. Promote nutrition: teach to include four basic food groups and increase intake of foods containing vitamin C (for healing) and protein (for tissue repair).
7. Emphasize need for adherence to medication regimen (take entire antibiotic series).

8. Teach to maintain cleanliness, personal hygiene.
9. Implement medical and nursing interventions for specific diagnosed infections.

B. Perineal infection
1. Teach to stay warm, but not to use hot water bottle in bed if chilled.
2. Assess site daily for decrease in redness, pain, and discharge.
3. Assist with sitz bath and perineal lamp 2 to 3 times daily; encourage meticulous perineum care.
4. Administer antibiotics and analgesics as prescribed.

C. Endometritis
1. Usually maintain bed rest (Fowler or semi-Fowler position) with bathroom privileges.
2. Palpate fundus and abdomen every 8 hours to assess pain and involution.
3. Administer antibiotics, usually IV, commonly using a saline lock (Table 6-22).

D. Parametritis
1. Promote lochial and uterine drainage by instructing client to use semi-Fowler position.
2. Determine amount and odor of lochia (heavy, foul-smelling lochia usually indicates anaerobic bacteria).
3. Monitor for development of pelvic thrombophlebitis: clot in ovarian vein will cause acute abdominal pain.
4. Administer IV antibiotics.

E. Peritonitis
1. Client is usually transferred to intensive care: *medical emergency*.
2. Give O₂ through mask.
3. Administer IV antibiotics.
4. Insert nasogastric tube for gastric decompression and prevention of vomiting caused by paralytic ileus.

5. Assess abdomen three times daily for tympany, distention, and bowel sounds.
6. Monitor and document I&O.

F. Mastitis
1. Obtain culture and sensitivity of breast milk.
2. Instruct client to breastfeed every 2 to 3 hours and to make sure breasts are emptied with each feed.
3. Do not let client cease breastfeeding abruptly unless health care provider so prescribes.
4. Tell client that she may have to discontinue breastfeeding if there is pus in breast milk or if antibiotic is contraindicated in breastfeeding. Mother should manually empty her breasts and discard the milk to maintain milk production and reduce congestion.
5. If the newborn develops diarrhea, contact health care provider regarding changing antibiotic.
6. Mastitis is usually treated at home by PO antibiotics.
7. Tell client to maintain bed rest for 48 hours.
8. Monitor client for abscess formation, need for incision and drainage.

G. Deep vein thrombophlebitis
1. See Medical Surgical Nursing for interventions, p. 98.
2. Administer anticoagulant therapy (heparin for 6 weeks; see Table 4-16, p. 97).

H. Cystitis and pyelonephritis
1. Collect urine for analysis and culture.
2. Avoid catheterization if at all possible.

I. STDs
1. See Medical-Surgical Nursing for interventions, p. 173.
2. Breastfeeding and rooming-in are affected when the mother has an STD (Table 6-23).

TABLE 6-22 Antibiotics

Drugs	Indications	Adverse Reactions	Nursing Implications
• Ampicillin (Ampicin, Ampilean)	• Broad-spectrum antibiotic used to treat postpartum endometritis, mastitis	• Rash, dermatitis • Nausea, vomiting • GI irritation	• Do not administer to clients with penicillin sensitivity • Does appear in breast milk, but may not cause neonate any discomfort
• Gentamicin sulfate (Garamycin)	• Aminoglycoside antibiotic used for serious puerperal infections	• GI irritation • Nephrotoxicity • Ototoxicity • Neurotoxicity • Possible hypersensitivity	• Do not mix with any other drug • Observe for ototoxicity: ataxia, tinnitus, headache • Observe for nephrotoxicity: elevated BUN and creatinine • Observe for neurotoxicity: paresthesia, muscle weakness • Monitor I&O closely

TABLE 6-23 Breastfeeding and Rooming-in Procedures for Mothers with Sexually Transmitted Diseases (STDs)

STDs	Rooming-in	Breastfeeding
AIDS/HIV positive	Yes	No
Cytomegalovirus (CMV)	Yes	No
Chlamydia	Yes	Yes
Gonorrhea (untreated)	No	No
Medication for 24 hours	Yes	Yes
Hepatitis	Yes	Yes
Herpes	Yes	Yes
Syphilis (untreated)	No	No
Medication × 24 hours	Yes	Yes
Trichomoniasis	Yes	Yes

HESI Hint • In most cases, a mother who is on antibiotic therapy can continue to breastfeed unless the health care provider thinks the neonate is at risk for sepsis by maternal contact. Sulfa drugs are used cautiously in lactating mothers because they can be transferred to the infant in breast milk.

HESI Hint • Many times mastitis can be confused with a blocked milk sinus, which is treated by nursing closer to the lump and by rotating the baby on the breast. Breastfeeding is not contraindicated for women with mastitis unless pus is in the breast milk, or the antibiotic of choice is harmful to the infant. If either of these occurs, milk production can still be fostered by manual expression.

HESI Hint • Clients taking anticoagulants can usually expect to have heavy menstrual periods.

HESI Hint • A nurse must be especially supportive of a postpartum client with infection because it usually implies isolation from newborn until organism is identified and treatment begun. Arrange phone calls to nursery and window viewing. Involve family, spouse, and significant others in teaching, and encourage other family members to continue neonatal attachment activities.

HESI Hint • The most common iatrogenic cause of a UTI is urinary catheterization. Encourage clients to void frequently and not ignore the urge. IV antibiotics are usually administered to clients with pyelonephritis.

HESI Hint • Remember, the risk for postpartum infections is higher in clients who experienced problems during pregnancy (e.g., anemia, diabetes) and who experienced trauma during labor and delivery.

POSTPARTUM HEMORRHAGE

A. It is a leading cause of maternal mortality that demands prompt recognition and intervention.

B. Hemorrhage can be caused by:
1. Uterine atony (poor muscle tone)
2. Lacerations of the vagina
3. Hematoma development in the cervix, perineum, or labia
4. Retained placental fragments
5. Full bladder

C. Predisposing factors include:
1. High parity
2. Dystocia, prolonged labor
3. Operative delivery: cesarean or forceps delivery; intrauterine manipulation
4. Overdistention of the uterus: polyhydramnios, multiple gestation, large neonate
5. Abruptio placentae
6. Previous history of postpartum hemorrhage
7. Infection
8. Placenta previa

Nursing Assessment

A. Excessive uterine bleeding during the first hour following delivery (hemorrhage more than one saturated pad every 15 minutes)

B. Excessive uterine bleeding during the postpartum period (more than one saturated pad per hour)

C. Blood loss of more than 500 ml during vaginal delivery; or loss of 1% or more of body weight (1 ml = 1 g)

D. Signs of hypovolemic shock:
1. Decreased BP
2. Weak, rapid pulse
3. Cool, clammy skin, colored ashen or gray

E. Signs of hematomas developing in perineum:
1. Intense perineal pain
2. Swelling and blue-black discoloration on perineum
3. Pallor, tachycardia, and hypotension (great blood loss); feeling of pressure in vagina, urethra, and bladder
4. Possible urinary retention, uterine displacement

F. Signs of bleeding from unrepaired laceration
1. Continuous trickle from vagina
2. Bleeding in spurts
3. Bleeding in presence of contracted fundus

G. Signs of bleeding from uterine atony
1. Soft, boggy uterus usually above umbilicus
2. Fundus that does not firm up with massage

Analysis (Nursing Diagnoses)

A. *Risk for deficient fluid volume* related to…

B. *Anxiety* related to…

C. *Risk for infection* related to…

Nursing Plans and Interventions

A. Early postpartum
1. Review chart for predisposing factors.
2. Monitor vital signs, fundus, lochia every 15 minutes for 1 hour; every 30 minutes for 1 hour; and every hour for the next 2 hours, or according to institution's policy.
3. Monitor level of consciousness.
4. Keep the bladder empty.
5. Call physician if atony or bleeding continues despite massage.
6. Anticipate increasing Pitocin (oxytocin) IV infusion and administering ergot preparation IM.
7. Count pads saturated and time required to saturate.
8. Monitor I&O (at least 30 ml/hr output); be sure to maintain fluid replacement.

B. Late postpartum
1. Anticipate quick hospitalization and determination of cause of bleeding.
2. Type and crossmatch for possible blood transfusion.
3. Administer oxytocic drugs and possibly ergot preparations as prescribed.

4. Administer antibiotics as prescribed.
5. Keep the client warm, and be alert for symptoms of shock.
6. Prepare client for possible surgical repair of laceration, evacuation of hematomas, or curettage for removal of placental fragments (most common reason for late postpartum hemorrhage).

C. Hematoma development
1. Apply ice pack to perineum to decrease swelling and pain.
2. Prepare client for surgical incision if hematoma is large.
3. Monitor vital signs closely. Because hemorrhage is covert, hypovolemia and anemia can occur without overt signs.
4. Administer analgesics and antibiotics as prescribed.
5. If severe hemorrhage and hypovolemic shock occur, notify physician immediately and:
a. Increase IV infusion to wide open.
b. Give O_2 at 10 L by facemask.
c. Monitor vital signs every 5 to 15 minutes.
d. Lower head of bed; position client supine.
e. Assist with insertion of central venous pressure (CVP) line or hemodynamic catheter.
f. Insert Foley catheter.

HESI Hint • During medical emergencies such as bleeding episodes, clients need calm, direct explanations and assurance that all is being done that can be done. If possible, allow support person at bedside.

HESI Hint • Risk factors for hemorrhage include dystocia, prolonged labor, overdistended uterus, abruptio placentae, and infection.

HESI Hint • What immediate nursing actions should be taken when a postpartum hemorrhage is detected?
• Perform fundal massage.
• Notify the health care provider if the fundus does not become firm with massage.
• Count pads to estimate blood loss.
• Assess and record vital signs.
• Increase IV fluids (additional IV line may be indicated).
• Administer oxytocin infusion as prescribed.

Review of Postpartum High-Risk Disorders

1. May women with a positive HIV antibody test breastfeed?
2. What are the common side effects of antibiotics used to treat puerperal infection?
3. How does the nurse differentiate the symptomatology of cystitis from that of pyelonephritis?
4. What are the signs of endometritis?
5. What are the nursing actions for endometritis and parametritis?
6. State four risk factors for or predisposing factors to postpartum infection.
7. State four risk factors for or predisposing factors to postpartum hemorrhage.
8. What immediate nursing actions should be taken when a postpartum hemorrhage is detected?
9. Must women diagnosed with mastitis stop breastfeeding?

Answers to Review

1. No. HIV has been found in breast milk. (*New England Journal of Medicine*, vol 325, August 1991).
2. GI adverse reactions: nausea, vomiting, diarrhea, and cramping. Hypersensitivity reactions: rashes, urticaria, and hives
3. Pyelonephritis has the same symptoms as cystitis (dysuria, frequency, and urgency) with the addition of flank pain, fever, and pain at costovertebral angle.
4. Subinvolution (boggy, high uterus); lochia returning to rubra with possible foul smell; temperature 100.4°F or higher; unusual fundal tenderness
5. Measures to promote lochial drainage; antipyretic measures (acetaminophen, cool cloths); administration of analgesics and antibiotics as prescribed; increase of fluids, with attention to high-protein and high-vitamin C diet.
6. Operative delivery, intrauterine manipulation, anemia or poor physical health, traumatic delivery, and hemorrhage
7. Dystocia or prolonged labor, overdistention of the uterus, abruptio placentae, and infection
8. Fundal massage. Notify health care provider if massage does not firm fundus. Count pads to estimate blood loss. Assess and record vital signs. Increase IV fluids and administer oxytocin infusion as prescribed.
9. No. Women who stop breastfeeding abruptly may make the situation worse by increasing congestion and engorgement and providing further media for bacterial growth. Client may have to discontinue breastfeeding if pus is present or if antibiotics are contraindicated for neonate.

Newborn High-Risk Disorders

MAJOR DANGER SIGNALS IN THE NEWBORN

A. Of neonates requiring special care at birth, 60% can be identified through the prenatal history and another 20% through a review of intrapartal risk factors.
B. Infants with Apgar scores of 7 to 10 rarely need resuscitative efforts; scores of 4 to 6 indicate mild to moderate asphyxia, and scores of 0 to 3 indicate severe asphyxia.
C. The family experiences extreme challenges in adapting to the crisis of a sick baby.

Danger Signs by System

A. Central nervous system: Lethargy, high-pitched cry, jitteriness, seizures, bulging fontanels
B. Respiratory system: Apnea (lack of breathing for 15 seconds), tachypnea, flaring nares, retractions, seesaw breathing, grunting, abnormal blood gases
C. Cardiovascular system: Abnormal rate and rhythm, persistent murmurs, differentials in pulse, dusky skin color, circumoral cyanosis
D. Gastrointestinal system: Absent feeding reflexes, vomiting, abdominal distention, changes in stool patterns, no stool
E. Metabolic system: Hypoglycemia, hypocalcemia, hyperbilirubinemia, labile temperature
F. Newborn weight is a major variable in determining survival
   1. Low birth weight (LBW): 2500 g or less
   2. Very low birth weight (VLBW): 1500 g or less

HESI Hint • "Jitteriness" is a clinical manifestation of hypoglycemia and hypocalcemia. Laboratory analysis is indicated to differentiate between the two causes.

HESI Hint • To avoid metabolic problems brought on by cold stress, the first step and number one priority in managing the newborn is to prevent loss of body heat; that is followed by the ABCs. Neonates produce heat by nonshivering thermogenesis, which involves the burning of brown fat. The neonate is easily stressed by hypothermia and develops acidosis as a result of hypoxia. Prevent chilling (keep under radiant warmer or in isolette). If an infant is cold, the first signs exhibited are prolonged acrocyanosis, skin mottling, tachycardia, and tachypnea. If an infant is cold-stressed, warm slowly over 2 to 4 hours because rapid warming may produce apnea. A neonate needs glucose; he or she has little glycogen storage and needs to be fed.

Nursing Plans and Interventions for Management of Newborn Resuscitation

A. Ventilations are done over mouth and nose using a size 1 mask for a term neonate, a size 0 for a preterm.

B. With neonates, initial ventilation with peak inflating pressures of 30 to 40 cm H_2O at a rate of 40 to 60 per minute is usually successful in unresponsive term infants

C. If the heart rate is under 60, compressions are done with thumbs side by side; hands encircle the thorax and cover the lower third of the sternum, to a depth of one third the anteroposterior chest diameter. The compression:ventilation ratio is 3:1 to achieve 120 events per minute (90 compressions plus 30 breaths).

D. Start IV fluids (usually in umbilical vein; may use peripheral vein).

E. Administer sodium bicarbonate or epinephrine as prescribed (Table 6-24).

F. Administer glucose as prescribed (stress rapidly causes hypoglycemia).

G. Assign someone to support parents during resuscitation.

H. Resuscitative efforts may be evaluated by the Silverman-Anderson Index of Respiratory Distress. Five criteria are graded:
   1. Upper chest synchronization
   2. Lower chest retractions
   3. Xiphoid retractions
   4. Nares dilation (flaring)
   5. Expiratory grunt

HESI Hint • The lower the score on the Silverman-Anderson Index of Respiratory Distress, the better the respiratory status of the neonate. A score of 10 indicates that a newborn is in severe respiratory distress. This is the exact *opposite* of the method used for Apgar scoring.

OXYGEN THERAPY FOR THE NEWBORN

Nursing Plans and Interventions

A. Principle: Always administer O_2 at the lowest concentration possible when correcting hypoxia. Use an O_2 analyzer to determine the exact O_2 concentration because O_2 is a "drug." Hypoxia and hyperoxia are both dangerous.

B. O_2 toxicity results in:
   1. Retinopathy of prematurity (retrolental fibroplasias, RLF).
   2. Bronchopulmonary dysplasia (BPD).

C. O_2 is prescribed in percentages and represents the FiO_2 (fraction of inspired O_2 in the "air"). Room air has an FiO_2 of 21%. O_2 can be prescribed at between 21% and 199%.

TABLE 6-24   Newborn Resuscitation

Drugs	Indications	Adverse Reactions	Nursing Implications
• Sodium bicarbonate	• Correction of severe metabolic acidosis in asphyxiated infants after adequate ventilation begun	• Fluid overload • Hypernatremia • Intracranial hemorrhage	• Do not mix with calcium solutions; causes precipitate • Use *pediatric* concentration of the drug • Infuse slowly and monitor I&O
• Epinephrine	• Asystole or severe bradycardia	• Tachydysrhythmias	• Make sure ventilation of newborn is adequate • Do not inject directly into artery • Monitor apical pulse or connect to ECG before use

D. Administration of O_2 to a newborn is done via:
1. Oxy-Hood: for concentrations up to 100%.
2. Nasal prongs: for low concentrations.
3. Continuous positive airway pressure (CPAP), which
   a. Reduces the work of breathing and keeps alveoli open to prevent atelectasis (works like the expiratory grunt).
   b. Is administered by nasal prongs or mechanical ventilator.

E. Surfactant administration, with natural bovine lung extract, beractant (Survanta), or artificial surfactant, colfosceril (Exosurf) is administered via endotracheal tube as an adjunct to oxygen and ventilation therapy to prevent and treat respiratory distress syndrome (RDS) in premature infants.
1. Prevention of RDS: Provided at birth to infants with clinical manifestations of surfactant deficiency or with a birth weight less than 1250 g.
2. Treatment of RDS: Administered to infants with confirmed diagnosis of RDS, preferably within 8 hours of birth.
3. Observe infant's condition for changes such as diuresis that may occur with improvement.
4. Ventilator settings may need changing as the infant's ability to oxygenate increases.

F. Adverse effects may include respiratory distress immediately after administration, bradycardia and oxygen desaturation. Extracorporeal membrane oxygenation (ECMO): blood is oxygenated outside the body through a bypass procedure.

G. Monitor for problems associated with neonatal hypoxia:
1. Respiratory acidosis
2. Organ damage
   a. Necrotizing enterocolitis (NEC). Hypoxic-ischemic injury to the mucosa of the intestinal tract results in abdominal distention, sepsis, and nutritional impairment.
   b. Patent ductus arteriosus (PDA). There is a return to fetal circulation in an attempt to provide O_2 to brain and large organs; it results in worsening respiratory distress and pulmonary edema due to increased blood flow to lungs.
   c. Intraventricular hemorrhage (IVH). Hypoxia causes vessel damage in the tiny periventricular capillaries, resulting in symptoms of increased intracranial pressure (IC) (e.g., seizures, decreased or absent reflexes, hypotonia, bulging fontanels, enlarged head circumference, setting-sun eyes, shrill cry, hypothermia, apnea, or bradycardia).

HESI Hint • Watch a newborn's Hct. It is difficult to oxygenate either an anemic newborn (lack of oxygen-carrying capacity) or a newborn with polycythemia (Hct >80%, thick, sluggish circulation).

H. Closely monitor the partial pressure of O_2 in the newborn's arterial blood (i.e., PO_2).
I. Monitor oxygenation status
1. Monitor arterial oxygen saturation level using pulse oximetry. It has a direct relationship to the partial pressure of O_2 in the arterial blood. Oxygen saturation should not fall below 90.
2. Monitor O_2 levels by placing a $TcPO_2$ (transcutaneous oxygen pressure monitor) on the newborn. $TcPO_2$ levels should range from 60 to 80 mm Hg.
3. Draw blood gas determinations from an arterial line every 3 to 4 hours. *Always* correlate O_2 saturation (SvO_2) and $TcPO_2$ readings with blood gases.
J. Criteria for mechanical ventilation: oxygen administration by other means does not reverse respiratory acidosis: pH <7.2, PO_2 <50, PCO_2 >60.

HESI Hint • The PO_2 should be maintained between 50 and 90 mm Hg. PO_2 <50 signifies hypoxia; PO_2 >90 signifies oxygen toxicity problems.

NEONATE WITH SEPSIS

Infections, especially in a preterm infant, can be overwhelming because of the immaturity of the immune system.

Nursing Assessment

A. Lethargy
B. Temperature instability
C. Difficulty feeding
D. Subtle color changes: mottling, duskiness
E. "Just acts funny"; subtle changes in behavior
F. Respiratory distress, apnea
G. Hyperbilirubinemia

Analysis (Nursing Diagnoses)

A. *Ineffective thermoregulation* related to...
B. *Risk for injury* related to...

Nursing Plans and Interventions

A. Prevent infection in the high-risk newborn
1. Meticulous handwashing: 3 minutes before day begins, 1 minute in between each baby

2. Apply triple-dye antimicrobial to cord.
3. Maintain sterile technique during procedures.
4. Avoid wearing rings and other jewelry in nursery and no artificial nails.
5. During contact with body secretions, *use universal precautions! Wear gloves!*
6. Document appearance of IV site every 30 to 60 minutes.
7. Watch skin integrity: use little tape; use sheepskin, waterbed, and range of motion (ROM).
8. Be alert for any staff member who has a herpes lesion that has not reached the crusting stage; such a person should *not* be in the nursery.
9. Maintain adequate nutrition: calculate calorie, protein and fluid needs according to weight.

B. If neonate develops signs of sepsis
1. Place in incubator or isolette and put in isolation room if possible.
2. Assist health care provider with a sepsis workup: blood cultures, spinal tap (CSF), urine collection, chest radiograph, chemistry, and CBC with differential.
3. Administer antibiotics as prescribed.

HESI Hint • Antibiotic dosage is based on the neonate's weight in kilograms. Peak and trough drug levels are drawn to evaluate whether therapeutic drug levels have been achieved. Closely monitor the neonate for adverse effects of all drugs.

PRETERM NEWBORN CARE

Definition: Supportive care for the neonate born at less than 38 weeks' gestation is based on the level of immaturity identified by gestational age and physical assessment.

Nursing Assessment

A. Respiratory distress due to:
1. Lung immaturity
2. Lack of surfactant lining alveoli (air sacs)
3. Immaturity of respiratory center in brain causing apnea and bradycardia
4. PDA, usually related to hypoxia
5. Results in a respiratory distress syndrome (RDS) (hypoxia and hypercarbia)

B. Temperature instability related to:
1. Insufficient subcutaneous fat
2. Larger ratio of body surface area to body weight
3. Extended, open body position
4. Immature hypothalamus

C. Nutrition problems related to:
1. Poorly developed suck
2. Small stomach

3. Immature digestion process: lacks some gastric and pancreatic enzymes (no bile salts)
4. Hypoglycemia: decreased glycogen storage in liver
5. Anemia: lack of fetal iron
6. Hyperbilirubinemia: inability of immature liver to handle bilirubin metabolism

D. Fluid and electrolyte problems related to:
1. Limited concentration/excretion ability of kidneys
2. Metabolic acidosis: decreased buffering capacity
3. Hypocalcemia (<7 mg/dl): inability to store and absorb calcium

E. Immunologic immaturity due to:
1. No IgM antibodies
2. No phagocytosis
3. Thin skin barrier
4. Intraventricular hemorrhage (IVH): weak, fragile capillaries in ventricles of brain

HESI Hint • Sepsis can be indicated by both a temperature increase and a temperature decrease.

Analysis (Nursing Diagnoses)

A. *Impaired gas exchange* related to…
B. *Ineffective thermoregulation* related to…
C. *Imbalanced nutrition: less than body requirements* related to…
D. *Infection* related to…

Nursing Plans and Interventions

A. Provide and monitor O_2 therapy.
B. Monitor thermoregulation.
1. Place infant under radiant warmer.
2. Cover infant with plastic wrap to reduce insensible water loss.
3. Warm all things that touch newborn: hands, equipment, O_2, and surfaces.
4. Maintain abdominal skin temperature at 98° to 98.9°F (use skin temperature probe taped over liver), and report any temperature <97°F or >99°F (both increase energy expenditure).
C. Monitor fluid and electrolytes. Observe for signs of:
1. Hypoglycemia: jitteriness, tremors, lethargy, hypotonia, apnea, weak or high-pitched cry, eye-rolling, and seizures
2. Hypocalcemia: jitteriness, apnea, increased muscle tone, edema, abdominal distention, feeding intolerance, and Chvostek sign (twitching over tapped parotid gland)
3. Excessive fluid volume: edema, tachycardia, bulging fontanels, and rales in lungs

4. Deficient fluid volume: sunken fontanels, poor skin turgor, and dry mucous membranes

D. If infant weighs <1500 g, report weight loss >12% (180 g) in first few days of life.

E. Weigh diapers daily.
1. Record diaper weight before putting it on infant.
2. Weigh diaper after infant has voided (1 ml urine = 1 g of weight).

F. Maintain urine output of 1 ml/kg/hr and specific gravity of 1.005 to 1.012.

G. Prevent intracranial hemorrhage (increased risk in VLBW).
1. Monitor vital signs, fontanels, muscle tone, and activity.
2. Monitor Hct level.
3. Follow minimal-stimulation protocol.

H. Maintain nutrition: breast milk is best.
1. Maintain 110 to 150 calories/kg/day; 140 to 160 ml/kg/day
2. Give oral nipple feedings if neonate:
   a. Observe infant: can suck well, has gag reflex, and has a coordinated suck-swallow ability.
   b. Observe that infant >34 weeks' gestation is gaining 20 to 30 g/day.
   c. Observe that infant consumes feeding for 20 minutes or longer without signs of fatigue or tachycardia.

I. Use modified "preemie" formulas: provide 24 calories/oz (increase calories without increasing fluid).

J. Institute gavage feeding if necessary: indicated to avoid aspiration resulting from a weak suck, an uncoordinated suck, and respiratory distress (Box 6-5 and Fig. 6-19).

K. Provide total parenteral nutrition (TPN): for preterm or postsurgical neonate who cannot handle or cannot metabolize enteral feedings (Box 6-6).
1. Monitor glucose, serum and urine.
2. Administer any IV fluid with a dextrose content above 12.5% through a central line.
3. Monitor lab values daily; may include Hct and serum electrolytes.
4. Administer calcium supplement and vitamin D to prevent rickets.
5. Vitamin E (tocopherol) supplement is given as antioxidant to enhance cellular integrity (i.e., prevent oxygen toxicity and red cell destruction).

L. Prevent injury resulting from hyperbilirubinemia (see Nursing Care of Newborn with Hyperbilirubinemia, p. 318).

M. Support family and parental adjustment.
1. Refer to Box 6-7.
2. Initiate early visitation, and accompany parents on first visit to ICU.
3. Provide information to parents daily.
4. Teach care-giving skills
5. Continue to enhance parent-infant bonding.

N. Plan for discharge using multidisciplinary approach.

BOX 6-5 *Gavage Feeding*

Newborn Client

- Gather equipment: sterile feeding tube (5 to 8 Fr); calibrated syringe for formula; stethoscope; sterile syringe without needle; paper tape; formula and medications if prescribed.
- Position newborn with head slightly elevated and towel under shoulders.
- Measure distance from bridge of the infant's nose to the earlobe and then to a point halfway between the xiphoid process and the umbilicus.
- Pass tube along back of tongue, advancing as newborn swallows.
- Test placement:
  - Inject 0.5 ml air using a sterile syringe while simultaneously listening for air "bubble" into stomach with stethoscope over epigastrium.
  - Aspirate a small amount of stomach contents and check pH to verify gastric contents (<3).

HESI HINT • If tube passes into trachea, newborn can make no noise (i.e., no crying). Newborn may gag, cough, or become cyanotic.

- Aspirate and measure any residual stomach contents and reduce volume of feeding by amount of residual obtained (if health care provider so prescribes).
- Attach large feeding syringe to tube with plunger removed; pour in warmed formula or breast milk and allow to flow by gravity. Hold 6 to 8 inches above newborn's head for slow feeding: 20 minutes or 1 ml/min.
- Stop flow at neck of syringe by pinching tubing.
- Clear tubing with small amount of sterile water (1 to 2 ml).
- Pinch tubing and withdraw quickly to avoid administering the feeding nasopharyngeally.
- Infant may be burped.
- Position infant on right side to minimize possibility of regurgitation and aspiration.
- Postpone any treatments for 1 hour so feeding is retained.
- Record amount of residual; the type and amount of the feeding; the time the feeding was started and the time the feeding ended; and the newborn's response to the feeding.

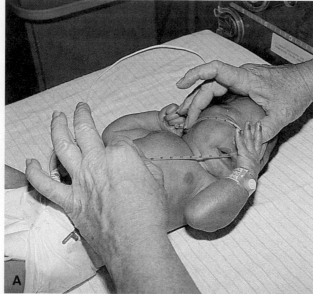

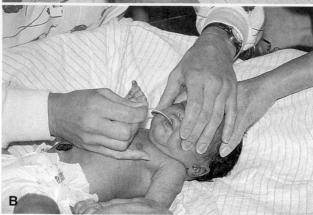

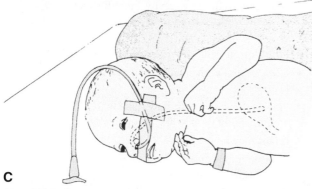

FIGURE 6-19 Gavage feeding. *A,* Measurement of gavage feeding tube from tip of nose to earlobe and then to midpoint between end of xiphoid process and umbilicus. Tape may be used to mark correct length on tube. *B,* Insertion of gavage tube using orogastric route. *C,* Indwelling gavage tube, nasogastric route. After feeding by orogastric or nasogastric tube, infant is propped on right side or placed prone (preterm infant) for 1 hour to facilitate emptying of stomach into small intestine. Note rolled towel for support. (*A* and *B,* courtesy Marjorie Pyle, RNC, Lifecircle, Costa Mesa, CA. *C,* from Lowdermilk DL, Perry SE: *Maternity nursing,* ed 9. St. Louis, 2010, Mosby.)

> **BOX 6-6** *Total Parenteral Nutrition*
>
> - Solutions are administered via a central intravenous access site or a peripherally inserted central venous catheter (PICC).
> - Potential complications associated with total parenteral nutrition (TPN) include hyperglycemia, electrolyte imbalance, infection, and dehydration.

> **BOX 6-7** *Emotional Aspects Related to Care of High-Risk Neonates*
>
> - Without adequate attention to the emotional and developmental needs of the sick neonate, the following may occur:
>   - Failure to thrive (slow or absent growth)
>   - Avoidance of eye contact with people
>   - Absent or weak crying; infant is trying to say, "I give up."
> - A baby who has been overstimulated with procedures or activities will need time out from interaction.
> - Sick neonates need developmentally appropriate stimulation and may need the services of occupational and physical therapists for developmental assessment and intervention.
> - Nurses may cuddle, swaddle, sing to, and offer pacifiers to infant and may put mobiles and decals in crib if baby is not on minimal-stimulation protocol to prevent intraventricular hemorrhage (IVH).

HESI Hint • Drugs used to treat neonatal infections can be ototoxic and nephrotoxic. Close monitoring of therapeutic levels and observation for side effects are required.

HESI Hint • Renal immaturity in a preterm infant makes the monitoring of the administration IV fluids and drug therapy crucial. Closely monitor BUN and creatinine levels when administering the -mycin antibiotics to treat infections in a neonate.

HYPERBILIRUBINEMIA

Definition: Excessive accumulation of bilirubin (usually unconjugated) in the blood due to red blood cell hemolysis

Nursing Assessment

A. Predisposing risk factors
1. Rh incompatibility

2. ABO incompatibility
3. Induction using oxytocin (Pitocin) because of IUGR
4. Prematurity
5. Sepsis
6. Perinatal asphyxia
7. Maternal diabetes mellitus or intrauterine infections
8. Cephalhematoma

B. Jaundice: sclera, skin (If whole body is yellow or palms are yellow, there is a danger of kernicterus [bilirubin encephalopathy] resulting from bilirubin deposition in brain.)

C. Total bilirubin determinations
1. Level increasing more than 5 mg/day
2. Term: level >12 mg/dl
3. LBW: level 10 to 12 mg/dl or greater
4. Preterm: level >5 mg/dl (Infant is more sensitive to kernicterus at lower bilirubin concentrations.)

D. Positive direct Coombs test (This result indicates presence of maternal antibody in the fetal RBC, an indication of sensitization. If >1:64, an exchange transfusion is indicated.)

E. Increased reticulocyte count (This usually indicates ABO incompatibility.)

F. Anemia

G. Urine and stools may be dark.

Analysis (Nursing Diagnoses)

A. *Risk for injury* related to…

B. *Impaired gas exchange* related to…

C. *Anxiety (parental)* related to…

Nursing Plans and Interventions

A. Notify health care provider of any abnormal assessment factors present.

B. Implement orders for phototherapy. (Phototherapy decomposes bilirubin in the skin through oxidation.)
1. Place unclothed neonate 18 inches below a bank of lights as prescribed until bilirubin levels fall to prescribed levels.
2. Place opaque mask over eyes to prevent retinal damage.
3. Monitor skin temperature.
4. Cover genitals with a small diaper or mask to catch urine and stool while leaving skin surface open to light.
5. Turn every 2 hours to avoid skin breakdown.
6. Turn off the lights for 5 to 15 minutes every 8 hours to assess for conjunctivitis.
7. Monitor for signs of dehydration.

C. Maintain hydration: nipple, gavage feedings, and IV fluids.

D. Assist with exchange transfusion.

E. Promote excretion of bilirubin by feeding in order to produce more stooling.

F. Provide a fiber-optic blanket for rooming-in or home phototherapy.

> **HESI Hint** • To assess for skin jaundice, apply pressure with thumb over bony prominences to blanch skin. After removing thumb, area will look yellow before normal skin color reappears. The best areas for assessment are the nose, forehead, and sternum. In dark-skinned infants, observe conjunctival sac and oral mucosa.

> **HESI Hint** • Lab tests measure total and direct (conjugated, excretable, non-fat-soluble) bilirubin levels. The dangerous bilirubin is the unconjugated, indirect (fat-soluble) type, which is measured by subtracting the direct from the total bilirubin.

> **HESI Hint** • Maintenance of hydration is crucial for all infants. A preterm infant is already at risk for fluid and electrolyte imbalances caused by increased body surface area resulting from extended body positioning and larger body area in relation to body weight. Phototherapy treatment for hyperbilirubinemia increases the risk for dehydration.

Effects on the Neonate of Substance Abuse

The effects on the neonate of maternal substance abuse are related to the substance as well as to the amount of the substance abused.

CIGARETTE SMOKING

Nursing Assessment

A. Neonate is small.

B. IUGR; retardation increases with the number of cigarettes smoked.

C. Neonates of mothers who are exposed to smoke-filled environments are also at risk.

Nursing Plans and Interventions

A. Teach the antepartum client that IUGR can be minimized or eliminated when smoking is stopped early in pregnancy.

B. Treat infant as a small-for-gestational-age infant.

NARCOTICS USE

Nursing Assessment of Neonatal Narcotic Withdrawal Syndrome

A. Irritability, hyperactivity

B. High-pitched cry

C. Coarse, flapping tremors

D. Poor feeding, frantic sucking, vomiting and diarrhea

E. Nasal stuffiness

Nursing Plans and Interventions

A. Swaddle and minimize handling.

B. Decrease environmental stimuli.

C. Provide pacifier.

D. Place in prone position with sheepskin.

E. Cover elbows and knees to prevent skin breakdown.

F. Keep bulb syringe close at hand.

ALCOHOL INTAKE

Nursing Assessment

A. Fetal alcohol syndrome (FAS):
1. Microcephaly
2. Growth retardation
3. Short palpebral fissures
4. Maxillary hypoplasia
5. Strabismus
6. Abnormal palmar creases, irregular hair, whorls
7. Poor suck, cleft lip, cleft palate, small teeth

B. Long-term complications of FAS:
1. Mental retardation, hyperactivity, developmental delays, attention deficits
2. Poor coordination
3. Facial abnormalities
4. Behavioral deviations (irritability)
5. Cardiac and joint abnormalities

C. The combined effects of cigarette smoking and alcohol consumption during pregnancy cause greater fetal anomalies than the sum of their individual effects.

Nursing Plans and Interventions

A. Determine how much and how often the mother drank alcoholic beverages during pregnancy or while breastfeeding. (Alcohol intake has serious harmful effects on the fetus, especially when consumed during the sixteenth to eighteenth weeks of pregnancy.)

B. Decrease environmental stimuli.

C. Provide enteral feedings if neonate has incoordinate sucking and swallowing.

Review of Newborn High-Risk Disorders

1. List the major CNS danger signals that occur in the neonate.

2. A baby is delivered blue, limp, and with a heart rate <100. The nurse dries the infant, suctions the oropharynx and gently stimulates the infant while blowing O_2 over the face. The infant still does not respond. What is the next nursing action?

3. What does the Silverman-Anderson index measure?

4. What are the two major complications of O_2 toxicity?

5. Necrotizing enterocolitis results from _____ and is manifested by _____. Ischemia/hypoxia results in _____.

6. Intraventricular hemorrhage is more common in _____ and results in symptoms of _____.

7. What conditions make oxygenation of the newborn more difficult?

8. In order to prevent problems with oxygenating the newborn, what parameters can the nurse observe?

9. What are the cardinal symptoms of sepsis in a newborn?

10. A premature baby is born and develops hypothermia. State the major nursing interventions to treat hypothermia.

11. Nurses often weigh diapers in order to determine exact urine output in the high-risk neonate. Explain this procedure.

12. What factors does a nurse look for in determining a newborn's ability to take in nourishment by nipple and mouth?

13. What complications are associated with total parenteral nutrition (TPN)?

14. In order to prevent rickets in the preterm newborn, what supplements are given?

15. List four nursing interventions to enhance family and parent adjustment to a high-risk newborn.

16. List the risk factors for hyperbilirubinemia.

17. List the symptoms of hyperbilirubinemia in the neonate.

18. Write one nursing diagnosis generated from the data pertinent to hyperbilirubinemia.

19. List three nursing interventions for the neonate undergoing phototherapy.

20. List the symptoms of neonatal narcotic withdrawal.

21. Neonates who are "sick" are prone to receive too much stimulation in the form of invasive procedures and handling and too little developmentally appropriate stimulation and affection. How might such an infant respond?

22. How should a nurse determine the length of a tube needed for the oral gavage feeding of a newborn?

23. What are the two best ways to test for correct placement of the gavage tube in the infant's stomach?

24. What characteristics would the nurse expect to see in a neonate with fetal alcohol syndrome?

Answers to Review

1. Lethargy, high-pitched cry, jitteriness, seizures, and bulging fontanels

2. Begin oxygenation by bag and mask at 30 to 50 breaths per minute. If heart rate is <60, start cardiac massage at 120 events per minute (30 breaths and 90 compressions). Assist health care provider in setting up for intubation procedure.

3. Respiratory difficulty

4. Retrolental fibroplasias and bronchopulmonary dysplasia

5. Ischemic hypoxia, abdominal distention, sepsis, and a lack of absorption from intestines; injury to the intestinal mucosa

6. Premature neonates and VLBW babies; increased intracranial pressure

7. Respiratory distress syndrome: alveolar prematurity and lack of surfactant; anemia; and polycythemia

8. PO_2 50 to 90; SvO_2 60 to 80 mm Hg

9. Lethargy, temperature instability, difficulty feeding, subtle color changes, subtle behavioral changes, and hyperbilirubinemia

10. Place under radiant warmer or in incubator with temperature skin probe over liver. Warm all items touching newborn. Place plastic wrap over neonate.

11. Diaper is weighed in grams before being applied to infant. Diaper is weighed after infant has wet it. Each gram of added weight is calculated and recorded as 1 ml of urine.

12. Infant has good suck, has coordinated suck-swallow, takes less than 20 minutes to feed, gains 20 to 30 g/day.

13. Hyperglycemia, electrolyte imbalance, dehydration, and infection

14. Calcium and vitamin D

15. Initiate early visitation at ICU. Provide daily information to family. Encourage participation in support group for parents. Encourage all attempts at care-giving (enhances bonding).

16. Rh incompatibility, ABO incompatibility, prematurity, sepsis, perinatal asphyxia

17. Bilirubin levels rising 5 mg/day, jaundice, dark urine, anemia, high reticulocyte (RBC) count, and dark stools

18. Risk for injury related to predisposition of bilirubin for fat cells in brain

19. Apply opaque mask over eyes. Leave diaper loose so stools and urine can be monitored but cover genitalia. Turn every 2 hours. Watch for dehydration.

20. Irritability, hyperactivity, high-pitched cry, frantic sucking, coarse flapping tremors, and poor feeding

21. Failure to thrive, absence of crying

22. Measure from the bridge of the nose to the earlobe and then to a point halfway between the xiphoid and the umbilicus.

23. Aspiration of stomach contents and pH testing; auscultation of an air bubble injected into the stomach

24. Microcephaly, strabismus, growth retardation, short palpebral fissures, maxillary hypoplasia, abnormal palmar creases, irregular hair, whorls, poor suck, cleft lip, cleft palate, small teeth

For more review, go to **http://evolve.elsevier.com/HESI/RN** for HESI's online study exams.

PSYCHIATRIC NURSING

7

Therapeutic Communication

Description: Verbal and nonverbal interactions between health care providers and clients for a goal-directed purpose

A. Communication is the primary tool used in the delivery of psychiatric nursing care and all nurse-client interactions (Table 7-1).

B. The focus of therapeutic interaction is to assist the client in gaining insight into thoughts, feelings, and behaviors (Table 7-2).

Coping Styles (Defense Mechanisms)

Description: Coping styles are automatic psychological processes that protect the individual against anxiety and from awareness of internal and external dangers and stressors. The individual may or may not be aware of these processes (Table 7-3).

Treatment Modalities

Description: Psychiatric and mental health treatment modalities used to promote mental health

TYPES OF TREATMENT MODALITIES

A. Milieu therapy
   1. The planned use of people, resources, and activities in the environment to assist in improving interpersonal skills, social functioning, and performing the activities of daily living
   2. The focus is on the here and now (i.e., assisting the client in dealing with the realities of today rather than focusing on situations and behaviors of the past).
   3. It uses limit setting.
   4. It involves the client in making decisions about her or his own care.

5. It uses activities that support group sharing, cooperation, and compromise (e.g., unit-governing groups).
6. Nursing interventions support client privacy and autonomy and provide clear expectations.

B. Behavior modification
   1. This process is used to change ineffective behavior patterns; it focuses on the consequences of actions rather than on peer pressure.
   2. Positive reinforcement is used to strengthen desired behavior (e.g., a client is praised or given a token that can be exchanged for a treat or desired activity).
   3. Negative reinforcement is used to decrease or eliminate inappropriate behavior (e.g., ignoring undesirable behavior, removing a token or privilege, giving a "time out").
   4. Role modeling and teaching new behaviors are important interventions.

C. Family therapy
   1. This form of group therapy identifies the entire family as the client.
   2. It is based on the concept of the family as a system of interrelated parts forming a whole.
   3. The focus is on the patterns of interaction within the family, not on any individual member.
   4. The therapist assists the family in identifying the roles assigned to each member based on family rules.
   5. Life scripts (living out parents' dreams) and self-fulfilling prophecies (unconsciously following what one thinks should happen, therefore setting it up to happen) are identified.
   6. Congruent and incongruent communication patterns and behaviors are identified.
   7. The goal is to decrease family conflict and anxiety and to develop appropriate role relationships.

D. Crisis intervention
   1. This form of therapy is directed at the resolution of an immediate crisis, which the individual is unable to handle alone.

TABLE 7-1 Helpful Techniques

Acknowledgment	Recognizing the client's opinions and statements without imposing your own values and judgment
Clarifying	The process of making sure you have understood the meaning of what was said
Confrontation	Calling attention to inconsistent behavior, information shared or not shared
Focusing	Assisting the client to explore a specific topic which may include sharing perceptions and theme identification
Information giving	Feedback about client's observed behavior
Open-ended questions	Questions that require more than a yes or no response
Reflecting/restating	Paraphrasing or repeating what the client has said (Be careful not to overuse; client will feel as though you are not listening.)
Silence	Can be therapeutic or can be used to control interaction; use carefully with paranoid client; may be misinterpreted or could be used to support paranoid ideation
Suggesting	Offering alternatives, e.g., "Have you ever considered...?"

HESI Hint • The purpose of therapeutic interaction with clients is to allow them the autonomy to make choices when appropriate. Keep statements value-free, advice-free, and reassurance-free. Remember, *just the facts! No opinions!*

HESI Hint • What action should the nurse take in a psychiatric situation when the client describes a physical problem? Assess, assess, assess! If a client in the psychiatric unit with paranoid schizophrenia complains of chest pain, take his or her blood pressure. If the OB client who has delivered a dead fetus complains of perineal pain, look at the perineal area (she may have a hematoma). Just because the focus of the client's situation is on his or her psychological needs, it does not mean that the nurse can ignore physiologic needs.

TABLE 7-2 Useful and Forbidden Phrases

Description	Examples
Useful Phrases	
• These are phrases that are useful in therapeutic interaction. • Keep the interaction open, genuine, and client-centered. • Keep the client as the focus. • Be aware of your own feelings and anxiety level.	• "Tell me about..." • "Go on..." • "I'd like to discuss what you're thinking..." • "What are your thoughts...?" • "Are you saying that...?" • "What are you feeling?" • "It seems as if..."
Forbidden Phrases	
• These are phrases that should *not* be used when interacting with clients. Avoid them at all costs (especially if they appear on an exam). • Avoid social interaction, clichés, and saying too much. • Avoid changing subjects. • Avoid words like *good, bad, right, wrong,* and *nice.*	• "You should..." • "You'll have to..." • "You can't..." • "If it were me, I'd..." • "Why don't you..." • "I think you..." • "It's the policy on this unit." • "Don't worry." • "Everyone..." • "Why...?" • "Just a second..." • "I know..."

HESI Hint • Remember, nurses are nice people, but they are also therapeutic.

HESI Hint • Basic communication principles can be applied to all clients:
• Establish trust.
• Demonstrate a nonjudgmental attitude.
• Offer self; be empathetic, not sympathetic.
• Use active listening.
• Accept and support client's feelings.
• Clarify and validate client's statements.
• Use matter-of-fact approach.

HESI Hint • Remember, a nurse's nonverbal communication may be more important than the verbal communication.

HESI Hint • A question concerning nurse-client confidentiality appears often on the NCLEX-RN. For the nurse to tell a client that he or she will not tell anyone about their discussion puts the nurse in a difficult position. Some information *must* be shared with other team members for the client's safety (e.g., suicide plan) and optimal therapy.

TABLE 7-3 Coping Styles (Defense Mechanisms)

Style	Description	Example
Denial	Unconscious failure to acknowledge an event, thought, or feeling that is too painful for conscious awareness	A woman diagnosed with cancer tells her family all the tests were negative.
Displacement	The transference of feelings to another person or object	After being scolded by his supervisor at work, a man comes home and kicks the dog for barking.
Identification	Attempt to be like someone or emulate the personality, traits, or behaviors of another person	A teenage boy dresses and behaves like his favorite singer.
Intellectualization	Using reason to avoid emotional conflicts	The wife of a substance abuser describes, in detail, the dynamics of enabling behavior yet continues to call her husband's workplace to report his Monday morning absences as an illness.
Introjection	Incorporation of values or qualities of an admired person or group into one's own ego structure	A young man deals with a business client in the same fashion his father deals with business clients.
Isolation	Separation of an unacceptable feeling, idea, or impulse from one's thought process	A nurse working in an emergency room is able to care for the seriously injured by isolating or separating her feelings and emotions related to the clients' pain, injuries, or death.
Passive-aggression	Indirectly expressing aggression toward others; a facade of overt compliance masks covert resentment.	An employee arrives late to a meeting and disrupts others after being reminded of the meeting earlier that day and promising to be on time.
Projection	Attributing one's own thoughts or impulses to another person	A student who has sexual feelings toward her teacher tells her friends the teacher is "coming on to her."
Rationalization	Offering an acceptable, logical explanation to make unacceptable feelings and behavior acceptable	A student who did not do well in a course says it was poorly taught and the course content was not important anyway.
Reaction formation	Development of conscious attitudes and behaviors that are the opposite of what is really felt	A person who dislikes animals does volunteer work for the Humane Society.
Regression	Reverting to an earlier level of development when anxious or highly stressed	After moving to a new home, a 6-year-old starts wetting the bed.
Repression	The *involuntary* exclusion of a painful thought or memory from awareness	A young man whose mother died when he was 12 years old cannot tell you how old he was or the year she died.
Sublimation	Substitution of an unacceptable feeling by a more socially acceptable one	A student who feels too small to play football becomes a champion marathon swimmer.
Suppression	The *intentional* exclusion of feelings and ideas	When about to lose Tara, Scarlet O'Hara says, "I'll think about it tomorrow."
Undoing	Communication or behavior done to negate a previously unacceptable act	A young man who used to hunt wild animals now chairs a committee for the protection of animals.

2. A crisis may develop when previously learned coping mechanisms are ineffective in dealing with the current problem.
3. The individual is usually in a state of disequilibrium.
4. If a client is in a panic state as a result of the disorganization, be very directive.
5. Focus on the problem, not the cause.
6. Identify support systems.
7. Identify fast-coping patterns used in other stressful situations.
8. The goal is to return individual to precrisis level of functioning.
9. Crisis intervention is usually limited to 6 weeks.

E. Cognitive therapy
1. It is directed at replacing a client's irrational beliefs and distorted attitudes.
2. It is focused, problem-solving therapy.
3. The therapist and client work together to identify and solve problems and overcome difficulties.
4. It is short-term therapy of 2 to 3 months' duration.
5. It involves cognitive restructuring.

F. Electroconvulsive therapy (ECT)
1. It involves the use of electrically induced seizures for psychiatric purposes. It is used with severely depressed clients who fail to respond to antidepressant medications and therapy. It may be used with extremely suicidal clients because 2 weeks are needed for antidepressants to take effect.
2. Nursing care prior to ECT
   a. Prepare client by teaching what the treatment involves.
   b. Avoid using the word "shock" when discussing the treatment with client and family.
   c. An anticholinergic (e.g., atropine sulfate) is usually given 30 minutes before treatment to dry oral secretions.
   d. A quick-acting muscle relaxant (e.g., succinylcholine [Anectine]) is given to client before the ECT. This helps to prevent bone or muscle damage.
   e. Have an emergency cart, suction equipment, and O_2 available in the room.
3. Nursing care after ECT
   a. Maintain patent airway; client is in an unconscious state immediately following ECT.
   b. Check vital signs every 15 minutes until client is alert.
   c. Reorient client after ECT (confusion is likely upon awakening).
   d. Common complaints after ECT include:
      (1) Headache
      (2) Muscle soreness
      (3) Nausea

HESI Hint • Nausea is a common complaint after ECT. Vomiting by an unconscious client can lead to aspiration. Because post-ECT clients are unconscious, the nurse must observe closely for the possibility of aspiration: *maintain a patent airway!*

G. Group intervention
1. This process is used with two or more clients who develop interactive relationships and share at least one common goal or issue.
2. The types of groups are as follows:
   a. The group may be closed (set group) or open (new members may join).
   b. The group may be small or large (>10 members).
   c. There are many types of groups (psychoeducation, supportive therapy, psychotherapy, self-help).
   d. Common nurse-led intervention groups include those that focus on medications, symptom management, anger management, and self-care.
3. The phases in groups are as follows:
   a. The initial, or orientation, phase is characterized by:
      (1) High anxiety
      (2) Superficial interactions
      (3) Testing the therapist to see if he or she can be trusted
   b. The middle, or working, phase is characterized by:
      (1) Problem identification
      (2) The beginning of problem solving
      (3) The beginning of the group sense of "we"
   c. The termination phase is characterized by:
      (1) Evaluation of the experience
      (2) The expression of feelings ranging from anger to joy
4. The advantages of groups are:
   a. The development of socializing techniques
   b. The opportunity to try new behaviors
   c. The promotion of a feeling of universality (i.e., not being alone with problems)
   d. The opportunity for feedback from the group, which may correct distorted perceptions
   e. The opportunity for clients to look at alternative ways of analyzing and dealing with problems

Review of Therapeutic Communication and Treatment Modalities

1. After the fourth group meeting, the informal leader makes the statement that she believes she can help the group more than the assigned facilitator and has better credentials. Identify the group dynamics and stage of development.
2. On an in-patient psychiatric unit, clients are expected to get up at a certain time, attend breakfast at a certain time, and arrive for their medications at the correct time. What form of therapy is incorporated into this unit?
3. The wife of a man killed in a motor vehicle accident has just arrived at the emergency department and is told of her husband's death. What nursing actions are appropriate for dealing with this crisis?
4. A 10-year-old is admitted to the children's unit of the psychiatric facility after stabbing his sister. His behavior is extremely aggressive with the other children on the unit. Using a behavior-modification approach with positive reinforcement, design a treatment plan for this child.
5. The 10-year-old, his sister, his mother, and the mother's live-in boyfriend are asked to attend a therapy meeting. Who is the "client" who will be treated during this session?
6. A 66-year-old woman is admitted to the psychiatric unit with agitated depression. She has not responded to antidepressants in the past. What would be the medical treatment of choice for this client?
7. Describe the nurse's role in preparing clients for ECT.
8. Describe the nursing interventions used to care for a client during and after ECT.

Answers to Review

1. The informal leader is "testing," which is a behavior indicative of a new group trying to establish trust. This group is still in the orientation phase of development.
2. Milieu
3. Take her to a quiet room, and ask her if there are family members, friends, or clergy you can call for her. Assess her need for medication and discuss it with health care provider. Stay with her, be firm and directive, and assess previous successful coping strategies.
4. Assess what activities he enjoys. Set up a token system; when he displays nonaggressive behavior, he earns a token good toward participating in the activity selected. He loses a token when he becomes aggressive.
5. The entire family
6. ECT
7. Give accurate, nonjudgmental information about the treatment. Explore client's concerns. Administer the following as prescribed: atropine sulfate to dry oral secretions, a quick-acting barbiturate to induce anesthesia such as Brevital Sodium, and a muscle relaxant such as Anectine. Check emergency equipment. Be sure suction equipment and O_2 are available.
8. Maintain patent airway. Check vital signs every 15 minutes until client is alert. Remain with client following treatment until client is conscious. Reorient if client is confused.

Anxiety

Description: Anxiety is unexplained discomfort, tension, apprehension, or uneasiness, which occurs when a person feels a threat to self. The threat may be real or imagined and is a very subjective experience.

LEVELS OF ANXIETY

A. Mild anxiety
   1. Is associated with daily life; motivates learning
   2. Produces increased levels of sensory awareness and alertness
   3. Allows for thoughts that are logical; client is able to concentrate and problem solve
   4. Allows client to appear calm and in control
B. Moderate anxiety
   1. Continues to motivate learning
   2. Allows client to be attentive and able to focus and problem solve
   3. Dulls perceptions of sensory stimuli; client becomes hesitant
   4. Causes client's speech rate and volume to increase; client becomes wordy
   5. Causes client to become restless (frequent body movements and gestures)

6. May be converted into physical symptoms, such as headaches, nausea, or diarrhea

C. Severe anxiety
  1. Stimulates fight-or-flight response
  2. Causes sensory stimuli input to be disorganized
  3. May cause perceptions to be distorted
  4. Impairs concentration and problem-solving ability
  5. Results in selective attention, focusing on only one detail
  6. Results in the verbalization of emotional pain (e.g., "I need help. I can't stand this")
  7. Causes tremors, increased motor activity (e.g., pacing, wringing hands)

D. Panic
  1. Causes perceptions to be grossly distorted; client is unable to differentiate real from unreal
  2. Causes client to be unable to concentrate or problem-solve; causes loss of rational, logical thinking
  3. Causes client to feel overwhelmed, helpless
  4. Causes loss of control, inability to function
  5. Can elicit behavior that may be angry and aggressive or withdrawn, with clinging and crying
  6. Requires immediate intervention

HESI Hint • Common physiologic responses to anxiety include increased heart rate and blood pressure; rapid, shallow respirations; dry mouth and tight feeling in throat; tremors and muscle tension; anorexia; urinary frequency; and palmar sweating.

HESI Hint • Anxiety is very contagious and is easily transferred from client to nurse and from nurse to client. First, the nurse must assess his or her own level of anxiety and remain calm. A calm nurse helps the client to gain control, decrease anxiety, and increase feelings of security.

Anxiety Disorders

GENERALIZED ANXIETY DISORDERS

Description: Unrealistic, excessive, or persistent (lasting 6 months or longer) anxiety and worry about two or more life circumstances. Previously learned coping mechanisms are inadequate to deal with this level of anxiety. Multiple theories exist concerning cause, including (but not limited to) neurobiochemical and psychodynamic theories.

Nursing Assessment

A. Severe anxiety
B. Motor tension
  1. Restlessness
  2. Quickly fatigued
  3. Feelings of "shakiness"
  4. Tension
C. Autonomic hyperactivity
  1. Shortness of breath
  2. Heart palpitations
  3. Dizziness
  4. Diaphoresis
  5. Frequent urination
D. Vigilance and scanning
  1. Difficulty concentrating
  2. Sleep disturbance
  3. Irritability, quick to become angry
E. On edge, appearance of being nervous
F. Low self-esteem

Analysis (Nursing Diagnoses)

A. *Anxiety* related to …
B. *Ineffective coping* related to …
C. *Disturbed sleep pattern* related to …
D. *Imbalanced nutrition: less than/more than body requirements* related to …

Nursing Plans and Interventions

A. Assess client so as to recognize anxiety and label the feeling (e.g., "What are you feeling now?").
B. Help client to identify the relationship between the stressor and the level of anxiety.
C. Provide opportunities to learn and test various adaptive coping responses.
D. Encourage exercise, deep-breathing techniques, visualization, relaxation techniques, and biofeedback.
E. Decrease environmental stimuli.

PANIC DISORDERS AND PHOBIAS

A. There are discrete periods of intense fear or discomfort that are unexpected and may be incapacitating.
B. It is characterized by an irrational fear of an external object, activity, or situation.
C. It is a chronic condition that has exacerbations and remissions.
D. The client transfers anxiety or fear from its source to a symbolic object, idea, or situation.
E. The client recognizes that the fear is excessive and unrealistic but "can't help it."

Common Phobias

A. Acrophobia: fear of heights
B. Agoraphobia: fear of crowds or open places
C. Claustrophobia: fear of closed-in places
D. Hydrophobia: fear of water
E. Nyctophobia: fear of the dark
F. Thanatophobia: fear of death

Nursing Assessment

A. Coping styles used (see Table 7-3):
   1. Displacement
   2. Projection
   3. Repression
   4. Sublimation
B. Autonomic hyperactivity
C. Panic attacks that usually peak at 10 minutes but can last up to 30 minutes, with a gradual return to normal functioning
D. Disruption in personal life as well as work life
E. Possible use of alcohol and drugs to decrease anxiety

Analysis (Nursing Diagnoses)

A. *Ineffective coping* related to...
B. *Social isolation* related to...

HESI Hint • When a client describes a phobia or expresses an unreasonable fear, the nurse should acknowledge the feeling (fear) and refrain from exposing the client to the identified fear. After trust is established, a desensitization process may be prescribed. Desensitization is the nursing intervention for phobia disorders. The nurse should:
- Assist client to recognize the factors associated with feared stimuli that precipitate a phobic response.
- Teach and practice with client alternative adaptive coping strategies, such as the use of thought substitution (replacing a fearful thought with a pleasant thought) and relaxation techniques. (Role-playing is useful when the client is in a calm state.)
- Expose client progressively to feared stimuli, offering support with the nurse's presence.
- Provide positive reinforcement whenever a decrease in phobic reaction occurs.
- *Note:* In all likelihood, the desensitization process will be overseen by a mental health practitioner (NP, psychological CNS, or psychologist).

HESI Hint • The nurse should place an anxious client where there are reduced environmental stimuli (a quiet area of the unit, away from the nurses' station).

Nursing Plans and Interventions

A. Establish trust; listen, use a calm approach and direct, simple questions. Remain with client; do not leave alone.
B. Provide a safe environment.
C. Draw client's attention away from feared object or situation.
D. Discuss with the client alternative coping strategies and encourage use of such alternatives.
E. Suggest substitution of positive thoughts for negative ones.
F. Assist in desensitizing client.
G. Gradually and systematically introduce the client to the anxiety-producing stimuli.
H. Pair the anxiety-producing stimuli with another response such as relaxation or exercise.
I. Encourage the sharing of fears and feelings with others.
J. Administer antianxiety medications as prescribed (Table 7-4).
K. Administer selective serotonin reuptake inhibitors (SSRIs) or other medications as prescribed (see Table 7-6).
L. Teach to decrease intake of caffeine and nicotine.

OBSESSIVE-COMPULSIVE DISORDER

Description: Anxiety associated with repetitive thoughts (obsession) or irresistible impulses (compulsion) to perform an action; fear of losing control is a major symptom of this disorder.

Nursing Assessment

A. Use of coping styles to control anxiety (see Table 7-3)
   1. Repression
   2. Isolation
   3. Undoing
B. Magical thinking (belief that one's thoughts or wishes can control other people or events)
C. Evidence of destructive, hostile, aggressive, and delusional thought content
D. Difficulty with interpersonal relationships
E. Interference with normal activities (e.g., a client who "must" wash her hands all morning and cannot take her children to school)
F. Safety issues involved in repetitive performance of the ritualistic activity (e.g., dermatitis occurring as a result of the continuous washing of hands)
G. Recurring intrusive thoughts
H. Recurring, repetitive behaviors that interfere with normal functioning

TABLE 7-4 Antianxiety Drugs

Drugs	Indications	Reactions	Nursing Implications
Benzodiazepines			
• Chlordiazepoxide HCl (Librium) • Diazepam (Valium) • Prazepam (Centrax) • Oxazepam (Serax) • Alprazolam (Xanax) • Clorazepate dipotassium (Tranxene) • Lorazepam (Ativan)	• Reduce anxiety • Induce sedation, relax muscles, inhibit convulsions • Treat alcohol and drug withdrawal symptoms • Safer than sedative-hypnotics	• Sedation • Drowsiness • Ataxia • Dizziness • Irritability • Blood dyscrasias • Habituation and increased tolerance	• Administer at bedtime to alleviate daytime sedation. • Greatest harm occurs when combined with alcohol or other CNS depressants. • Instruct to avoid driving or working around equipment. • Gradually taper drug therapy due to withdrawal effects; do not stop suddenly. • Used only as short-term drug and as supplement to other medications
Nonbenzodiazepines			
• Buspirone (BuSpar)	• Do not exhibit muscle relaxant or anticonvulsant activity • Are not effective for management of substance use	• Dizziness	• Takes several weeks for antianxiety effects to become apparent • Intended for short-term use
• Zolpidem (Ambien)	• Used for short-term treatment of insomnia	• Daytime drowsiness	• Give with food 1 to 1½ hours before bedtime

Analysis (Nursing Diagnoses)

A. *Social isolation* related to...

B. *Ineffective coping* related to...

Nursing Plans and Interventions

A. Provide for client's physical needs.

B. Allow performance of the compulsive activity with attention given to safety (e.g., skin integrity of a hand washer).

C. Explore meaning and purpose of the behavior with client.

D. Avoid punishing and criticizing.

E. Establish routine to avoid anxiety-producing changes.

F. Assist client with learning alternative methods of dealing with stress.

G. Avoid reinforcing compulsive behavior.

H. Limit the amount of time for performance of ritual, and encourage client to gradually decrease the time.

I. Administer antianxiety medications as prescribed (see Table 7-4).

J. Administer SSRIs and tricyclic antidepressants as prescribed (see Table 7-6).

HESI Hint • The best time for interaction with a client is at the completion of the performed ritual. The client's anxiety is lowest at this time; therefore, it is an optimal time for learning.

HESI Hint • Compulsive acts are used in response to anxiety, which may or may not be related to the obsession. It is the nurse's responsibility to help alleviate anxiety.

Interfering will increase anxiety. These acts should be allowed as long as the client's acts are free of violence. The nurse should:
• Actively listen to the client's obsessive themes.
• Acknowledge the effects that ritualistic acts have on the client.
• Demonstrate empathy.
• Avoid being judgmental.

POSTTRAUMATIC STRESS DISORDER

Description: Severe anxiety, which results from a traumatic experience (e.g., war, earthquake, rape, incest)

Nursing Assessment

A. Anxiety; level proportional to the perceived degree of threat experienced by the client

B. Anxiety manifested in symptomatic behaviors
1. Intrusive thoughts
2. Flashbacks of the experience
3. Nightmares
4. Emotional detachment

C. Responses to anxiety such as
1. Shock
2. Anger
3. Panic
4. Denial

D. Self-destructive behavior, such as suicidal ideation and substance abuse

E. Visible reminders of trauma (e.g., scars, physical disabilities)

Analysis (Nursing Diagnoses)

A. *Posttrauma syndrome* related to ...

B. *Ineffective coping* related to ...

C. *Risk for other-directed/self-directed violence* related to ...

Nursing Plans and Interventions

A. Provide consistent, nonthreatening environment.

B. Implement suicidal and homicidal precautions if assessment indicates risk.

C. Listen to client's details of events to identify the most troubling aspect of events.

D. Assist client to develop objectivity in perceiving event and identify areas of no control.

E. Assist client to regain control by identifying past situations that have been handled successfully.

F. Administer antianxiety and antipsychotic medications as prescribed so as to decrease anxiety, manage behavior, and provide rest (see Table 7-8; and see Table 7-3).

HESI Hint • For clients with posttraumatic stress disorder, the nurse should:
- Actively listen to client's stories of experiences surrounding the traumatic event.
- Assess suicide risk.
- Assist client to develop objectivity about the event and problem-solve regarding possible means of controlling anxiety related to the event.
- Encourage group therapy with other clients who have experienced the same or related traumatic events.

Review of Anxiety Disorders

1. State five autonomic responses to anxiety.
2. Identify the coping style used by a person who feels guilty about masturbating as a child and develops a hand-washing compulsion as an adult.
3. Identify anxiety-reducing strategies the nurse can teach.
4. Which levels of anxiety facilitate learning?
5. A Vietnam veteran is plagued by nightmares and is found trying to strangle his roommate one night. List, in order of priority, the appropriate nursing interventions.
6. A client displays a phobic response to flying. Describe the desensitization process that would probably be implemented.
7. A client is in the middle of an extensive ritual that focuses on food during lunch. However, the client is scheduled for group therapy, which is about to start. What action should the nurse take?

Answers to Review

1. Shortness of breath, heart palpitations, dizziness, diaphoresis, frequent urination
2. Undoing
3. Deep breathing techniques, visualization, relaxation techniques, exercise, biofeedback
4. Mild to moderate
5. Protect roommate from harm. Stay with client. If the client is agitated, administer antianxiety medications as prescribed. Arrange for private room. Place client on homicidal precautions at night.
6. Talk about planes. Look at pictures of planes. Make plans to accompany client during a visit to airport. Accompany client onto a plane. Allow the client to board a plane alone. Accompany the client on a short flight while listening to a relaxation tape.
7. Allow client to complete the ritual. Discuss with the group leader the possibility of allowing the client to enter the group late. Arrange for client to begin lunch earlier so that the ritual can be completed prior to scheduled activities.

Somatoform Disorders

A. A group of disorders characterized by the expression of unexplained physical symptoms that have no physical basis.

B. The physical symptom is thought to be an unconscious expression of an internal conflict.

C. Somatoform disorders occur more often in women and begin before 30 years of age.

D. Children may learn that physical complaints are an acceptable coping strategy and are rewarded by receiving attention for this behavior. This is referred to as a secondary gain.

E. These clients may abuse analgesics without relief from pain or discomfort. They may accumulate prescriptions by "doctor shopping" to relieve physical symptoms.

TYPES OF SOMATOFORM DISORDERS

A. Somatization disorder
   1. Recurrent somatic complaints for which frequent medical attention is sought but no medical pathology is present
   2. Example: a client who complains of chest pains but has a normal ECG and normal cardiac enzymes

B. Hypochondriasis
   1. The belief in and fear of having a disease, including misinterpretation of physical signs as "proof" of the presence of the disease
   2. Example: A client has a rash that is quite minor but insists that he has a serious disease such as lupus.

C. Conversion disorder
   1. A disorder characterized by transferring a mental conflict into a physical symptom for which there is no organic cause
   2. Example: blindness, paralysis, seizures, deafness, and pseudocyesis (false pregnancy)

Nursing Assessment

A. Preoccupation with pain or bodily function for at least 6 months' duration

B. History of frequent "doctor shopping"

C. Absence of emotional concern regarding the physical impairment

D. May report excessive dysmenorrhea

E. Vital signs may be elevated as in a panic attack

F. Fear of having a serious disease

G. Excessive use of analgesics

H. Rumination about physical symptoms

I. Drug abuse; drug screening needed to determine presence of abuse and, if present, the level of abuse

J. Depression and presence of suicidal ideation

K. Social or occupational impairment

L. Presence of blindness, deafness, paralysis, or seizures suggestive of a neurologic disease

Analysis (Nursing Diagnoses)

A. *Chronic pain* related to …

B. *Ineffective coping* related to …

C. *Disturbed personal identity* related to …

Nursing Plans and Interventions

A. Convey a nonjudgmental attitude.

B. Record duration and intensity of pain with attention to factors that precipitate onset.

C. Encourage expression of angry feelings.

D. Implement suicide precautions if indicated.

E. No one medication is particularly recommended. Comorbid disorders such as anxiety and depression are treated with disorder-specific medications.

F. Focus interactions and activities away from self and pain.

G. Help client identify connection between pain and anxiety.

H. Increase time and attention given to client as reward for not focusing on self or physical symptoms.

I. Help client identify needs met by the sick role (e.g., attention and freedom from responsibility) (Table 7-5).

J. Encourage use of anxiety-reducing techniques such as deep breathing, visualization, meditation, exercise, and relaxation.

> **HESI Hint** • Be aware of your own feelings when dealing with this type of client. It is a challenge to be nonjudgmental. The pain is real to the person experiencing it. These disorders cannot be explained medically; they result from internal conflict. The nurse should:
> • Acknowledge the symptom or complaint.
> • Reaffirm that diagnostic test results reveal no organic pathology.
> • Determine the secondary gains acquired by the client.

TABLE 7-5 Terms Associated with Somatoform Disorders

Term	Definition
La belle indifference	Term used to describe the lack of concern over physical illness; seen in conversion reactions
Primary gain	A decrease in anxiety resulting from the ability to deal with a stressful situation
Secondary gain	The rewards obtained from the sick role, e.g., freedom from certain responsibilities; sympathy

Review of Somatoform Disorders

1. Describe the difference between primary and secondary gains.
2. Explain the difference between somatization and hypochondriasis.
3. An air traffic controller suddenly develops blindness. All physical findings are negative. The client's history reveals increased anxiety about job performance and fear about job security. What type of disorder is this? What purpose is the blindness serving? What nursing interventions are indicated?
4. A 29-year-old secretary, who is obese, has visited seven different doctors in the past year with a complaint of chest pain and shortness of breath. She is certain she is having a heart attack in spite of the health care provider's reassurance that all tests are normal. What type of disorder is this? What nursing actions are indicated?
5. Five years ago, a woman was involved in a motor vehicle accident that killed her friend who was a passenger in the car she was driving. Since that time, she has been unable to work because of severe back pain. The pain is unrelieved by prescribed medications. What type of disorder is this? What are the contributing causes? Describe the nursing care.

Answers to Review

1. The primary gain is a decrease in anxiety that results from some effort made to deal with stress. The secondary gain is the advantage, other than reduced anxiety, that occurs as a result of the sick role.
2. The term *somatization* is used to describe a person who has many recurrent complaints with no organic basis; a person with hypochondriasis has unrealistic or exaggerated physical complaints. The concerns of those who are experiencing somatization and of those who are hypochondriacal are so exaggerated that they interfere with social and occupational functioning.
3. Conversion reaction; decreases the anxiety about job; assist with activities of daily living (ADLs), encourage expression of anger, teach relaxation techniques, and assist with the identification of anxiety related to job security and performance.
4. Hypochondriacal disorder; decrease anxiety; teach relaxation techniques; explore relationship between the symptoms and past experiences with heart disease; focus interactions away from bodily concerns.
5. Somatization disorder; unresolved grief, anxiety; evaluate pain medication use or abuse; document duration and intensity of pain; assist client to identify precipitating factors related to request for medication.

Dissociative Disorders

A. These disorders involve alteration in the function of consciousness, personality, memory, or identity.
B. Dissociative disorders may be sudden and temporary or gradual and chronic.
C. Persons afflicted with these types of disorders handle stressful situations by "splitting" from the situation and going into a fantasy state.

TYPES OF DISSOCIATIVE DISORDERS

A. Psychogenic amnesia
  1. It is the sudden temporary inability to recall extensive personal information.
  2. It usually occurs after a traumatic event, such as a threat of death or injury, an intolerable life situation, or a natural disaster.
  3. It is the most common dissociative disorder.
B. Psychogenic fugue
  1. It is characterized by a person suddenly leaving home or work with the inability to recall his or her identity, so this involves flight as well as loss of memory.
  2. This disorder rarely occurs.
  3. Excessive use of alcohol may contribute to a fugue state.
C. Dissociative identity disorder
  1. It is the presence of two or more distinct personalities within an individual.
  2. The personalities emerge during stress.
D. Depersonalization
  1. It is characterized by a temporary loss of one's reality and the ability to feel and express emotions.
  2. Client expresses a fear of "going crazy."
  3. Client describes a sense of "strangeness" in the surrounding environment.

Nursing Assessment

A. Depression, mood swings, insomnia, potential for suicide

B. Varying degrees of orientation

C. Varying levels of anxiety

D. Impairment of social and occupational functioning

E. Alcohol or drug abuse (Drug screening is necessary to determine presence and level of abuse.)

Analysis (Nursing Diagnoses)

A. *Ineffective coping* related to …

B. *Potential for self-directed/other-directed violence* related to …

Nursing Plans and Interventions

A. Reduce environmental stimulation to decrease anxiety.

B. Stay with client during periods of depersonalization. (The client is often fearful, and the nurse's presence assists in providing support and comfort during fearful episode.)

C. Demonstrate acceptance of client's behavior during various experiences and personalities.

D. Document emergence of different personalities, if present.

E. Implement suicide precautions if assessment indicates risk.

F. Encourage client to identify stressful situations that cause a transition from one personality to another.

G. Help client to identify effective coping patterns used in other stressful situations.

H. Assist client in using new alternative coping methods.

> **HESI Hint** • The nurse should be aware that all behavior has meaning.

> **HESI Hint** • Avoid giving clients with dissociative disorders too much information about past events at one time. The various types of amnesia that accompany dissociative disorders provide protection from pain. Too much too soon may cause decompensation.

Review of Dissociative Disorders

1. Describe the difference between psychogenic amnesia and a psychogenic fugue.
2. What is a multiple personality disorder?
3. List three possible causes of psychogenic amnesia.
4. Describe depersonalization disorder.

Answers to Review

1. Psychogenic amnesia is the sudden inability to recall certain events in one's life. A psychogenic fugue state is characterized by the individual's leaving home and being unable to recall his or her identity or past.
2. The presence of two or more distinct personalities within an individual; the personalities emerge during stress.
3. A traumatic event such as a threat of death or injury; an intolerable life situation; a natural disaster
4. A temporary loss of one's reality; a loss of the ability to feel and express emotions; a sense of "strangeness" in the surrounding environment; individuals with this disorder express a fear of "going crazy."

Personality Disorders

CLUSTER A: PARANOID

Description: It is characterized by suspicious, strange behavior that may be precipitated by a stressful event. It may manifest as intense hypochondriasis.

A. Paranoid personality

1. Displays pervasive and long-standing suspiciousness
2. Mistrusts others; is suspicious, fearful
3. Projects blame for own problems onto others
4. Is in touch with reality
5. Verbally: uses hostile, accusatory dialogue that is reality-based

6. Nonverbally: appears suspicious, tense, distant, watchful, and angry
7. Example: a teacher who always suspects students of cheating during an exam or obtaining test questions prior to the exam

B. Schizoid personality
1. Is socially detached, shy, introverted
2. Avoids interpersonal relationships, lacks social skills
3. Is cold, quiet, and aloof; has few friends
4. Is emotionally detached, introverted, unresponsive, and has autistic thinking
5. Verbally: says little, appears withdrawn and seclusive
6. Nonverbally: is dull, humorless, and has little expression
7. Example: A computer programmer who works day and night, his only "relationship" being with his computer

C. Schizotypal personality
1. Has interpersonal deficits
2. Has eccentricities and odd beliefs
3. Is socially isolated
4. Example: A person who spends hours walking the streets and wears a hat with all kinds of things hanging from it and all sorts of mismatched clothing

Nursing Assessment

A. Determine degree of suspiciousness and mistrust of others.
B. Assess degree of anxiety.
C. Determine whether delusions are present:
1. Reference or control
2. Persecution
3. Grandeur
4. Somatic
D. Assess degree of insecurity.

Analysis (Nursing Diagnoses)

A. *Risk for self-directed violence* related to …
B. *Risk for other-directed violence* related to …
C. *Social isolation* related to …

Nursing Plans and Interventions

A. Establish trust.
B. Be truthful and honest; follow through on commitments.
C. Assist client to identify situations that provoke anxiety and aggressive behaviors.
D. Avoid confrontation with the client over delusions.
E. Help client to focus on the feelings that cause the delusions.
F. Assist in identifying thoughts, perceptions, and own conclusions about reality.

G. Avoid talking and laughing where client can see but not hear you.
H. Engage in noncompetitive activities that require concentration.
I. Involve client in treatment plan.
J. Promote family involvement in therapy, teaching, and medication compliance.

CLUSTER B: DRAMATIC, EMOTIONAL

A. Antisocial personality
1. Shows aggressive acting-out behavior pattern without any remorse
2. Is clever and manipulative in order to meet own self-centered needs
3. Lacks social conscience and ability to feel remorse; is emotionally immature and impulsive
4. Has ineffective interpersonal skills that impair the forming of close and lasting relationships
5. Verbally: is disparaging, humiliating, and belligerent toward those perceived as a threat
6. Nonverbally: is cold, callous, and insensitive to others; can display socially gracious behaviors in order to meet own needs
7. Example: a prison inmate who tries to get special privileges by bribing the guards (i.e., acting out the role of a con artist)

B. Borderline personality
1. Has disturbances regarding self-image and sexual, social, and occupational roles
2. Shows impulsive, self-damaging behavior; makes suicidal gestures
3. Is other-directed, overly dependent on others
4. Is unable to problem-solve or learn from experience
5. Tends to view others as either all good or all bad (e.g., "splitting" behavior)
6. Verbally: is self-critical, demanding, whiny, manipulative, and argumentative and can become verbally abusive
7. Nonverbally: has highly changeable and intense affect, impulsive behaviors
8. Example: a teenage girl who threatens to commit suicide when her boyfriend leaves, but in 6 weeks has new boyfriend and is clinging to him

C. Histrionic personality
1. Seeks attention by overreacting and exhibiting hyperexcitable emotions
2. Is overly dramatic, seeks attention, and tends to exaggerate
3. Has chaotic relationships, demonstrates angry outbursts or tantrums
4. Verbally: is loud, excitable, overreactive, attempts to draw attention to self

5. Nonverbally: is immature, self-centered, dependent on attention and care from others, seductive and flirty
6. Example: a hostess at a party who is overly excited to see the guests and welcomes them in a loud, showy manner that draws attention to herself

D. Narcissistic personality
1. Perceives self as all-powerful and important, is critical of others, arrogant
2. Has exaggerated feeling of self-importance and self-love
3. Needs attention and admiration
4. Is preoccupied with power and appearance
5. Exploits others
6. Verbally: talks about self incessantly and does whatever necessary to draw attention to self
7. Nonverbally: is inattentive and indifferent to others, appears concerned only with self
8. Example: a star football player whose success has gone to his head

CLUSTER C: ANXIOUS, FEARFUL

A. Avoidant personality
1. Is socially inhibited
2. Feels inadequate
3. Is hypersensitive to negative criticism, rejection
4. Longs for relationships
5. Example: a man who refuses to play on the employees' softball team because he is afraid his teammates will make fun of him

B. Dependent personality
1. Has unreasonable wishes and wants, and expresses needs in a demanding, whining manner while professing independence and denying dependent behavior
2. Is passive, without accepting responsibility for consequences of his or her own behavior
3. Has low self-esteem, sees self as stupid, unable to make decisions
4. Is dependent on others to meet his or her needs
5. Verbally: is self-depreciating, demanding others to meet needs
6. Nonverbally: appears dull, uninterested in others, dissatisfied with self
7. Example: An adult who exhibits adolescent-type behavior, wants others to take care of him or her while at the same time declaring independence

C. Obsessive-compulsive personality
1. Attempts to control self through the control of others or the environment
2. Shows inattention to new facts or different viewpoints
3. Is cold and rigid toward others
4. Is a perfectionist, inflexible, and stubborn
5. Acts with blind conformity and obedience to rules
6. Is excessively neat and clean
7. Is preoccupied with work efficiency and productivity
8. Verbally and nonverbally: expresses disapproval of those whose behaviors and standards are different from own
9. Example: a nurse who insists that all staff on his or her unit wear a freshly starched uniform every day and has no tolerance for those who are not as "professional" as he or she is

Nursing Assessment

A. Assess degree of social impairment.
B. Determine degree of manipulative behavior.
C. Assess degree of anxiety.
D. Determine the risk for self- or other-directed violence.

Analysis (Nursing Diagnoses)

A. *Disturbed personal identity* related to ...
B. *Ineffective coping* related to ...
C. *Social isolation* related to ...
D. *Risk for self-directed/other-directed violence* related to ...

Nursing Plans and Interventions

A. Establish trust; use straightforward approach.
B. Protect client from injury to self and others.
C. Assist client to recognize manipulative behavior.
D. Focus on client's strengths and accomplishments.
E. Set limits on manipulative behaviors when necessary.
F. Reinforce independent, responsible behaviors.
G. Assist client to recognize the need to respect the needs and rights of others.
H. Encourage socialization with others to improve skills.

HESI Hint • Personality disorders are long-standing behavioral traits that are maladaptive responses to anxiety and that cause difficulty in relating to and working with other individuals. NCLEX-RN® questions sometimes test personality disorder content by describing management situations.

HESI Hint • Persons with personality disorders are usually comfortable with their disorders and believe that they are right and the world is wrong. These individuals usually have very little motivation to change. Think of them as a challenge!

Review of Personality Disorders

Give an example of a behavior or a description of an individual who exhibits each of the following personality disorders:
1. Obsessive-compulsive
2. Antisocial
3. Borderline
4. Dependent
5. Narcissistic
6. Histrionic
7. Paranoid
8. Schizoid
9. Maladaptive

Answers to Review

1. Orderly, rigid
2. Unable to conform to social norms.
3. Needy, always in a crisis, self-mutilating, unable to sustain relationships, splitting behavior
4. Unable to make decisions for self, allows others to assume responsibility for his or her life
5. Feelings of self-importance and entitlement; may exploit others to get own needs met
6. Dramatic, flamboyant, needs to be the center of attention
7. Suspicious, mistrusts others, is watchful and secretive
8. Isolated and introverted, no close friends
9. Nothing he or she does is wrong (e.g., authorities are "out to get me")

Eating Disorders

ANOREXIA NERVOSA

A. This psychiatric disorder involves a voluntary refusal to eat and maintain minimal weight for height and age.
B. A distorted body image and fear of becoming obese drive the excessive dieting and exercise.
C. A reported 15% to 20% of those diagnosed die.
D. It is more common in females than in males.
E. It occurs primarily in adolescents and young adults.
F. It is often associated with parent-child conflicts about dependency issues. Children often feel as though their bodies and weight are their only areas of control.
G. Possible causes
  1. A dysfunctional family system
  2. Unrealistic expectations of perfection
  3. Ambivalence about maturation and the assumption of independence

Nursing Assessment

A. Weight loss of at least 15% of ideal or original body weight
B. Excessive exercise
C. Apathy about physical condition and inordinate pleasure in weight loss
D. Skeletal appearance (usually hidden by baggy clothes)
E. Distorted body image (usually sees self as fat)
F. Low self-esteem
G. Hair loss and dry skin
H. Irregular heartbeat, decreased pulse, and BP resulting from decreased fluid volume
I. Amenorrhea for at least 3 months
J. Delayed psychosexual development (adolescents) or disinterest in sex (adults)
K. Dehydration and electrolyte imbalance (decreased potassium, sodium, and chloride) resulting from:
  1. Diet pill abuse
  2. Enema and laxative abuse
  3. Diuretic abuse
  4. Self-induced vomiting

Analysis (Nursing Diagnoses)

A. *Imbalanced nutrition: less than body requirements* related to ...
B. *Disturbed personal identity* related to ...
C. *Interrupted family process* related to ...

Nursing Plans and Interventions

A. Monitor weight, vital signs, and electrolytes (especially potassium, thyroid levels, and calcium/phosphorus for osteoporosis).

B. Provide a structured, supportive environment, especially during mealtimes.

C. Set a time limit for eating.

D. Carefully monitor food and fluid intake.

E. Be alert to client's choosing low-calorie foods.

F. Be alert to possible discarding of food through others or in pockets, wastebaskets, or drawers.

G. Monitor client after meals for possible vomiting.

H. Monitor activity level to prevent excessive exercise.

I. Use positive reinforcement to build self-esteem and develop a realistic body image.

J. Devise a behavior-modification program if indicated.
   1. Include an established weight goal and weigh on a regular schedule.
   2. Weigh in same clothes, with back to scale; this prevents manipulation and arguing about exact weight.
   3. Praise weight gain rather than food intake.

K. Focus interactions away from food and eating.

L. Administer antidepressant medications as indicated (Table 7-6).

M. Teach client that sudden withdrawal from medications may cause seizures,

N. Encourage family therapy.

O. Provide snacks between meals.

P. Monitor activity and assess for weakness, fatigue, and pathologic fractures.

Q. Provide safe environment and assess for suicide ideation. Implement suicide precautions if necessary.

R. Assess for water loading prior to weighing.

> **HESI Hint** • People with anorexia gain pleasure from providing others with food and watching them eat. These behaviors reinforce their perception of self-control. Do not allow these clients to plan or prepare food for unit-based activities.

BULIMIA NERVOSA

A. An eating disorder characterized by eating excessive amounts of food followed by self-induced purging by vomiting, misuse of laxatives, diuretics or other medications, fasting, and/or excessive exercise.

B. Bulimic clients usually report a loss of control over eating during the bingeing.

Nursing Assessment

A. Refer to Anorexia Nervosa, Nursing Assessment.

B. Diarrhea or constipation, abdominal pain, and bloating

C. Dental damage due to excessive vomiting (Gastric hydrochloric acid erodes dental enamel.)

D. Sore throat and chronic inflammation of the esophageal lining, with possible ulceration

E. Financial stressors related to food budget

F. Concerns with body shape and weight; bulimics usually are not underweight.

Analysis (Nursing Diagnoses)

A. *Disturbed personal identity* related to …

B. *Interrupted family process* related to …

C. *Ineffective coping* related to …

D. *Risk for self-directed violence* related to …

Nursing Plans and Interventions

A. Monitor weight, vital signs, and electrolytes (especially potassium).

B. Provide a structured, supportive environment, especially around mealtime.

C. Monitor client after meals for possible vomiting.

D. Assist client to learn strategies, other than eating, for dealing with feelings.

E. Encourage client to express feelings of anger.

F. Discuss strategies to stop vomiting and laxative use.

G. Use positive reinforcement to build self-esteem and develop a realistic body image.

H. Administer antidepressant medications as indicated (see Table 7-6).

I. Promote family therapy.

> **HESI Hint** • Individuals with bulimia often use syrup of ipecac to induce vomiting. If ipecac is not vomited and is absorbed, cardiotoxicity may occur and can cause conduction disturbances, cardiac dysrhythmias, fatal myocarditis, and circulatory failure. Because heart failure is not usually seen in this age group, it is often overlooked. Assess for edema and listen to breath sounds.

> **HESI Hint** • Physical assessment and nutritional support are a priority; the physiologic implications are great. Nursing interventions should increase self-esteem and develop a positive body image. Behavior modification is useful and effective. Family therapy is most effective because issues of control are common in these disorders. (Therapy is usually long term.)

Review of Eating Disorders

1. Describe the clinical symptoms of anorexia nervosa.
2. State two psychodynamic differences between anorexia and bulimia.
3. A client with anorexia has her friend bring her several cookbooks so she can plan a party when she is discharged. What nursing intervention is appropriate in addressing this behavior?
4. Anorexia nervosa may be precipitated by what factors?
5. What might the initial treatment include for a client admitted to the hospital with a diagnosis of bulimia nervosa?

Answers to Review

1. Weight loss of at least 15% of ideal or original body weight; hair loss; dry skin; irregular heart rate; decreased pulse; decreased blood pressure; amenorrhea; dehydration; electrolyte imbalance
2. Anorexia nervosa deals with issues of control and a struggle between dependence and independence. Bulimia deals with loss of control (binge eating) and guilt (purging).
3. Discuss activities that don't involve food and that can take place after discharge. Discuss the cookbooks with the treatment team, and if the treatment plan so indicates, take the books from the client.
4. Mother-daughter conflicts usually focusing on independence/dependence issues; discomfort with maturation; need for control; desire for perfection.
5. Blood work to evaluate electrolyte status; replenishment of electrolytes and fluids as indicated; careful monitoring for evidence of vomiting.

Mood Disorders

Definition: Disturbances in mood manifested by extreme sadness or extreme elation

DEPRESSIVE DISORDERS

Definition: Pathologic grief reactions ranging from mild to severe states

Symptoms of Varying Degrees of Depression

A. Mild
1. Feelings of sadness
2. Difficulty concentrating and performing usual activities
3. Difficulty maintaining usual activity level
B. Moderate
1. Feelings of helplessness and powerlessness
2. Decreased energy
3. Sleep pattern disturbances
4. Appetite and weight changes
5. Slowed speech, thought, movement (may also be agitated and hyperactive)
6. Rumination on negative feelings
C. Severe
1. Feelings of hopelessness, worthlessness, guilt, shame
2. Despair
3. Flat affect
4. Indecisiveness
5. Lack of motivation
6. Change in physical appearance (slumped posture, unkempt)
7. Suicidal thoughts
8. Possible delusions and hallucinations
9. Sleep and appetite disturbances
10. Loss of interest in sexual activity
11. Constipation

HESI Hint • The most important signs and symptoms of depression are a depressed mood with a loss of interest in the pleasures in life. The client has sustained a loss. Other symptoms include:
- Significant change in appetite, often accompanied by a change in weight, either weight loss or gain
- Insomnia or hypersomnia (usually sleeping during the day, often because the client is not sleeping at night due to anxiety)
- Fatigue or lack of energy
- Feelings of hopelessness, worthlessness, guilt, or overresponsibility
- Loss of ability to concentrate or think clearly
- Preoccupation with death or suicide

Nursing Assessment

A. Determine type of depression.
  1. Exogenous: caused by a reaction to environmental or external factors
  2. Endogenous: caused by an internal biologic deficiency (biogenic amines at receptor sites in the brain)
B. Determine the degree of depression.
C. Determine current suicide risk (see Care of the Suicidal Client).
D. Arrange for lab tests.
  1. Dexamethasone-suppression test (DST)
    a. It is an indirect marker of depression.
    b. It is considered positive (abnormal) if post-DST cortisol level is greater than 5 mg/dl.
  2. Biogenic amines
    a. A decreased serotonin is indicative of depression.
    b. A decreased norepinephrine level is indicative of depression.

Analysis (Nursing Diagnoses)

A. *Risk for self directed violence* related to …
B. *Disturbed personal identity* related to …
C. *Self-care deficit (specify)* related to …
D. *Disturbed sleep pattern* related to …
E. *Imbalanced nutrition: less than/more than body requirements* related to …
F. *Activity intolerance* related to …
G. *Ineffective coping* related to …

Nursing Plans and Interventions

A. Directly ask client about feelings and plans to harm self.
B. Implement suicide precautions if assessment indicates risk (see Care of the Suicidal Client).
C. Monitor sleep, nutrition, and elimination patterns.
D. Assist client with ADLs.
E. Initiate interaction with client (use nondemanding approach).
F. Insist on participation in activities. Do not give the client a choice about participating in activities; (e.g., "It's time to go to the gym for basketball").
G. Observe for sudden elevation in mood; may indicate increased risk for suicide.
H. Assist client in identifying a support system.
I. Encourage discussion of feelings of helplessness, hopelessness, loneliness, and anger.
J. Administer antidepressant medication as indicated (see Table 7-6).
K. Sit in silence if client is nontalkative.
L. Spend time with client and return when promised.

HESI Hint • Depressed clients have difficulty hearing and accepting compliments because of their lowered self-concept. Comment on signs of improvement by noting the behavior (e.g., "I notice you combed your hair today" not, "You look nice today").

HESI Hint • The nurse knows depressed clients are improving when they begin to take an interest in their appearance or begin to perform self-care activities that were previously of little or no interest to them.

CARE OF THE SUICIDAL CLIENT

Suicide Precautions

A. Obtain history; a previous suicide attempt is a most significant risk factor. Other risk groups include those with biologic and organic causes of depression, such as substance abuse, organic brain disorders, or other medical problems.
B. Be aware of the major warning signs of an impending suicide attempt:
  1. A client begins giving away his or her possessions.
  2. A previously depressed client becomes happy. He or she has made the decision to commit suicide, is no longer debating the possibility, and has figured out how to accomplish the suicide.

Evaluate Intent

A. Directly ask the client about his or her intent. Example: "Do you ever think about harming yourself?"
B. If a client is currently contemplating suicide, ask about his or her plans for carrying out the attempt. Example: "Do you have a plan for harming yourself?"
C. Identify the method chosen; the more lethal the method, the higher the probability that an attempt is imminent. "What is your plan for harming yourself?" Example: A client mentions a shotgun and plans to put it to his head and pull the trigger.
D. Determine the availability of the method chosen. If the method is readily available, the attempt is more likely. Example: The client has a loaded shotgun in his room, so it is readily available.

Nursing Interventions

A. Express concern for the client. Example: "I am very concerned that you are feeling so bad that you want to harm yourself."

TABLE 7-6   Antidepressant Drugs

Drugs	Indications	Adverse Reactions	Nursing Implications
Tricyclics			
• Amitriptyline HCl (Elavil) • Desipramine HCl (Norpramin) • Imipramine HCl (Tofranil) • Nortriptyline HCl (Aventyl) • Protriptyline HCl (Vivactil) • Maprotiline (Ludiomil)	• Depression • Clients with morbid fantasies do not respond well to these drugs.	• Anticholinergic effects: dry mouth, blurred vision, constipation, and urinary retention • CNS effects: sedation, psychomotor slowing, and poor concentration • Cardiovascular effects: tachycardia, orthostatic, hypotension, quinidine-like effect on the heart (assess history of MI) • GI effects: nausea and vomiting • Narrow therapeutic index (can be lethal in overdose)	• Administer at bedtime to minimize sedative effect. • Takes 2 to 6 weeks to achieve therapeutic effects. • 1 to 3 weeks should elapse between discontinuing tricyclics and initiating MAO inhibitors. • Teach client to avoid alcohol. • Avoid concurrent use of antihypertensive drugs. • Carefully evaluate suicide risk.
MAO-Inhibitors (monoamine oxidase inhibitors)			
• Isocarboxazid (Marplan) • Phenelzine sulfate (Nardil) • Tranylcypromine sulfate (Parnate)	• Depression • Phobias • Anxiety	• Tachycardia • Urinary hesitancy, constipation • Impotence • Dizziness • Insomnia • Muscle twitching • Drowsiness • Dry mouth • Fluid retention • *Hypertensive crisis:* severe hypertension, severe headache, chest pain, fever, sweating, nausea and vomiting	• Must *not* be used with tricyclics (cause *hypertensive crisis*). • Major concern is need for dietary restrictions—*certain drug and food interactions can cause hypertensive crisis.* • Instruct client *not* to eat foods with high tyramine content: aged cheese, red wine, beer, beef and chicken, liver, yeast, yogurt, soy sauce, chocolate, bananas. • Teach client *not* to take over-the-counter drugs without physician approval. • Teach the warning signs of hypertensive crisis: headaches, palpitations, increased BP. • Teach client to use caution around machinery.
SSRIs (Selective serotonin reuptake inhibitors)			
• Fluoxetine HCl (Prozac) • Paroxetine (Paxil) • Sertraline (Zoloft) • Fluvoxamine (Luvox) • Citalopram (Celexa)	• Depression • Anxiety • Panic disorder • Aggression • Anorexia nervosa • OCD	• Drowsiness • Dizziness, light-headedness • Headache • Insomnia • Depressed appetite	• Effective 2 to 4 weeks after treatment is initiated. • Should *not* be used with MAO inhibitors: cause hypertensive crisis (violent reaction). • Should wait at least 14 days between discontinuing MAO inhibitor and starting Prozac.

TABLE 7-6 Antidepressant Drugs—cont'd

Drugs	Indications	Adverse Reactions	Nursing Implications
• Escitalopram (Lexapro)		• Serotonin syndrome • Sexual dysfunction • Allergic reaction or rash; withhold drug if occurs	• At least 5 weeks should lapse between discontinuing Prozac and initiating an MAO inhibitor. • May be given in evening if sedation occurs. • Monitor for serotonin syndrome (defined by at least 3 symptoms): → Rapid onset of altered mental states → Agitation → Myoclonus → Hyperreflexia → Fever → Shivering → Diaphoresis → Ataxia → Diarrhea • Caution client about OTC use of St. John's Wort.
Newer antidepressant drugs (atypical antidepressants)			
• Trazodone (Desyrel) • Mirtazapine (Remeron) • Bupropion (Wellbutrin)	• Depression • With trazodone: insomnia, dementia with agitation	• Safer than tricyclics and MAO inhibitors in terms of side effects	• Effective 2 to 4 weeks after treatment is initiated.
S/NRIs (serotonin/norepinephrine reuptake inhibitors)			
• Duloxetine (Cymbalta) • Venlafaxine (Effexor)	• Depression • Anxiety • Panic disorder • Aggression • Anorexia nervosa • OCD	• Nausea • Dry mouth • Insomnia • Headache • Fatigue • Depressed appetite • Increased sweating • Sexual dysfunction • Withdrawal symptoms with abrupt cessation (agitation, tremors, headache, nightmares)	• Should not be used with MAO inhibitors: cause hypertensive crisis (violent reaction). • Should wait at least 14 days between discontinuing MAO inhibitor and starting S/NRIs. • Take baseline blood pressure and monitor periodically (can cause slight drop in BP). • Monitor for worsening of pretreatment symptoms and inform client of possibility. • (Nursing Implications for SSRIs, p. 327).

B. Tell the client that you will share this information with the staff. Example: "I need to share this with the staff so that we can provide for your safety until you are feeling better."

C. Offer the client hope. Example: "You're feeling bad at this moment, but these feelings will pass. We have medications and treatments that can help you through the bad times."

D. Stay with the client. Never leave a suicidal client alone. Legally, the nurse should follow the policy of the institution regarding suicidal clients and should be able to demonstrate that these policies were carried out. Follow the agency policy regarding the removal of potentially hazardous objects such as razors, etc.

HESI Hint • The nurse should suspect an imminent suicide attempt if a depressed client becomes "better" (i.e., happy or even elated). Be aware: a happy affect may signify that the client feels relieved that a plan has been made and is prepared for the suicide attempt.

HESI Hint • When dealing with a depressed client, the nurse should assist with personal hygiene tasks and encourage the client to initiate grooming activities even when he or she does not feel like doing so. This helps promote self-esteem and a sense of control.

HESI Hint • An important nursing intervention for the depressed client is to sit quietly with the client. When answering NCLEX-RN® questions, remember that you are working at Utopia General and there is plenty of time and staff to provide ideal nursing care. Do not let the realities of clinical situations deter you from choosing the best nursing intervention. The best intervention is to sit quietly with the client, offering support with your presence.

HESI Hint • There are always questions about drugs on the NCLEX-RN. Here are some tips: Know the common side effects of drug groups. For example:
• Antianxiety drugs: sedation, drowsiness
• Antidepressant drugs: anticholinergic effects, postural hypotension
• MAO inhibitors: hypertensive crisis
  Know specific problems and concerns in drug therapy. For example:
• Lithium requires renal function assessment and monitoring.
• Phenothiazines cause extrapyramidal effects (EPS); tardive dyskinesia can be permanent if client is not assessed regularly for signs of tardive dyskinesia!
  Know specific client teachings about drug therapy. For example:
• Phenothiazines cause photosensitivity, so client must wear protective clothing and sunglasses.
• MAO inhibitors require dietary restrictions to prevent hypertensive crisis.

BIPOLAR DISORDER, OR MANIC-DEPRESSIVE ILLNESS

A. It is an affective disorder that is manifested by mood swings involving euphoria, grandiosity, and an inflated sense of self-worth. This disorder may or may not include sudden swings to depression.
B. In order to be diagnosed with a bipolar disorder, according to the DSM-IV-TR classification, a client must have at least one episode of major depression. A client may cycle, going from elevation to depression, with periods of normal activity in between.

Characteristics of Varying Degrees of Mania
A. Mild
  1. Feeling of being on a high
  2. Feelings of well-being
  3. Minor alterations in habits
  4. Usually does not seek treatment because of pleasurable effect
B. Moderate
  1. Grandiosity
  2. Talkativeness
  3. Pressured speech
  4. Impulsiveness
  5. Excessive spending
  6. Bizarre dress and grooming
C. Severe
  1. Extreme hyperactivity
  2. Flight of ideas
  3. Nonstop activity (e.g., running, pacing)
  4. Sexual acting out; explicit language
  5. Talkativeness
  6. Overresponsiveness to external stimuli
  7. Easily distracted
  8. Agitation and possibly explosiveness
  9. Severe sleep disturbance
  10. Delusions of grandeur or persecution

Nursing Assessment
A. Determine level of depression exhibited (Symptoms of Varying Degrees of Depression, p. 338).
B. Determine level of mania exhibited (Characteristics of Varying Degrees of Mania, p. 342).
C. Assess nutrition and hydration status.
D. Assess level of fatigue.
E. Assess danger to self and others in relation to level of impulse impairment present.

Analysis (Nursing Diagnoses)
A. *Risk for self-directed/other-directed violence* related to…
B. *Self-care deficit (specify)* related to…

Nursing Plans and Interventions

A. Maintain client's physical health: provide nutrition, rest, and hygiene.

B. Provide safe environment (grandiose thinking and poor impulse control can result in accidents and/altercations with other clients).

C. Decrease environmental stimulation (e.g., place in private room or seclusion room).

D. Implement suicide precautions if assessment indicates risk.

E. Use consistent approach to minimize manipulative behavior.

F. Use frequent, brief contacts to decrease anxiety.

G. Implement constructive limit setting.

H. Avoid giving attention to bizarre behavior (e.g., dress and language).

I. Try to meet needs as soon as possible to keep client from becoming aggressive.

J. Provide small, frequent feedings of food that can be carried (e.g., small finger sandwiches).

K. Engage in simple, active, noncompetitive activities.

L. Avoid distracting or stimulating activities in the evening to help promote sleep and rest.

M. Praise self-control, acceptable behavior.

N. Promote family involvement in therapy, teaching, and medication compliance.

O. Administer lithium, sedatives, and antipsychotics as prescribed (Table 7-7).

TABLE 7-7 Mood Stabilizing Drugs

Drugs	Indications	Adverse Reactions	Nursing Implications
• Lithium carbonate (Carbolith)	• Bipolar disorders, especially the manic phase	• Nausea, fatigue, thirst, polyuria, and fine hand tremors • Weight gain • Hypothyroidism • Early signs of toxicity: diarrhea, vomiting, drowsiness, muscle weakness, lack of coordination	• Lithium is excreted by the kidney. Maintain adequate serum levels. • Assess electrolytes, especially sodium. • Baseline studies of renal, cardiac and thyroid status must be obtained before lithium therapy is begun. • Teach client *early* symptoms of lithium toxicity. If drug is continued, coma, convulsions, and death may occur. • Instruct client to keep salt usage consistent. • Use with diuretics is contraindicated. Diuretic-induced sodium depletion can increase lithium levels, causing toxicity.
Anticonvulsant Mood Stabilizers			
• Valproic acid (Depakene)	• Used in bipolar disorder alone or with lithium	• GI distress: nausea, anorexia, vomiting • Hepatotoxicity • Neurologic symptoms: tremor, sedation, headache, dizziness	• Administer with food. • Monitor blood levels. • Maintain serum levels 50 to 125 µg/ml.
• Carbamazepine (Tegretol)	• Used in bipolar disorders • Used as alternative to lithium	• Dizziness • Ataxia • Blood dyscrasias	• Maintain serum levels at 8 to 12 g/ml. • Stop drug if WBC drops below 3000/mm³ or neutrophil count goes below 1500/mm³. • Monitor hepatic and renal function.
• Lamotrigine (Lamictal)	• Used in bipolar disorder alone or with other mood stabilizers	• Headache • Dizziness • Double vision • Rash	• To minimize risk of severe rash, give low dosage, 25 to 50 mg/day initially, then gradually increase to maintenance dose of 200 mg/day (used alone) or 100 mg/day (with Valproate) or 400 mg/day (with Carbamazepine).

HESI Hint • Atypical antipsychotic drugs are also indicated for mania (risperidone, olanzapine, quetiapine, aripiprazole, and ziprasidone; Table 7-8).

HESI Hint • Monitor serum lithium levels carefully. The therapeutic range is between 0.5 and 1.5 mEq/L. The therapeutic and toxic levels are very close to each other on the readings. Signs of toxicity are evident when lithium levels are more than 1.5 mEq/L. Blood levels should be drawn 12 hours after *last* dose.

HESI Hint • Manic clients can be very caustic toward authority figures. Be prepared for personal putdowns. Avoid arguing or becoming defensive.

HESI Hint • What activities are appropriate for a manic client? Noncompetitive physical activities that require the use of large muscle groups.

HESI Hint • Where should a manic client be placed on the unit?

Make every attempt to reduce stimuli in the environment. Place the client in a quiet part of the unit.

HESI Hint • What interventions should the nurse use if a client becomes abusive?
- Redirect negative behavior or verbal abuse in a calm, firm, nonjudgmental, nondefensive manner.
- Suggest a walk or other physical activity.
- Set limits on intrusive behavior. For example, "When you interrupt, I cannot explain the procedure to the others; please wait your turn."
- If necessary, seclude or administer medication if client becomes totally out of control. Always remember to use compassion because nurses are "nice" people.

Review of Mood Disorders

1. Identify the physiologic changes that commonly occur with depression.
2. A client who has been withdrawn and tearful comes to breakfast one morning smiling and interacting with her peers. Prior to breakfast she gave her roommate her favorite necklace. What actions should the nurse take and why?
3. Name the components of a suicide assessment.
4. A client on your unit refuses to go to group therapy. What is the most appropriate nursing intervention?
5. A client is standing on a table loudly singing "The Star-Spangled Banner" and is encircled by sheets, which have been set afire. In order of priority, describe appropriate nursing actions.

Answers to Review

1. Weight change (loss or gain), constipation, fatigue, lack of sexual interest, somatic complaints, and sleep disturbances
2. Assess for suicidal ideation, plan, and means of carrying out plan. Place on precautions as indicated. A sudden change in mood and giving away possessions are two possible signs that a suicide plan has been developed.
3. Existence of a plan, existence of a method, availability of method chosen, lethality of method chosen, identified support system, and history of previous attempts
4. Accompany client to the group; do not give client option. Client needs to be mobilized.
5. Remove client and other persons in the vicinity to a safe area and activate hospital fire plan. When area is safe, place client in quiet environment with low stimulation and medicate as indicated.

Thought Disorders

SCHIZOPHRENIA

Description: Psychiatric disorder characterized by thought disturbance, altered affect, withdrawal from reality, regressive behavior, difficulty with communication, and impaired interpersonal relationships (see Types of Schizophrenia)

Types of Schizophrenia

A. Catatonic
   1. Stupor (decrease in reaction to the environment) or mutism
   2. Rigidity (maintenance of a posture against efforts to be moved)
   3. Posturing (waxy flexibility)
   4. Negativism (resistance to instructions)
   5. Excitement (severely agitated, out of control)
   6. Potential for violence to self or others during stupor or excitement

B. Disorganized
   1. Incoherence
   2. Flat or inappropriate affect
   3. Disorganized, uninhibited behavior
   4. Unusual mannerisms
   5. Socially withdrawn
   6. No delusions present

C. Paranoid
   1. Systematized delusions, hallucinations related to a single theme, or both
   2. Ideas of reference (misconstruing trivial events and remarks by giving them personal significance)
   3. Potential for violence if delusions are acted upon

D. Residual
   1. Socially withdrawn
   2. Inappropriate affect
   3. Eccentric or peculiar behavior
   4. Absence of prominent delusions and hallucinations
   5. No current psychotic behavior exhibited

E. Undifferentiated
   1. Prominent delusions and hallucinations
   2. Incoherence and grossly disorganized behaviors
   3. Failure to meet any of the criteria for the other types

> **HESI Hint** • When evaluating client behaviors, consider the medications the client is receiving. Exhibited behaviors may be manifestations of schizophrenia *or* a drug reaction.

> **HESI Hint** • There are five types of schizophrenia specified in the DSM-IV-TR, which is a diagnostic manual prepared by the American Psychiatric Association that provides diagnostic criteria for all psychiatric disorders.

Nursing Assessment

A. Assess for disturbance in thought process.
   1. Interpret content of internal and external stimuli.
      a. Symbolism: meaning given to words by client to screen thoughts and feelings that would be difficult to handle if stated directly
      b. Delusions: fixed false beliefs that may be persecutory, grandiose, religious, or somatic in nature
      c. Ideas of reference: belief that conversations or actions of others have reference to the client
   2. Note form: construction of verbal communication.
      a. Looseness of association: lack of clear connection from one thought to the next
      b. Tangential or circumstantial speech: failing to address the original point, giving many nonessential details
      c. Echolalia: constantly repeating what is heard
      d. Neologism: creating new words
      e. Preservation: repeating same word or phrase in response to different questions
      f. Word salad: speaking a jumbled mixture of real and made-up words
   3. Note process: flow of thoughts.
      a. Blocking: gap or interruption in speech due to absent thoughts
      b. Concrete thinking: thinking based on fact versus abstract and intellectual points

B. Assess for disturbance in perception.
   1. Hallucinations: false sensory perception, usually auditory or visual in nature
   2. Illusions: misinterpretation of external environment
   3. Depersonalization: perceives self as alienated or detached from real body
   4. Delusions: false, fixed beliefs that cannot be changed by reason

C. Assess for disturbance in affect (feelings or mood).
   1. Blunted or flat
   2. Inappropriate
   3. Incongruent with context of situation or event

D. Assess for disturbance in behavior.
  1. Incoherent and disorganized
  2. Impulsive, uninhibited
  3. Posturing, unusual mannerisms
  4. Social withdrawal, neglect of personal hygiene
  5. Exhibiting echopraxia: repetition of another person's movements
E. Assess for disturbance in interpersonal relationships.
  1. Difficulty establishing trust
  2. Difficulty with intimacy
  3. Fear and ambivalence toward others

Analysis (Nursing Diagnosis)

A. *Disturbed sensory perception* related to ...

Nursing Plans and Interventions

A. Establish trust.
B. Sit with mute clients.
C. Provide safe and secure environment.
D. Assist with physical hygiene and ADLs.
E. Use matter-of-fact, nonjudgmental approach.
F. Use clear, simple, concrete terms when talking with client.
G. Accept and support client's feelings; use clarification.
H. Reinforce congruent thinking. Stress reality.
I. Avoid arguing and avoid agreeing with inaccurate communications.
J. Set limits on behavior.
K. Avoid stressful situations.
L. Structure time for activities so as to limit time for withdrawal.
M. Encourage client to identify positive characteristics related to self.

N. Praise socially acceptable behavior.
O. Avoid fostering a dependent relationship.
P. Promote family involvement in therapy, teaching, and medication compliance.

> **HESI Hint** • Use Bleuler's four As to help remember the important characteristics of schizophrenia:
> • Autism (preoccupied with self)
> • Affect (flat)
> • Associations (loose)
> • Ambivalence (difficulty making decisions)

DELUSIONAL DISORDERS

Description: Characterized by suspicious, strange behavior, which may be precipitated by a stressful event. May manifest as intense hypochondriasis.

Nursing Assessment

A. Determine degree of suspiciousness and mistrust of others.
B. Assess degree of anxiety.
C. Determine whether delusions are present.
  1. Reference or control
  2. Persecution
  3. Grandeur
  4. Somatic
D. Assess degree of insecurity.

Analysis (Nursing Diagnoses)

A. *Risk for self-directed and/or other-directed violence* related to ...
B. *Social isolation* related to ...

Nursing Interventions for Delusional and Hallucinating Clients

Client Is Delusional	Client Is Hallucinating
A. Encourage recognition of distorted reality. B. Divert focus from delusional thought to reality; do not permit rumination on false ideas. C. Do not agree with or support delusions. D. Avoid arguing about the delusion. Be very matter-of-fact. E. Avoid physically touching client, especially if delusions are persecutional. F. Administer antipsychotic drugs (Table 7-8). G. Monitor and treat side effects of psychotropic drugs (Table 7-9). H. Administer antiparkinsonian drugs. (Table 7-10).	A. Protect client from injury that might result from responding to commands of the voices; pay attention to the content. B. Avoid denying or arguing with client about the hallucination. C. Discuss your observations with client (e.g., "You appear to be listening to something"). D. Make frequent but brief remarks to interrupt the hallucinations. E. Administer antipsychotic drugs (Table 7-8). F. Monitor and treat side effects of psychotropic drugs (Table 7-9). G. Administer antiparkinsonian drugs (Table 7-10).

HESI Hint • Observe for increased motor activity and/or erratic response to staff and other clients. The client may be experiencing an increase in command hallucinations. When this occurs, there is an increased potential for aggressive behavior. THINK PRN!

HESI Hint • Do not argue with a client about the delusions. Logic does not work; it only increases the client's anxiety. Be matter-of-fact and divert delusional thought to reality. Trust is the basis for all interactions with these clients. Be supportive and nonjudgmental. Stress increases anxiety and the need for delusions and hallucinations. Do not agree that you hear voices (you should be the client's contact with reality), but acknowledge your observation of the client; for example, "You look like you're listening to something."

TABLE 7-8 Antipsychotic Drugs

Traditional Drugs	Indications	Adverse Reactions	Nursing Implications

• Phenothiazines
• Chlorpromazine HCl (Thorazine)
• Trifluoperazine HCl (Stelazine)
• Thioridazine HCl (Mellaril)
• Perphenazine (Trilafon)
• Triflupromazine (Vesprin)
• Loxapine (Loxitane)
• Molindone (Moban)
	• To control psychotic behavior: hallucinations, delusions, and bizarre behavior	• Drowsiness
		• Orthostatic hypotension
		• Weight gain
		• Anticholinergic effects
		• Extrapyramidal effects
		  → Pseudo-parkinsonism
		  → Akathisia
		  → Dystonia
		  → Tardive dyskinesia
		• Photosensitivity
		• Blood dyscrasias: granulocytosis, leukopenia
		• Neuroleptic malignant syndrome
			• Extrapyramidal effects are *major* concern.
			• Monitor elderly clients closely.
			• Takes 2 to 3 weeks to achieve therapeutic effect.
			• Keep client supine for 1 hour after administration and advise to change positions slowly because of effects of orthostatic hypotension.
			• Teach client to avoid:
			  → Alcohol
			  → Sedatives (potentiate effect of CNS depressants)
			  → Antacids (reduce absorption of drug)

• Fluphenazine HCl (Prolixin)	• To control psychotic behavior • Useful in treatment of psychomotor agitation associated with thought disorders	• Same as other phenothiazines	• Absorbed slowly. • Used with noncompliant clients because it can be administered IM once every 14 days.
Nonphenothiazines			
• Haloperidol (Haldol) • Chlorprothixene (Taractan) • Thiothixene HCl (Navane) • Pimozide (Orap)	• To control psychotic behavior • Less sedative than phenothiazines	• Severe extrapyramidal reactions • Leukocytosis • Blurred vision • Dry mouth • Urinary retention	• Teach client to avoid alcohol. • Orap is used only for Tourette's syndrome.
Long Acting			
• Fluphenazine decanoate (Prolixin Decanoate) • Haloperidol decanoate (Haldol Decanoate)	• Clients who require supervision with medication regimens	• Similar to Prolixin and Haldol	• Similar to Haldol and Prolixin. • Prolixin can be given every 7 to 28 days. • Haldol can be given every 4 weeks. • Requires several months to reach steady-state drug levels.

(Continued)

TABLE 7-8 Antipsychotic Drugs—cont'd

Traditional Drugs	Indications	Adverse Reactions	Nursing Implications
Atypical Antipsychotic Drugs			
• Risperidone (Risperdal) • Olanzapine (Zyprexa) • Quetiapine (Seroquel) • Aripiprazole (Ability) • Ziprasidone (Geodon) • Clozapine (Clozaril) • Aripiprazole (Abilify)	• Treat positive and negative symptoms of schizophrenia without significant EPS • Clients who have not responded well to typical antipsychotics or have side effects with typical antipsychotics • Fewer side effects • Clozapine has superior efficacy in clients who have been treatment resistant.	• Risperdal: neuroleptic malignant syndrome (NMS), EPS, dizziness, GI symptoms (nausea, constipation), anxiety • Zyprexa: drowsiness, dizziness, EPS, agitation • Seroquel: drowsiness, dizziness, headache, EPS, weight gain, anticholinergic effects • Clozaril: agranulocytosis, drowsiness, dizziness, GI symptoms, neuroleptic malignant syndrome	• Monitor WBC weekly for first 6 months, then biweekly. • Baseline VS and ECG; report abnormal VS. • Monitor for symptoms of NMS and EPS. • Teach to change positions slowly. • Abilify is a new class of antipsychotic drugs dopamine system stabilizers (DSSs) for schizophrenia and acute bipolar mania. • Seroquel monitor lipids especially for obese, diabetic, or hypertensive clients.

TABLE 7-9 Side Effects of Psychotropic Drugs and Nursing Interventions

Side Effects	Characteristics	Nursing Interventions
Blood dyscrasias		
• Agranulocytosis: occurs in first weeks of treatment • Thrombocytopenia: decreased platelets	• Sore throat, fever, chills	• Protect from infections. • Provide comfort measures: gargle for sore throat, use lozenges and analgesics.
	• Bruises easily, petechia	• Teach client safety measures.
Extrapyramidal effects		
• Parkinsonism: occurs within 1 to 4 weeks after initiation of treatment • Akathisia: occurs within 1 to 6 weeks after initiation of treatment • Dystonia: occurs within 1 to 2 days after initiation of treatment • Tardive dyskinesia: develops late in treatment	• Rigidity, shuffling gait, pill rolling hand movements, tremors, dyskinesia, mask-like face	• Administer anticholinergics drugs, i.e., Cogentin, Artane. Other drugs for EPS include Benadryl, Symmetrel, Ativan, Klonopin; Inderal for akathisia and vitamin E for tardive dyskinesia.
	• Restlessness, agitation, and pacing. Sudden difficulty sitting still (can be confused with tardive dyskinesia).	• Rule out anxiety. Can ask client, "Are you feeling so restless that you can't sit still?"
	• Limb and neck spasms, uncoordinated, jerky movements, difficulty speaking and swallowing, rigidity and muscle spasms	• Emergency treatment is with IM anticholinergics drug. *Have respiratory emergency equipment available.*
	• Involuntary tongue and lip movements, blinking, choreiform movements of limbs and trunk.	• Permanent side effect; antiparkinsonian drugs are of no help in decreasing symptoms. Teach client and family to report side effects *early.*

TABLE 7-9   Side Effects of Psychotropic Drugs and Nursing Interventions—cont'd

Side Effects	Characteristics	Nursing Interventions
• Photosensitivity	• Sunlight: exposed skin turns blue and color changes occur in eyes but does not cause vision impairment	• Teach client to stay out of sun, wear protective clothing and sunglasses. • Skin discoloration will disappear within 6 months after drug is discontinued.
• Neuroleptic malignant syndrome	• Life-threatening emergency: high fever, tachycardia, stupor, increased respirations, severe muscle rigidity	• Increased risk with phenothiazines. • Early recognition is important; transfer to medical facility for hydration, nutritional support and treatment of possible respiratory failure and renal failure.
• Serotonin syndrome	• Confusion, disorientation, autonomic dysfunction.	• Notify health care provider, stat. • Provide systems support.
• Anticholinergic effects	• Dry mouth, blurred vision, tachycardia, nasal congestion, constipation, urinary retention, orthostatic hypotension	• Encourage sips of water, chewing sugarless gum or hard candy. • Increase fiber in diet. • Change positions slowly to avoid dizziness. • Report urinary retention to physician. • Tolerance to these side effects will usually occur.

HESI Hint • Know the side effects of drugs commonly used to treat schizophrenia since client behavioral changes may be due to drug reactions instead of schizophrenia.

TABLE 7-10   Antiparkinsonian Drugs

Drugs	Indications	Adverse Reactions	Nursing Implications
• Trihexyphenidyl HCl (Artane) • Benztropine mesylate (Cogentin) • Amantadine (Symmetrel)	• Acts on the extrapyramidal system to reduce disturbing symptoms	• Anticholinergic effects • Drowsiness • Headaches • Urinary hesitancy • Memory impairment	• Usually given in conjunction with antipsychotic drugs

Review of Thought Disorders

1. A client is sitting alone talking quietly. There is no one around. What nursing action should be taken?
2. A client dials 222-2222 and asks for his fiance, Candice Bergen. This is an example of what type of thought disorder?
3. A client has been sitting in the same position for 2 hours. He is mute. What type of schizophrenia is this client experiencing? Describe appropriate nursing interventions for this client.
4. A client is very agitated. He believes that the CIA has tapped the phone and is sending messages through the television and that you are an agent who has been planted by the agency. In order of priority, list the appropriate nursing actions when intervening in this situation. What type of delusion is this client experiencing?
5. The nurse asks the client, "What brought you to the hospital?" The client's response is, "The bus." What type of thinking is this client exhibiting?

Answers to Review

1. Quietly approach client and note the behavior. Assess the content of the hallucinations (e.g., "I noticed you talking. Are you hearing voices? Can you tell me about the voices you are hearing?")
2. Delusion of grandeur
3. Catatonic; spend time with client; assist with ADLs; be alert to potential for violence toward self or others; be aware of fluid and nutrition needs.
4. Approach client and offer solitary activity as distraction. Assess need for medication. Encourage verbalization of feelings and promote outlet for expression. The delusion is paranoid disorder with delusions of reference (CIA).
5. Concrete

Substance Abuse

Description: Regular use of substances that affect the central nervous system, resulting in behavioral changes; the chemicals involved produce physiologic and psychological dependence.

ALCOHOLISM

This is a drinking pattern that interferes with physical, social, familial, vocational, and emotional functioning.

Nursing Assessment

A. Patterns indicative of alcoholism:
   1. Episodic drinking (binges)
   2. Continuous drinking
   3. Morning drinking
   4. Increase in family fighting about drinking
   5. Increase in absences from work or school, especially Mondays
   6. Blackouts
   7. Hiding drinking pattern
   8. Legal problems (DUIs)
   9. Health problems such as gastritis
B. Family history of alcoholism or substance abuse
C. Dependency, yet resentfulness of authority
D. Impulsive, abusive behavior
E. Impaired judgment, memory loss
F. Incoordination, slurred speech
G. Mood varying between euphoria and depression
H. Intoxication as determined by blood alcohol level (BAL; 0.10% or greater is considered intoxication.)
I. Previous experience with treatment centers or Alcoholics Anonymous (AA)
J. Alcohol withdrawal symptoms:
   1. Begin shortly after drinking stops, as early as 4 to 6 hours after
   2. Anxiety, nausea, insomnia, tremors, hyper-alertness, and restlessness
   3. Sudden or gradual increase in all vital signs
   4. Delirium tremens (DTs); may appear 12 to 36 hours after last drink:
      a. Tachycardia, tachypnea, diaphoresis
      b. Marked tremors
      c. Hallucinations
      d. Paranoia
   5. Grand mal seizures (possible)
K. Chronic alcohol-related illnesses:
   1. Chronic gastritis
   2. Cirrhosis and hepatitis
   3. Korsakoff syndrome: organic syndrome that frequently follows delirium tremens; associated with chronic alcoholism
   4. Wernicke syndrome: a severe disorder (encephalopathy) occurring in chronic alcoholics; probably due to a deficiency of vitamin B_1 (thiamin); may escalate Korsakoff syndrome; is treated with thiamine chloride
   5. Malnutrition and dehydration
   6. Pancreatitis
   7. Peripheral neuropathy

Analysis (Nursing Diagnoses)

A. *Risk for injury* related to...
B. *Ineffective family coping* related to...

TABLE 7-11 Alcohol Deterrent

Drugs	Indications	Adverse Reactions	Nursing Implications
• Disulfiram (Antabuse)	• Treatment of alcoholism; aversion therapy • Interferes with breakdown of alcohol causing an accumulation of acetaldehyde (a byproduct of alcohol in the body)	• *Severe side* effects occur if alcohol is consumed: • Nausea and vomiting • Hypotension, headaches • Rapid pulse and respirations • Flushed face and bloodshot eyes • Confusion • Chest pain • Weakness, dizziness	• Teach client what to expect if alcohol is consumed while taking the drug. • Be aware that some alcoholic clients use the side effects as a means of "punishing" themselves or as a form of masochism, and if a client repeatedly consumes alcohol while taking the drug, the healthcare provider should be notified. • Persons with serious heart disease, diabetes, epilepsy, liver impairment, or mental illness should not take Antabuse.

HESI Hint • What medications can the nurse expect to administer to chemically dependent clients? In treating alcohol withdrawal, Librium or Ativan are commonly used. Antabuse is often used as a deterrent to drinking alcohol. Client teaching should include the effects of consuming any alcohol while on Antabuse. Encourage client to read all labels of over-the-counter medications and food products that may contain small amounts of alcohol.

C. *Imbalanced nutrition: less than body requirements* related to …

D. *Situational low self-esteem* related to …

Nursing Plans and Interventions

A. Maintain safety, nutrition, hygiene, and rest.

B. Implement suicide precautions if assessment indicates risk.

C. Provide care during withdrawal.
  1. Monitor vital signs, I&O, electrolytes.
  2. Observe for impending delirium tremens.
  3. Prevent aspiration; implement seizure precautions.
  4. Reduce environmental stimuli.
  5. Medicate with antianxiety medication, usually Librium or Ativan (see Table 7-4).
  6. Provide high-protein diet and adequate fluid intake (limit caffeine).
  7. Provide vitamin supplements, especially B$_1$ and B complex.
  8. Provide emotional support.

D. Rehabilitation:
  1. Use direct, matter-of-fact, nonjudgmental attitude.
  2. Confront denial and rationalization (main coping styles used by alcoholics).
  3. Confront manipulations; set firm limits on behavior.
  4. Set short-term, realistic goals.
  5. Help increase self-esteem.

  6. Explore ways to increase frustration tolerance without alcohol.
  7. Identify ways to decrease loneliness.
  8. Encourage client to accept responsibility for own behavior.
  9. Identify availability of support systems (family, friends, church, AA).
  10. Identify activities and friendships not related to drinking.
  11. Provide group and family therapy; refer family to Al-Anon family groups or Al-Ateen.

E. Provide client and family teaching regarding the side effects of Antabuse if it is used as a deterrent to drinking (Table 7-11).

DRUG ABUSE

Description: State of dependency produced by repeated use of a substance that causes altered perception or mood, or both

Nursing Assessment

A. Pattern of drug use
  1. What drugs are used?
  2. What is the drug of choice?
  3. How much is used and how often?
  4. How long has the drug been used?

B. Physical evidence of drug usage
  1. Needle track marks
  2. Cellulitis at puncture site
  3. Poor nutritional status
  4. Inflammation of nasal passages

TABLE 7-12 Drug Withdrawal and Overdose Symptoms

Drugs	Withdrawal	Overdose	Effect
Opiates			
• Heroin • Morphine • Codeine • Opium • Methadone	• Watery eyes, runny nose, dilated pupils • Anxiety • Diaphoresis, fever • Nausea, vomiting, and diarrhea • Achiness • Abdominal cramps • Insomnia • Tachycardia	• Respiratory depression leading to respiratory arrest • Circulatory depression leading to cardiac arrest • Unconsciousness leading to coma • Death	• General physical and mental deterioration • Rapid tolerance • Impaired judgment
• Cocaine	• Depression • Fatigue • Disturbed sleep • Anxiety • Psychomotor agitation	• Tachycardia • Pupillary dilatation • Increased BP • Cardiac arrhythmias • Perspiration, chills • Nausea, vomiting	• Psychological dependence • Tolerance within hours or days
• Amphetamines	• Depression • Fatigue • Disturbed sleep	• Restlessness • Tremors • Rapid respiration • Confusion • Assaultive behavior • Hallucinations • Panic	• Paranoid delusions
• Hallucinogenic	• No withdrawal	• Panic • Psychosis	• Flashbacks • Impaired judgment
Antianxiety drugs			

• Benzodiazepines:
  • Valium
  • Serax
  • Ativan
	• Tremors
	• Agitation
	• Anxiety
	• Abdominal cramps
	• Grand mal seizures
		• Drowsiness
		• Confusion
		• Hypotension
		• Coma → death
			• Withdrawal occurs if there is abrupt cessation
			• Temporary psychosis

HESI Hint • What type of therapy is used with chemically dependent clients? Group therapy is effective, as are support groups such as Alcoholics Anonymous and Narcotics Anonymous.

HESI Hint • Harm reduction is a community health strategy designed to reduce the harm of substance abuse to families, individuals, community, and society. Examples: More compassionate drug treatment options, including abstinence and drug-substitution models; HIV-related interventions such as needle exchanges; directed drug-use management should the client wish to continue use; changes in laws concerning possession of paraphernalia and drug use.

C. Possible causes of drug dependency
  1. Desire to escape reality and problems
  2. Low self-esteem
  3. Peer or culture pressure
  4. Inherent susceptibility to drug dependence
D. Symptoms of withdrawal and overdose are particular for the drug used (Table 7-12).

Analysis (Nursing Diagnoses)

A. *Risk for injury* related to …

B. *Risk for infection* related to …
C. *Disturbed personal identity* related to …

Nursing Plans and Interventions

A. Assess level of consciousness and vital signs. (Rapid withdrawal can be fatal for persons addicted to barbiturates, antianxiety medications, and hypnotics.)
B. Monitor I&O and electrolytes.

C. Implement suicide precautions if assessment indicates risk.

D. Provide adequate nutrition, hydration, and rest.

E. Administer medications according to detoxification protocol of medical unit.

F. Phenothiazines may be used to decrease the discomfort of withdrawal.

G. Confront denial (main coping style used by substance abusers).
   1. Focus on substance abuse problem.
   2. Confront the placing of blame on external problems.

H. Reinforce reality in simple, concrete terms.

I. Encourage verbal expression of anger and depression.

J. Assist with identification of stressors and areas of conflict.

K. Encourage exploration of alternative coping strategies.

L. Positively reinforce insight into behavior patterns.

M. Help identify an appropriate support system.

N. Provide support to significant others.

O. Teach danger of AIDS and other blood-related diseases.

HESI Hint • Know what defense mechanisms are used by chemically dependent clients. Denial and rationalization are the two most common coping styles used. Their use must be confronted so the client's accountability for his or her own behavior can be developed.

HESI Hint • What basic needs take priority when working with chemically dependent clients? Nutrition is a priority. Alcohol and drug intake has superseded the intake of food for these clients.

HESI Hint • What behaviors are expected during withdrawal? In the alcoholic, delirium tremens (DTs) occurs 12 to 36 hours after the last intake of alcohol. Know the symptoms. In drug abuse, withdrawal symptoms are specific to the type of drug.

Review of Substance Abuse

1. Three days ago, a client was admitted to the medical unit for a GI bleed. His BP and pulse rate gradually increased, and he developed a low-grade fever. What assessment data should the nurse obtain? What kind of anticipatory planning should the nurse develop?
2. What physical signs might indicate that a client is abusing intravenous medications?
3. What behaviors would indicate to the nurse manager that an employee has a possible substance abuse problem?

4. A client becomes extremely agitated, abusive, and very suspicious. He is currently undergoing detoxification from alcohol with Librium 15 mg every 6 hours. What nursing actions are indicated?
5. A client in the third week of a cocaine rehabilitation program returns from an unsupervised pass. The nurse notices that he is euphoric and is socializing with the other clients more than he has in the past. What nursing actions are indicated?

Answers to Review

1. Obtain a drug and alcohol consumption assessment, including type, frequency, and time of last dose or drink. Call the health care provider and report findings. Anticipate withdrawal and delirium tremens. Provide a quiet, safe environment. Place on seizure precautions. Anticipate giving a medication like Librium.
2. Needle track marks; cellulitis at puncture site; poor nutritional status
3. Change in work performance, withdrawal, increase in absences (especially Mondays and Fridays), increase in number of times tardy, long breaks, lateness returning from lunch

4. Notify the health care provider immediately and anticipate an increase in dose or frequency of Librium. Provide a quiet, safe environment. Approach in a quiet, calm manner. Avoid touching client.
5. Notify health care provider of observed behavior change. Get a urine drug screen as prescribed. Confront client with observed behavior change.

Abuse

CHILD ABUSE

Description: Includes physical and mental injury, sexual abuse, and neglect

Nursing Assessment

A. Most important indicators of child abuse:
1. Injuries not congruent with the child's developmental age or skills
2. Injuries not correlated with the stated cause
3. Delay in seeking medical care
B. Bruises in unusual places and in various stages of healing
C. Bruises, welts caused by belts, cords, etc.
D. Burns (cigarette, iron); immersion burns (symmetrical in shape)
E. Whiplash injuries caused by being shaken
F. Bald patches where hair has been pulled out
G. Fractures in various stages of healing
H. Failure to thrive, unattended-to physical problems
I. Torn, stained, bloody underclothes
J. Lacerations of external genitalia
K. Bedwetting, soiling
L. Sexually transmitted diseases
M. Parent seeing child as "different" from other children
N. Parent using child to meet own needs
O. Parent seldom touching or responding to child; may be very critical of child
P. Child appearing frightened and withdrawn in the presence of parent or other adult
Q. Family history of frequent moves, unstable employment, marital discord, and family violence
R. One parent answering all the questions

Analysis (Nursing Diagnoses)

A. *Fear* related to…
B. *Impaired parenting* related to…
C. *Interrupted family process* related to…

Nursing Plans and Interventions

A. *Nurses are legally required to report all cases of suspected child abuse to the appropriate local or state agency.*
B. Take color photographs of injuries.
C. Document factual, objective statements about child's physical condition, child-family interactions, and interviews with family.
D. Establish trust, and care for the child's physical problems; these are the primary and immediate needs of these children.

E. Recognize own feelings of disgust and contempt for the parents.
F. Utilize principles of crisis intervention.
G. Assist child and family to develop self-esteem.
H. Teach basic child development and parenting skills to family.
I. Support the need for family therapy.

> **HESI Hint** • Select only one nurse to care for an abused child. Abused children have difficulty establishing trust. The child will be less anxious with one consistent caregiver.

INTIMATE-PARTNER VIOLENCE

A. It is a criminal act of physical, emotional, economic, or sexual abuse between an assailant and a victim, who most commonly are, or were, in an intimate relationship (may be marital or dating).
B. Abuse is usually a tension-releasing action as well as a lack of impulse control.
C. Assailant may come from a family in which battering and physical violence were present.
D. Persons act more violently when drinking or using drugs.
E. The relationship is usually characterized by extreme jealousy and issues of power and control.
F. Women in a battering relationship may lack self-confidence and feel trapped. They may be embarrassed about their situation, which results in isolation and dependency on the abuser.
G. Abuse often begins during pregnancy or occurs more frequently during pregnancy.

Nursing Assessment

A. Delay between time of injury and time of treatment
B. Anxious when answering questions about injury
C. Abdominal injuries during pregnancy
D. Looks to abuser for answers to questions related to injuries
E. Depression or suicidal ideation
F. Feeling of responsibility for "provoking" partner
G. Low self-esteem
H. Abrasions, cuts, lacerations, sprains, black eyes
I. Psychosomatic (somatoform) complaints
J. Concurrent use of alcohol, drugs

Analysis (Nursing Diagnoses)

A. *Disturbed personal identity* related to…
B. *Disabled family coping* related to…
C. *Fear* related to…

D. *Risk for injury* related to …

E. *Powerlessness* related to …

Nursing Plans and Interventions

A. Establish trust; use nonjudgmental approach.

B. Treat physical wounds and injuries.

C. Document factual, objective statements about client's physical condition, injuries, and interaction with partner or family.

D. Determine potential for further violence.

E. Provide crisis intervention.

F. Assist with referral to shelter if necessary or desired, with adult's consent.

G. Assist client with contacting authorities if charges are to be pressed.

H. Interview abused partner when the abuser is not present.

> **HESI Hint** • Women who are abused may rationalize the spouse's behavior and unnecessarily accept blame for his actions. The woman may or may not choose to press charges. Be sure to give her the number of a shelter or help line for future occurrences and help her to develop a safety plan.

ELDER ABUSE

A. It is an act that causes physical, verbal, financial, or psychosocial injury or exploitation as well as the physical neglect of an aged adult.

B. Abuse of the elderly is underreported; the estimated number varies from 1% to 10% of the elderly population.

C. The majority of the abuse is committed by spouses and children but other caregivers are guilty too.

Nursing Assessment

A. Bruises on the upper arms (bilaterally, resulting from being shaken)

B. Broken bones caused by falls (resulting from being pushed)

C. Dehydration or malnourishment

D. Overmedication

E. Poor physical hygiene, improper medical care

F. Withdrawn behavior, feelings of hopelessness, helplessness

G. Behavior that may be demanding, belligerent, and aggressive

H. Repeated visits to health care agency for injuries and falls

I. Injuries that do not correlate with stated cause

J. Misuse of money by children or legal guardians

Analysis (Nursing Diagnoses)

A. *Fear* related to …

B. *Interrupted family process* related to …

C. *Risk for injury* related to …

Nursing Plans and Interventions

A. Establish trust; use nonjudgmental approach.

B. Meet physical needs, treat wounds and injuries.

C. Document factual, objective statements about client's physical condition, injuries, and interaction with significant other and family.

D. Report suspected abuse to the appropriate local or state authorities.

E. Arrange community resources to provide "respite care" for the caregiver.

F. Arrange visiting nurses, nutrition services, or adult day care if possible.

> **HESI Hint** • It is difficult for an elderly person to admit abuse for fear of being placed in a nursing home or being abandoned. Therefore, it is imperative to establish a trusting relationship with the elderly client.

RAPE AND SEXUAL ASSAULT

Definition: Crime involving lack of consent, force, and sexual penetration; an act of aggression, *not* passion

Nursing Assessment

A. Physical assessment with careful documentation of injuries

B. Emotional status: self-blame, anxiety, fear, humiliation, disbelief, and anger

C. Coping behaviors

D. Identification of support system

E. Details of the assault

Analysis (Nursing Diagnoses)

A. *Rape-trauma syndrome* related to …

B. *Powerlessness* related to …

C. *Fear* related to …

D. *Risk for injury* related to …

Nursing Plans and Interventions

A. Communicate nonjudgmental acceptance.

B. Provide physical care to treat injuries.

C. Give clear, concise explanations of all procedures to be performed.

D. Document factual objective statements of physical assessment; record client's *exact* words in describing the assault.

E. Notify police and encourage victim to prosecute.

F. Collect and label evidence carefully in the presence of a witness.

G. Notify rape crisis team or counselor if available in the community.

H. Allow discussion of feelings about the assault.

I. Advise of potential for venereal disease, pregnancy, and HIV.

J. Provide information about medical care available.

K. Support client, family, and friends.

> **HESI Hint** • Rape victims are at high risk for posttraumatic stress disorder (PTSD). Immediate intervention to diminish distress is vital. The nurse should also assess for and intervene for sequelae such as unwanted pregnancy, sexually transmitted diseases, and HIV risk.

> **HESI Hint** • Questions on the NCLEX-RN exam regarding physical and sexual abuse usually focus on three aspects:
> 1. Physical manifestations of abuse
> 2. Client safety
> 3. Legal responsibilities of the nurse. In children, the nurse is legally responsible for reporting all suspected cases of abuse. In intimate-partner abuse, it is the adult's decision; the nurse should be supportive of the decision. Remember to document objective factual assessment data and the client's exact words in cases of sexual abuse and rape.

Review of Abuse

1. What family dynamics are often seen in child abuse cases?
2. What behavior might the nurse observe in a child who is abused?
3. Identify nursing interventions for dealing with an abused child.
4. When does battering of women often begin or escalate?
5. What dynamics prevent a battered spouse from leaving the battering situation?
6. Why is elder abuse so underreported?
7. What types of abuse are seen in the elderly?
8. Identify nursing interventions for working with a rape survivor.

Answers to Review

1. Parent sees child as "different" from other children. Parent uses child to meet his or her own needs. Parent seldom touches or responds to child. Parent may be very critical of child. There is a family history of frequent moves, unstable employment, marital discord, and family violence. One parent answers all the questions.
2. Child may appear frightened and withdrawn in the presence of parent or adult.
3. All cases of suspected abuse must be reported to appropriate local and state agencies. Take color photographs of injuries. Document factual, objective statements of child's physical condition, child-family interactions, and interviews with family. Establish trust, and care for the child's physical problems. These are the primary and *immediate* needs of these children. Recognize own feelings of disgust and contempt for the parents. Teach basic child development and parenting skills to family.
4. During pregnancy
5. A woman in a battering relationship may lack self-confidence and feel trapped. She is often embarrassed to tell friends and family, so she becomes isolated and dependent upon the abuser.
6. It is difficult for an elderly person to admit abuse for fear of being placed in a nursing home or being abandoned.
7. Abuse can be physical, verbal, psychosocial, exploitive, or physical neglect.
8. Communicate nonjudgmental acceptance. Provide physical care to treat injuries. Give clear, concise explanations of all procedures to be performed. Notify police; encourage victim to prosecute. Collect and label evidence carefully in the presence of a witness. Document factual, objective statements about physical condition; record client's exact words in describing the assault. Notify rape crisis team or counselor if available in the community. Allow discussion of feelings about the assault. Advise of potential for venereal disease, HIV, or pregnancy, and describe medical care available.

Organic Disorders

Description: Abnormal psychological or behavioral signs and symptoms that occur as a result of cerebral disease, systemic dysfunction, or use of or exposure to exogenous substances.

DELIRIUM AND DEMENTIA

Delirium	Dementia

Description: Acute process that, if treated, is usually reversible. It is recognized by its sudden onset.
A. It occurs in response to a specific stressor, such as:
  1. Infection
  2. Drug reaction
  3. Substance intoxication or withdrawal
  4. Electrolyte imbalance
  5. Head trauma
  6. Sleep deprivation
B. The treatment of choice is the correction of the causative disorder.
	Description: Cognitive impairments characterized by gradual, progressive onset; it is irreversible. Judgment, memory, abstract thinking, and social behavior are affected.
	A. It is most commonly seen in:
	  1. Alzheimer disease (Table 7-13)
	  2. Multiinfarctions (brain)
	B. It also occurs in:
	  1. Huntington chorea
	  2. Parkinson disease
	  3. Multiple sclerosis and brain tumors
	  4. Wernicke-Korsakoff syndrome (chronic alcoholics)

HESI Hint • The basic difference between delirium and dementia is that delirium is acute and reversible, whereas dementia is gradual and permanent.

Nursing Assessment

A. Limited attention span, easily distracted
B. Confusion and disorientation, impaired judgment
C. Delusions, visual hallucinations, or sensory illusions
D. Labile affect; sudden anger
E. Anxiety and depression
F. Loss of recent and remote memory
G. Confabulation (making up responses, stories to fill in lost memory)
H. Impaired coordination
I. Increased psychomotor activity
J. Slurring of speech
K. Decreased personal hygiene
L. Sleep deprivation, day-night reversal
M. Incontinence and constipation

Analysis (Nursing Diagnosis)

A. *Dressing/grooming self-care deficit* related to …

Nursing Plans and Interventions

A. Provide safe, consistent environment.
B. Maintain health, nutrition, safety, hygiene, and rest.
C. Assist with ADLs.
D. Provide support to client and family.
E. Provide routine in daily activities.
F. Mark the bathroom clearly.
G. Reorient the client as needed.
H. Use simple, direct statements.
I. See Dementia in Gerontologic Nursing, p. 370, for additional interventions.

HESI Hint • Confusion in the elderly is often accepted as being part of growing old. However, the confusion may be due to dehydration with resulting electrolyte imbalance. Think "sudden change" when obtaining a history. Such changes are usually due to a specific stressor, and treatment of the causative stressor will usually result in correcting the confusion.

HESI Hint • Confabulation is not lying. It is used by the client to decrease anxiety and protect the ego.

TABLE 7-13   Alzheimer Medications

Drugs	Adverse Reactions	Nursing Implications
Acetyl cholinesterase inhibitors		
• Tacrine HCl (Cognex) • Donepezil HCl (Aricept) • Rivastigmine (Exelon) • Galantamine (Reminyl) • Extended release (Concerta) • Amphetamine mixture (Adderall)	• Overall—nausea and diarrhea • Cognex: considerable GI distress elevated liver enzymes	• Teach clients that they should take *no* anticholinergic medication. • Medications should not be used in cases of severe liver impairment. • Take with meals to avoid GI upset. • Do not discontinue abruptly.

HESI Hint • One may also use atypical antipsychotics such as risperidone, quetiapine, olanzapine. Clozaril is not a front-line agent because of side effects. One may also give mood stabilizers and antianxiety medications as indicated.

HESI Hint • Nursing interventions for the confused elderly should focus on:
• Maintaining the client's health and safety.
• Encouraging self-care.
• Reinforcing reality orientation (e.g., saying, "Today is Monday," and calling the client by name).
• Providing a consistent, safe environment; engaging client in simple tasks and activities to build self-esteem.

HESI Hint • Providing a consistent caregiver is a priority in planning nursing care for the confused older client. Change increases anxiety and confusion.

Review of Organic Disorders

1. List five causes of delirium.
2. Describe the nursing care for a client with Alzheimer disease.
3. Identify three or more causes of dementia.

Answers to Review

1. Infection, alcohol withdrawal, electrolyte imbalance, sleep deprivation, brain injury (i.e., subdural hematoma).
2. Provide a safe, consistent environment. (Do not make changes, if possible. Change increases anxiety and confusion.) Stick to routines. If client wanders, make sure he or she has a name tag. Provide assistance as needed with ADLs. Make sure bathroom is clearly labeled.
3. Alzheimer disease, multiinfarcts (brain), Huntington chorea, multiple sclerosis, Parkinson disease.

Childhood and Adolescent Disorders

ATTENTION-DEFICIT (HYPERACTIVITY) DISORDER (ADD/ADHD)

Description: Developmentally inappropriate attention, impulsiveness, and hyperactivity

Nursing Assessment

A. Physical assessment
B. More prevalent in boys
C. Failure to listen to and follow instructions
D. Difficulty playing quietly and sitting still
E. Disruptive, impulsive behavior
F. Distractibility to external stimuli

TABLE 7-14 Stimulants

Drugs	Indications	Adverse Reactions	Nursing Implications
• Dextroamphetamine sulfate (Dexedrine) • Methylphenidate HCL (Ritalin) • Pemoline (Cylert)	• Treat ADD/ADHD • Methylphenidate is also used to treat narcolepsy	• May interact with MAO inhibitors producing fever and hypertensive crisis • Nervousness, and insomnia; dizziness • Tourette syndrome • Tachycardia, palpitations, angina, dysrhythmias • Anorexia, weight loss, nausea, and abdominal pain	• Short-acting, 2 to 4 hours. • Teach to take last dose at least 6 hours before bedtime if insomnia occurs. • Administer 1 to 3 doses daily. • Administer with or after meals to avoid appetite suppression. • Monitor heart rate, rhythm, and BP. • Monitor height and weight to detect growth suppression.

G. Excessive talking

H. Shifting from one unfinished task to another

I. Underachievement in school performance

Analysis (Nursing Diagnoses)

A. *Risk for injury: trauma* related to …

B. *Social isolation* related to …

C. *Interrupted family process* related to …

Nursing Plans and Interventions

A. Decrease environmental stimuli.

B. Set limits on behavior when indicated.

C. Provide a safe, comfortable environment.

D. Initiate a behavior contract to help child manage own behavior.

E. Administer medications as prescribed (Table 7-14).

CONDUCT AND OPPOSITIONAL DEFIANT DISORDERS

Definition: Conduct disorder is an antisocial behavior characterized by violation of laws, societal norms, and the basic rights of others without feelings of remorse or guilt.

Definition: Oppositional defiant disorder is characterized by behavior that fails to adhere to established norms, but does not violate the rights of others.

Nursing Assessment: Conduct Disorder

A. Physical fighting

B. Running away from home

C. Lying, stealing

D. Cruelty to animals

E. Frequent truancy

F. Vandalism, arson

G. Use of alcohol, drugs

Nursing Assessment: Oppositional Defiant Disorder

A. Argumentativeness

B. Blaming others for own problems

C. Defying rules and authority

D. Using obscene language

E. Acting resentful, vindictive

Analysis (Nursing Diagnoses): Conduct and Defiant Disorders

A. *Risk for other-directed violence* related to …

B. *Chronic low self-esteem* related to …

C. *Ineffective family coping* related to …

Nursing Plans and Interventions: Conduct and Defiant Disorders

A. Assess verbal and nonverbal cues for escalating behavior so as to decrease outbursts.

B. Use a nonauthoritarian approach.

C. Avoid asking "why" questions.

D. Initiate a "show of force" with a child who is out of control.

E. Use a "quiet room" when external control is needed.

F. Clarify expressions or jargon if meanings are unclear.

G. Teach to redirect angry feelings to safe alternative, such as a pillow or punching bag.

H. Implement behavior modification therapy if indicated.

I. Role-play new coping strategies with client.

HESI Hint • Children also experience depression, which often presents as headaches, stomachaches, and other somatic complaints. Be sure to assess suicide risk, especially in the adolescent.

HESI Hint • The client's lack of remorse or guilt about the antisocial behavior represents a malfunction of the superego, or conscience. The id functions on the basic instinct level and strives to meet immediate needs. The ego is in touch with external reality and is the part of the personality that makes decisions.

HESI Hint • Important points to remember when answering NCLEX-RN questions:
- A child in this situation may be involved in a self-fulfilling prophecy (e.g., "Mom says that I'm a trouble-maker therefore, I must live up to Mom's expectations").
- Confront the client with his or her behavior (e.g., lying). This gives the client a sense of security.
- Provide consistent interventions; this helps to prevent manipulation. Inconsistency does not help the client develop self-control.

Review of Childhood and Adolescent Disorders

1. A 7-year-old boy is disruptive in the classroom and is described by his parents as being hyperactive. What is the most probable psychiatric disorder? What are the signs and symptoms of this disorder? What drug is usually prescribed for this disorder?

2. A 15-year-old boy is threatening to drop out of school. His parents, both alcoholics, say they can't stop him. He has just been arrested for stealing a car and breaking into a house. What is the most probable disorder? Develop nursing diagnoses and interventions for this disorder.

Answers to Review

1. Attention deficit disorder (ADD/ADHD). More prevalent in boys; failure to listen to or follow instructions; difficulty playing quietly; disruptive behavior; impulsive behavior; difficulty sitting still; distractibility to external stimuli; excessive talking; shifting from one unfinished task to another; and underachievement in school performance. Ritalin.

2. Conduct disorder.
    A. Risk for violence related to …, depending on client.
    B. Disturbed self-esteem related to …, depending on client.
    C. Ineffective family coping related to …, depending on client.
    D. Assess verbal and nonverbal cues for escalating behavior so as to decrease outbursts. Use a nonauthoritarian approach. Avoid asking "why" questions. Initiate a show of force with a child who is out of control. Initiate suicide precautions when assessment indicates risk. Use a quiet room when external control is needed. Clarify expressions or jargon if meanings are unclear. Teach to redirect angry feelings to a safe alternative, such as a pillow or punching bag. Implement behavior modification therapy if indicated. Role-play new coping strategies.

For more review, go to **http://evolve.elsevier.com/HESI/RN** for HESI's online study exams.

GERONTOLOGIC NURSING

A. Aging is an individual process that affects each person differently.

B. For the purpose of data collection, those 65 years of age and older are considered older adults ("elderly").

C. The number of older adults is increasing in the United States; by the year 2020 it is expected that 20% of the population will be over the age of 65.

D. Of older adults, 80% have one or more chronic illnesses, and 50% have two or more chronic illnesses.

E. Older adults are the greatest users of health care.

F. Only 5% of older adults live in institutional settings.

Theories of Aging

SOCIOLOGIC THEORIES

A. Disengagement theory: progressive social disengagement occurs with aging

B. Activity theory: successful aging (as measured by the individual's satisfaction with life) depends on maintaining a high level of activity and involvement

BIOLOGIC THEORIES

A. Wear-and-tear theory: after repeated use and damage, body structures and functions wear out because of stress.

B. Free-radical theory: oxidation releases chemicals that affect the cell membranes and DNA replication; relates aging to environmental pollutants.

C. Immune theory: the aging process affects the immune system, causing a decrease in T cells and a rise in the incidence of infection.

PSYCHOLOGIC THEORIES

A. Short-term memory suffers an age-related decline.

B. Long-term memory undergoes minimal change.

C. Memory is affected by changes in the environment (e.g., moving, changes in caregivers).

HESI Hint • Either a lack of stimulation or an overload of changes can result in confusion. Provide as much consistency and routine as possible when caring for older adults in order to reduce the possibility of creating confusion.

Physiologic Changes

A. The aged are vulnerable to disease because of decreased physiologic reserve, less flexible homeostatic processes, and less effective body defenses.

B. Aging is characterized by the concept of loss.
   1. Physiologic and psychosocial losses occur even in "healthy" aging people.
   2. Increased longevity contributes to the demand placed on the health care system.
   3. Diseases in older adults do not always present classic signs and symptoms.
   4. Chronic illness becomes more prevalent as one ages.
   5. Resistance to stressors diminishes as one ages.
   6. The *frail elderly* (those over 75 years of age) are the fastest growing segment of the population and the highest users of health care.

HESI Hint • Changes in the heart and lungs result in less efficient utilization of O_2, which reduces an individual's capacity to maintain physical activity for long periods of time. Physical training for older persons can significantly reduce blood pressure and increase aerobic capacity. NCLEX-RN® questions ask about teaching and designing rehabilitation programs for older adults. The answers should contain something about exercise and nutrition.

HESI Hint • Older persons often complain that they cannot get to sleep at night and do not sleep soundly even after they fall asleep. This is because they have shorter stages of sleep, particularly shorter cycles between stages 1 and 4 and REM sleep (stage 4 is deep sleep). They are easily awakened by environmental stimuli. They often compensate by napping during the day, which leads to further disruptions of night sleep. A common response is the use of prescription sleeping pills, which can create still further problems of disorientation, etc.

CARDIOVASCULAR SYSTEM

A. Age-related changes in the cardiovascular system predispose the older person to developing dysrhythmias and other cardiac problems.

B. Cardiac output decreases as a result of a decrease in heart rate and stroke volume (heart rate slows with age, resting heart rate remains unchanged).

C. Cardiac output decreases because vessels lose elasticity. The heart's contractility decreases in response to increased demands.

D. Diastolic murmurs are present in over one half of older adults because the mitral and aortic valves become thick and rigid.

E. Dysrhythmias (bradycardia, tachycardia, atrial fibrillation, and heart block) become more common as one ages, in part because of higher systolic blood pressure (BP) and increased size of the atria.

F. Significant increases in systolic BP occur as a result of altered distribution of blood flow and increased peripheral resistance.

G. Arteriosclerosis increases with age and can cause cardiovascular problems.
1. Peripheral vascular disease
2. Edema
3. Coronary artery disease: acute coronary insufficiency, myocardial infarction (MI), dysrhythmias, heart failure (HF)

HESI Hint • Both systolic and diastolic blood pressures tend to increase with normal aging, but the elevation of the systolic is greater. Remember the physiology of blood pressure, which is expressed as a ratio of systolic to diastolic pressure. Systolic refers to the level of blood pressure during the contraction phase, whereas diastolic refers to the stage when the chambers of the heart are filling with blood.

Nursing Assessment

A. Dizziness or blackouts with sudden position change (orthostatic hypotension)

B. Diuresis after lying down

C. Feelings of heart palpitations

D. Swelling in hands and feet (rings and shoes have become tight)

E. Weight gain without changes in eating pattern

F. Difficulty breathing at night (ask older persons if they are using an increased number of pillows at night)

G. Confusion, personality changes resulting from O_2 deficit.

Analysis (Nursing Diagnoses)

A. *Activity intolerance* related to…

B. *Ineffective tissue perfusion (specify)* related to…

C. *Acute/chronic pain* related to…

D. *Decreased cardiac output* related to…

Nursing Plans and Interventions

A. Monitor blood pressure in lying, sitting, and standing positions.

B. Teach to avoid fatigue.

C. Encourage regular, low-level exercise.

D. Teach to change positions slowly to avoid falls and injuries.

E. Take apical and radial pulse; note deficits or rhythm abnormalities.

F. Teach to avoid extreme hot and cold because of decreased peripheral sensation.

G. Teach to avoid sitting with feet in a dependent position.

H. Weigh daily if indicated.

I. Encourage frequent rest periods.

J. Encourage strict adherence to medication regimen; no over-the-counter drugs (may interfere with digitalis).

K. Determine support system for follow-up.

HESI Hint • Dysrhythmias in older adults are particularly serious because older persons cannot tolerate decreased cardiac output, which can result in syncope, falls, and transient ischemic attacks (TIAs). Pulse may be rapid, slow, or irregular.

HESI Hint • Angina symptoms may be absent in older adults or they may be confused with gastrointestinal symptoms.

RESPIRATORY SYSTEM

A. Many older adults, along with the normal changes brought on by increased age, have respiratory diseases.

B. Respiratory muscles become rigid and lose strength, thereby restricting ventilation and decreasing vital capacity.

C. Lessened ability to cough and breathe deeply.

D. Lungs lose elasticity, become rigid (greatest change occurs in persons 70 years and older), decreasing pulmonary circulation.

E. Although total lung capacity and tidal volume are unaffected by age, gas exchange is reduced. Po_2 decreases to 75 mm Hg at age 70. Pco_2 is unchanged by age.

> **HESI Hint** • With aging, the muscles that operate the lungs lose elasticity so that respiratory efficiency is reduced. Vital capacity (the amount of air brought into the lungs at one time) decreases. Breathing may become more difficult after strenuous exercise or after climbing up several flights of stairs. The rate of decline has been found to be slower in more active persons. The nurse should encourage older persons to remain physically active for as long as possible. Declining muscle strength may impair cough efficiency. This fact makes older persons more susceptible to chronic bronchitis, emphysema, and pneumonia.

Nursing Assessment

A. Confusion (may be the first sign of respiratory infection)

B. Respiratory infection (an acute emergency in an older person)

C. Pneumonia (a major cause of death in the older generation)

D. Breathlessness

E. Dyspnea and fatigue (chronic obstructive pulmonary disease [COPD])

F. Cough present and sputum produced

Analysis (Nursing Diagnoses)

A. *Ineffective breathing pattern* related to…

B. *Impaired gas exchange* related to…

C. *Ineffective airway clearance* related to…

D. *Activity intolerance* related to…

> **HESI Hint** • COPD is the major cause of respiratory disability in older adults.

Nursing Plans and Interventions

A. Encourage clients to receive pneumonia vaccine every 5 years and an influenza vaccine yearly.

B. Remember that hypoxia can manifest as confusion. Encourage client to get assistance with medication regimen to prevent hypoxia.

C. If client is a smoker, encourage him or her to stop. (Regardless of age, cardiovascular and respiratory status does improve with smoking cessation and exercise.)

D. For older postoperative clients, turning, deep breathing, and use of incentive spirometer are imperative to prevent complications.

E. Encourage deep breathing. Teach breathing techniques such as pursed-lip breathing to facilitate respirations.

F. Some ventilatory assistance techniques such as postural drainage pose hazards for older adults.

GASTROINTESTINAL SYSTEM

A. Age-related changes are bothersome but are rarely a direct cause of death.

B. Relaxation of the lower esophageal sphincter results in delayed emptying and an increased risk for aspiration.

C. Decreased peristalsis and impaired absorption contribute to constipation problems.

D. The incidence of hiatal hernia increases with age.

E. Delayed gastric emptying makes digestion of large amounts of food difficult.

F. With age, hunger sensations decrease.

G. With age, the production of pepsin and hydrochloric acid decreases.

H. With age, the absorption of calcium decreases.

I. With age, the absorption of vitamins B_1 and B_2 decreases.

J. Diverticulosis in the sigmoid colon occurs in one third of those over age 60.

K. Decreased enzyme production in the liver affects drug metabolism and detoxification processes.

L. A decrease in the amount of bile in the gallbladder causes increased difficulty in emptying.

M. Loss of teeth is common, resulting in decreased ability to chew food adequately.

> **HESI Hint** • Changes that contribute to chronic constipation with age:
> • The number of enzymes in the small intestine is reduced, and simple sugars are absorbed more slowly, resulting in decreased efficiency of the digestive process.
> • The smooth-muscle content and the muscle tone of the wall of the colon decrease. Anatomic changes in the large intestine result in decreased intestinal motility.
> • Psychological factors, as well as abuse of over-the-counter laxatives, are factors.
> • Decreases in fluid intake and mobility contribute to constipation.

Nursing Assessment

A. Brittle teeth due to thinning enamel

B. Receding gums resulting from periodontal disease (the major cause of tooth loss after the age of 30)

C. Decrease in taste sensation

D. Dry mouth due to a decrease in saliva production

E. Poor tolerance of high-fat meals and poor absorption of fat-soluble vitamins

F. Decreased glucose tolerance

> **HESI Hint** · Tooth loss is not a normal aging process. Good dental hygiene, good nutrition, and dental care can prevent tooth loss.

Analysis (Nursing Diagnoses)

A. *Constipation* related to…

B. *Risk for deficient/imbalanced fluid volume* related to…

C. *Impaired oral mucous membrane* related to…

D. *Imbalanced nutrition: less than/more than body requirements* related to…

Nursing Plans and Interventions

A. Encourage good oral hygiene; encourage client to use soft toothbrush.

B. Assess dentures for proper fit.

C. Promote adequate bowel functioning.
   1. Determine what is normal GI functioning for each individual.
   2. Encourage client to increase fiber and bulk in the diet.
   3. Provide adequate hydration.
   4. Encourage regular exercise.
   5. Encourage eating small, frequent meals.
   6. Discourage the use of laxatives and enemas.
   7. Document bowel movements: frequency and consistency.

D. Encourage use of different spices to increase taste sensation.

E. Educate older clients about hidden sodium (canned soups, antacids, over-the-counter medications).

> **HESI Hint** · Older people appear to eat small quantities of food at mealtimes. This is because the digestive system of older persons features a decrease in the contraction time of the muscles, and more time is needed for the cardiac sphincter to open. Therefore, it takes more time for the food to be transmitted to the stomach. Thus, the sensation of fullness may occur before the entire meal is consumed.

GENITOURINARY SYSTEM

Normal aging does not impact continence or sexual functioning, but mental, physical, and cognitive changes can have a significant impact.

Analysis (Nursing Diagnoses)

A. *Disturbed personal identity* related to…

B. *Impaired urinary elimination* related to…

C. *Sexual dysfunction* related to…

> **HESI Hint** · Older persons have a higher risk for developing renal failure because normal age-related changes result in compromised renal functioning. The nurse should pay careful attention to urinary output in older clients because it is the first sign of loss of renal integrity.

Kidney

Nursing Assessment

A. Size of kidney decreases due to reduced renal tissue growth.

B. Glomerular filtration rate decreases due to a decrease in renal blood flow resulting from lower cardiac output. Decreased renal clearance of drugs is the result.

C. Tubular function diminishes.
   1. Lower specific gravity occurs because the tubules are less capable of concentrating urine.
   2. Proteinuria of 1+ is common.
   3. Blood urea nitrogen (BUN) is slightly increased.

D. Glucose reabsorption decreases.
   1. Classic symptoms of diabetes mellitus may not appear in older adult clients.
   2. Symptoms of diabetes mellitus in older adults may include fatigue, infection, and sensory changes caused by neuropathy.

E. Chronic diseases such as atherosclerosis and hypertension also decrease renal functioning in older adults.

Nursing Plans and Interventions

A. Observe for signs of dehydration or electrolyte imbalance.

B. Encourage an intake of at least 2 to 3 liters of fluid daily.

C. Instruct client about importance of completing antibiotics until entire prescription is gone, even if symptoms go away.

D. Write out antibiotic schedule, including any special instructions. Print in large letters.

Bladder

Nursing Assessment

A. The capacity of the bladder decreases by one half, resulting in urinary frequency and nocturia.

B. Emptying the bladder becomes difficult because of a weakening of the bladder and perineal muscles and because of a decrease in sensation of urge to void. (This sets up a propensity for urinary tract infections [UTIs] due to residual urine in the bladder.)

C. Increased frequency and dribbling occur in men because of a weakened bladder and an enlarged prostate.

D. Prostatic enlargement may cause urinary retention and bladder infection in males.

E. Women may experience stress incontinence.

Nursing Plans and Interventions

A. Initiate a bladder-training program if indicated.

B. Encourage older women to void at first urge when possible.

C. Initiate a skin-care program if incontinence is present.

D. Provide methods of dealing with incontinence. Kegel exercises can help.

E. Teach to avoid sleeping pills and sedation, which may cause nocturnal incontinence.

F. Teach to avoid caffeine because it promotes diuresis.

> **HESI Hint** • Kegel exercises consist of tightening and relaxing the vaginal and urinary meatus muscles. These exercises have been very successful in reducing the incidence of incontinence. They must be done consistently, and they can be done unobtrusively at home.

> **HESI Hint** • Older adults with incontinence may seek isolation, thereby predisposing themselves to loneliness.

> **HESI Hint** • From 15% to 30% of community-based older adults and almost 50% of older adults living in nursing homes suffer from difficulties with bladder control. Older persons may be more sensitive to alcohol and caffeine since these substances inhibit the production of antidiuretic hormone (ADH). An assessment of sensitivity to bladder problems is essential when planning nursing care.

> **HESI Hint** • **MEDICATION ALERT!**
> As one ages, the total number of functioning glomeruli decreases until renal function has been reduced by nearly 50%. This decrease in the filtration efficiency of the kidneys has grave implications for persons who are taking medication. Of particular importance are penicillin, tetracycline, and digoxin, which are cleared from the bloodstream primarily by the kidneys. These drugs remain active longer in an older person's system. Therefore, they may be more potent, indicating a need to adjust the dose and frequency of administration.

REPRODUCTIVE SYSTEM

Female Reproductive Organs

Nursing Assessment

A. Perineal muscle weakness and atrophy of the vulva occur with age.

B. Estrogen production decreases when menopause occurs.

C. Vaginal mucous membrane becomes dry, elasticity of tissue decreases, surface becomes smooth, and secretions become reduced and more alkaline

D. Incidence of vaginitis increases.

E. Libido does not change.

Nursing Plans and Interventions

A. Observe for signs of vaginitis; report and treat if present.

B. Perineal care should be promoted.

C. Note: Elderly rape victims sustain particularly extensive penetration trauma.

D. Prescription creams can help with vaginal dryness.

Male Reproductive Organs

Nursing Assessment

A. Testosterone production decreases.

B. Testicular size decreases.

C. Libido does not change.

Nursing Plans and Interventions

A. Encourage annual digital examination for early identification of prostate cancer.

NEUROLOGIC SYSTEM

A. Neurologic disease is the major cause of disability in older adults. Alzheimer disease, cerebral vascular accidents, and Parkinson disease are the major disorders in this category (see Medical Surgical Nursing, p. 143).

B. Brain
   1. Cerebral blood flow and oxygen utilization decrease

2. Neurons do not regenerate; therefore, neurologic losses are permanent.

C. Peripheral nerves
  1. Decreased ability to respond to multiple stimuli because of a decrease in both autonomic and sympathetic nervous system functioning

> **HESI Hint** · Alzheimer disease is the most common irreversible dementia of old age. It is characterized by deficits in attention, learning, memory, and language skills. Discuss the problems family members have in dealing with clients with Alzheimer disease in relation to the following disease manifestations:
> * Depression
> * Night wandering
> * Aggressiveness or passiveness
> * Failure to recognize family members

Nursing Assessment

A. Headache; determine type and difference from previous headaches.

B. Transient ischemic attacks (TIAs) manifested as:
  1. Weakness.
  2. Difficulty speaking.
  3. Blackouts.

C. Tremors in hands while at rest

D. Decrease of arm swing while walking

E. Gait disturbances resulting from less efficient kinesthetic senses

F. Delay in reflex response to noxious stimuli (hot surfaces, bumping into objects, etc.)

Analysis (Nursing Diagnoses)

A. *Risk for ineffective cerebral tissue perfusion* related to...

B. *Disturbed sensory perceptions* related to...

C. *Impaired verbal communication* related to...

Nursing Plans and Interventions

A. Perform a complete mental status exam and test cognitive thinking.

B. Record level of consciousness.

C. Record sensory awareness (vision, hot and cold sensations, pain).

D. Place food within visual field.

E. Provide alternative method of communication if indicated.

F. Arrange environment for optimum safe self-care. Reorient older person to environment as needed.

G. Provide activities based on cognitive level of functioning.

H. Keep precautionary respiratory equipment at bedside (higher risk for choking aspiration).

I. Decrease noise and clutter in environment; keep environment as consistent as possible.

J. Enhance orientation with windows, calendars, and clocks. Reorient by asking specific questions in a calm, direct way.

K. Ask about life history events; this is a good way to begin the reorientation process.

L. Allow as much autonomy as possible.

M. Provide assistive devices as needed for ambulation.

N. Minimize potential sources of injury in environment.

> **HESI Hint** · Strokes resulting from cerebral thrombosis are more common in older persons than are strokes from cerebral hemorrhage. Clots tend to develop when patient is awake or just arising.

> **HESI Hint** · Normal loss of brain cells is compounded by alcohol, smoking, and breathing polluted air. In relation to such losses, the nurse should teach older clients to shop at noncrowded times in stores that are familiar to them, slow down well in advance of traffic signals, stay in the slower lane of the freeway, avoid freeways during rush hours, and leave for appointments well ahead of time.

ENDOCRINE SYSTEM

Nursing Assessment

A. Thyroid activity decreases (see Medical Surgical Nursing, Hypothyroidism, p. 122). Symptoms commonly go undiagnosed in the older adult because they are attributed to being "normal for age."

B. T_3 level decreases.

C. Metabolic rate slows.

D. Aldosterone blood level and urinary excretion decrease.

E. Estrogen production ceases with menopause; ovaries, uterus, and vaginal tissue atrophy.

F. Gonadal secretion of progesterone and testosterone decreases.

G. Glucose intolerance may occur with aging.

Analysis (Nursing Diagnoses)

A. *Activity intolerance* related to...

B. *Fatigue* related to...

Nursing Plans and Interventions

A. Encourage thyroid testing for older clients who seem depressed. Hypothyroidism is often "dismissed" as depression.

B. Refer to Medical-Surgical Nursing, Hypothyroidism, p. 122.

C. Elderly clients may have difficulty with "lifelong" medication regimens. Develop memory cues for medications and caution against abrupt withdrawal.

D. See Medical-Surgical Nursing, Diabetes, p. 124.

> **HESI Hint** • The most common endocrine disorders in the older adult are thyroid dysfunctions and diabetes.

MUSCULOSKELETAL SYSTEM

Description: Age-related changes in the musculoskeletal system are gradual but have significant impact on levels of mobility, which put older adults at risk for falls and fractures.

Analysis (Nursing Diagnoses)

A. *Acute/chronic pain* related to…

B. *Risk for disuse syndrome* related to…

C. *Risk for injury* related to…

Bone

Nursing Assessment

A. Bone loss begins at about age 40.

B. Bone loss is more common in women than in men.

C. Osteoporosis occurs more often in women. (See Medical-Surgical Nursing, p. 132.)

Nursing Plans and Interventions

A. See Medical-Surgical Nursing, Osteoporosis, p. 133.

B. Teach that adequate calcium intake may help lessen osteoporotic changes (recommend 1000 mg daily or more, with vitamin D).

C. Establish muscle-strengthening program (small weights, aquatic therapy).

Muscle

Nursing Assessment

A. Muscle cells are lost and not replaced.

B. Older persons fatigue more easily because of changes in enzyme activity.

C. Lean body mass decreases with increased body fat.

Nursing Plans and Interventions

A. Prevent accidents by ensuring a safe environment.

B. Remove all hazards so that pathways are clear.

C. Provide adequate lighting day and night to prevent falls.

D. Teach clients not to back up, but to turn around to move in the direction they wish to go.

E. Encourage regular exercise.

Joints

Nursing Assessment

A. Cartilage erosion occurs.

B. Range of motion of joints decreases.

Nursing Plans and Interventions

A. Teach that multiple medications, especially diuretics and sedatives, contribute to falls.

B. Encourage older persons to change positions slowly to prevent orthostatic hypotension.

> **HESI Hint** • Impaired mobility, impaired skin integrity, decreased peripheral circulation, and a lack of physical activity place older adults at risk for developing decubitus ulcers.

> **HESI Hint** • Ways to help prevent or decrease the occurrence of falls:
> • Install adequate lighting.
> • Paint the edges of stairs a bright color.
> • Place a bell on any resident cats; cats move quickly and can get underfoot.
> • Wear proper footwear that supports the foot and contributes to balance; shoes should be made of nonslippery materials.

> **HESI Hint** • Fractured hips and hip replacements are common in older persons. Teach clients the proper way to sit and rise after hip replacement so that the body-to-lap angle is never less than 90 degrees. They should not lean forward while sitting because that can cause dislocation of the prosthesis.

INTEGUMENTARY SYSTEM

Description: Skin, hair, and nail changes occur with aging and can cause problems concerning discomfort and self-esteem.

Nursing Assessment

A. Thin skin: provides a less effective barrier to trauma. Varicosities (brown or blue discolorations): indicate poor circulation.
   1. Less effectiveness in retaining water
   2. Decreased ability of the skin to detect and regulate temperature
   3. Dry skin resulting from a decrease in endocrine secretion
   4. Loss of elastin and increased vascular fragility

B. Hair loss; increased facial hair in women

C. Decrease in number and size of sweat glands

D. Brittle and thick nails

Analysis (Nursing Diagnoses)

A. *Impaired skin integrity* related to...
B. *Risk for injury* related to...
C. *Risk for infection* related to...

Nursing Plans and Interventions

A. Encourage use of oils or lubricants on skin at least twice a day.
B. Discourage use of powder, which can be drying.
C. Teach to avoid overexposure to sunlight.
D. Encourage good nutrition and increased fluid intake.
E. Teach to maintain adequate humidity in the environment.
F. Teach to avoid temperature extremes.
G. Teach good foot care.
H. Observe bony prominences for signs of pressure.
I. Teach that poor peripheral circulation may retard the healing of foot and hand lesions.

> **HESI Hint** • Peripheral circulation decreases as one ages. Regular assessment of the feet is very important because it increases the opportunity to discover and treat skin care problems early. These problems could become more serious because of decreased circulation.

> **HESI Hint** • Older persons have dry, wrinkled skin because they lose subcutaneous fat and the second layer of skin, the dermis, becomes less elastic.

SENSORY SYSTEM

Description: Changes in the sensory system, which affects vision, hearing, taste, touch, smell, and balance, occur gradually and are often unnoticed.

Analysis (Nursing Diagnoses)

A. *Disturbed sensory perception* related to...
B. *Risk for injury* related to...
C. *Social isolation* related to...

Vision

Nursing Assessment

A. Reduced tear production
B. Presbyopia: age-related decrease in the ability of the eye to accommodate for near vision
C. Arcus senilis: glossy white ring encircling the periphery of the cornea (appears either partially or completely)

D. Cataracts: an abnormal progressive clouding or opacity of the lens of the eye (a common vision problem affecting older adults)
E. Glaucoma: Primary open-angle glaucoma (80% to 90% of cases) is a chronic progressive disease involving increased intraocular pressure (IOP), usually bilaterally, that can lead to permanent damage of the optic nerve and is asymptomatic until very late in the disease, when there is a noticeable loss of peripheral vision, causing tunnel vision. Acute angle-closure glaucoma, which is an emergency characterized by a rapid rise in IOP accompanied by redness and pain in and around the eye, severe headache, nausea and vomiting, and blurring of vision when the path of the aqueous humor is blocked and IOP builds to greater than 50 mm Hg. If untreated, blindness can occur in 2 days, but an iridectomy, can ease the pressure.

Nursing Plans and Interventions

A. Provide interventions to supplement loss of sensory input.
B. Encourage social interaction.
C. Use bright colors and large print for written materials.
D. Describe environment verbally to the visually impaired to increase orientation and decrease confusion.
E. Arrange for glasses if appropriate.
F. Maximize visual and nonvisual aids, such as large-print books, recorded books, and lighted mirror.
G. Encourage use of artificial tears; teach to avoid rubbing, picking at eyes (risk for infection).
H. Encourage regular eye exams; assist with administering eye drops.

> **HESI Hint** • Diminished eyesight results in:
> • A loss of independence (driving and the ability to perform activities of daily living [ADLs]).
> • A lack of stimulation.
> • The inability to read.
> • The fear of blindness.

Hearing

Nursing Assessment

A. Presbycusis is the age-related decrease in hearing acuity, auditory threshold, pitch and tone discrimination, and speech intelligibility (ability to understand another person's speech).
B. Hearing of high pitches diminishes first.
C. Ability to discriminate tones is lost.

Nursing Plans and Interventions

A. Provide auditory cues to supplement loss of sensory input.

B. Supply written materials to the hearing-impaired to reinforce what may not have been heard.

C. Directly face hearing-impaired individuals when talking to them so they can read lips and interpret facial expressions; this also lessens suspicion.

D. Decrease background noises.

E. Arrange for hearing aids if appropriate.

> **HESI Hint** • Lower the tone of your voice when talking to an older person who is hearing-impaired. High-pitched tones (i.e., women's voices) are the first to become difficult to hear; therefore, lowering the pitch of your voice increases the likelihood that an older person with a hearing loss will be able to hear you speak.

> **HESI Hint** • Presbycusis (age-related hearing loss) can result in decreased socialization, avoidance of friends and family, decreased sensory stimulation, and hazardous conditions when driving.

Gustation (Taste) and Olfaction (Smell)

Nursing Assessment

A. Taste buds decrease in number and atrophy, resulting in decreased sensitivity to taste.

B. It is not known whether the sense of smell is affected by aging.

Nursing Plans and Interventions

A. Use stronger spices, if tolerated, to increase the taste of foods. Use substitutes for salt and sugar.

B. Adapt ethnic favorites to dietary and taste limitations.

> **HESI Hint** • Use frequent touch to decrease the sense of isolation and to compensate for visual and auditory sensory loss.

Psychosocial Changes

LOSS

Nursing Assessment

A. Loss of spouse, children, friends

B. Loss of role in the workplace and in the family
   1. This affects status and prestige; can produce feelings of uselessness and nonparticipation
   2. Withdrawal or disengagement from the mainstream of life may occur after retirement.

C. Loss of socioeconomic status
   1. Decreased income usually occurs.
   2. Those on fixed incomes experience the effects of inflation more profoundly than the rest of the population.
   3. Loss of income affects the quality of health care available to the individual.

D. Loss of physical capacity

> **HESI Hint** • Older persons undergo a great many changes, which are usually associated with loss (loss of spouse, friends, career, home, health, etc.). Therefore, older persons are extremely vulnerable to emotional and mental stress.

Analysis (Nursing Diagnoses)

A. *Situational low self-esteem* related to...

B. *Powerlessness* related to...

Nursing Plans and Interventions

A. Determine the losses older clients are currently having and have had in the past 2 years.

B. Evaluate level of depression and suicidal risk.

C. Determine alcohol usage.

D. Promote activities that allow the individuals to use past experiences and knowledge, thereby promoting a feeling of self-worth and increased self-esteem.

E. Promote reminiscing about significant life experiences.

> **HESI Hint** • Integrity vs. despair is Erikson's final stage of growth and development. Reminiscing is a means of setting one's life in order (accepting life and self), which is the task of this stage, according to Erikson's development theory. The goal of this stage is to feel a sense of the meaning of one's life, rather than to feel despair or bitterness that one's life has been wasted. The major task of old age is to redefine self in relation to a changed role. Those persons who had been in charge of situations most of their lives may now find themselves in dependent positions. This role adjustment is a major task of old age.

> **HESI Hint** • Think about the following situations and discuss the nursing care for each:
> • A nursing supervisor who has had a stroke and is sent to a long-term facility for rehabilitation
> • An oil company executive who retires after 42 years with the company to travel in his recreational vehicle with his wife and dog
> • Shortly after their fifty-third wedding anniversary, a woman who has never worked outside the home loses her husband to brain cancer

Dementia

> **HESI Hint** • There are many conditions that can imitate dementia in the older adult. A key role of the nurse is to make a complete assessment so as to rule out other possible causes of particular behavior.

Description: Permanent, progressive impairment in cognitive functioning manifested by memory loss (both long-term and short-term) and accompanied by impairment in judgment, abstract thinking, and social behavior.

A. The two most common types of dementia are multi-infarct dementia and Alzheimer disease.
   1. Multiinfarct dementia results from repeated strokes, which can cause complete deterioration of the cerebral tissue.
   2. Alzheimer disease is characterized by brain atrophy, a progressive physical and mental deterioration that lasts 5 to 14 years before death occurs.
B. The incidence is as follows:
   1. There are 1.2 million cases in the United States in people over the age of 65.
   2. This amounts to between 10% and 20% of older adults population.
C. It is the leading reason for institutionalization of older adults; nearly two thirds of the institutionalized older adults have some form of cognitive impairment.
D. Approximately 20% of those diagnosed with dementia actually have pseudodementia, which is reversible. Possible causes of false dementias include:
   1. Drug side effects, interactions, and adverse reactions (Lithium, barbiturates, atropine, and bromides are known to have dementia as a side effect.)
   2. Depression
   3. Nutritional deficits
   4. Metabolic disorders, hypothyroidism, anemia, hypoglycemia
E. Irreversible dementia has a gradual onset and a progressive downward course. Alzheimer disease is the most common type.

NURSING ASSESSMENT

A. Slow, insidious onset that is unrelated to a specific cause, condition, or situation
B. Personality changes that are often accompanied by withdrawal
C. Confusion, often unnoticed by the client
D. Memory loss:
   1. Client is usually aware of memory loss.
   2. Memory loss begins with recent memory loss and progresses to total memory loss.
E. Risk factors:
   1. Family history of dementia
   2. Family history of Down syndrome
   3. Enzyme deficiency
   4. Immune system deficiency
   5. Aluminum toxicity
   6. Acetylcholine (a neurotransmitter) deficiency

ANALYSIS (NURSING DIAGNOSES)

A. *Self-care deficit (specify)* related to…
B. *Risk for injury* related to…

NURSING PLANS AND INTERVENTIONS

A. Keep client functioning and actively involved in social and family activities as long as possible.
B. Maintain an orderly, almost ritualistic schedule to promote a sense of security.
C. Maintain a regularly scheduled reality orientation on a daily basis.
   1. Keep client oriented as to time, place, and person (repeatedly).
   2. Keep a calendar and clock within sight at all times.
      a. Display a calendar and clock that can be read by older persons (i.e., a clock with large numbers and a calendar that can be read by those with deteriorating vision).
      b. Be sure the date and time are accurate (i.e., keep the calendar current and the clock in working order).
D. Encourage family to bring pictures of family members from home. Familiar objects promote a sense of continuity and security.
E. Administer prescribed drugs to reduce emotional lability, agitation, and irritability or prescribed antidepressant, as indicated.
   1. Medications for Alzheimer: Cholinesterase inhibitors (ChEIs) that act by stopping or slowing the action of acetylcholinesterase to break down acetylcholine, increasing available acetylcholine. Acetylcholine is thought to be a neurotransmitter important in the neurons of the hippocampus and cerebral cortex for memory.
      a. tacrine (Cognex)
      b. donepezil (Aricept)
      c. rivastigmine (Exelon)
      d. galantamine (Razadyne)
F. Speak in a slow, calm voice; avoid excitement.
G. Provide support and education to family and long-term caregivers.

Health Maintenance and Preventive Care

NURSING PLANS AND INTERVENTIONS

A. Encourage periodic health appraisal and counseling to prevent illness.
   1. ECG to detect subtle heart abnormalities
   2. Chest radiograph to detect tuberculosis or lung cancer
   3. Pulmonary function tests to detect chronic bronchitis and emphysema
   4. Tonometer test to measure intraocular pressure as a test for glaucoma
   5. Blood glucose to detect diabetes mellitus
   6. Pap smear to detect cancer of cervix; digital rectal examination to detect cancer of prostate
   7. Hearing and vision testing to detect sensory deprivation
   8. Breast self-examination monthly

B. Promote accident prevention.
   1. Prevent falls.
   2. Maintain physical and mental activities to help client improve confidence and mobility.
   3. Teach to rise to upright position slowly because of the possibility of postural hypotension (orthostatic hypotension).
   4. Encourage regular exercise.

C. Protect against infectious diseases.
   1. Teach client to avoid individuals who are ill.
   2. Encourage immunization against influenza and pneumonia.
   3. Encourage nutritious diet and plenty of fluids.

D. Avoid temperature extremes; prevent hypothermia.

E. Encourage older persons to stop smoking; it is *never* too late.

F. Educate clients about proper foot care.

G. Encourage proper nutrition and weight control.

H. Encourage use of support services (Meals-on-Wheels) and support groups (church).

I. Discourage the use of over-the-counter medication. Review all medications yearly and encourage the client to throw away outdated drugs and prescriptions.

J. Diseases and conditions that affect older adults are the same ones that affect younger adults. However, in older adults, the signs and symptoms of pathology may be subtle, slow to develop, and quite different from those seen in younger persons (Table 8-1).

TABLE 8-1 Diseases and Conditions in the Elderly

Disease or Condition	Description in Terms of the Elderly	Nursing Implications
Delirium	• Confused states develop over short periods of time if caused by systemic illness or medications. • This state can develop suddenly.	• Establish a meaningful environment. • Help maintain body awareness. • Help client cope with confusion, delusions, and illusions. • See Nursing Interventions for Dementia, p. 370.
Cardiac dysrhythmias	• Incidence increases with age. • More serious in older adults because of lower tolerance of decreased cardiac output (can result in syncope, falls, TIAs, and confusion). • Symptoms result from compromised circulation and O_2 deficit.	• Assess, prevent, and manage dysrhythmias. • Advise smoking cessation. • Encourage exercise and weight control.
Cataracts	• Often a result of normal aging changes. • Most common pathologic problem affecting the eyesight of older adults. • Treatment is surgical removal.	• Teach instillation of eye drops. • Reduce glare in environment. • Assistance is required postoperatively because affected eye is covered, and disorientation may occur.
Glaucoma	• Risk of acquiring increases with age.	• Loss of sensory input can result in confusion.

(Continued)

TABLE 8-1   Diseases and Conditions in the Elderly—cont'd

Disease or Condition	Description in Terms of the Elderly	Nursing Implications
Cerebrovascular accident (CVA)	• Interruption of cerebral circulation; it is caused by occlusion or hemorrhage in the brain. • Risk increases with age.	• Prevent deterioration of client's condition. • Maximize functional abilities (occupational therapy). • Assist client in accepting physical deficits. • Check gag reflex before client receives food or fluids. • Prevent injuries to paralyzed limbs.
Decubitus ulcer	• Immobility puts older adults at risk for developing decubitus ulcers.	• Reposition frequently. • Massage bony prominences. • Provide adequate nutrition.
Hypothyroidism	• It usually occurs after age 50. • Symptoms are often similar to normal aging changes, and they have an insidious onset, making it difficult to detect in older adults. • Elderly are at greater risk for developing myxedema coma, which is life-threatening.	• Often diagnosed as depression; with treatment, signs of depression disappear. • Caution against abruptly discontinuing medication.
Thyrotoxicosis (Graves' disease)	• Symptoms may be absent or attributed to other, more common diseases in older adults. • Weight loss and HF may be predominant symptoms.	• It is precipitated by stressful events such as trauma, surgery, or infection. Be alert for signs and symptoms. • Can be fatal if untreated.
COPD	• It is a major cause of respiratory disability in older adults. • Most older persons exhibit both chronic bronchitis and chronic emphysema. • Fatigue is a common result because of the increased work required to breathe (dyspnea).	• Encourage to stop smoking. • Keep in mind older person's state of confusion when teaching about treatment regimen. • Plan rest periods to allow patient to maintain oxygen levels.
Urinary tract infections (UTIs)	• Their incidence increases with age. • Older persons are often asymptomatic or exhibit vague, ill-defined symptoms. • With infections, older persons often become confused.	• Suspect UTI when client's voiding habits change.

END-OF-LIFE CARE

Description: This period of life is important because the type of medical care often shifts from invasive intervention aimed at prolonging life to supportive intervention that focuses on control of symptoms. From an insurance and hospice point of view, the end-of-life stage begins 6 months before death. The major problem with this definition is the difficulty in predicting the period of client survival. Physicians are likely to overestimate survival time, which probably is one reason that the average client lives only 24 days after being admitted to hospice.

A. Pain management is a priority in end-of-life care because untreated or undertreated pain consumes energy, interferes with function, affects quality of life and social interactions, and contributes to sleep disturbances, hopelessness, and loss of control.

B. Dyspnea (distressing shortness of breath) may be related to pulmonary, cardiac, neuromuscular, or metabolic disorders, obesity, anxiety, and spiritual distress. Of concern to families in particular is the gurgling sound, ("death rattle") that occurs close to the end of life. Alleviating dyspnea can contribute to the client's comfort and decrease the family's anxiety.

C. Anxiety, a subjective feeling of apprehension, tension, insecurity, and uneasiness, can range from mild to severe. At end of life, anxiety may be associated with various physical and emotional factors including dyspnea, a lifelong pattern of responding to stress, or a preexisting anxiety disorder. To allow the client some peace, anxiety should be brought under control, using first nonpharmacological interventions (relaxation techniques, visual imagery, music therapy, empathetic listening, reassurance, and reinforcement of previously successful anxiety-reducing methods) followed by pharmacological agents as needed.

D. Gastrointestinal symptoms can take many forms including nausea, vomiting, gastritis, constipation, and diarrhea. If not controlled, gastrointestinal symptoms can negatively impact the client's comfort and quality of life.

E. Psychiatric symptoms of depression and delirium are very common at end of life and if unrecognized can rob clients nearing death of the quality of life and quality of care they deserve.

Spirituality is recognized by both health care professionals and clients as an important element at the end of life. *Spirituality* is a broad concept that encompasses the search for meaning in life experiences and relationships with others, and religion is that aspect of spirituality that is associated with a sense of connectedness to a personal deity. Both spirituality and religion help to create a sense of purpose and meaning that makes life worthwhile. Recognition of spirit distress is important to help the dying client come to terms with the end of life.

F. Support for family caregivers is important because for many persons at end of life, family caregivers may do everything from assisting with ADLs to giving medications and managing medical equipment and treatments. They often are the ones who serve as go-betweens for the client and health care providers. Although caregivers may find great satisfaction in their role, they often experience stress and diminished physical health.

G. Family support during bereavement period is essential because following the loss through death of a significant person, the survivor (especially with older adults) is at increased risk for illness or death. Normal responses to grief can be physical, psychological, cognitive, and/or spiritual, a dynamic, pervasive, and a highly individualized process (uncomplicated grief). Complicated grief is persistent maladaptive behaviors that occur following loss that intensifies to the level where the individual is overwhelmed, or remains interminably in the state of grief without progression through the mourning process to completion. When the nurse identifies complicated grief it should be reported so a referral for help can be made to the correct provider, such as a bereavement counselor.

Review of Gerontologic Nursing

1. What are normal memory changes that occur as one ages?
2. What symptoms might the nurse expect to see in an older person who has had an overload of changes as well as a respiratory infection?
3. Why can the blood pressure of older adults be expected to increase?
4. What is the major cause of respiratory disability in older adults?
5. List five nursing interventions to promote adequate bowel functioning for older persons.
6. How can a female nurse increase the older client's ability to hear her speak?
7. What is the most common visual problem occurring in older adults?
8. Describe the following conditions that occur in older adults:
   A. Presbyopia
   B. Arcus senilis
   C. Presbycusis
9. Describe the onset of Alzheimer disease.
10. What is the purpose of a reality-orientation group?
11. What are two factors that cause a decrease in the excretion of drugs by the kidneys?
12. What areas of care are important for end-of-life care?

Answers to Review

1. Short-term memory declines, whereas long-term memory undergoes minimal change.
2. Confusion
3. Heart work increases in response to increased peripheral resistance.
4. COPD
5. Determine what is "normal" GI functioning for each individual, increase fiber and bulk in the diet, provide adequate hydration, encourage regular exercise, and encourage eating small meals frequently.
6. Lower the pitch or tone of her voice
7. Cataracts
8. Describe the following:

A. Decreased ability of the eye to accommodate to close work
B. Glossy white ring encircling the periphery of the cornea
C. Decrease in hearing acuity, auditory threshold, pitch and tone discrimination, and speech intelligibility
9. Slow, insidious onset and a progressive downward course
10. To keep the client oriented to time, place, and person
11. Decrease in glomerular filtration and slowed organ functioning
12. Pain, dyspnea, anxiety, gastrointestinal symptoms, psychiatric symptoms, spirituality, support for family caregivers, family support during bereavement period

For more review, go to **http://evolve.elsevier.com/HESI/RN** for HESI's online study exams.

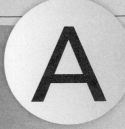

Test	Adult	Child	Infant/Newborn	Elder	Nursing Implications
			HEMATOLOGIC		
Hgb Hemoglobin: g/dl	Male: 14–18 Female: 12–16 Pregnant: >11	1–6 yr: 9.5–14 6–18 yr: 10–15.5	Newborn: 14–24 0–2 weeks: 12–20 2–6 months: 10–17 6 mo-1 yr: 9.5–14	Values slightly decreased	High-altitude living increases values. Drug therapy can alter values. Slight Hgb decreases normally occur during pregnancy.
Hct Hematocrit: %	Male: 42–52 Female: 37–47 Pregnant: >33	1–6 yr: 30–40 6–18 yr: 32–44	Newborn: 44–64 2–8 weeks: 39–59 2–6 months: 35–50 6 mo-1 yr: 29–43	Values slightly decreased	Prolonged stasis from vasoconstriction secondary to the tourniquet can alter values. Abnormalities in RBC size may alter Hct values.
RBC Red blood cell count: million/mm^3	Male: 4.7–6.1 Female: 4.2–5.4	1–6 yr: 4–5.5 6–18 yr: 4.5–5	Newborn: 4.8–7.1 2–8 weeks: 4–6 2–6 months: 3.5–5.5 6 mo-1 yr: 3.5–5.2	Same as adult	Never draw specimen from an arm with an infusing IV. Exercise and high altitudes can cause an increase in values. Pregnancy values are usually lower. Drug therapy can alter values.
WBC White blood cell count: 1000/mm^3	Both sexes: 5–10	≤2 yr: 6.2–17 ≥2 yr: 5–10	Newborn, term: 9–30	Same as adult	Anesthetics, stress, exercise, and convulsions can cause increased values. Drug therapy can decrease values for 24 to 48 hr postpartum; it is normal to have a count as high as 25.
Platelet count: 1000/mm^3	Both sexes: 150–400	150–400	Premature infant: 100–300 Newborn: 150–300 Infant: 200–475	Same as adult	Values may increase if living at high altitudes, exercising strenuously, or taking oral contraceptives. Values may decrease due to hemorrhage, DIC, reduced production of platelets, infections, prosthetic heart

Test	Adult	Child	Infant/ Newborn	Elder	Nursing Implications
					valves, and drugs (acetaminophen, aspirin, chemotherapy, H_2-blockers, INH, Levaquin, streptomycin, sulfonamides, thiazide diuretics).

HESI Hint · The laboratory values that are most important to know for the NCLEX-RN® examination are Hgb, Hct, WBCs, Na, K, BUN, blood glucose, ABGs (blood gases), bilirubin for newborn, and therapeutic range for PT/INR and PTT.

Test	Adult	Child	Infant/ Newborn	Elder	Nursing Implications
SED rate, ESR Erythrocyte sedimentation rate: mm/hr	Male: up to 15 Female: up to 20 Pregnant: ↑ all trimesters	up to 10	Newborn: 0–2	Same as adult	Rate is elevated during pregnancy.
PT Prothrombin time: seconds	Both sexes: 11–12.5 Pregnant: Slight ↓	Same as adult	Same as adult	Same as adult	Used in regulating Coumadin therapy. Therapeutic range is 1.5 to 2 times normal/control.
INR International Normalized Ratio	Both sexes 2–3.5	Same as adult	Same as adult	Same as adult	Used to monitor anticoagulation therapy
PTT Partial thromboplastin time: seconds (see APTT)	Both sexes: 60–70 Pregnant: Slight ↓	Same as adult	Same as adult	Same as adult	It is used in regulating heparin therapy. Therapeutic range is 1.5 to 2.5 times normal or control.
APTT Activated partial thromboplastin time: seconds	Both sexes: 30–40	Same as adult	Same as adult	Same as adult	It is used in regulating heparin therapy. Therapeutic range is 1.5 to 2.5 times normal or control.

BLOOD CHEMISTRY					
Alkaline phosphatase: IU/L	Both Sexes: 30–120	2–8 yr: 65–210 9–15 yr: 60–300 16–21 yr: 30–200	<2 yr: 85–235	Slightly higher than adults	Hemolysis of specimen can cause a false elevation in values.
Albumin: g/dl	Both sexes: 3.5 to 5 Pregnant: slight ↑	4.5–9	Premature infant: 3–4.2 Newborn: 3.5–5.4 Infant 6–6.7	Same as adult	No special preparation is needed.
Bilirubin total: mg/dl	Total: 0.3–1 Indirect: 0.2–0.8 Direct: 0.1–0.3	Same as adult	Newborn: 1–12	Same as adult	Client is to be NPO except for water for 8 to 12 hr prior to testing.

(Continued)

Test	Adult	Child	Infant/ Newborn	Elder	Nursing Implications
					Prevent hemolysis of blood during venipuncture. Do *not* shake tube; it can cause inaccurate values. Protect blood sample from bright light.
Calcium: mg/dl	Both sexes: 9–10.5	8.8–10.8	<10 days: 7.6–10.4 Umbilical: 9–11.5 10 days-2 yr: 9–10.6	Values tend to decrease	No special preparation is needed. Use of thiazide diuretics can cause increased calcium values.
Chloride: mEq/L	Both sexes: 98–106	90–110	Newborn: 96–106 Premature Infant: 95–110	Same as adult	Do not collect from an arm with an infusing IV solution.
Cholesterol: mg/dl	Both Sexes: <200	120–200	Infant: 70–175 Newborn: 53–135	Same as adult	Do not collect from an arm with an infusing IV solution.
High-density lipoprotein [HDL] (alpha lipoproteins), which are predominantly protein with a small amount of cholesterol	Male: >45 Female : >55	1 to 9 yr: 53–56 10 to 14 yr: 52–55 15 to 19 yr: 46–52	Newborn: 35	Same as adult	
Low-density lipoprotein [LDL] (beta lipoproteins), which are primarily cholesterol		1 to 9 yr: 93–100 10 to 14 yr: 97 15 to 19 yr: 94–96	Newborn: 29	Same as adult	
CPK Creatine phosphokinase: IU/L	Male: 55–170 Female: 30–135	Same as adult	Newborn: 65–580	Same as adult	Specimen must not be stored prior to running test.
Creatinine: mg/dl	Male: 0.6–1.2 Female: 0.5–1.1	Child: 0.3–0.7 Adolescent: 0.5–1	Newborn: 0.2–0.4 Infant: 0.3–1.2	Decrease in muscle mass may cause decreased values	It is preferred but not necessary to be NPO 8 hr prior to testing. A ratio of 20:1, BUN to creatine, indicates adequate kidney functioning.

Test	Adult	Child	Infant/ Newborn	Elder	Nursing Implications
Glucose: mg/dl	Both sexes: 70–100	≤2 yr: 60–100 >2 yr: 70–110	Cord: 45–96 Premature infant: 20–60 Newborn: 30–60 Infant: 40–90	Increase in normal range after age 50	Client to be NPO except for water 8 hr prior to testing. Caffeine can caused increased values.
HCO_3: mEq/L	Both sexes: 21–28	Same as adult	Infant: 20–28 Newborn: 13–22	Same as adult	None
Iron: mcg/dl	Male: 80–180 Female: 60–160	50–120	Newborn: 100–250	Same as adult	It is preferred but not necessary to be NPO 8 hr prior to testing.
TIBC Total iron binding capacity: mcg/dl	Both sexes: 250–460	Same as adult	Same as adult	Same as adult	None
LDH Lactic dehydrogenase: IU/L	Both sexes: 100–190	60–170	Infant: 100–250 Newborn: 160–450	Same as adult	No IM injections are to be given 8 to 12 hr prior to testing. Hemolysis of blood will cause false positive.
Potassium: mEq/L	Both sexes: 3.5–5	3.4–4.7	Infant: 4.1–5.3 Newborn: 3–5.9	Same as adult	Hemolysis of specimen can result in falsely elevated values. Exercise of the forearm with tourniquet in place may cause an increased potassium levels.
Protein total: g/dl	Both sexes: 6.4–8.3	6.2–8	Premature infant: 4.2–7.6 Newborn: 4.6–7.4 Infant: 6–6.7	Same as adult	It is preferred but not necessary to be NPO 8 hr prior to testing.
AST/SGOT Aspartate amino-transferase: IU/L	0–35 Female slightly lower than adult males	3–6 yr: 15–50 6–12 yr: 10–50 12–18 yr: 10–40	0–5 days: 35–140 <3 yr: 15–60	Slightly higher than adult	Hemolysis of specimen can result in falsely elevated values. Exercise may cause an increased value.
ALT/SGPT Alanine amino-transferase: IU/ml	Both sexes: 4–36	Same as adult	Infant may be twice as high as an adult	Slightly higher than adult	Hemolysis of specimen can result in falsely elevated values. Exercise may cause an increased value.
Sodium: mEq/L	Both sexes: 136–145	136–145	Infant: 134–150 Newborn: 134–144	Same as adult	Do not collect from an arm with an infusing IV solution.

(Continued)

Test	Adult	Child	Infant/ Newborn	Elder	Nursing Implications
Triglycerides: mg/dl	Male: 40–160 Female: 35–135	6–11 yr: 31–108 12–15 yr: 36–138 16–19 yr: 40–163	0–5 yr: 30–86	Same as adult	Client is to be NPO 12 hr before testing. No alcohol for 24 hr before test.
Urea nitrogen: mg/dl	Both sexes: 10–20	5–18	Infant: 5–18 Newborn: 3–12 Cord: 21–40	Slightly higher	None
Thyroid-stimulating hormone (TSH, thyrotropin)	Both sexes: 2–10	Same as adult	Newborn: 3–18 Cord: 3–12	Same as adult	The TSH test is used to differentiate primary and secondary hypothyroidism. TSH levels are subject to a diurnal variation. Some drugs that may cause increased levels (antithyroid medications, lithium, potassium iodide, and TSH injection). Some drugs may cause decreased levels (aspirin, nonsteroidal antiarthritics dopamine, heparin, steroids, and T_3). No food or drink restrictions are necessary.
Triiodothyronine (T_3)	Both sexes: 70–205	1–5 yr: 105–270 6–10 yr: 95–240 ng/dL 11–15 yr: 80–215 ng/dL 16–20 yr: 80–210 ng/dL	Newborn: 100–740 Infant: 105–245	40–180	Primarily to diagnose hyperthyroidism Total T_3 values are increased in pregnancy, because serum proteins are increased at that time.

Test	Adult	Child	Infant/ Newborn	Elder	Nursing Implications
Thyroxine (T_4)	Male: 4–12 Female: 5–12	1–5 yr: 7–15 5–10 yr: 6–13 10–15 yr: 5–12	Newborn: 1–3 days: 11–22 1–2 weeks: 10–16 Infant: 8–16	5–11	Newborns are screened to detect hypothyroidism, so mental retardation can be prevented with early diagnosis. A heel stick is used to collect the blood. Slight increase in T_4 levels during pregnancy. Stop taking exogenous T_4 medication 1 month before testing
ARTERIAL BLOOD CHEMISTRY					
pH	Both sexes: 7.35–7.45	Same as adult	Infant: 5–18 Newborn: 3–12 Cord: 21–40	Same as adult	Specimen must be heparinized. Specimen must be iced for transport. All air bubbles must be expelled from sample. Direct pressure to puncture site must be maintained.
P_{CO_2}: mmHg	Both sexes: 35–45	Same as adult	<2 yr: 26–41	Same as adult	Specimen must be heparinized. Specimen must be iced for transport. All air bubbles must be expelled from sample. Direct pressure to puncture site must be maintained.
P_{O_2}: mmHg	Both sexes: 80–100	Same as adult	Newborn: 60–70	Same as adult	Specimen must be heparinized. Specimen must be iced for transport. All air bubbles must be expelled from sample. Direct pressure to puncture site must be maintained.

(Continued)

Test	Adult	Child	Infant/ Newborn	Elder	Nursing Implications
HCO_3: mEq/L	Both sexes: 21–28	Same as adult	Infant/Newborn: 16–24	Same as adult	Specimen must be heparinized. Specimen must be iced for transport. All air bubbles must be expelled from sample. Direct pressure to puncture site must be maintained.
O_2 saturation: %	Both sexes: 95–100	Same as adult	Newborn: 40–90	95	Specimen must be heparinized. Specimen must be iced for transport. All air bubbles must be expelled from sample. Direct pressure to puncture site must be maintained.

URINALYSIS (UA)

Characteristic	Normal	Nursing Implications
Appearance	Clear	May be a midstream, clean-catch specimen. Cloudy urine may be caused by the presence of pus (necrotic WBCs), RBCs, or bacteria, or ingestion of certain foods. Urine that has been refrigerated for longer than 1 hr can become cloudy
Color	Yellow to amber	Pale yellow to amber color because of the pigment urochrome (product of bilirubin metabolism). The color indicates the concentration of the urine (dilute urine- straw colored; concentrated urine; deep amber and varies with specific gravity). Color can change with ingestion of certain foods or medications. Urine darkens with prolonged standing.
Odor	Aromatic	Diabetic ketoacidosis has the strong, sweet smell of acetone. UTI, the urine may have a foul odor. When urine stands for a long time and starts to decompose, it has an ammonia-like smell.
pH	4.6–8.0 (average, 6.0)	Bacteria, UTI, or a diet high in citrus fruits or vegetables may cause increased urine pH. Urine pH becomes alkaline on standing. The urine pH of an uncovered specimen will become alkaline. A first-voided specimen is best for testing urine specific gravity.

Characteristic	Normal	Nursing Implications
Protein	0–8 mg/dl 50–80 mg/24 hr (at rest) <250 mg/24 hr (during exercise)	Proteinuria indicator of renal disease Test the urine of all pregnant women for proteinuria, an indicator of preeclampsia. If significant protein is noted at urinalysis, a 24-hr urine specimen should be collected so that the quantity of protein can be measured. Transient proteinuria may be associated with severe emotional stress, excessive exercise, and cold baths. A first-voided specimen is best to test for protein.
Specific gravity	Adult: 1.005–1.030 (usually, 1.010–1.025) Elderly: values decrease with age Newborn: 1.001–1.020	Renal disease tends to diminish concentrating capability. Specific gravity is a measurement of hydration status, with overhydration the urine is more dilute, with dehydration the urine is more concentrated. Drugs that may cause increased specific gravity include dextran and sucrose.
Leukocyte esterase	Negative	Positive results indicate UTI. False-positive results may occur in specimens contaminated by vaginal secretions (heavy menstrual discharge, trichomonas infection, parasites) that contain WBCs. False-negative results may occur in specimens containing high levels of protein or ascorbic acid.
Nitrites	None	Chemical testing is done with a dipstick containing a reagent that reacts with nitrites to produce a pink color. A positive test result indicates the need for a urine culture.
Ketones	None	Ketones spill over into the urine when blood glucose levels in diabetic patients are elevated. Ketonuria is associated with poorly controlled diabetes. Ketonuria may occur with acute febrile illnesses, especially in infants and children. Special diets (carbohydrate-free, high-protein, high-fat) and some drugs may cause ketonuria. Testing for ketones can be performed immediately after urine collection. Dip a reagent stick (Ketostix) into the urine specimen. Read the strip in 15 seconds by comparing it with the color chart.
Bilirubin	None	Obstruction of the bile duct by a gallstone causes conjugated hyperbilirubinemia, and unlike the unconjugated form, conjugated bilirubin is water soluble and can be excreted into the urine. Bilirubin is not stable in urine, especially when exposed to light.
Crystals	None	Crystals found on microscopic examination indicate that renal stone formation is imminent, if not already present. Radiographic contrast media may cause precipitation of urinary crystals.
Casts	None	For casts to form, the pH must be acidic and the urine concentrated. Two types of casts: Hyaline casts are conglomerations of protein, and cellular casts are conglomerations of degenerated cells.
Glucose	Fresh specimen: none 24-hr specimen: 50–300 mg/24 hr	Glucose is not excreted by the kidney unless blood levels exceed approximately 180 mg/dL, so can reflect the degree of glucose elevation in the blood. Collect a fresh double-voided specimen. In pregnancy glycosuria is common, but persistent and significantly high levels may indicate gestational diabetes.

(Continued)

Characteristic	Normal	Nursing Implications
White blood cells (WBCs)	0–4 per low-power field	The presence of five or more WBCs in the urine indicates a UTI involving the bladder or kidneys, or both. A clean-catch urine culture should be done for further evaluation. Vaginal discharge may contaminate the urine specimen and factitiously cause WBCs in the urine.
WBC casts	None	WBC casts are most frequently found in infections of the kidney, poststreptococcal glomerulonephritis or inflammatory nephritis.
Red blood cells (RBCs)	≤2	Hematuria can be microscopic or gross. Bladder, ureteral, and urethral diseases are the most common causes of RBCs in the urine. The most common cause of RBCs in the urine is from contamination of menses, so before collection of the sample, determine whether the patient is having a period. Traumatic urethral catheterization may cause RBCs in the urine.
RBC casts	None	RBC casts suggest glomerulonephritis interstitial nephritis, acute necrosis, pyelonephritis, renal trauma, or renal tumor. Strenuous physical exercise may cause RBC casts.
Volume		24-hr specimen is required. If a 24-hr urine collection is needed, refrigerate urine during the collection period.

Source: Pagana KD, Pagana TJ: Mosby's diagnostic and laboratory test reference, ed 8. St Louis, 2007, Mosby.

RECOMMENDED DAILY REQUIREMENTS AND FOOD SOURCES

FOOD GROUPS AND SERVINGS PER DAY

Food Group	Child	Adult	Pregnant	Lactating
Dairy	3 or more servings	3 or more servings	3 or more servings	3 or more servings
Protein—meat, poultry, fish, dry beans, eggs, nuts	2 or more servings	2 or more servings	3 servings	2 servings
Vegetables	3–5 servings	3–5 servings	3–5 servings	3–5 servings
Fruits	2–4 servings	2–4 servings	2–4 servings	2–4 servings
Bread, cereal, rice, and pasta	6–11 servings (serving size may be reduced)	6–11 servings	6–11 servings	6–11 servings

FAT-SOLUBLE VITAMINS

Vitamin	Food Source
A	Liver Egg yolks, fortified margarine, and butter Dark green and deep orange fruits and vegetables, e.g., apricots, broccoli, cantaloupe, carrots, pumpkin, winter squash, sweet potatoes, and spinach
D	Fortified and full-fat dairy products Fish oil Can be synthesized in the skin when exposed to sunlight
E	Vegetable oils and their products such as salad oils, margarine, nuts, seeds, avocado, and mango
K	Green leafy vegetables (such as lettuce, cabbage, spinach), peas, asparagus, meat, milk, and soybean oil

FOODS HIGH IN SODIUM

Vegetables	Condiments	Miscellaneous
Canned vegetables	Bouillon cubes	Bacon
Carrots, particularly canned	Mustard, prepared	Cheeses
Tomatoes, particularly canned	Olives, pickled, canned or bottled	Ready-to-eat breakfast cereals
Tomato catsup	Pickles, cucumber, dill	Peanut butter
Tomato juice	Salad dressings, commercially prepared	Soups, commercially prepared, canned
	Soy sauce	Corned beef

WATER-SOLUBLE VITAMINS	
Mineral	**Food Sources**
C	Citrus fruits, cantaloupes, strawberries, tomatoes, potatoes, broccoli, green peppers, and spinach
B_1 (thiamine)	Pork, beef, liver, whole grains, legumes, and wheat germ
B_2 (riboflavin)	Liver, milk, milk products, soybeans, and enriched cereals
B_e (nicotinic acid)	Meat, poultry, fish, peanuts, and enriched grains
B_6 (pyridoxine)	Meat, poultry, grains, seeds, and seafood
Folic acid	Liver, beans, peas, spinach, and yeast
B_{12}	Shellfish, liver, fish, and lean meat

MINERALS	
Mineral	**Food Sources**
Calcium	Milk, cheese, dark green vegetables, dried figs, soy, and legumes
Phosphorus	Milk, liver, legumes, fish, and soy
Magnesium	Whole grains, green leafy vegetables, tea, nuts, and fruit
Iron	Meats, eggs, legumes, whole grains, green leafy vegetables, and dried fruits
Iodine	Marine fish, shellfish, dairy products, iodized salt, and some breads
Potassium	Citrus fruits and dried fruits, bananas, watermelon, potatoes, legumes, tea, and peanut butter
Zinc	Meats, seafood, and whole grains

INDEX

Page numbers followed by "*f*" indicate figure(s); "*t*" indicate table(s); "*b*" indicate box(es).

Arterial blood gases
  acid-base disorders, 44t
  analysis of, 44t
  normal values for, 28t, 70
Arterial bypass, 96
Arterial pressures, 31t
Arthrectomy, 88
Arthritis. *See* Rheumatoid arthritis
Ascites, 115
Ascorbic acid. *See* Vitamin C
Asparaginase, 159t
Aspartate aminotransferase, 379
Aspirin, 131t
Assault, 12, 355–356
Assertive communication, 16
Assessment, 3t
Assignments, 14
Asterixis, 115
Asthma, 69t, 196
Astramorph PF. *See* Morphine sulfate
Asynchronous pacemakers, 101
Atelectasis, 52t
Atenolol, 88t, 94t
Ativan. *See* Lorazepam
Atorvastatin, 89t
Atovaquone, 56t
Atrial fibrillation, 99, 100f
Atrial flutter, 99, 100f
Atrial septal defect, 201, 201f
Atropine sulfate (Atropisol), 89t, 102t, 152t
Atrovent. *See* Ipratropium
Attention-deficit disorder, 207, 358–359
Attention-deficit/hyperactivity disorder, 207, 358–359
Authority, 17
Automated external defibrillator, 35
Autonomic dysreflexia, 148
Autosomal recessive, 224
Avandia. *See* Rosiglitazone
Avapro. *See* Irbesartan
Aventyl. *See* Nortriptyline hydrochloride
Avoidant personality, 335
Avonex. *See* Interferon beta-1a
Avulsion fracture, 136t
Axid. *See* Nizatidine
Axillary body temperature, 285
Azactam, 67t
Azithromycin, 67t
Azmacort. *See* Triamcinolone
Azopt. *See* Brinzolamide

B

Babinski reflex, 282t
Back, 280t
Bacterial meningitis, 211–212
Bacterial vaginosis, 292t
Bactrim. *See* Trimethoprim/sulfamethoxazole
Barrel chest, 70
Base excess, 28t
Basic life support, 35–36
Bathing of newborn, 285

Battery, 12, 241
Beclomethasone dipropionate, 72t
Behavior modification, 322
Benadryl. *See* Diphenhydramine hydrochloride
Benazepril, 95t
Benign prostatic hyperplasia, 85–86
Benzathine penicillin, 66t
Benzodiazepines, 329t, 352t
Benztropine mesylate, 152t, 349t
Bereavement, 373
Beta blockers, 88t, 94t
Beta-adrenergic agonists, 196, 197t
Beta-adrenergic receptor–blocking agents, 140t
Betapace. *See* Sotalol
Betaseron. *See* Interferon beta-1b
Bethanechol chloride, 216t
Biaxin. *See* Clarithromycin
Bicarbonate, 314t
  in acid-base disorders, 44t
  acidosis and, 36
  carbonic acid and, 43, 44f
  chemical buffer function of, 43
  normal values for, 28t, 379, 382
Bicillin L-A. *See* Benzathine penicillin
Biguanides, 127t
Bile sequestrants, 89t
Bilirubin
  hyperbilirubinemia, 318–319
  normal levels of, 377–378
  in urine, 383
Bilirubin delta optical density assessment, 246
Bimatoprost, 140t
Biofeedback, 61t
Biogenic amines, 339
Biologic response modifiers, 82, 83t, 161t–162t
Biophysical profile, 246, 252
Bioterrorism, 21, 22t–25t
Bipolar disorder, 342–344
Bisacodyl, 273t
Bisoprolol, 94t
Bisphosphonates, 133
Bladder, 365
Bleomycin sulfate (Blenoxane), 159t
Blocadren. *See* Timolol maleate
Blood chemistry tests, 377–381
Blood dyscrasias, 348t
Blood lead level test, 194
Blood pressure
  elevated. *See* Hypertension
  in newborn, 278t
  physiology of, 91
  in pregnancy, 239, 242
Blood products, 32t–33t
Blood transfusions
  reactions associated with, 32t–33t
  shock treated with, 32t–33t
Blood urea nitrogen, 39t, 380
Blue bloater, 70
Bodily injury, 184
Body temperature, 278t, 285

Body weight
    fluid retention determinations and, 80
    maternal gain, in pregnancy, 242
    newborn, 278t, 313
Bone mineral density, 133
Borderline personality, 334
Bottle-feeding, 284
Botulism, 22t–23t
Bowel cancer. *See* Colorectal cancer
Bowel management program, 144b
Brachytherapy, for prostate cancer, 172
Bradycardia, 248–249
Brain attack, 153–155
Brain tumors, 149, 212–213
Braxton Hicks contractions, 237, 254
Brazelton Neonate Behavioral Assessment Scale, 277
Breach of duty, 11
Breast(s)
    infection of, 309–310, 311t
    lactating, 269, 272t
    postpartum changes, 269, 271
    self-examination of, 170, 271b
Breast cancer, 169–171
Breastfeeding
    description of, 272, 272t
    maternal alcohol ingestion during, 320
    sexually transmitted diseases and, 310, 311t
Breath sounds
    assessment of, 73
    bronchial, 65
Breathing
    assessment of, 35–36
    during labor, 259
    in older adults, 363
Breech position, 256f
Brethine. *See* Terbutaline sulfate
Bretylium tosylate (Bretylol), 102t
Brinzolamide, 140t
Bromocriptine mesylate, 152t
Bronchial breath sounds, 65
Bronchiolitis, 198–199
Bronchitis, chronic, 65, 69t
Bronchodilators, 72t
Bronuometer. *See* Isoetharine
Brown fat, 240, 314
Brudzinski sign, 211
Budesonide, 72t
Buerger disease, 95
Bulimia nervosa, 337–338
Bumetanide (Bumex), 93t
BUN. *See* Blood urea nitrogen
Bupropion, 341t
Burns
    care for, 176–177
    in children, 192–193
    description of, 176
    first-degree, 176
    fluid therapy for, 179, 193
    full-thickness, 176, 176f, 193
    infection risks, 179

Burns *(Continued)*
    inhalation, 177
    Lund and Browder chart for, 176, 178t, 193
    nursing assessment of, 177–178
    nursing plans and interventions for, 178–181
    partial-thickness, 176, 176f, 193
    physiologic responses to, 179f
    rehabilitation for, 181
    rule of nines for, 176, 177f
    second-degree, 176
    superficial, 176, 176f
    third-degree, 176
Burst fracture, 135t
Buspirone (BuSpar), 329t
Busulfan, 159t
Butorphanol tartrate, 265t
Buttocks, 280t

C

Calan. *See* Verapamil hydrochloride
Calcium
    food sources of, 387
    imbalances of, 40t–41t
    normal levels of, 378
    pregnancy intake of, 244
Calcium channel blockers, 88t, 95t
Calculi
    renal, 84
    urinary, 145
Camptosar. *See* Irinotecan
Cancer. *See also* Oncologic disorders
    breast, 169–171
    cervical, 168–169
    colorectal, 113–114
    definition of, 165
    laryngeal, 73–74
    lung, 76–78
    ovarian, 169
    prostate, 171–173
    signs of, 165
    testicular, 171
Candida albicans, 174t, 293t
Candidiasis
    oral, 55t
    vaginal, 174t
Cane, 134
Capreomycin (Capastat), 75t
Captopril (Capoten), 95t
Carafate. *See* Sucralfate
Carbamazepine, 208t, 211, 343t
Carbapenems, 67t
Carbolith. *See* Lithium carbonate
Carbonic acid, 43, 44f
Carbonic anhydrase inhibitors, 140t
Carcinoembryonic antigen, 113
Carcinoma, 165
Cardiac arrest, 35–36
Cardiac catheterization, 203
Cardiac conduction system, 48f

Diamox. *See* Acetazolamide
Diapering of newborn, 285
Diaphragm, 275*t*
Diarrhea, 191–192
Diastole, 48
Diazepam, 329*t*, 352*t*
DIC. *See* Disseminated intravascular coagulation
Diclofenac, 131*t*
Dicloxacillin sodium, 66*t*
Didanosine, 56*t*
Differentiation, 165
Digibind. *See* Digoxin-immune Fab
Digitalis, 105*t*
Digitoxin, 102*t*, 105*t*
Digoxin, 102*t*, 105*t*, 204*b*
Digoxin-immune Fab, 105*t*
Dilantin. *See* Phenytoin sodium
Dilation and curettage, 166
Dilaudid. *See* Hydromorphone
Diltiazem hydrochloride, 88*t*, 95*t*
Diovan. *See* Valsartan
Diphenhydramine hydrochloride, 162*t*
Diphtheria, tetanus, and pertussis vaccine, 186*f*, 188*t*
Dipyridamole, 97*t*
Direct Coombs test, 319
Disaster nursing
    bioterrorism, 21, 22*t*–25*t*
    levels of prevention, 19
    nurse's role in, 19
    triage, 19–21, 20*t*, 21*f*
Discoid lupus erythematosus, 131–132
Disopyramide phosphate, 102*t*
Disorganized schizophrenia, 345
Displaced fracture, 135*t*
Displacement, 324*t*
Disseminated intravascular coagulation, 33–35
Dissociative disorders, 332–333
Dissociative identity disorder, 332–333
Distraction, 61*t*
Disulfiram, 351*t*
Ditropan. *See* Oxybutynin
Diuretics, 93*t*, 147*t*, 212*t*
Diverticular diseases, 111–112
Diverticulitis, 111
Diverticulosis, 111, 363
Docetaxel, 160*t*
Docusate sodium, 273*t*
Domestic abuse. *See* Intimate-partner violence
Donepezil hydrochloride, 358*t*
Dopamine, 152*t*
Dornase alfa, 197
Dorzolamide, 140*t*
Dosage calculations, 197*t*
Down syndrome, 206, 206*f*
Doxazosin, 94*t*
Doxorubicin hydrochloride, 159*t*
Doxycycline hyclate, 66*t*
Drug abuse, 351–353
DTaP vaccine. *See* Diphtheria, tetanus, and pertussis vaccine
Dual-energy x-ray absorptiometry, 133
Duchenne muscular dystrophy, 213

Dulcolax suppository. *See* Bisacodyl
Duloxetine, 341*t*
Dumping syndrome, 110
Duragesic. *See* Fentanyl citrate
Duramorph. *See* Morphine sulfate
Dysarthria, 154
Dysmenorrhea, 166
Dysphagia, 154
Dysphasia, 154
Dyspnea, 372
Dysrhythmias, 99–101, 100*f*, 371*t*
Dystocia, 296–297
Dystonia, 348*t*

E

Ear(s)
    infection of. *See* Otitis media
    newborn, 280*t*
Early decelerations, 250
Eating disorders, 336–338
ECG. *See* Electrocardiogram
Echolalia, 345
Eclampsia, 298
Ectopic pregnancy, 287–288
Edrophonium test, 151
Efavirenz, 56*t*
Effexor. *See* Venlafaxine
Eisenmenger syndrome, 200
EKG. *See* Electrocardiogram
Elavil. *See* Amitriptyline hydrochloride
Eldepryl. *See* Selegiline
Elder abuse, 355
Elderly. *See* Older adult
Electrocardiogram, 46–49, 47*b*, 47*f*, 100*f*
Electroconvulsive therapy, 325
Electroencephalograph, 146
Electrolytes. *See also specific electrolyte*
    balance of. *See* Fluid and electrolyte balance
    imbalances in, 40*t*–41*t*
    renal disorders' effect on, 79
Electronic fetal monitoring, 247*f*–251*f*, 247–250
Elspar. *See* Asparaginase
Emancipated minors, 13
Embolectomy, 96
Embolytic stroke, 153
Emergency admission, 12
Emergency care, 14
Emergency delivery, 304–305
Eminase. *See* Anistreplase
Emphysema, 65, 69*t*
Enalapril maleate, 95*t*
End stage renal disease, 81–82
Endarterectomy, 96
Endocarditis, 104–106
Endocrine disorders
    Addison disease, 122–123
    Cushing syndrome, 124
    diabetes mellitus. *See* Diabetes mellitus
    hyperthyroidism, 120*f*, 120–121
    hypothyroidism, 122, 227, 372*t*

HIV encephalopathy, 55*t*
Hivid. *See* Zalcitabine
HMG-CoA reductase inhibitors, 89*t*
Hodgkin disease, 164–165
Holter monitor, 46, 101
Homan sign, 98
Homeostasis, 38
Hormone replacement therapy, 133
Hospitalization
  admission, 12
  rights during, 12
Human chorionic gonadotropin, 239
Human immunodeficiency virus. *See* HIV
Human papillomavirus
  description of, 168, 174*t*
  maternal, 291
  vaccine for, 187*f*
Hycamtin. *See* Topotecan
Hydatidiform mole, 287
Hydralazine, 94*t*
Hydration, 319
Hydrocephalus, 209–210
Hydrochlorothiazide, 93*t*
Hydrochlorothiazide/amiloride, 93*t*
Hydrochlorothiazide/spironolactone, 93*t*
Hydrochlorothiazide/triamterene, 93*t*
Hydrocortisone, 123*t*
Hydromorphone, 60*t*
Hydrophobia, 328
Hydroxyurea (Hydrea), 158, 159*t*
Hygroton. *See* Chlorthalidone
Hyperbilirubinemia, 283–284, 318–319
Hypercalcemia, 41*t*
Hypercarbia, 65
Hyperemesis gravidarum, 302
Hyperglycemia, 126, 128*t*
Hyperkalemia, 40*t*, 80
Hypermagnesemia, 41*t*
Hypernatremia, 40*t*
Hyperphosphatemia, 41*t*
Hypertension
  gestational, 298
  systemic, 91, 93, 93*t*–95*t*
Hypertensive disorders of pregnancy, 298–300
Hyperthyroidism, 120*f*, 120–121
Hypertonic solutions, 42*t*
Hyperventilation, 259
Hypocalcemia, 40*t*, 121, 121*f*, 316
Hypochondriasis, 331–332
Hypoglycemia, 126, 128*t*, 283, 316
Hypoglycemics, 303
Hypokalemia, 40*t*
Hypomagnesemia, 41*t*
Hyponatremia, 40*t*
Hypophosphatemia, 41*t*
Hypospadias, 217–218
Hypothermia, 283
Hypothyroidism
  congenital, 227
  description of, 122, 372*t*
Hypotonic solutions, 42*t*

Hypovolemic shock, 29, 30*t*, 312
Hypoxemia, 65
Hypoxia, neonatal, 315
Hysterectomy, 166, 168
Hytrin. *See* Terazosin hydrochloride

I

Ibuprofen, 131*t*
Idarubicin (Idamycin), 159*t*
Identification (defense mechanism), 324*t*
Identification (of patient), 13
Ileostomy, 114
Illusions, 345
Imidazole carboxamide, 159*t*
Imipenem, 67*t*
Imipramine hydrochloride, 340*t*
Immobilization, 145
Immune theory, 361
Immunizations, 185, 186*f*–187*f*, 188*t*–189*t*
Immunosuppression, 157, 163
Impacted fracture, 136*t*
Implementation, 3*t*
Inability to stand trial, 13
Inactivated poliovirus vaccine, 186*f*–187*f*, 188*t*
Incident reports, 11
Incomplete fracture, 134, 135*t*, 229
Increased intracranial pressure, 146–147, 209
Increased intraocular pressure, 139
Indapamide, 93*t*
Inderal. *See* Propranolol hydrochloride
Indinavir, 56*t*
Indomethacin (Indocin), 131*t*, 201, 295*t*–296*t*
Inevitable/incomplete miscarriage, 287
Infant. *See also* Children; Newborn
  body temperature of, 278*t*, 285
  cardiac disease in, 300–302
  foreign body airway obstruction in, 37
  growth and development of, 182–183
  hemoglobin levels in, 223
  HIV in, 57
  hydration in, 319
  hydrocephalus in, 209–210
  oxygen administration in, 197*b*
  phenylketonuria screening in, 227, 284
Infection
  burn wound, 179
  newborn prevention, 283
  opportunistic, 53–54, 55*t*
  perineal, 309–310
  postpartum, 309–311, 310*t*–311*t*
  during pregnancy, 290, 291*t*–293*t*
  urinary tract. *See* Urinary tract infections
Infectious heart disease, 104–106
Infective endocarditis, 105–106
Inflammatory bowel diseases, 110–112
Inflammatory heart disease, 104–106
Infliximab, 231*t*
Influenza vaccine, 186*f*–187*f*
Information giving, 323*t*
Informed consent, 13

INH. *See* Isoniazid
Inhalation burns, 177
Inhalation tularemia, 23t–24t
Injury
    acceleration-deceleration, 146, 146f
    bodily, 184
    head, 145–147, 146f
    spinal cord, 147–149
Inocor. *See* Amrinone
Insanity, 13
Insulin-dependent diabetes mellitus. *See* Type 1 diabetes mellitus
Integrilin. *See* Eptifibatide
Integumentary system. *See also* Skin
    age-related changes in, 367–368
    in newborn, 279t
    postpartum changes in, 270
Intellectualization, 324t
Intentional torts, 12
Interferon alfa-2a, 162t
Interferon alfa-2b, 162t
Interferon beta-1a, 161t
Interferon beta-1b, 161t
Interleukin-2, 162t
International normalized ratio, 377
Intestinal obstruction, 112–113
Intimate-partner violence, 354–355
Intracellular fluid, 38
Intracranial hemorrhage, 317
Intracranial pressure, increased, 146–147
Intradural block, 266
Intraoperative care, 51
Intrapartum nursing care, 254–269, 294, 301
Intrauterine device, 275t
Intrauterine growth restriction, 245, 298
Intravenous analgesics, 265
Intravenous lines, 164t
Intravenous therapy, 41–43, 42t
Intraventricular hemorrhage, 315
Introjection, 324t
Intron A. *See* Interferon alfa-2b
Intussusception, 112, 221
Invanz. *See* Ertapenem
Invasion of privacy, 12
Invirase. *See* Saquinavir
Involuntary admission, 12
Iodine, 387
Ipratropium, 72t
Ipratropium/albuterol, 72t
Irbesartan, 94t
Irinotecan, 160t
Iron
    administration of, 157t
    deficiency of, 190, 191t, 290t
    food sources of, 191t, 387
    normal levels of, 379
    pregnancy intake of, 244
Isocarboxazid, 340t
Isoetharine, 72t
Isolation, 324t
Isoniazid, 75t, 76

Isoproterenol hydrochloride (Isuprel), 72t
Isoptin. *See* Verapamil hydrochloride
Isosorbide dinitrate (Isordil), 88t
Isosorbide mononitrate (Imdur), 88t
Isotonic solutions, 38, 42t
IUD. *See* Intrauterine device

J

Jaundice, 115, 284, 319
Jaw-thrust maneuver, 35
"Jitteriness," 313
Job analysis studies, 3–4
Joint Commission, 14
Joint replacement, 136–137
Juvenile rheumatoid arthritis, 233

K

Kabikinase. *See* Streptokinase (Streptase)
Kaletra. *See* Ritonavir
Kanamycin (Kantrex), 75t
Kaposi's sarcoma, 55t
Keflex. *See* Cephalexin
Kefzol. *See* Cefazolin
Kegel exercises, 272
Kernicterus, 319
Kernig sign, 211
Ketoacidosis, diabetic, 228
Ketones, 383
Ketorolac tromethamine, 131t
Kidney(s)
    acid-base balance functions of, 44
    age-related changes in, 364–365
    cardiovascular system and, 87
    fluid and electrolyte balance role of, 38
    immaturity of, in preterm infant, 318
    urine output by, 79
Kidney stones, 84
Klonopin. *See* Clonazepam
Korsakoff syndrome, 350
Kyphosis, 232f
Kytril. *See* Granisetron

L

La belle indifference, 331t
Labetalol, 94t
Labor. *See also* Pregnancy
    analgesia or anesthesia during, 264–267
    breathing techniques in, 259
    cardinal movement of the mechanism of, 259f
    cesarean birth, 305–306
    complications during
        dystocia, 296–297
        preterm labor, 294, 295t–296t, 301
    emergency delivery, 304–305
    episiotomy during, 262, 271, 271b
    false, 254
    fetal positions in, 255–256, 257f
    fetal presentation in, 255, 256f, 267

Reminyl. *See* Galantamine
Renal calculi, 84
Renal dialysis. *See* Dialysis
Renal disorders
    acute renal failure, 79–81, 80*t*
    benign prostatic hyperplasia, 85–86
    in children
        acute glomerulonephritis, 214, 215*t*
        hypospadias, 217–218
        nephrotic syndrome, 214–215, 215*t*
        urinary tract infections, 215, 216*t*
        vesicoureteral reflex, 217
        Wilms tumor, 217
    chronic renal failure, 81–82
    medications for, 216*t*
    urinary tract infections, 52*t*, 82–84, 149
    urinary tract obstruction, 84–85
Renal failure
    acute, 79–81, 80*t*
    chronic, 81–82
Renal transplantation, 82, 83*t*
Repaglinide, 127*t*
Repression, 324*t*
Reproduction, 235–240
Reproductive disorders
    breast cancer, 169–171
    cervical cancer, 168–169
    cystocele, 167–168
    ovarian cancer, 169
    prostate cancer, 171–173
    rectocele, 167–168
    sexually transmitted diseases, 173–175, 174*t*, 291*t*, 310, 311*t*
    testicular cancer, 171
    uterine prolapse, 167–168
    uterine tumors, 166–167
Reproductive system
    age-related changes in, 365
    postpartum changes, 269
Rescriptor. *See* Delavirdine
Residual schizophrenia, 345
Respiratory acidosis, 44*t*–45*t*
Respiratory alkalosis, 44*t*–45*t*, 259
Respiratory disorders
    in children
        asthma, 196
        bronchiolitis, 198–199
        cystic fibrosis, 196–198
        epiglottitis, 198
        otitis media, 199
        signs of, 195–196
        tonsillitis, 199
    chronic airflow limitations, 65, 68–73
    chronic bronchitis, 65, 69*t*
    emphysema, 65, 69*t*
    laryngeal cancer, 73–74
    lung cancer, 76–78
    pneumonia, 64–65, 66*t*–68*t*
    tuberculosis. *See* Tuberculosis
Respiratory distress, 195–196
Respiratory distress syndrome, 315
Respiratory failure, 27–29

Respiratory rates
    in children, 196*t*
    in newborn, 278*t*
Respiratory syncytial virus, 198
Respiratory system, 362–363
Responsibility, 17
Restraints, 15
Resuscitation
    cardiac arrest, 35–36
    newborn, 36, 314, 314*t*
    pediatric, 36–37
Reteplase (Retavase), 92*t*
Retinal detachment, 142
Retinol. *See* Vitamin A
Retrovir. *See* Zidovudine
Reye syndrome, 212
Rheumatoid arthritis, 130–131
    juvenile, 233
Rh$_O$ (D) immune globulin (RhoGAM), 273*t*
Riboflavin. *See* Vitamin B$_2$
Ricin, 24*t*–25*t*
Rifampin (Rifadin), 75*t*, 76
Riopan. *See* Aluminum hydroxide/magnesium hydroxide
Risperidone (Risperdal), 348*t*
Ritalin. *See* Methylphenidate hydrochloride
Ritodrine hydrochloride, 295*t*–296*t*
Ritonavir, 56*t*
Rituximab (Rituxan), 161*t*
Rivastigmine, 358*t*
Robaxin. *See* Methocarbamol
Rocephin. *See* Ceftriaxone
Roferon-A. *See* Interferon alfa-2a
Rooting reflex, 282*t*
Rosiglitazone, 127*t*
Rotavirus vaccine, 186*f*
RR interval, 48
Rubella
    characteristics of, 190
    maternal, 292*t*
    teratogenicity of, 292*t*
    vaccine for, 186*f*–187*f*, 188*t*, 273*t*
Rubeola, 190
Rule of nines, 176, 177*f*
Rythmol. *See* Propafenone

S

Salmeterol, 72*t*
Saquinavir, 56*t*
Sarcoma, 165
Sarin, 24*t*–25*t*
Schizoid personality, 334
Schizophrenia, 345–346
Schizotypal personality, 334
School-age child, 184, 196*t*
Scoliosis, 231–232, 232*f*
Secondary gain, 331*t*
Seizures
    description of, 210–211
    eclamptic, 300
Selective estrogen receptor modulators, 133

NOTES

NOTES

NOTES

NOTES

NOTES

NOTES